Management of Metastatic Disease to the Musculoskeletal System

Management of Metastatic Disease to the Musculoskeletal System

EDITED BY

John P. Heiner, M.D.

Professor, Department of Orthopedics and Rehabilitation,
University of Wisconsin Medical School, Madison, Wisconsin

Timothy J. Kinsella, M.D.

Professor and Chairman, Department of Radiation Oncology,
Case Western Reserve University School of Medicine, Cleveland, Ohio

Thomas A. Zdeblick, M.D.

Professor, Department of Orthopedics and Rehabilitation,
University of Wisconsin Medical School, and Director, University of
Wisconsin Spine Center, Madison, Wisconsin

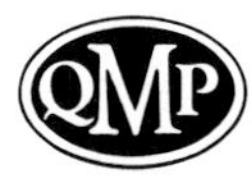

Quality Medical Publishing, Inc.

ST. LOUIS, MISSOURI   2002

Printed in the United States of America.

This book presents current scientific information and opinion pertinent to medical professionals.
It does not provide advice concerning specific diagnosis and treatment of individual cases and
is not intended for use by the layperson. The authors and publisher will not be responsible
or liable for actions taken as a result of the opinions expressed in this book.

PUBLISHER   Karen Berger
ASSOCIATE EDITOR   Michelle Leaman
PROJECT MANAGER   Book Production, Inc.
COVER DESIGN   David Berger

Quality Medical Publishing, Inc.
11970 Borman Drive, Suite 222
St. Louis, Missouri 63146
Telephone: 1-800-348-7808
Web site: http://www.qmp.com

LIBRARY OF CONGRESS CATALOGING-IN-PUBLICATION DATA

Management of metastatic disease to the musculoskeletal system / edited by John P.
Heiner, Timothy J. Kinsella, Thomas A. Zdeblick.
     p.   ; cm.
   Includes bibliographical references and index.
   ISBN 1-57626-088-7
     1. Musculoskeletal system—Cancer. 2. Bone metastasis. 3. Metastasis. I. Heiner, John
P., 1955-   . II. Kinsella, Timothy J. III. Zdeblick, Thomas A.
     [DNLM: 1. Bone Neoplasms—secondary. 2. Muscle Neoplasms—secondary. 3.
Neoplasm Metastasis—therapy. WE 258 M2668 2001]
   RC280.M83 M36 2001
   616.99'47—dc21

                                                                    2001019409

BPI/WW/WW
5   4   3   2   1

Contributors

William A. Abdu, M.D., M.S.
Associate Professor of Orthopaedic Surgery, Dartmouth Hitchcock Medical Center, Lebanon, New Hampshire

Fadi W. Abdul-Karim, M.D.
Professor of Pathology, Case Western Reserve University School of Medicine, and Director of Anatomic Pathology, University Hospitals of Cleveland, Cleveland, Ohio

Mark R. Albertini, M.D.
Assistant Professor, Department of Medicine, University of Wisconsin Medical School, Madison, Wisconsin

Jesse Aronowitz, M.D.
Associate Professor, Department of Radiation Oncology, Health Science Center, State University of New York, Syracuse, New York

Azhar M. Awan, M.D.
Clinical Associate Professor, Department of Radiation and Cellular Oncology, University of Chicago, Chicago, Illinois; Medical Director, Department of Radiation Oncology, LaGrange Memorial Treatment Pavilion, LaGrange, Illinois

Howard H. Bailey, M.D.
Assistant Professor, Departments of Medicine and Obstetrics and Gynecology, University of Wisconsin Medical School, Madison, Wisconsin

Laurence H. Baker, D.O.
Professor of Internal Medicine, Division of Hematology/ Oncology, University of Michigan, and Deputy Director and Director for Clinical Research, University of Michigan Comprehensive Cancer Center, Ann Arbor, Michigan

Joseph Benevenia, M.D.
Associate Professor and Vice-Chairman, Department of Orthopaedics, Division of Musculoskeletal Oncology, University of Medicine and Dentistry of New Jersey, Newark, New Jersey

Edgar Ben-Josef, M.D.
Associate Professor, Department of Radiation Oncology, Karmanos Cancer Institute, Wayne State University, and Harper Hospital, Detroit, Michigan

J. Sybil Biermann, M.D.
Assistant Professor, Department of Orthopaedic Surgery, University of Michigan, Ann Arbor, Michigan

Eduardo Bruera, M.D.
Professor of Medicine and F.T. McGraw Chair in the Treatment of Cancer, Department of Symptom Control and Palliative Care, The University of Texas M.D. Anderson Cancer Center, Houston, Texas

Charles S. Cathcart, M.D.
Assistant Professor, Department of Radiology, University of Medicine and Dentistry of New Jersey, Newark, New Jersey

Mary M. Checovich, M.S.
Associate Researcher, Department of Surgery, University of Wisconsin Medical School, Madison, Wisconsin

Christina W. Chin, M.D.
Pain Management Specialist and Physician, Department of Anesthesiology, Muhlenberg Regional Medical Center, Plainfield, New Jersey

Timothy A. Damron, M.D.
Associate Professor, Department of Orthopedic Surgery, and Adjunct Associate Professor, Department of Neuroscience and Physiology, Upstate Medical Center, State University of New York, Syracuse, New York

Randy F. Davis, M.D.
Assistant Professor, Department of Orthopedics and Neurosurgery, Johns Hopkins University, Baltimore, Maryland

John L. Eady, M.D.
Professor and Chairman, Department of Orthopaedic Surgery, University of South Carolina School of Medicine; Director of Orthopaedic Education, Palmetto Richland Memorial Hospital; and Director of Orthopaedic Education, WJB Dorn Veterans Administration Medical Center, Columbia, South Carolina; Adjunct Professor of Orthopaedics, Medical University of South Carolina, Charleston, South Carolina

Rodney J. Ellis, M.D.
Assistant Professor, Department of Radiology and Radiation Oncology, Case Western Reserve University School of Medicine, Cleveland, Ohio

Patrick J. Getty, M.D.
Assistant Professor, Department of Orthopaedic Surgery, Case Western Reserve University School of Medicine, and University Hospitals of Cleveland, Cleveland, Ohio

Theresa A. Guise, M.D.
Associate Professor, Department of Medicine, Division of Endocrinology, University of Texas Health Science Center at San Antonio, San Antonio, Texas

Leonard L. Gunderson, M.D.
Professor and Chair of Oncology, Mayo Medical School and Mayo Clinic, Rochester, Minnesota

Michael G. Haddock, M.D.
Assistant Professor of Oncology, Mayo Medical School, and Consultant, Division of Radiation Oncology, Mayo Clinic, Rochester, Minnesota

Paul M. Harari, M.D.
Associate Professor, University of Wisconsin Comprehensive Cancer Center, Madison, Wisconsin

Stephen P. Hardy, M.D.
Clinical Associate Professor of Plastic Surgery, University of Wisconsin Medical School, Madison, Wisconsin

Gregory K. Hartig, M.D.
Assistant Professor of Otolaryngology, Department of Surgery, University of Wisconsin Medical School, Madison, Wisconsin

John P. Heiner, M.D.
Professor, Department of Orthopedics and Rehabilitation, University of Wisconsin Medical School, Madison, Wisconsin

John G. Heller, M.D.
Professor of Orthopaedic Surgery, Emory University School of Medicine, Atlanta, Georgia

Stephen M. Horowitz, M.D.
Associate Professor and Chief of Orthopedic Oncology, Hahnemann University Hospital, Philadelphia, Pennsylvania; South Jersey Orthopedic Associates, Voorhees, New Jersey

Steven P. Howard, M.D., Ph.D.
Assistant Professor of Human Oncology, University of Wisconsin Medical School, Madison, Wisconsin

Christy Manker Kesslering, M.D.
Department of Radiation Oncology, University of Wisconsin Medical School, Madison, Wisconsin

Scott E. Kilpatrick, M.D.
Assistant Professor, Department of Pathology and Laboratory Medicine, University of North Carolina, and University of North Carolina Hospitals, Chapel Hill, North Carolina

Timothy J. Kinsella, M.D.
Professor and Chairman, Department of Radiation Oncology, Case Western Reserve University School of Medicine, Cleveland, Ohio

Joseph M. Kowalski, M.D.
Assistant Professor, Department of Orthopaedic Surgery, School of Medicine and Biomedical Sciences, State University of New York, Buffalo, New York

Richard D. Lackman, M.D.
Magnuson Associate Professor and Chairman, Department of Orthopaedic Surgery, University of Pennsylvania School of Medicine, Philadelphia, Pennsylvania

Gerald J. Lang, M.D.
Assistant Professor, Department of Orthopedics and Rehabilitation, University of Wisconsin Medical School, Madison, Wisconsin

David L. Larson, M.D.
Professor and Chairman, Department of Plastic and Reconstructive Surgery, Medical College of Wisconsin, Milwaukee, Wisconsin

Walter L. Longo, M.D.
Professor, Department of Medicine, University of Wisconsin Hospital and Clinics, Madison, Wisconsin

John C. McDermott, M.D.
Professor of Radiology and Chief of Angiography and Interventional Radiology, University of Wisconsin Hospital and Clinics, and Professor of Radiology, William S. Middleton Veterans Memorial Hospital, Madison, Wisconsin

Douglas J. McDonald, M.D.
Professor of Orthopedic Surgery, Washington University School of Medicine, St. Louis, Missouri

Minesh P. Mehta, M.D.
Interim Chair and Associate Professor, Department of Human Oncology, University of Wisconsin Medical School, Madison, Wisconsin

Wilson C. Mertens, M.D.
Medical Director of Cancer Services, North Oakland Medical Centers, Pontiac, Michigan

Thomas J. O'Brien, M.D.
Spine Surgeon, Premier Orthopedics, Nashville, Tennessee

Michael J. O'Connell, M.D.
Professor of Oncology, Mayo Medical School, and Consultant in Medical Oncology, Mayo Clinic, Rochester, Minnesota

Regis J. O'Keefe, M.D., Ph.D.
Associate Professor of Orthopaedic Oncology and Metabolic Bone Disease, University of Rochester and Strong Memorial Hospital, Rochester, New York

Kurt R. Oettel, M.D.
Oncology Fellow, Department of Medicine, University of Wisconsin Medical School, Madison, Wisconsin

Doreen M. Oneschuk, M.D.
Assistant Professor, Department of Oncology, Division of Palliative Medicine, University of Alberta, and Palliative Care Physician Consultant, Regional Palliative Care Program, Edmonton, Alberta, Canada

William M. Parrish, M.D.
Assistant Professor, Department of Orthopaedics and Rehabilitation, Pennsylvania State University College of Medicine, Hershey, Pennsylvania

Terrance D. Peabody, M.D.
Assistant Professor, Department of Surgery, Section of Orthopaedic Surgery and Rehabilitation Medicine, University of Chicago, Chicago, Illinois

Scott B. Perlman, M.D.
Associate Professor of Radiology, Section of Nuclear Medicine, and Director, University of Wisconsin PET Imaging Center, University of Wisconsin Hospital and Clinics, Madison, Wisconsin

Arthur T. Porter, M.D.
Professor, Department of Radiation Oncology, Wayne State University; President and Chief Executive Officer, The Detroit Medical Center; Department of Radiation Oncology, Harper Hospital, Detroit, Michigan; President, American College of Radiation Oncology, Oakbrook, Illinois

Douglas J. Pritchard, M.D.
Professor of Orthopedics and Oncology, Department of Orthopedic Surgery, Mayo Foundation, Rochester, Minnesota

Matthew T. Provencher, M.D.
Resident, Department of Orthopaedic Surgery, Naval Medical Center, San Diego, California

Juluru P. Rao, M.D.
Director of Orthopaedic Resident Education, Department of Orthopaedic Surgery, Jersey City Medical Center, Jersey City, New Jersey; Clinical Professor, Department of Orthopaedics, University of Medicine and Dentistry of New Jersey, Newark, New Jersey

Santi Rao, M.D.
Orthopaedic Surgeon, The Specialists Orthopedic Corporation, Fairfield, California

Douglas Reintgen, M.D.
Professor of Surgery, University of South Florida, Tampa, Florida

Gregory H. Ripple, M.D.
Southern Vermont Cancer Center, Bennington, Vermont

Randy N. Rosier, M.D., Ph.D.
Chairman, Department of Orthopaedics, and Professor of Oncology, Biochemistry, and Biophysics, University of Rochester, Rochester, New York

James R. Ryan, M.D.
Professor, Department of Orthopaedic Surgery, Wayne State University; Chief of Orthopaedic Oncology, Department of Orthopaedic Surgery, Hutzel Hospital; and Director of Musculoskeletal Service, Karmanos Cancer Center, Detroit, Michigan

Michael A. Samuels, M.D.
Assistant Professor of Radiation Oncology, Case Western Reserve University School of Medicine, Cleveland, Ohio

Julian C. Schink, M.D.
Professor and Vice Chair, Department of Obstetrics and Gynecology, University of Wisconsin Medical School, Madison, Wisconsin

Craig A. Schulz, M.D.
Resident, Department of Human Oncology, University of Wisconsin Hospital and Clinics, Madison, Wisconsin

Franklin H. Sim, M.D.
Professor of Orthopedic Surgery, Mayo Clinic, Rochester, Minnesota

James A. Stewart, M.D.
Professor, Department of Medicine, Section of Medical Oncology, University of Wisconsin Medical School; University of Wisconsin Comprehensive Cancer Center, Madison, Wisconsin

Murali Sundaram, M.D., F.R.C.R.
Professor of Radiology, St. Louis University Health Sciences Center, St. Louis, Missouri

Charles R. Thomas, Jr., M.D.
Associate Professor and Vice-Chairman, Department of Radiation Oncology; Adjunct Associate Professor, Division of Medical Oncology, Department of Medicine, University of Texas Health Science Center at San Antonio; Member, Cancer Therapy and Cancer Research Center and San Antonio Cancer Institute, San Antonio, Texas

Katsuro Tomita, M.D., Ph.D.
Professor and Chairman, Department of Orthopaedic Surgery, Kanazawa University School of Medicine, Kanazawa, Japan

Michael J. Tuite, M.D.
Associate Professor, Department of Radiology, University of Wisconsin Medical School, Madison, Wisconsin

Andrew T. Turrisi III, M.D.
Professor and Chairman, Department of Radiation Oncology, Medical University of South Carolina, Charleston, South Carolina

Lynn Van Ummersen, M.D.
Assistant Professor, Department of Medicine, University of Wisconsin Hospital and Clinics, and University of Wisconsin Comprehensive Cancer Center, Madison, Wisconsin

Ray Vanderby, Jr., Ph.D.
Associate Professor, Departments of Orthopedic Surgery and Biomedical Engineering, University of Wisconsin Medical School, Madison, Wisconsin

William G. Ward, M.D.
Associate Professor, Department of Orthopaedic Surgery, Wake Forest University, Winston Salem, North Carolina

James N. Weinstein, D.O., M.S.
Professor of Surgery and Community and Family Medicine and Director, Surgical Outcomes Assessment Program, Center for the Evaluative Clinical Sciences, Dartmouth Medical School; Director, Spine Center, Department of Orthopaedic Surgery, Dartmouth Hitchcock Medical Center, Lebanon, New Hampshire

George Wilding, M.D.
Anderson Professor of Medicine, and Head of Medical Oncology Section, University of Wisconsin Hospital and Clinics, Madison, Wisconsin

Todd E. Williams, M.D.
Assistant Professor, Department of Radiation Oncology, Medical University of South Carolina, Charleston, South Carolina

Wen-hsien Wu, M.D.
Professor, Department of Anesthesia and Pain Medicine, University of Medicine and Dentistry of New Jersey, and Department of Anesthesiology, University Hospital, Newark, New Jersey

Alan W. Yasko, M.D.
Associate Professor of Surgery and Chief, Section of Orthopaedic Oncology, Department of Surgical Oncology, The University of Texas M.D. Anderson Cancer Center, Houston, Texas

Thomas A. Zdeblick, M.D.
Professor, Department of Orthopedics and Rehabilitation, University of Wisconsin Medical School, and Director, University of Wisconsin Spine Center, Madison, Wisconsin

Metastatic disease to the skeleton is a
common endpoint for a number of malignant diseases.
In the practice of oncology we encounter a large number of patients
battling the pain and disability that is an all too common component of this
disease. Amazingly these patients consistently exhibit courage
and humor despite the ominous circumstances
in which they have been placed.

This book is dedicated to these patients
who have taught us a lot about appreciating life
and facing death with dignity. Hopefully this book will improve
the treatment of these patients and allow us to improve
the quality of their lives.

Foreword

Metastatic disease to the musculoskeletal system is accompanied by severe pain, impaired mobility, and progressive disability. The quality of life of the patients in whom this complication develops often becomes much worse. Proper management will markedly improve that quality of life, decrease pain, and improve mobility. The management of this complication entails a multidisciplinary approach. Up until now there has been no single reference text that provides the broad scope of diagnosis, management, and specific disease-related discussions. This book edited by Drs. John Heiner, Timothy Kinsella, and Thomas Zdeblick is unique. The 42 chapters contain useful information for the cancer specialist, radiotherapist, and orthopedic surgeon, who often work together to manage the various clinical manifestations of bone metastases.

Of particular note are the 27 chapters that not only deal with specific cancers but also present discussions of specific axial and peripheral bone metastases. These include skull base, orbit, spinal pelvis, femurs, arm, shoulder, and soft tissue sites. The focus here is on solving problems of anatomical sites. The final chapters deal with possible complications of the therapies, such as fixation failure and wound healing following radiation.

This text will be a valuable resource for the oncologist, radiotherapist, surgeon, and internist who are challenged to make the right diagnosis and treatment choices for their patients.

Paul P. Carbone, M.D., M.A.C.P.
Professor of Medicine Emeritus
University of Wisconsin Medical School
Madison, Wisconsin

Preface

With the advances in cancer therapy, the survival and quality of life have markedly changed for a large number of patients with cancer. With the longer survival of these patients, late metastatic disease to the skeleton has become an increasingly common problem. It is not unusual for patients to now survive for years with metastatic disease to the bones, especially those patients with breast and prostate cancer. Keeping the patients ambulatory and independent is now the goal.

Multiple modalities are used in most patients to try to minimize bone pain and pathologic fractures. The research into metastatic skeletal disease is growing exponentially along with clinical trials of various osteoclast inhibitors to reduce pathologic fractures. Radiation therapy and surgery are coordinated to give optimal local control of disease, especially in the spine and long bones. Unfortunately, although much progress has been made in metastatic disease, we still have a long way to go. Many patients with lung cancer and gastrointestinal malignancies usually have a rapidly progressive downhill course after the advent of metastatic skeletal disease. Some of the lesions are difficult to control locally with both surgery and radiation and ultimately require amputation.

This text attempts to give the reader a broad overview of musculoskeletal metastatic disease. Authors from many of the major cancer centers across the country have contributed their knowledge, with several contributors from outside the United States. Each author brings a unique perspective that adds to this multi-institutional approach for these patients. The chapters are organized to provide information about site-specific disease as well as information about the prognosis and treatment of specific tumors. Each lead author has assembled a multidisciplinary team to assist in writing most disease and site-specific chapters. Hopefully, oncologists, internists, radiation therapists, and orthopedic surgeons will all find the topics and discussions helpful in the daily management of these patients. As we found when assembling this book, many of the chapters have little information in the peer-reviewed literature, so it is our hope that readers will be encouraged to add to the research in the area of metastatic disease of the skeleton. This book is our initial attempt to compile a large amount of information from diverse sources to help the clinicians who care for the patient with musculoskeletal metastatic disease, and we hope the readers find the text informative and practical.

In Appreciation

We owe a tremendous amount of thanks to Andrea Schmick for all of her patience and help in organizing and collecting the chapters for this book. We would also like to thank Karen Berger and Michelle Leaman at Quality Medical Publishing for their support of this book. Their editing comments were invaluable.

John P. Heiner, M.D.
Timothy J. Kinsella, M.D.
Thomas A. Zdeblick, M.D.

Contents

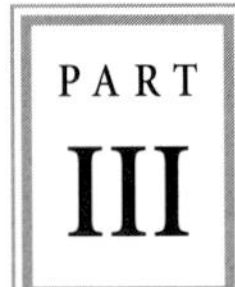

PART III

Therapeutic Approaches

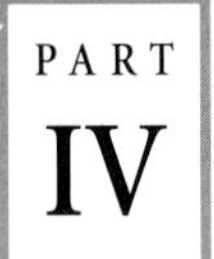

PART IV

Management of Specific Metastatic Tumors

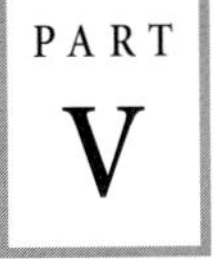

PART

V

Management of Specific Metastatic Sites

Axial Skeleton

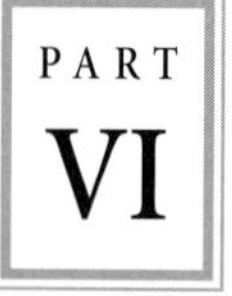

PART

VI Special Problems

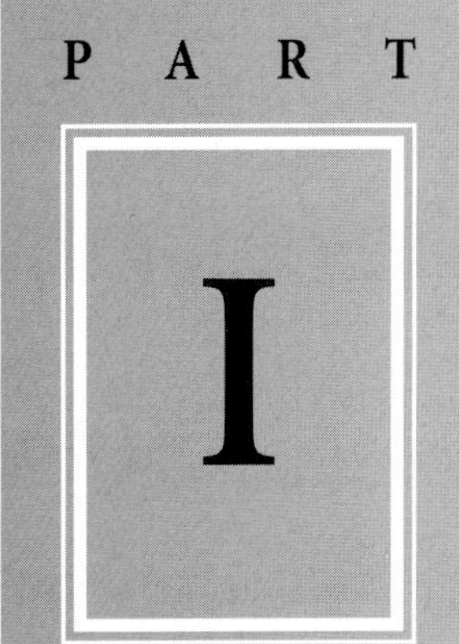

Fundamentals

1 History and Epidemiology

Timothy A. Damron, M.D.

History
Prevalence
Improving Survival Rates
Impact on Society

HISTORY

Evidence of metastatic skeletal disease has been discovered in some of the earliest remains of human civilization. In addition, the history of metastatic disease is closely interwoven into the rich early history of medicine, cancer, and surgery, with physicians from Hippocrates to Paget, Schwann, von Recklinghausen, and Virchow involved in its lore.[1] The earliest evidence of metastatic disease stems from excavations of 415 mummies and skeletons from the large necropolis of Thebes West, Upper Egypt.[2] It is estimated that these specimens were deposited between 1500 and 500 BC. Four cases of malignant tumors affecting the skeleton were identified among these parts. Radiographs in two of the cases showed multiple mixed lytic and blastic lesions, suggesting metastatic carcinoma. In two other individuals' bones, radiographs showed multiple lytic defects in the vertebrae, pelvis, and skull, which were considered suggestive of multiple myeloma.[2] From the authors' calculations of age- and sex-adjusted tumor prevalence based on the four cases discovered among 325 adults, skeletal malignant tumors were somewhat more common in Egypt more than 2500 years ago than they were in an English population from 1901 to 1905 and somewhat less common than they are today.

Other reports of metastatic disease in the skull and facial bones of Egyptian mummies have been reported.[3] Disseminated melanin-containing deposits consistent with metastatic malignant melanoma were discovered in the skull and bones of the extremities in two pre-Columbian Inca mummies estimated by radioactive carbon dating to be 2400 years old.[4] Metastatic prostate cancer deposits were discovered in the skeleton of a mature man from the Middle Ages excavated in Svendborg, Denmark.[5] Clearly, skeletal metastatic disease was a prevalent health problem even in historic populations, and factors affecting the varying prevalence were at work even then.[2]

Hippocrates (460-377 BC) is the first investigator to have recorded a recognition of malignant neoplasms and metastatic disease.[6-9] He described the invasion of tumors into both bone and soft tissue. The term "metastasis" was first used in the Hippocratic corpus, *On the Nature of the Human Being,* to refer to evacuation and shifting of an abnormal humor from one internal organ to another.[10] The prevailing theory of diseases at that time was based on the doctrine of Empedocles (ca. 495-435 BC) that there were four elements: fire, water, earth, and air.[1,10,11] Hippocratic medicine turned this doctrine into the concept of four body fluids: warm, dry blood; cold, dry yellow bile; warm, wet black bile; and cold, wet mucus. Diseases were thought to be caused by an imbalance of these fluids. According to this "humoralist" theory, tumors were attributed to an excess of black bile.[3] Galen, a Greek physician born around 130 AD, extended these humoralist views into a doctrine that dominated medical understanding for centuries.[1] Galen refined the term "metastasizing" to refer to the condition in which diseases move from one part of the body to another.[10]

More than a millennium passed before the next written evidence of the concept of metastatic disease. During the fifteenth century, the sudden occurrence of a pathologic fracture was considered by some to be the result of divine or satanic intervention for either inordinate pride or inadequate religious zeal.[12] In 1735, de Gorter suggested that "cancereuse stoffe" may enter the blood circulation and make "een metastasis van de eene glandule op de andere" (a metastasis from one glandule to another).[1] During the Age of Enlightenment in the eighteenth century, Galen's humoralist concepts began to be questioned.

In the 1820s, when optically corrected microscope lenses began to be manufactured, Johannes Müller began to study tumors under the microscope.[10] Müller's student, Theodor Schwann, suggested in the first of three landmark papers published during 1838 that the cell theory for animal tissues, already accepted in botany, could be applied to the study of tumors.[10] Müller and Schwann championed this cell theory throughout the 1850s. In keeping with the long-standing tradition of the humoralist theory, the origin of the cells, both normal and diseased, was initially theorized to be a rudimentary, pleuripotential fluid "blastema." Metastases were attributed to dissemination of diseased blastema.[1] Sir James Paget stated, "A rudimental liquid, an unformed cancerous blastema, mingled with the blood, may be as effectual as any germs." Müller, siding with the developing "solidistic" theory of disease, speculated that, in fact, cells might be the essential component of metastases: "Once cells with a productive tendency have arisen, it can readily be seen how the uptake of germnuclei into the circulation can lead to their spread via the circulation to a soil suitable for their development, and thus give rise to secondary tumors."[10] In 1840, Bernhard von Langenbeck provided objective support to the cellular metastatic theory when he identified aggregates of cancer cells within the pelvic veins, the right side of the heart, the pulmonary artery, and the subpleural region in two women with uterine cancer.[10] Dunglinson's medical dictionary of 1842 reflects the current thinking and controversy at that time.[10] Metastasis was defined then as a "change in the seat of a disease; attributed by the Humorists, to the translation of the morbific matter to a part different from that which it had previously occupied; and by the Solidists, to the displacement of the irritation."

It was not until 1865 that the cellular basis of metastasis began to gain acceptance with the reports by Thiersch[13] that epithelial cells were the origin of carcinoma. In 1889, Stephen Paget, of London, emphasized the importance of the "soil" in allowing growth of embolic tumor cells by noting the propensity for liver metastases and the paucity of splenic metastases in 735 cases of breast cancer.[1]

During the early and middle parts of the twentieth century, metastases were considered a relatively passive process resulting from growth of the primary tumor, anoxia, reduced cell-to-cell cohesiveness, and resultant detachment of cells.[14,15] Surgical treatment of metastatic disease to bone, up to and during this period, was limited, and apathy prevailed in the care of these unfortunate patients because of their poor overall prognosis. To a large extent, apathy remained the norm until the 1960s and 1970s, when Harrington, Sim, and others[16-18] demonstrated that the addition of bone cement to internal fixation techniques improved longevity of the implants in the face of severely diseased bone and translated into decreased pain and improved function for the patients.

During the 1970s and 1980s a greater understanding of the multistep process of tumor invasiveness and metastasis was achieved.[3] At the same time, surgical techniques evolved as more versatile internal fixation devices and prostheses became widely available. The Zickel nail, originally the standard for pathologic proximal femur fractures, began to be supplanted by the locked reconstruction intramedullary nail.[19-22] Modular segmental replacement prostheses, originally developed as custom implants for limb salvage after bone sarcomas, began to be used in metastatic disease.[23] During the 1990s and the beginning of the new millennium, the focus in metastatic disease has shifted to specific signaling networks and cell-cycle control pathways that are unique to metastasizing cells and that may serve as targets for drug or gene therapy. Prevention of the skeletal complications of metastatic disease has already begun to be achieved through the use of bisphosphonates to counteract the actions of the cellular mediator of osteolysis, the osteoclast. These drugs have become the current norm in the treatment of breast cancer, prostate cancer, lung cancer, and symptomatic myeloma.[24-26] Despite these impressive steps forward, metastatic disease remains a prevalent problem with significant impact on society.

PREVALENCE

During the year 2000, there will be an estimated 1,220,100 new cancer cases in the United States, based on data from the U.S. Bureau of the Census and age-specific cancer rates from the National Cancer Institute's Surveillance, Epidemiology, and End Results (SEER) program.[27] From 20% to 85% of patients with these cancers may develop bone marrow involvement.[3,28-30] These estimates vary considerably on the basis of the methods from which they are derived. Autopsy estimates, despite the inherent difficulty of accurately documenting skeletal metastases by this technique, have suggested the highest prevalence.[29,31] Estimates based on nuclear medicine studies are higher than estimates based on plain radiographs alone.[28-30,32,33] Bone has traditionally been the third most common site of metastatic disease, after lung and liver.[3,34] In contrast to the high prevalence of metastatic disease to bone, during 2000 there will be only an estimated 1400 new cases of bone sarcoma.[27]

The total number of estimated new cancer cases has increased from the 930,000 new cases cited when the last major text on metastatic disease to bone was published in 1988.[3] This increase primarily reflects our ever increasing population because the incidence rates for all cancers peaked in 1992 and declined by approximately 2.2% per year from 1992 through 1996.[27]

Although any malignancy has the potential to involve bone, there are specific primary carcinomas, called "osteophilic" carcinomas, that have a propensity to involve bone.[3,34] The five most common osteophilic tumors are, in order of decreasing prevalence, breast, prostate, lung, kidney, and thyroid. The numbers of estimated new cases and deaths in the year 2000 for these five sites are shown in Table 1-1. These sites will account for an estimated minimum of 42% of the new cancer cases in women and 36% in men during the year 2000.[27] During the same year, cancers to these sites will account for more than 42% of estimated cancer deaths in men and 40% in women.

Breast, prostate, lung, and kidney primary carcinomas account for at least 75% of adult skeletal metastases.[34] For men, the prostate and lung are the most common sites of primary tumors. The prostate is the site of 29% of new cases of cancer in men but has also been estimated to account for 60% of skeletal metastases in men.[27,34] For women, the breast and lung are the most common sites of primary tumors. Breast carcinoma accounts for 30% of new cases of cancer in women and 70% of skeletal metastases in women.[27,34] Lung primary carcinomas account for 14% of new cancer cases in men and 12% in women.[27]

"Osteophobic" tumors are those with a particularly low prevalence of skeletal involvement.[34] Primary cancers of the skin, oral cavity, esophagus, cervix, stomach, and colon have been classically considered osteophobic.[35] However, with improved survival of patients with these cancers, combined with widespread use of more sensitive imaging tests, skeletal metastases to many of these sites are being reported with increasing frequency.[36-51] Despite these reports, typically no more than 2% of patients with these types of cancers will have clinically apparent skeletal metastases. Some unusual tumors, such as nasopharyngeal carcinoma, not classically included in the short list of osteophilic sources, appear also to have a relative affinity for bone as a site of metastasis.[52,53]

IMPROVING SURVIVAL RATES

The improving survival for cancer patients began to be well documented during the 1990s. The improving trends in the United States estimated 5-year survival rates for the most osteophilic bone tumors are shown in Table 1-2. Age-adjusted cancer death rates between 1990 and 1996 showed a consistent downward trend for breast, prostate, and lung cancer for the first time since initiation of such record keeping in 1930.[27] Death rates for women with breast cancer have declined an average

Table 1-1 Estimated new cancer cases and deaths for the year 2000 in the United States

Primary source	New cases	Deaths
Breast	184,200	41,200
Prostate	180,400	31,900
Lung	164,100	156,900
Kidney	31,200	11,900
Thyroid	18,400	1,200

Excerpted from Greenlee RT, Murray T, Bolden S, Wingo PA. Cancer statistics, 2000. CA Cancer J Clin 50:7-33, 2000.

Table 1-2 Five-year relative United States cancer survival rates (%) for osteophilic primary sites by year of diagnosis

Primary site	1974-1976	1980-1982	1989-1995
Breast	75	76	85
Prostate	67	73	92
Lung	13	13	14
Kidney	52	52	60
Thyroid	92	94	95

Excerpted from Greenlee RT, Murray T, Bolden S, Wingo PA. Cancer statistics, 2000. CA Cancer J Clin 50:7-33, 2000.

of 1.8% per year between 1990 and 1996.[27] During the same period there was an average 1.6% decline per year in the death rates for men with prostate and lung-bronchus cancers. Annual breast cancer deaths in the United States were highest in 1995 at 43,844 and declined to 41,943 in 1997.[27] Prostate cancer deaths peaked in 1994 at 34,902 and declined to 32,891 in 1997. Deaths from lung and bronchus cancer in men peaked at 92,493 in 1993 and declined to 91,278 in 1997.[27]

IMPACT ON SOCIETY

Despite the encouraging trends in survival for many cancers, cancer and therefore metastatic disease remain major health problems. Cancer remains the second leading cause of death in the United States, accounting for an estimated 539,577 deaths (23.3% of all deaths) during 1997.[27] Only the death rate for heart disease, which accounted for an estimated 726,974 deaths (31.4% of all deaths) during the same period, is higher. The death rate for cancer is 164.1 per 100,000 population. The next most frequent cause of death in the United States, cerebrovascular disease, has a death rate less than one fourth that of cancer.[27]

The improving survival rate for cancer patients has important implications in the care of patients with metastatic disease to bone. Complications of skeletal metastatic disease, including bone pain, pathologic fracture, hypercalcemia, immobility, and even spinal cord syndromes, are a more sustained source of morbidity for the cancer patient who is now living longer with metastatic disease. Such patients require more prolonged treatment after the development of metastatic disease. Problems that in the past have been associated with terminal events must now be treated for years. Medications to counteract the damaging effects of metastatic disease on bone, such as the bisphosphonates, may be required for prolonged periods. Fracture fixation constructs may be expected to survive for years rather than just a few months—and often in the face of segmentally deficient bone. To improve the quality of life for these patients, better biologically based treatments of metastatic disease are needed to reduce pain and suffering. Novel therapies to prevent the development, dissemination, proliferation, and growth of metastatic

deposits are necessary. Approaches to pathologic fractures should be focused on improving healing rather than relying on metal and bone cement reconstruction. When necessary, reconstructive alternatives for pathologic fractures, spinal involvement, and acetabular destruction will need to survive for increasingly long periods. Continued multidisciplinary work from both a clinical and a research standpoint is crucial.

REFERENCES

1. De Moulin D. A Short History of Breast Cancer. Boston: Martinus Nijhoff Publishers, 1983.
2. Zink A, Rohrbach H, Szeimies U, et al. Malignant tumors in an ancient Egyptian population. Anticancer Res 19:4273-4277, 1999.
3. Frassica FJ, Sim FH. Pathogenesis and prognosis. In Sim FH, ed. Diagnosis and Management of Metastatic Bone Disease: A Multidisciplinary Approach. New York: Raven Press, 1988, pp 1-6.
4. Urteaga O, Pack GT. On the antiquity of melanoma. Cancer 19:607-610, 1966.
5. Tkocz I, Bierring F. A medieval case of metastasizing carcinoma with multiple osteosclerotic bone lesions. Am J Phys Anthropol 65:373-380, 1984.
6. Adams F. The Genuine Works of Hippocrates. London: Sydenham Society, 1849.
7. Keil H. The historical relationship between the concept of tumor and the ending -oma. Bull Hist Med 24:352-377, 1950.
8. Long ER. A History of Pathology. New York: Dover Publications, 1965, pp 63-75.
9. Osler W. The Evolution of Modern Medicine. New Haven: Yale University Press, 1921.
10. Rather LJ. The Genesis of Cancer: A Study in the History of Ideas. Baltimore: The Johns Hopkins University Press, 1978.
11. Haeger K. The rise of Western surgery. In Haeger K, ed. The Illustrated History of Surgery. New York: Bell Publishing Company, 1988, pp 35-68.
12. Brant S. Das Narrenschiff [The Ship of Fools], 1494.
13. Thiersch C. Der Epithelialkrebs namentlich der Haut: Eine anatomisch-Klinische Untersuchung. Leipzig: W Engelmann, 1865.
14. Tyzzer EE. Factors in the production and growth of tumor metastases. J Med Res 28:309-333, 1913.
15. Eaves G. The invasive growth of malignant tumours as a purely mechanical process. J Pathol 109:233-237, 1973.
16. Harrington KD, Sim FH, Enis JE, Johnston JO, Diok HM, Gristina AG. Methylmethacrylate as an adjunct in internal fixation of pathologic fractures. J Bone Joint Surg Am 58: 1047-1055, 1976.
17. Harrington KD. The use of methylmethacrylate as an adjunct in the internal fixation of malignant neoplastic fractures. J Bone Joint Surg Am 54:1665-1676, 1972.
18. Sim FH, Daugherty TW, Ivins JC. The adjunctive use of methylmethacrylate in fixation of pathological fractures. J Bone Joint Surg Am 56:40-48, 1974.

19. Zickel RE, Mouradian WH. Intramedullary fixation of pathological fractures and lesions of the subtrochanteric region of the femur. J Bone Joint Surg Am 58:1061-1066, 1976.

20. Mickelson MR, Bonfiglio M. Pathological fractures in the proximal part of the femur treated by Zickel-nail fixation. J Bone Joint Surg Am 58:1067-1070, 1976.

21. Sangeorzan BJ, Ryan JR, Salciccioli GG. Prophylactic femoral stabilization with the Zickel nail by closed technique. J Bone Joint Surg Am 68:991-999, 1986.

22. Weikert DR, Schwartz HS. Intramedullary nailing for impending pathological subtrochanteric fractures. J Bone Joint Surg Br 73:668-670, 1991.

23. Lane JM, Sculco TP, Zolan S. Treatment of pathological fractures of the hip by endoprosthetic replacement. J Bone Joint Surg Am 62:954-959, 1980.

24. Kristensen B, Ejlertsen B, Groenvold M, Hein S, Loft H, Mouridsen HT. Oral clodronate in breast cancer patients with bone metastases: A randomized study. J Intern Med 246:67-74, 1999.

25. Blomqvist C, Elomaa I. Bisphosphonate therapy in metastatic breast cancer. Acta Oncol 35:81-83, 1996.

26. Bloomfield DJ. Should bisphosphonates be part of the standard therapy of patients with multiple myeloma or bone metastases from other cancers? An evidence-based review [see comments]. J Clin Oncol 16:1218-1225, 1998.

27. Greenlee RT, Murray T, Bolden S, Wingo PA. Cancer statistics, 2000. CA Cancer J Clin 50:7-33, 2000.

28. Mercer SW, Duthrie RB. Orthopedic Surgery. Baltimore: Williams & Wilkins, 1964.

29. Jaffe HL. Tumors and Tumorous Conditions of Bones and Joints. Philadelphia: Lea & Febiger, 1958.

30. Johnston AD. Pathology of metastatic tumors in bone. Clin Orthop 73:8-32, 1970.

31. Abrams HL, Sprio R, Goldstein N. Metastases in carcinoma: Analysis of 1000 autopsied cases. Cancer 3:74, 1950.

32. Galasko CSB. The value of scintigraphy in malignant disease. Cancer Treat Rev 2:225, 1975.

33. Tofe AJ, Francis MD, Harvey WJ. Correlation of neoplasms with incidence and localization of skeletal metastases: An analysis of 1,355 diphosphonate bone scans. J Nucl Med 16:986-989, 1975.

34. Robbins SG, Lane JM, Healey JH, Cornell CN. Metastatic bone disease: Epidemiology, biology, diagnosis, and treatment. In Lane JM, Healey JH, eds. Diagnosis and Management of Pathologic Fractures. New York: Raven Press, 1993, pp 83-98.

35. Sim FH. Metastatic bone disease and myeloma. In Ewarts CMC, ed. Surgery of the Musculoskeletal System, vol. 11. New York: Churchill Livingstone, 1983, p 393.

36. Coker DD, Elias EG, Viravathana T, McCrea E, Hafiz M. Chemotherapy for metastatic basal cell carcinoma. Arch Dermatol 119:44-50, 1983.

37. DeBoer DK, Schwartz HS, Thelman S, Reynolds VH. Heterogeneous survival rates for isolated skeletal metastases from melanoma. Clin Orthop Feb(323):277-283, 1996.

38. Kleinberg C, Penetrante RB, Milgrom H, Pickren JW. Metastatic basal cell carcinoma of the skin: Metastasis to the skeletal system producing myelophthisic anemia. J Am Acad Dermatol 7:655-659, 1982.

39. Stewart WR, Gelberman RH, Harrelson JM, Seigler HF. Skeletal metastases of melanoma. J Bone Joint Surg Am 60:645-649, 1978.

40. Vigorita VJ, Vitale A, Sclafani S, Pinnapureddy PR. Case report 403: Extramammary Paget disease of the skin with disseminated skeletal metastases. Skeletal Radiol 15:680-684, 1986.

41. Yousem DM, Magid D, Scott WW Jr, Fishman EK. Treated invasive cervical carcinoma: Utility of computed tomography in distinguishing between skeletal metastases and radiation necrosis. Clin Imaging 13:147-153, 1989.

42. du Toit JP, Grove DV. Radioisotope bone scanning for the detection of occult bony metastases in invasive cervical carcinoma. Gynecol Oncol 28:215-219, 1987.

43. Kim RY, Weppelmann B, Salter MM, Brascho DJ. Skeletal metastases from cancer of the uterine cervix: Frequency, patterns, and radiotherapeutic significance. Int J Radiat Oncol Biol Phys 13:705-708, 1987.

44. Nitzan DW, Livni N, Marmary Y, Ben-Baruch N, Sela J, Catane R. The use of monoclonal anti-CEA antibody immunohistochemistry in detecting the origin of oral cavity metastasis. Int J Oral Maxillofac Surg 19:162-164, 1990.

45. Singh HK, Silverman JF, Ballance WA Jr, Park HK. Unusual small bone metastases from epithelial malignancies: Diagnosis by fine-needle aspiration cytology with histologic confirmation. Diagn Cytopathol 13:192-195, 1995.

46. Schultz SR, Bree RL, Schwab RE, Raiss G. CT detection of skeletal muscle metastases. J Comput Assist Tomogr 10:81-83, 1986.

47. Narvaez JA, Narvaez J, Clavaguera MT, Juanola X, Valls C, Fiter J. Bone and skeletal muscle metastases from gastric adenocarcinoma: Unusual radiographic, CT and scintigraphic features. Eur Radiol 8:1366-1369, 1998.

48. Jacobsen S, Stephensen SL, Paaske BP, Lie PG, Lausten GS. Skeletal metastases of unknown origin: A retrospective analysis of 29 cases. Acta Orthop Belg 63:15-22, 1997.

49. Carstens SA, Resnick D. Diffuse sclerotic skeletal metastases as an initial feature of gastric carcinoma. Arch Intern Med 140:1666-1668, 1980.

50. Besbeas S, Stearns MW Jr. Osseous metastases from carcinomas of the colon and rectum. Dis Colon Rectum 21:266-268, 1978.

51. Rougraff BT, Kneisl JS, Simon MA. Skeletal metastases of unknown origin: A prospective study of a diagnostic strategy. J Bone Joint Surg Am 75:1276-1281, 1993.

52. Sham JS, Cheung YK, Chan FL, Choy D. Nasopharyngeal carcinoma: Pattern of skeletal metastases. Br J Radiol 63:202-205, 1990.

53. Khor TH, Tan BC, Chua EJ, Chia KB. Distant metastases in nasopharyngeal carcinoma. Clin Radiol 29:27-30, 1978.

Molecular Mechanisms of Metastasis

Randy N. Rosier, M.D., Ph.D., and
Regis J. O'Keefe, M.D., Ph.D.

The prevention of metastatic cancer is one of the greatest challenges facing medicine. Although advances in local treatments for cancer and its early detection have improved outcomes in many patients, it remains true that once metastasis of a cancer has occurred, the likelihood of cure diminishes profoundly. The essential characteristic of all cancers is their ability to migrate to organ sites remote from the primary tumor and generate secondary tumors at these sites, which essentially defines the process of metastasis. Fundamentally, it is this ability that segregates malignant from benign neoplasms, and the property of metastasis is what makes cancer a lethal disease. In the example of primary musculoskeletal cancers, or sarcomas, limb salvage procedures, modern imaging, and multimodality treatments have improved local control rates of 95%; yet one third to half of all patients with sarcoma still succumb to metastatic disease. Clearly, improved scientific understanding of metastasis is essential to making further major advances in improving survival of patients with cancer.

Metastasis is an incredibly complex biologic phenomenon and yet is remarkable in the universality of its component processes across an enormous diversity of tumor types. Although the basic process is common to all cancers, it has long been recognized that patterns of metastasis have many features that are specific to the tumor type. We are only beginning to understand some of the molecular events that are common to all metastatic tumors, as well as those factors that account for the specificity of particular patterns of dissemination. The "seed and soil" hypothesis, first advanced by Paget in 1889, finds increasing support as new findings regarding the molecular and cellular biology of metastasis evolve.[1,2] The tenets of this hypothesis are that, to metastasize, the tumor cell, or "seed," must possess specific properties conferring the ability to migrate to a remote site and proliferate into a secondary tumor; the "soil," referring to the host tissue and its cellular components, must produce an environment where implantation, proliferation, and development of supporting functions, such as vasculature, are accommodated. The importance of host–tumor cell interactions in the metastatic process is becoming more apparent as the molecular controlling events and factors are better defined.

Examples of the specificity of the host–tumor cell interactions are numerous: metastatic sarcomas almost always involve the lungs; many carcinomas tend to metastasize to bone and preferentially involve the axial and proximal appendicular skeleton; certain soft tissue tumors involve lymph nodes and others do not; and colonic carcinomas metastasize to the liver, even though some carcinomas rarely involve this organ. Some of these patterns may relate to anatomic factors, such as vascular and lymphatic supply, that allow access to a given site.[2] Trapping of tumor cells that enter the venous circulation in the pulmonary capillary bed has long been assumed to account for the high incidence of metastasis to the lungs by many tumor types. The propensity for hepatic metastasis of colonic carcinomas is accounted for in part by the vascular patterns of these organs. Similarly, the lack of nodal metastasis by bone tumors may relate to the absence of lymphatic vessels within bone, decreasing the accessibility of this route to those tumors. Another example is the propensity of primary tumors within pelvic organ systems to metastasize preferentially to the spine and pelvic bones, hypothesized to be related to the potential for bidirectional blood flow in the valveless veins within Batson's plexus along the spine.[2] These geographic anatomic factors are undoubtedly important; however, it is becoming increasingly apparent that local tumor cell–host interactions may provide additional targeting mechanisms that confer secondary site specificity. In an interesting experiment that highlights the importance of such interactions, Kuratsu et al.[3] used an osteosarcoma metastasis animal model. When injected intravenously, osteosarcoma cells would metastasize preferentially to the lungs, mimicking the clinical situation with this tumor type. The investigators removed pieces of lung and implanted them ectopically in the subcutaneous tissue. On intravenous injection, the osteosarcoma cells were then found to metastasize both to the lungs and to the lung explants. Furthermore, when lung tissue was digested to obtain just the cells without the organ architecture, and these cells were implanted ectopically in the subcutaneous tissue, remarkably the osteosarcoma cells metastasized to the cell pellets. This result demonstrates dramatically the importance of host tissue–tumor cell interactions as a major determinant in the patterns of metastatic spread.

METASTATIC EVENTS AND MODELS

A specific series of coordinated events is required for metastasis to occur, and these events provide new targets for cancer treatment. The sequence of events and the tumor cell properties essential to metastasis include the following: (1) cell motility, (2) expression of proteases allowing degradation of extracellular matrix and basement membranes, (3) intravasation, (4) endothelial attachment and interaction at a remote site, (5) extravasation at a remote site, involving again the use of proteolytic mechanisms, (6) attachment to host tissues by means of tumor cell–host interactions, (7) proliferation of cells to form a secondary tumor, (8) induction of angiogenesis to develop blood supply to support further tumor growth and local invasion, and (9) potential further metastasis from the secondary site by repetition of the sequence of events.

The metastatic process and its key steps are depicted in Fig. 2-1. These events are further modulated by participation of the host immune cells in tumor cell destruction and inflammatory responses. Defining the rate-limiting steps of this sequence is essential to the development of new approaches to circumventing metastasis of cancers. This has been made difficult by the diversity of tumor types and behaviors, however, and by the problems associated with the creation of valid models to study the metastatic process. Parameters that have been studied in vitro include cell growth, tumor–host cell interactions, cell attachment factors, chemotaxis mechanisms, invasiveness, protease expression and regulation, and the effects of cytokines and growth factors on cell behavior. Some insights have also been gained by study of the expression of factors important to metastasis, such as matrix metalloproteinases (MMPs), growth factors, and oncogenes, in tissue specimens or blood samples from cancer patients.[4-7] Many aspects of metastasis, however, can be studied only with in vivo models, and

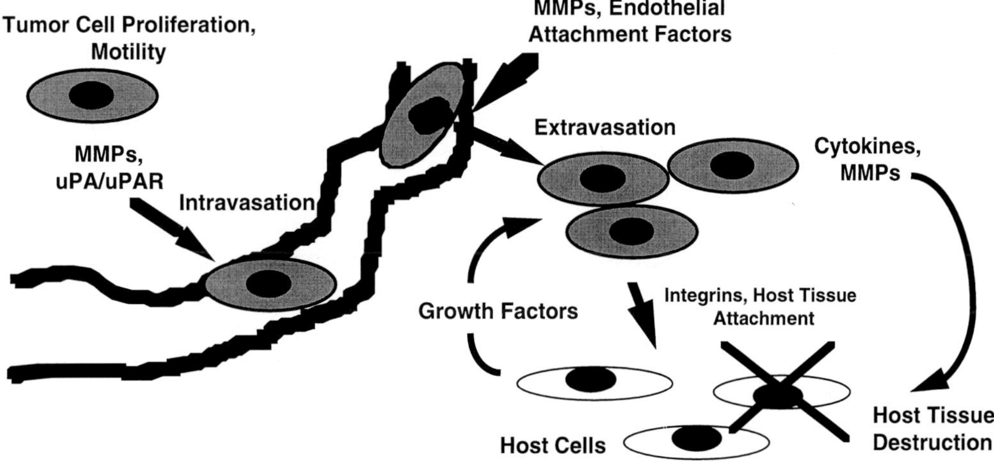

Fig. 2-1   Summary of the process of metastasis. Tumor cells proliferate at the primary site and exhibit the property of motility through expression of specific cytoskeletal genes. For cells to penetrate the basement membrane of vascular or lymphatic channels, expression of MMPs, in particular MMP9 (gelatinase B), is required, in conjunction with expression of uPA and the uPA receptor, uPAR. Presumably the expression of uPA and uPAR functions to activate and concentrate MMP activities at the invading margin of the cell. After intravasation the cells migrate to distant capillaries, where they attach to endothelial cells by specific mechanisms and employ similar proteolytic mechanisms for extravasation into the target organ or tissue. The tumor cells recognize specific attachment factors in the host tissue matrix or cell surfaces, such as integrin ligands. In addition, locally produced growth factors may stimulate tumor proliferation and factors necessary for invasion. Cytokines and MMPs regulated by cytokines result in local host tissue destruction and tumor progression.

the models used have many limitations. Frequently, animal models rely on the introduction of tumor cells intravenously or intra-arterially, with evaluation of subsequent sites of extravasation and secondary tumor formation.[3,8,9] These types of models, although useful, fall short of including the early events of actual metastasis (i.e., intravasation). Studies of cells introduced experimentally into the circulation have shown that as many as 80% of cells may extravasate, a percentage that is probably far greater than during the physiologic process.[9] Nevertheless, the similarity of target organ specificity to natural metastasis in many of these models, as in the osteosarcoma model described previously,[3] does indicate the usefulness of studying some aspects of tumor-host interaction. The introduction of tumor cells directly into the target site can also yield valuable information about local tumor establishment and progression in terms of host-tumor interactions. An example is breast cancer implantation in bone, which has been productive in elucidating factors controlling tumor cell–bone interactions and the critical role of osteoclasts in bone metastasis.[10] In a number of animal models of natural metastasis, implanted tumor cells will migrate to other organ sites in a predictable manner and form secondary tumors.[11,12] These models facilitate study of some of the earlier events in the process. Many animal tumors, however, differ significantly from their human equivalents in their behavior. Substantial efforts have therefore been focused on the study of human tumors, using immunologically compromised mice, such as nude mice or mice with severe, combined immunodeficiency, in which xenogenic tumor growth and metastasis can be evaluated.[13,14] An alternative similar type of in vivo model used recently is the chick embryo chorioallantoic membrane, which, when implanted with human tumor cells, results in remote metastases.[15,16] This model is used at a developmental stage that precedes immune system formation, allowing successful xenografting.[16] Although these types of models incorporate the intravasation, extravasation, remote site targeting, and angiogenesis aspects of the metastatic process, the lack of a normal immune system eliminates the inflammatory responses and immunologic modulation of natural metastasis, which may be critical. Although the majority of the models used to study

metastasis are clearly imperfect, they have contributed important insights into the molecular mechanisms.

Until recently, there have been few data to evaluate the possible rate-limiting steps in the overall process of metastasis. This is due in part to the limitations of the available metastatic models in defining the discrete phases of this process and enabling manipulation of specific phases. A recent study has provided some important new insights in this regard.[16] Metastatic potential has been associated with specific MMPs and their activators, one of which is urokinase-type plasminogen activator (uPA) and its cell surface receptor (uPAR).[4-6,17,18] The uPA/uPAR system appears to function to generate and localize plasmin activity to the immediate environment of the tumor cell plasma membrane. The activity of plasmin is important in proteolytically activating many MMPs, which can then function to degrade extracellular matrix and allow basement membrane invasion. Using the embryonic chick chorioallantoic membrane model to evaluate human tumor metastasis, Kim et al.[16] showed that only cells that expressed two specific elements were capable of intravasation: uPAR and MMP9 (also known as gelatinase B). This is an important finding because in other types of models, such as in vivo intravenous injection or in vitro invasiveness assays that assess penetration of basement membrane–like materials, normal cells or nonmetastatic tumor cells can extravasate or invade, indicating a lack of sensitivity of the model systems to the rate-limiting steps involved in true metastasis. In the chorioallantoic membrane model, a minute fraction of cells inoculated (on the order of 0.05%) actually intravasate, in comparison with much higher rates that can extravasate in other types of models. Furthermore, with this model, normal cells or malignant cells that do not express both uPAR and MMP9 cannot metastasize, which begins to separate out some of the critical requirements for metastasis and points to intravasation as one of the rate-limiting steps in metastasis.

ONCOGENES

Oncogenes are genes involved in growth regulation that have been implicated in the transformation of tumors to a malignant phenotype. Mutations in numerous regulatory genes involved in control of cell proliferation can result in loss of growth control and have been associated with malignancy and metastatic potential. A large number of genes have been identified in which mutations are associated with specific types of cancer. Oncogenes are classified as either proto-oncogenes or anti-oncogenes. Proto-oncogenes are normal growth-regulating genes in which mutations stimulate cell proliferation. Proto-oncogenes were initially identified from viruses that induced malignant transformations in cells or caused tumors in animals. Some viruses can incorporate an oncogene through recombinant events, and overexpression of this gene when the virus infects a cell leads to uncontrolled cell proliferation, or malignant transformation. Some proto-oncogenes associated with human cancers include erb-B1 (squamous carcinomas), c-*myc* (lymphoma), *brca*-1 and *brca*-2 (breast cancer), L-*myc* (lung cancer), *bcl*-2 (lymphoma), *ras* (lung cancer), c-*fos* (osteosarcoma, chondrosarcoma), and c-*src* (colon cancer).[19] Antioncogenes, also called tumor suppressor genes, include the *RB* and p53 genes. These genes normally inhibit cell proliferation, but mutations can interfere with their function and allow excessive cell division. *RB* gene mutations have been associated with retinoblastoma, breast cancer, lung cancer, and osteosarcoma. Mutations of the p53 genes have been found in nearly 50% of human cancers and are common in osteosarcoma, colon cancer, and breast cancer.[7,19] Mutations can occur either in somatic cells or in germline cells, as a result of errors during replication or of environmental mutagens such as toxic chemicals (carcinogens) or radiation. Germline mutations are heritable, whereas somatic mutations are not. The Li-Fraumeni cancer syndrome is the result of a germline mutation in p53 that causes a strong hereditary predisposition to a number of cancers, including colonic carcinoma and osteosarcoma.[19]

Because of the redundancy of the growth regulatory proteins, frequently more than one gene must be altered before a cell can become malignant, particularly in the case of tumor suppressor genes. The need for multiple "hits" to express a fully malignant phenotype is well accepted. In some cases, such as when the *RB* gene is present, a combination of a germline mutation that confers susceptibility does not lead to a malignancy until a second somatic mutation occurs that affects the other *RB* allele.

Rare instances in which a malignant tumor spontaneously regresses or disappears have been hypothesized to result from a further somatic mutation that interferes with cell proliferation or enhances apoptosis.[19] Although proto-oncogene mutations are clearly implicated in the growth dysregulation associated with malignant transformation, relatively little is known about their role in conferring metastatic capability. The *ras* proto-oncogene, which is associated with several cancers, has been found to correlate with metastatic potential in some cells.[19-21] Specific *ras* mutations that stimulate ras-1 mitogen-activated protein kinase (MEK) and its activation target, the extracellular-regulated kinase (ERK) pathway, lead to metastatic tumors, whereas mutations that do not activate the MEK/ERK pathways are tumorigenic but not metastatic.[20] Commutations of *ras* and c-*myc* have also been associated with increased expression of a metastatic phenotype.[21] However, further definition of the specific roles of proto-oncogene mutations in enabling tumor metastasis apart from their growth-dysregulating functions, is currently lacking. This is an important area for further investigation if we are to understand the regulation of tumor metastasis.

CELL MOTILITY

Tumor cells must be motile to be capable of migrating to distant sites and achieving ingress to vascular or lymphatic channels. Under the proper conditions, most cells exhibit the cytoskeletal elements necessary for motility, especially in the in vitro environment of cell culture. Cytoskeletal proteins are essential for numerous cellular functions, including mitosis, cell motility, and intracellular movement and organization of organelles. The cytoskeleton is composed of three major types of polymeric protein filaments: actin filaments, microtubules of tubulin, and the intermediate filaments vimentin or lamin. Cell surface movements are controlled by interactions of the actin molecules with myosins in the cytoplasm, enabling contractility and cell movement. Actin fiber formation is regulated by the Rho family of G proteins, which controls polymerization of the actin proteins. Numerous cytoplasmic proteins associate with the cytoskeletal proteins and control their structure, contractility, and stability. Cell-cell and cell-matrix interactions may be important modulators of cell motility. In addition, chemotaxis may play a significant role in stimulation of motility, as demonstrated for migration of leukocytes in inflammation.[22]

The gene *nm23* (nonmetastatic-23) was originally identified as being expressed at high levels in melanoma cells that did not metastasize and at low levels in cells capable of metastasis. There has been extensive literature and some controversy over the role of *nm23* in metastasis of human cancers.[23,24] Two isoforms of the human gene, *nm23H1* and *nm23H2,* have been identified. Expression of *nm23* correlated with a better prognosis and a lower rate of metastasis in some studies, and a number of studies have also shown that transfection and overexpression of *nm23* experimentally inhibit metastasis. The gene functions as a nucleoside diphosphate kinase and is also homologous to a transcription factor called Puf. Not all studies have shown *nm23* expression to correlate with metastasis, however, and *nm23* remains controversial as a prognostic marker.[25] Recent evidence suggests that the function of *nm23* is to decrease cell motility, and it may be in this manner that the gene influences metastasis.[26,27] This may also explain the lack of correlation in many studies with metastatic potential, because many normal cells or benign tumor cells can exhibit motility without demonstrating metastatic capability. Thus motility is likely a necessary but not a sufficient condition for metastasis.

A second gene that has been identified as a marker or predictor of metastasis is *mts1* (metastasin). It recently has been shown to be a member of the calcium-binding regulatory protein family called the S100 proteins, specifically S100A4.[28] This protein associates with cytoskeletal elements, such as myosin, that control motility and may regulate this cellular function. Metastatic phenotype has been conferred on benign tumors by transfection with S100A4,[29] suggesting that the regulation of motility may be essential in metastasis. The S100A4 protein also binds and sequesters p53, which may have additional effects on tumor growth regulation.[28] A recent study has also documented the formation of "invadopodia" along the advancing edges of malignant cells, where MMP and cell attachment mechanisms may be concentrated.[30] The formation of such structures is undoubtedly dependent on involvement of the cytoskeleton and a specialized aspect of cell motility in malignancy.

MATRIX METALLOPROTEINASES

For cancer cells to invade locally or transgress basement membranes to gain access to lymphatic or vascular channels for dissemination, there is a critical requirement for enzymes capable of degrading the extracellular matrix, or MMPs. A growing number of MMP family members have been identified, although they have certain characteristic features in common. MMPs are secreted proteins produced by both normal and malignant cells. These enzymes have a unique structure conferring metal dependence, with two zinc atoms coordinately bound by conserved histidine groups, one a catalytic and the other a structural site[31-33] (Fig. 2-2). In addition, two calcium-binding sites are also conserved. The enzymatic activity of the MMPs is dependent on the appropriate cation interactions with these sites. All MMPs are secreted in a latent or propeptide form, with part of the peptide folded in such a manner as to block the catalytic sites from substrate access.[32] The folding is controlled by a conformational mechanism called a cysteine switch. Proteolytic activity cleaves the propeptide, allowing MMP enzymatic activity. MMPs can cleave one another in a cascade fashion, amplifying an initial proteolytic event, and tend to have rather broad substrate specificity for various proteins of the extracellular matrix. MMPs were initially characterized according to their molecular weights by the technique of zymography, which involves electrophoresis of cell protein extracts or secreted proteins on a gel containing gelatin. Incubation with appropriate divalent cations causes degradation of the gelatin, and the gel is then stained with Coomassie blue, which binds to the gelatin in the gel wherever the MMP degradation of the gelatin has not occurred. The resulting clear bands against the blue background indicate the relative amounts of activity and molecular weights of the proteases present (Fig. 2-3). Latent forms of MMPs can be activated in vitro by mercuric compounds such as aminophenylmercuric acetate, which results in loss of the propeptide and a change in migration on zymograms to the characteristic molecular weight of the active protein.[34]

Collagenases (MMP1, MMP8, and MMP13), stromelysins (MMP3, MMP10, and MMP11), and gelatinases (MMP2 and MMP9) are some of the major subgroups of MMPs that have been studied

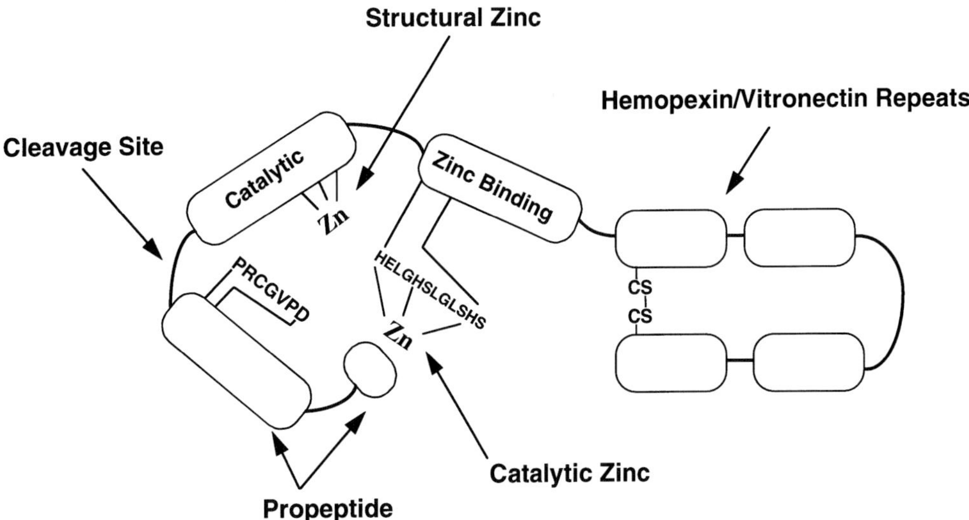

Fig. 2-2   Matrix metalloproteinase structure. All MMPs exhibit a conserved structure. The propeptide region interacts with the catalytic zinc binding site, maintaining the enzyme in an inactive configuration. The zinc binding site employs a conserved amino acid sequence with three coordinating histidine residues. After proteolytic cleavage of the propeptide, the enzyme becomes active, with exposure of the catalytic zinc site. A second conserved zinc binding site is necessary for proper structural conformation for proteolytic activity. In addition, there are two conserved calcium-binding domains (not shown). The enzymes also contain hemopexin and vitronectin repeat modules, which may confer substrate specificity, although their function is uncertain.

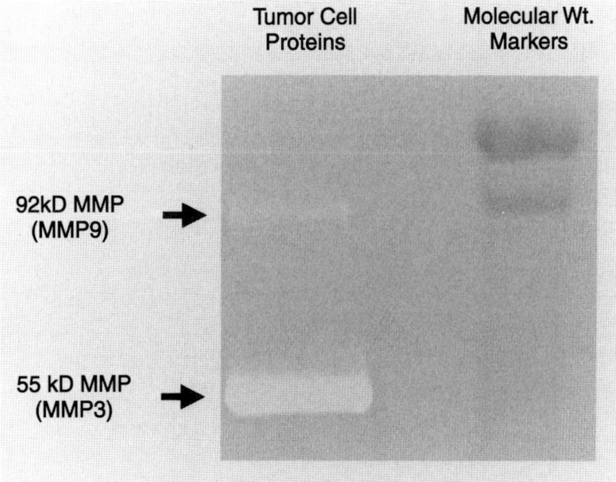

Fig. 2-3   Zymogram. Tumor cell extracts are processed on a mildly denaturing sodium dodecyl sulfate gel into which gelatin is incorporated. Molecular weight markers are processed in parallel. The gel is then incubated with divalent cations at 37° C to allow enzymatic activity, and the gelatin is digested wherever there is proteolytic enzyme present in the gel. Subsequently the gel is stained with Coomassie blue, which stains the gelatin protein diffusely throughout the gel, except wherever it has been digested by the MMPs. The MMP identity is determined by the molecular weight of the clear bands where the gelatin has been digested.

in relation to metastasis, and essentially all tumor cells have been demonstrated to produce one or more of these enzymes.[35] Other types of proteases that may be involved in malignant tumor invasion and metastasis include serine proteases and cathepsins. Serpins are serine protease inhibitors analogous to tissue inhibitor of metalloproteinases (TIMPs), which may play a role in the balance of proteolytic activity in metastasis. Table 2-1 shows some of the more widely studied MMPs.[32] In addition to producing MMPs, tumor cells can induce the expression of MMPs in adjacent host stromal cells. Some MMPs are bound to the plasma membrane after secretion, and these are termed membrane-type MMPs (MT-MMPs).[36] Elevated levels of both secreted MMPs and MT-MMPs have been associated with a wide range of human cancers, and MMP expression is becoming an accepted marker for metastatic potential.[4-6,35] All cells that produce MMPs also produce natural inhibitory proteins of MMP activity, or TIMPs.[37-40] So far, four isoforms of TIMP have been identified. TIMP1 and TIMP2 have been the most extensively studied in cancers and in musculoskeletal remodeling processes. TIMP3 is a matrix-bound form with a prob-

able function in extracellular matrix remodeling and homeostasis. TIMPs bind stoichiometrically to latent MMPs, maintaining them in an inactive form. Dissociation of TIMP from MMPs enables catalytic activity to occur.[37,40] The MMPs that have been most commonly reported to be elevated in metastatic cancers include MMP1, MMP2, MMP3, and MMP9.[35] Thus it is the balance of TIMP and MMP production that controls the overall amount of proteolytic activity. The ratios of the expression of MMP1 to TIMP1 and MMP2 to TIMP2 have been implicated as prognostic markers for local recurrence and metastasis in chondrosarcoma.[41] Transfection with TIMPs has been shown to decrease markedly the metastatic potential of tumor cells in vitro and in vivo, and recombinant TIMP has also been shown to have antimetastatic activity.[38,39]

MMPs are critical to normal processes such as development, growth, tissue remodeling, and tissue homeostasis. In most resting adult tissues they are expressed at low levels, but under pathologic conditions such as inflammation, neoplasia, or injury and repair, the MMP levels are increased.[31,32] Because MMPs are clearly necessary for metastasis,

Table 2-1   Matrix metalloproteinase terminology and substrates

MMP	Name	Substrates
MMP1	Interstitial collagenase	Collagens I, II, III, VII, VIII, X, proteoglycan
MMP2	Gelatinase A	Collagens I, IV, V, VII, X, XI, elastin
MMP3	Stromelysin 1	Proteoglycans, fibronectin, laminin, collagen IV, V, IX, X, elastin, procollagen
MMP7	Matrilysin (PUMP1)	Fibronectin, laminin, collagen IV, gelatin
MMP8	Neutrophil collagenase	Collagen I, II, III, VII, VIII, X, proteoglycans
MMP9	Gelatinase B	Collagen IV, V, elastin, proteoglycans
MMP10	Stromelysin 2	Same as stromelysin 1
MMP11	Stromelysin 3	Serpin
MMP12	Elastase	Elastin
MMP13	Collagenase 3	Fibrillar collagens
MMP14	MT-MMP	Progelatinase A
MMP15	MT2-MMP	Unknown
MMP16	MT3-MMP	Progelatinase A
MMP17	MT4-MMP	Unknown
MMP18		Unknown

they are an appealing therapeutic target for the treatment or prevention of metastasis. The conserved structure of the MMPs also makes it possible to disrupt function pharmacologically by using inhibitors with metal chelating properties, which can interfere with the critical cation interactions with the catalytic sites of the enzymes, and allows broad specificity for different MMPs. Tetracyclines and hydroxamic acids are some of the types of drugs that have been shown to inhibit MMP enzymatic activity through their metal chelating properties, and they have demonstrated some antimetastatic potential in several animal model systems.[42,43] In addition, tetracyclines have been used in periodontal disease and arthritis models to inhibit MMP activity and have been shown to have therapeutic benefit in some studies.[44,45] Hydroxamates such as batimastat and marimastat have demonstrated antitumor activity in animal models and some clinical trials, and several hydroxamates are being investigated as antimetastatic agents in current clinical trials.[42,46]

Several agents that regulate MMP expression, such as retinoids, growth factors, modulators of cyclic adenosine monophosphate, and modulators of arachidonic acid metabolism, have also been investigated.[12,47-50] Retinoic acid regulates collagenase expression and has been shown in several studies to have antitumor activity with lung, breast, and squamous cell tumors.[49,51] Although its antitumor activity has been thought to be related to a differentiating effect, effects on MMP expression are also present.[49] The regulatory elements in the MMP9 gene promoter have recently been characterized, and DNA binding sequences for transcription factors, including NFκB, SP-1, Ets, AP-1, and RB, have been identified.[52] Thus the NFκB pathway, which regulates many cytokines, and the AP-1 pathway of the c-*fos* and c-*jun* family members, which mediates a wide variety of growth factor and hormonal responses, proliferation, and differentiation of many cell types, may be two key regulatory pathways for MMP9 expression. Tumor necrosis factor alpha (TNF-α), which stimulates the NFκB pathway, is known to up-regulate MMP9 expression.[48] MMP9, as mentioned previously, not only is strongly correlated with metastasis in a number of studies but also appears to be essential to the critical metastatic step of intravasation.[16]

UROKINASE-TYPE PLASMINOGEN ACTIVATOR AND ITS RECEPTOR

Increased plasminogen activation and plasmin production correlate with metastasis, probably because of enhancement of the proteolytic cascade of MMP activities. uPA is bound to a specific cell surface receptor, uPAR, which appears to localize the plasmin-generating activity of the uPA to the immediate environment of the tumor cell. Plasmin is an activator of MMP9, among others, and may contribute to metastasis through this function.[17,18] Two endogenous protein inhibitors of uPA, uPAI1 and uPAI2, have also been identified. Paradoxically the expression of uPAI correlates positively with metastasis and poor prognosis in cancers.[53,54] The reason for this positive correlation is presently unclear. Increased uPA activity has been shown in studies of metastatic malignancies, as has increased uPAR expression. The interaction of the uPAI inhibitors, uPA, and uPAR is incompletely understood, but the expression of uPA and uPAR is a critical element of intravasation.[16] Inhibition of uPA or blockade of uPAR can prevent metastasis, and, conversely, overexpression enhances metastatic potential.[55] uPA expression correlates with prognosis in soft tissue sarcomas and breast cancer.[54,56] However, multiple pathways are clearly operant in metastasis, because mice genetically deficient in plasminogen, although demonstrating retarded nodal metastasis of a lung carcinoma, showed no difference from normal mice in pulmonary metastasis.[57] It is possible that the uPA-uPAR system may operate on as yet unidentified proteases to enhance their activity and function in the metastatic process.

ATTACHMENT FACTORS

Another important step in controlling target site selection and secondary tumor growth is the attachment or interaction of the metastatic cells with the host tissue and cells. A number of attachment factors have been implicated in the metastatic spread of tumor cells. Interactions of the cell with surrounding matrix are mediated through the cytoskeleton. One mechanism that links cells to matrix is the integrin family of cell surface receptors, which interact with matrix proteins containing a specific sequence of amino acids, arginine-glycine-aspartate, or RGD. Many extracellular matrix proteins, including collagens, contain RGD sequences, which can interact with integrin receptors. Integrins are transmembrane heterodimeric signaling molecules composed of α and β subunits, which associate in specific combinations in different cell types.[58] All mesenchymal cells express specific subsets of integrin receptors on the cell surface, and more than 20 heterodimers have been identified between 9 types of β subunits and 14 types of α subunits. The various heterodimers possess differing and sometimes overlapping specificity for particular matrix RGD-containing proteins. Integrin receptors have relatively lower affinities for their ligands than growth factor and hormone receptors and are 10 to 100 times more abundant on cell surfaces. The β subunit contains a binding domain that interacts with the cytoskeletal proteins talin and α-actinin and, on ligand binding, causes formation of linkages to the actin cytoskeleton.[59] These areas of focal receptor-cytoskeletal contact can activate kinases such as the focal adhesion kinase or the tyrosine kinase product of the *src* gene. This activation in turn leads to a signal cascade, which can result in changes in gene expression.[60] Integrins have been identified as important regulators of tumor cell attachment to host tissue matrix, such as in metastasis to bone. Metastasis can be inhibited in some tumor models by using synthetic RGD peptides to saturate integrin binding sites.[61] Adhesion to platelets can also affect tumor metastasis.[19] In the circulation, metastatic tumor cells lodge in end-organ capillaries, where they associate with a fibrin clot. Platelet aggregation also occurs, and the platelets can release growth factors, such as platelet-derived growth factor and transforming growth factor beta (TGF-β), that may stimulate tumor cell functions, potentially enhancing growth or extravasation. Proteins called disintegrins have been shown to have antimetastatic activity on melanomas by binding to platelet integrins and blocking them from interaction with tumor cells.[62]

Another class of adhesion molecules is the hyaluronan receptor family, which recognizes hyaluronate-like carbohydrate groups in extracellular matrix. This is also known as the CD44 receptor group, and a number of different isoforms have been identified. CD44 has been implicated in the attachment of tumor cells to matrix in target tissues during metastasis.[58] CD44 is concentrated in the advancing pseudopodia, or invading tumor cells ("invadopodia"), and co-localizes with

MMP9.[63] Thus the tumor cell may coordinate attachment to matrix with its localized digestion.

A family of attachment factors that have homology to the immunoglobulins are the cell-cell adhesion molecules (CAMs). These CAMs mediate cell-cell contact events rather than cell-matrix interactions. Intercellular CAM putatively allows attachment of tumor cells to endothelium and has been associated with metastasis of melanoma cells; use of blocking peptides can inhibit metastasis.[58] Cadherins and selectins are other families of cell-cell attachment proteins. Cadherins and CAMs are homophilic receptors (i.e., binding to a like receptor on a different cell to mediate signaling events). CAMs can have both prometastatic and antimetastatic properties; CAMs may hold cells together in a primary tumor and prevent cell migration, or they can facilitate tumor cell attachment to other cell types, such as endothelial cells or target tissue cells, thereby enhancing the metastatic process.[58]

ANGIOGENESIS

Another important aspect of secondary tumor development at metastatic sites is the ability of the tumor to induce a vascular supply for itself to provide the requisite nutrients and oxygen for further growth. A number of angiogenic factors have been identified that may contribute to the induction of tumor vasculature.[64] These factors include members of the fibroblast growth factor (FGF) family, particularly FGF2, and vascular endothelial growth factor (VEGF). In addition, proteins have been identified that inhibit vascularization, such as angiostatin and endostatin.[65,66] Observations that sudden growth of metastases occasionally follows removal of a primary tumor led Folkman and coworkers (Cao et al.[65]) to isolate a substance from the urine of patients with primary tumors. This substance, called angiostatin, potently suppresses the development of new blood vessels. It was subsequently identified as a fragment of plasmin, and a second protein, called endostatin, with similar function has been identified as a fragment of collagen type XIII.[65,66] Thus these protein degradation products may be produced by the primary tumors to suppress competition for the host by the metastatic tumors. Angiostatin and endostatin have been reported to cause regression of metastatic melanoma in animal models and are being pursued as possible antimetastatic and antitumor agents.

VEGF receptors have also been shown to be important for tumor progression and may confer responsiveness to tumor-secreted VEGF by metastases.[64] A number of pharmacologic agents targeted at inhibiting angiogenesis are under development and have shown antimetastatic and antitumor activity in preclinical studies.

THE IMMUNE SYSTEM

The interplay of the immune system and cancer metastasis is another area in which basic knowledge is limited. It is well established that immune recognition and natural killer T-cell function are involved in the destruction of malignant cells, and neoplastic surveillance is therefore one of the important functions of the immune system. Immunotherapies to stimulate the immune system to recognize and kill tumor cells are being developed as new therapeutic modalities to fight cancer, with some evidence of success in both animal and clinical studies.[67] Further, an increasing amount of data implicates cytokines, important regulatory proteins produced by both tumor cells and host immune cells, as playing a significant role in tumor progression and metastasis. Because many of these cytokines can be manipulated pharmacologically, administered therapeutically as recombinant proteins, blocked by administration of recombinant binding proteins or antibodies, or controlled in immune cells with various molecular immunotherapies, they provide a new potential therapeutic target in the metastatic process.

CYTOKINES

Cytokines are normal modulators of inflammatory and immunologic processes. These factors were originally described in cells of immune or hematopoietic lineages, and the largest families are the colony-stimulating factors and the interleukins. Interleukins 1 and 6 (IL-1 and IL-6) and tumor necrosis factor alpha (TNF-α) are all characterized as proinflammatory cytokines, which enhance the inflammatory response. These factors are balanced by a number of anti-inflammatory cytokines, including IL-4, IL-10, and IL-12. The expression of TNF and IL-6 has been associated with increased metastatic potential, whereas expression of IL-10 inversely correlates with metastasis.[68-70] Transfection or exogenous addition of IL-10 and IL-12 has been found to have an antimetastatic effect.[70,71]

TNF stimulates MMP expression,[48] and TNF activity is in turn dependent on MMP expression because TNF is secreted in a membrane-bound form and requires cleavage by an MT-MMP to have activity.[72] Thus TNF may amplify its prometastatic effect through MMP regulation. TNF regulation and function are complex, however. TNF can cause apoptosis of cells, including tumor cells, through a receptor-mediated mechanism involving the TNF type 1 receptor (also called CD95). Therefore, TNF can also have antitumor activity[73] and has even been studied therapeutically in some clinical trials. IL-1 and IL-6 have also been shown to stimulate MMP expression, whereas proteolytic activity is inhibited by IL-10 expression.

GROWTH FACTORS

Growth factors are ubiquitous secreted proteins present in both normal and neoplastic cells that regulate cell growth and differentiation in complex ways. Transforming growth factor beta (TGF-β) is overexpressed in a number of tumors and has been reported to correlate negatively with prognosis in breast and prostate cancers.[74,75] TGF-β may function to enhance angiogenesis by metastatic tumors,[74] although its effects on cells are numerous. TGF-β has also been shown to stimulate MMP expression,[37] and its stimulation of osteoblastic bone formation has been proposed to play a role in the blastic response of bone to metastatic prostate cancer.[76] Bone morphogenetic proteins (BMPs) and FGFs have also been identified as growth factor products of prostate carcinoma cells, which may contribute to the excessive bone formation observed in blastic prostate metastases.[77,78] Epidermal growth factor also stimulates metastasis in several carcinoma types.[79] A growth factor that is produced by mesenchymal cells but acts primarily on cells of epithelial origin is hepatocyte growth factor. This factor is also called scatter factor because it causes cancer cells to disaggregate, or "scatter," in vitro and may be a prometastatic growth factor.[80]

BONE METASTASIS

On the basis of presumed host tissue–tumor cell interactions, there are five common carcinomas with a high propensity to metastasize to bone: prostate, breast, lung, kidney, and thyroid carcinoma. Of these, prostate, breast, and lung cancers are the most common malignancies, accounting for more than half a million new cases per year in this country alone. Autopsy studies demonstrate bone metastases in 50% to 90% of patients who succumb to these malignancies.[2,76] Therefore bone metastasis is an enormous clinical problem both epidemiologically and economically. These bone-metastasizing tumors cause severe morbidity and contribute to the death of patients with cancer through bone pain, pathologic fractures, bone marrow suppression, and hypercalcemia. Aggressive treatment of bone metastasis and prophylactic fixation of impending pathologic fractures can markedly improve the quality of life for patients with cancer and have become a standard approach in the treatment of this problem. However, an increased understanding of the pathogenesis of these lesions and of the metastatic process in general has the potential to markedly improve methods of treatment and metastatic prevention in this patient population.

Recent data provide new insights into the destruction of bone by metastatic tumors. Lytic metastases contain increased numbers of osteoclasts, as do lytic primary tumors such as lymphoma. Magnetic resonance imaging and immunohistochemical studies of primary lymphoma of bone, which frequently is manifested by a large extraosseous soft tissue mass at presentation, demonstrated channels through the cortex excavated by osteoclasts, associated with high levels of expression of osteoclastic-stimulating cytokines by the tumor cells.[81] Similarly, increased expression of the bone-resorptive cytokines (IL-1, IL-6, and TNF) has been found in lytic lesions of metastatic carcinoma.[82] In an animal model of metastatic breast cancer, tumor deposits introduced into the bone were incapable of causing bone destruction in osteopetrotic animals that lacked functional osteoclasts.[83] These studies document the essential nature of the osteoclast in mediating bone destruction and the stimulatory role of bone resorptive cytokine expression by the tumor cells.

Parathyroid hormone–related protein (PTHrP) has also recently been shown to be a key regulator of bone metastasis in breast and prostate cancers.[8,84,85] PTHrP acts through the PTH/PTHrP receptor to stimulate protein kinase signaling responses and is important in the local regulation of endochondral bone formation and osteoblastic function. PTHrP stimulates bone resorption, and signaling of osteoclastic stimulation occurs through the osteoblast. In a series of breast cancers it was demonstrated that only those which expressed PTHrP metastasized to bone.[85] Similarly, in an animal model of metastatic breast cancer, blocking antibody to PTHrP caused a dramatic suppression of the ability of the tumor to cause bone metastases.[8] Metastasis of prostate tumors to bone has also been associated with high levels of PTHrP expression.[84] Thus PTHrP may be a key regulator of the interaction of tumor cells with bone, facilitating metastasis to this site by specific tumors that express this growth factor. The interactions between bone cells and tumor cells are summarized in Fig. 2-4. PTHrP is discussed more extensively in Chapter 9, "Therapy Affecting Bone Resorption and Deposition."

The availability of antiresorptive agents that inhibit osteoclast function has enabled application of these agents, developed initially for the treatment of Paget's disease and osteoporosis, to metastatic bone disease. These drugs bind to hydroxyapatite mineral in bone and are therefore concentrated in this tissue. They inhibit osteoclast function relatively effectively by interfering with mevalonate metabolism, which prevents prenylation (a type of lipid modification) of proteins and leads to apoptosis of the osteoclasts.[86] In animal models, bisphosphonates inhibit the development and progression of metastasis, potentially through both osteoclastic suppression and an interference with tumor adhesion to bone.[87,88] Furthermore, survival can be improved with bisphosphonate therapy in animal models.[87] Early clinical trials with first-generation bisphosphonates, such as etidronate, did not show convincing efficacy in the prevention of bone destruction and fractures. However, with the development of newer bisphosphonate agents that effectively inhibit osteoclast activity without impairing bone mineralization, increasing numbers of clinical trials have demonstrated efficacy in decreasing morbidity and pathologic fractures in patients with metastatic cancers. Risedronate, pamidronate, clodronate, olpadronate, and alendronate, and other bisphosphonates, have been used with similar findings among these agents. The incidence of pathologic fractures can be reduced by approximately 50%, and some studies have

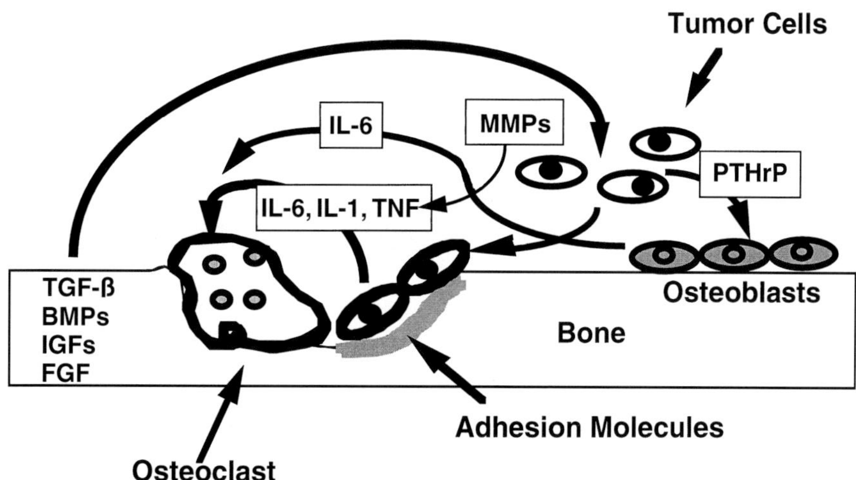

Fig. 2-4 Interactions between tumor and bone cells. Osteoclasts resorb bone matrix, releasing stored growth factors such as TGF-β, BMPs, IGFs, and FGFs. These factors normally are activated and induce local mesenchymal cell proliferation and differentiation into mature osteoblasts but, in the presence of tumor cells, can activate these cells as well. The tumor cells attach to the bone surface through integrins and CD44 receptors, which recognize ligands in the resorption surface of the bone matrix. Tumor cells elaborate bone resorptive cytokines such as IL-6, IL-1, and TNF, which further stimulate osteoclastic differentiation and bone resorption. In addition, the tumor cells may secrete factors, such as PTHrP, that cause osteoblasts in the local area to release such bone resorptive cytokines as IL-6 as well, further augmenting bone destruction. The cytokines enhance MMP secretion by the tumor and stromal cells, which may enhance release of TNF, as well as causing local matrix tissue damage and invasion of bone marrow.

also demonstrated improved survival.[89-92] Recently, clodronate was found to suppress not only bone metastasis of breast cancer but soft tissue progression as well.[92]

Another effect observed with bisphosphonates is rapid ossification of lytic areas in bone within a few months after the start of therapy (Fig. 2-5). Presumably, this results from the release of anabolic growth factors such as TGF-β and BMPs from bone matrix being resorbed by the tumor-stimulated osteoclasts. On sudden blockade of osteoclastic activity by the bisphosphonate therapy, the regional osteoblastic stimulus caused by the released growth factors can be expressed and the lytic areas can rapidly fill in with bone (see Fig. 2-4). A significant part of the observed response in bone lesions of metastatic carcinoma to local radiotherapy could also be due to suppression of osteoclasts and their precursors, which are radiosensitive. Because of the overwhelming support for bisphosphonate therapy in metastatic bone disease in the literature, this

modality has rapidly been adopted by oncologists and is becoming a standard adjuvant in treatment of patients with bone metastases. The most common approach is use of pamidronate intravenously on a monthly basis, a regimen originally used for treatment of hypercalcemia. However, there is ample support for the use of orally active agents such as risedronate, clodronate, and alendronate as well. The optimal drug-dosing regimens for these various agents have not yet been studied systematically. Chapter 9 discusses these treatment options in greater depth.

Future directions of antimetastatic therapy will undoubtedly include multiple concomitant strategies for disrupting molecular mechanisms of metastasis. Such approaches could include MMP inhibition, antiresorptive agents, cytokine-modulating agents, cell attachment blockade, antiangiogenic agents, and uPA-uPAR inhibition. Modulation of TIMP expression by transfection in combination with bisphosphonate therapy has demonstrated a

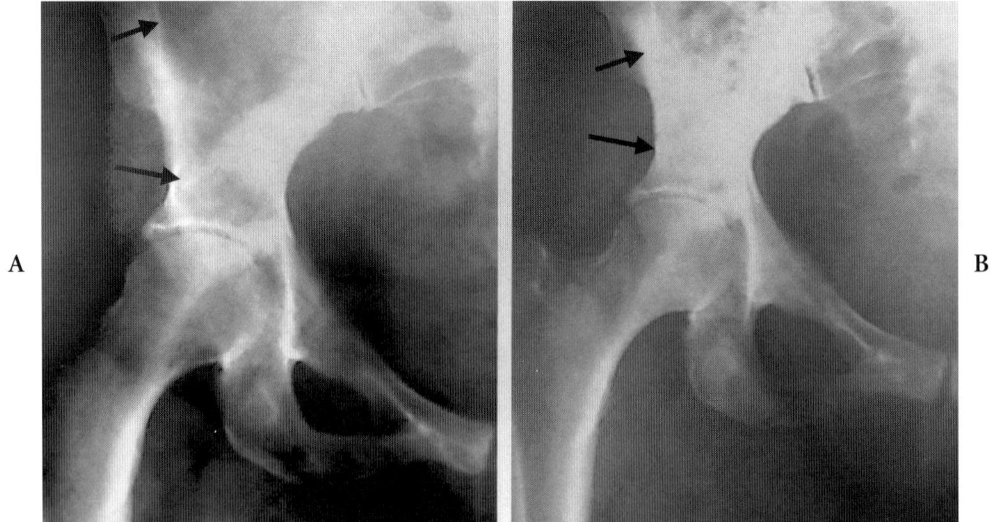

Fig. 2-5 Treatment of metastatic bone disease with bisphosphonates. **A,** Patient had extensive mixed lytic and blastic metastasis of lung carcinoma, with large, painful lytic areas in the pelvis and acetabulum. **B,** After 3 months of treatment with orally administered alendronate, dense ossification of the lytic regions was observed. This is consistent with osteoblastic stimulation by the released growth factors from the massive bone resorption after inhibition of bone resorption by the bisphosphonate. The patient also had resolution of pain at these sites.

significant additive effect in an animal model.[93] However, on a cautionary note, further research is needed before rational combinatorial therapeutic strategies can be developed. The complexities of the pathways that regulate metastasis can potentially produce antagonistic effects of combined antimetastatic agents. Such effects have been shown in an animal metastasis model using retinoids and tetracyclines, in which the up-regulation of TIMP expression by retinoids was abrogated by the MMP inhibitor minocycline, resulting in less antimetastatic efficacy of the agents used in combination than of either agent used alone.[94] These concerns also apply to pharmacologic manipulation of cytokines, because agents such as IL-6 and TNF have been shown to have both antitumor and prometastatic effects. However, the rapidly accumulating new information on the molecular mechanisms involved in the metastatic process will undoubtedly lead to many new therapeutic approaches, effectively changing current cancer treatment paradigms that have been targeted at disruption of cell proliferation to those which include inhibition of metastasis.

REFERENCES

1. Paget S. The distribution of secondary growths in cancer of the breast. Lancet 1:571-573, 1889.
2. Berrettoni BA, Carter JR. Current concepts review: Mechanisms of cancer metastasis to bone. J Bone Joint Surg Am 68:308-312, 1986.
3. Kuratsu S, Uchida A, Araki N. Mechanism of organ selectivity in the determination of metastatic patterns of Dunn osteosarcoma. Trans Orthop Res Soc 17:196, 1992.
4. Baker T, Tickle S, Wasan H, Docherty A, Isenberg D, Waxman J. Serum metalloproteinases and their inhibitors: Markers for malignant potential. Br J Cancer 70:506-512, 1994.
5. Naylor MS, Stamp GW, Davies BD, Balkwill FR. Expression and activity of MMPs and their regulators in ovarian cancer. Int J Cancer 58:50-56, 1994.
6. Onisto M, Riccio MP, Scannapieco P, Caenazzo C, Griggio L, Spina M, Stetler-Stevenson WG, Garbisa S. Gelatinase A/TIMP-2 imbalance in lymph-node–positive breast carcinomas, as measured by RT-PCR. Int J Cancer 63:621-626, 1995.
7. Noguchi S, Koyama H, Kasugai T, Tsuji N, Tsuda H, Akiyama F, Motomura K, Inaji H. The possible prognostic significance of p53 immunostaining status of the primary tumor in patients developing local recurrence after breast-conserving surgery. Oncology 55:450-455, 1998.
8. Guise TA, Yin JJ, Taylor SD, Kumagai Y, Dallas M, Boyce BF, Yoneda T, Mundy GR. Evidence for a causal role of parathyroid hormone–related protein in the pathogenesis of human breast cancer–mediated osteolysis. J Clin Invest 98:1544-1549, 1996.

9. Luzzi KJ, MacDonald IC, Schmidt EE, Kerkvliet N, Morris VL, Chambers AF, Groom AC. Multistep nature of metastatic inefficiency: Dormancy of solitary cells after successful extravasation and limited survival of early micrometastases. Am J Pathol 153:865-873, 1998.

10. Clohisy DR, Ogilvie CM, Carpenter RJ, Ramnaraine ML. Localized, tumor-associated osteolysis involves the recruitment and activation of osteoclasts. J Orthop Res 14(1):2-6, 1996.

11. Cerosaletti KM, Blieden TM, Harwell LW, Welsh KM, Frelinger JG, Lord EM. Alteration of the metastatic potential of line 1 lung carcinoma cells: Opposite effects of class I antigen induction by interferons versus DMSO or gene transfection. Cell Immunol 127:299-310, 1990.

12. Schneider MR, Schirner M, Lichtner RB, Graf H. Antimetastatic action of the prostacyclin analogue cicaprost in experimental mammary tumors. Breast Cancer Res Treat 38:133-141, 1996.

13. Chang SG, Kim JI, Jung JC, Rho YS, Lee KT, An Z, Wang X, Hoffman RM. Antimetastatic activity of the new platinum analog [Pt(*cis-dach*)(DPPE).2NO3] in a metastatic model of human bladder cancer. Anticancer Res 17:3239-3242, 1997.

14. Lyu MA, Choi YK, Park BN, Kim BJ, Park IK, Hyun BH, Kook YH. Over-expression of urokinase receptor in human epidermoid-carcinoma cell line (Hep3) increases tumorigenicity on chorio-allantoic membrane and in severe-combined deficiency immunodeficient mice. Int J Cancer 77:257-263, 1998.

15. Kobayashi T, Koshida K, Endo Y, Imao T, Uchibayashi T, Sasaki T, Namiki M. A chick embryo model for metastatic human prostate cancer. Eur Urol 34:154-160, 1998.

16. Kim J, Yu W, Kovalski K, Ossowski L. Requirement for specific proteases in cancer cell intravasation as revealed by a novel semiquantitative PCR-based assay. Cell 94:353-362, 1998.

17. Andreasen PA, Kjoller L, Christensen L, Duffy MJ. The urokinase-type plasminogen activator system in cancer metastasis: A review. Int J Cancer 72:1-22, 1997.

18. Rabbani SA, Xing RH. Role of urokinase (uPA) and its receptor (uPAR) in invasion and metastasis of hormone-dependent malignancies. Int J Oncol 12:911-920, 1998.

19. Springfield DS, Bolander ME, Friedlaender GE, Lane N. Molecular and cellular biology of inflammation and neoplasia. In Simon SR, ed. Orthopaedic Basic Science. Rosemont, Ill.: American Academy of Orthopaedic Surgeons, 1994, pp 219-276.

20. Webb CP, VanAelst L, Wigler MH, Woude GF. Signaling pathways in Fas-mediated tumorigenicity and metastasis. Proc Natl Acad Sci USA 95:8773-8778, 1998.

21. Bernhard EJ, Hagner B, Wong C, Lubenski I, Muschel RJ. The effect of E1A transfection on MMP-9 expression and metastatic potential. Int J Cancer 60:718-724, 1995.

22. Alberts B, Bray D, Lewis J, Raff M, Roberts K, Watson JD. The cytoskeleton. In The Molecular Biology of the Cell, 3rd ed. New York: Garland Publishing, 1994, pp 787-861.

23. Freije JM, MacDonald NJ, Steeg PS. Differential gene expression in tumor metastasis: Nm23. Curr Top Microbiol Immunol 213(Pt 2):215-232, 1996.

24. Freije MJ, MacDonald NJ, Steeg PS. Nm23 and tumour metastasis: Basic and translational advances. Biochem Soc Symp 63:261-271, 1998.

25. Charpin C, Garcia S, Bonnier P, Martini F, Andrac L, Horschowski N, Lavaut MN, Allasia C. Prognostic significance of Nm23/NDPK expression in breast carcinoma, assessed on 10-year follow-up by automated and quantitative immunocytochemical assays. J Pathol 184:401-407, 1998.

26. Wagner PD, Steeg PS, Vu ND. Two-component kinase-like activity of nm23 correlates with its motility-suppressing activity. Proc Natl Acad Sci USA 94:9000-9005, 1997.

27. Russell RL, Pedersen AN, Kantor J, Geisinger K, Long R, Zbieranski N, Townsend A, Shelton B, Brunner N, Kute TE. Relationship of nm23 to proteolytic factors, proliferation and motility in breast cancer tissues and cell lines. Br J Cancer 78:710-717, 1998.

28. Sherbet GV, Lakshmi MS. S100A4 (MTS1) calcium binding protein in cancer growth, invasion and metastasis. Anticancer Res 18:2415-2421, 1998.

29. Lloyd BH, Platt-Higgins A, Rudland PS, Barraclough R. Human S100A4 (p9Ka) induces the metastatic phenotype upon benign tumour cells. Oncogene 17:465-473, 1998.

30. Ford HL, Zain SB. Interaction of metastasis associated Mts1 protein with nonmuscle myosin. Oncogene 10:1597-1605, 1995.

31. Woessner JF Jr. Literature on vertebrate matrix metalloproteinases and their tissue inhibitors. In Birkedal-Hansen H, Werb Z, Welgus HG, Van Wart HE, eds. Matrix Metalloproteinases and Inhibitors. Matrix Special Suppl. 1. Stuttgart: Gustav Fischer, 1992, pp 425-501.

32. Woessner JF Jr. The family of matrix metalloproteinases. Ann NY Acad Sci 732:11-19, 1994.

33. Gooley PR, Johnson BA, Marcy AI, Cuca GC, Salowe SP, Hagmann WK, Esser CK, Springer JP. Secondary structure and zinc ligation of human recombinant short-form stromelysin by multidimensional heteronuclear NMR. Biochemistry 32:13098-13108, 1993.

34. Shapiro SD, Fliszar CJ, Broekelmann TJ, Mecham RP, Senior RM, Welgus HG. Activation of the 92-kDa gelatinase by stromelysin and 4-aminophenylmercuric acetate: Differential processing and stabilization of the carboxyl-terminal domain by tissue inhibitor of metalloproteinases (TIMP). J Biol Chem 270:6351-6356, 1995.

35. Cockett MI, Murphy G, Birch ML, O'Connell JP, Crabbe T, Millican AT, Hart IR, Docherty AJ. Matrix metalloproteinases and metastatic cancer. Biochem Soc Symp 63:295-313, 1998.

36. Sato H, Seiki M. Membrane-type matrix metalloproteinases (MT-MMPs) in tumor metastasis. J Biochem 119:209-215, 1996.

37. Overall CM. Regulation of tissue inhibitor of matrix metalloproteinase expression. Ann NY Acad Sci 732:51-64, 1994.

38. Wang M, Liu YE, Greene J, Sheng S, Fuchs A, Rosen EM, Shi YE. Inhibition of tumor growth and metastasis of human breast cancer cells transfected with tissue inhibitor of metalloproteinase 4. Oncogene 14:2767-2774, 1997.

39. Watanabe M, Takahashi Y, Ohta T, Mai M, Sasaki T, Seiki M. Inhibition of metastasis in human gastric cancer cells transfected with tissue inhibitor of metalloproteinase 1 gene in nude mice. Cancer 77(8 Suppl):1676-1680, 1996.

40. Apte SS, Olsen BR, Murphy G. The gene structure of tissue inhibitor of metalloproteinases (TIMP)-3 and its inhibitory activities define the distinct TIMP gene family. J Biol Chem 270:14313-14318, 1995.

41. Berend KR, Toth AP, Harrelson JM, Layfield LJ, Hey LA, Scully SP. Association between ratio of matrix metalloproteinase-1 to tissue inhibitor of metalloproteinase-1 and local recurrence, metastasis, and survival in human chondrosarcoma. J Bone Joint Surg Am 80:11-17, 1998.

42. Zervos EE, Norman JG, Gower WR, Franz MG, Rosemurgy AS. Matrix metalloproteinase inhibition attenuates human pancreatic cancer growth in vitro and decreases mortality and tumorigenesis in vivo. J Surg Res 69:367-371, 1997.

43. Masumori N, Tsukamoto T, Miyao N, Kumamoto Y, Saiki I, Yoneda J. Inhibitory effect of minocycline on in vitro invasion and experimental metastasis of mouse renal adenocarcinoma. J Urol 151:1400-1404, 1994.

44. Rifkin BR, Vernillo AT, Golub LM. Blocking periodontal disease progression by inhibiting tissue-destructive enzymes: A potential therapeutic role for tetracyclines and their chemically modified analogs. J Periodontol 64(8 Suppl):819-827, 1993.

45. Greenwald RA, Moak SA, Ramamurthy NS, Golub LM. Tetracyclines suppress matrix metalloproteinase activity in adjuvant arthritis and, in combination with flurbiprofen, ameliorate bone damage. J Rheumatol 19:927-938, 1992.

46. Nemunaitis J, Poole C, Primrose J, Rosemurgy A, Malfetano J, Brown P, Berrington A, Cornish A, Lynch K, Rasmussen H, Kerr D, Cox D, Millar A. Combined analysis of studies of the effects of the matrix metalloproteinase inhibitor marimastat on serum tumor markers in advanced cancer: Selection of a biologically active and tolerable dose for longer-term studies. Clin Cancer Res 4:1101-1109, 1998.

47. Tanaka K, Iwamoto Y, Ito Y, Ishibashi T, Nakabeppu Y, Sekiguchi M, Sugioka Y. Cyclic AMP–regulated synthesis of the tissue inhibitors of metalloproteinases suppresses the invasive potential of the human fibrosarcoma cell line HT1080. Cancer Res 55:2927-2935, 1995.

48. Mann EA, Hibbs MS, Spiro JD, Bowik C, Wang XZ, Clawson M, Chen LL. Cytokine regulation of gelatinase production by head and neck squamous cell carcinoma: The role of tumor necrosis factor-alpha. Ann Otol Rhinol Laryngol 104:203-209, 1995.

49. Nakajima M, Lotan D, Baig MM, Carralero RM, Wood WR, Hendrix MJC, Lotan R. Inhibition by retinoic acid of type IV collagenolysis and invasion through reconstituted basement membrane by metastatic rat mammary adenocarcinoma cells. Cancer Res 49:1698-1706, 1989.

50. Cocoran ML, Stetler-Stevenson WG, Brown PD, Wahl LM. Interleukin-4 inhibition of prostaglandin E2 synthesis blocks interstitial collagenase and 92 kDa type IV collagenase/gelatinase production by human monocytes. J Biol Chem 267:515-519, 1992.

51. Budd GT, Adamson PC, Gupta M, Homayoun P, Sandstrom SK, Murphy RF, McLain D, Tuason L, Peereboom D, Bukowski RM, Ganapathi R. Phase I/II trial of all-trans retinoic acid and tamoxifen in patients with advanced breast cancer. Clin Cancer Res 4:635-642, 1998.

52. Himelstein BP, Lee EJ, Sato H, Seiki M, Muschel RJ. Transcriptional activation of the matrix metalloproteinase-9 gene in an H-*ras* and v-*myc* transformed rat embryo cell line. Oncogene 14:1995-1998, 1997.

53. Bajou K, Noel A, Gerard RD, Masson V, Brunner N, Holst-Hansen C, Skobe M, Fusenig NE, Carmeliet P, Collen D, Foidart JM. Absence of host plasminogen activator inhibitor 1 prevents cancer invasion and vascularization. Nature Med 4:923-928, 1998.

54. Knoop A, Andreasen PA, Andersen JA, Hansen S, Laenkholm AV, Simonsen AC, Andersen J, Overgaard J. Prognostic significance of urokinase-type plasminogen activator and plasminogen activator inhibitor-1 in primary breast cancer. Br J Cancer 77:932-940, 1998.

55. Ignar DM, Andrews JL, Witherspoon SM, Leray JD, Clay WC, Kilpatrick K, Onori J, Kost T, Emerson DL. Inhibition of establishment of primary and micrometastatic tumors by a urokinase plasminogen activator receptor antagonist. Clin Exp Metastasis 16:9-20, 1998.

56. Choong PF, Ferno M, Akerman M, Willen H, Langstrom E, Gustafson P, Alvegard T, Rydholm A. Urokinase-plasminogen-activator levels and prognosis in 69 soft-tissue sarcomas. Int J Cancer 69:268-272, 1996.

57. Bugge TH, Kombrinck KW, Xiao Q, Holmback K, Daugherty CC, Witte DP, Degen JL. Growth and dissemination of Lewis lung carcinoma in plasminogen-deficient mice. Blood 90:4522-4531, 1997.

58. Miyasaka, M. Cancer metastasis and adhesion molecules. Clin Orthop 312:10-18, 1995.

59. Alberts B, Bray D, Lewis J, Raff M, Roberts K, Watson JD. The cytoskeleton. In The Molecular Biology of the Cell, 3rd ed. New York: Garland Publishing, 1994, pp 995-999.

60. Bergan R, Kyle E, Nguyen P, Trepel J, Ingui C, Neckers L. Genistein-stimulated adherence of prostate cancer cells is associated with the binding of focal adhesion kinase to beta-1-integrin. Clin Exp Metastasis 14:389-398, 1996.

61. Komazawa H, Fujii H, Kojima M, Mori H, Ono M, Itoh I, Azuma I, Saiki I. Combination of anti-cell adhesive synthetic Arg-Gly-Asp-Ser analogue and anticancer drug doxorubicin heightens their original antimetastatic activities. Oncol Res 7:341-351, 1995.

62. Beviglia L, Stewart GJ, Niewiarowski S. Effect of four disintegrins on the adhesive and metastatic properties of B16F10 melanoma cells in a murine model. Oncol Res 7:7-20, 1995.

63. Bourguignon LY, Gunja-Smith Z, Iida N, Zhu HB, Young LJ, Muller WJ, Cardiff RD. CD44v(3,8-10) is involved in cytoskeleton-mediated tumor cell migration and matrix metalloproteinase (MMP-9) association in metastatic breast cancer cells. J Cell Physiol 176:206-215, 1998.

64. Zetter BR. Angiogenesis and tumor metastasis. Annu Rev Med 49:407-424, 1998.

65. Cao Y, O'Reilly MS, Marshall B, Flynn E, Ji RW, Folkman J. Expression of angiostatin cDNA in a murine fibrosarcoma suppresses primary tumor growth and produces long-term dormancy of metastases. J Clin Invest 101:1055-1063, 1998.

66. Sasaki T, Fukai N, Mann K, Gohring W, Olsen BR, Timpl R. Structure, function and tissue forms of the C-terminal globular domain of collagen XVIII containing the angiogenesis inhibitor endostatin. EMBO J 17:4249-4256, 1998.

67. Kim S, Haas GP, Hillman GG. Development of immunotherapy for the treatment of malignancies refractory to conventional therapies. Cytokines Cell Mol Ther 2:13-19, 1996.

68. Orosz P, Kruger A, Hubbe M, Ruschoff J, Von Hoegen P, Mannel DN. Promotion of experimental liver metastasis by tumor necrosis factor. Int J Cancer 60:867-871, 1995.

69. Di Carlo E, Modesti A, Castrilli G, Landuzzi L, Allione A, de Giovanni C, Musso T, Musiani P. Interleukin 6 gene-transfected mouse mammary adenocarcinoma: Tumour cell growth and metastatic potential. J Pathol 182:76-85, 1997.

70. Kundu N, Beaty TL, Jackson MJ, Fulton AM. Antimetastatic and antitumor activities of interleukin 10 in a murine model of breast cancer. J Natl Cancer Inst 88:536-541, 1996.

71. Fujiwara H, Hamaoka T. Antitumor and antimetastatic effects of interleukin 12. Cancer Chemother Pharmacol 38(Suppl):S22-S26, 1996.

72. Gearing AJ, Beckett P, Christodoulou M, Churchill M, Clements J, Davidson AH, Drummond AH, Galloway WA, Gilbert R, Gordon JL, et al. Processing of tumour necrosis factor-alpha precursor by metalloproteinases. Nature 370 (6490):555-557, 1994.

73. Ashkenazi A, Dixit VM. Death receptors: Signaling and modulation. Science 281:1305-1308, 1998.

74. Connolly JM, Rose DP. Angiogenesis in two human prostate cancer cell lines with differing metastatic potential when growing as solid tumors in nude mice. J Urol 160:932-936, 1998.

75. Farina AR, Coppa A, Tiberio A, Tacconelli A, Turco A, Colletta G, Gulino A, Mackay AR. Transforming growth factor-beta-1 enhances the invasiveness of human MDA-MB-231 breast cancer cells by up-regulating urokinase activity. Int J Cancer 75:721-730, 1998.

76. Mundy GR, Yoneda T. Facilitation and suppression of bone metastasis. Clin Orthop 312:34-44, 1995.

77. Harris SE, Harris MA, Mahy P, Wozney J, Feng JQ, Mundy GR. Expression of bone morphogenetic protein messenger RNAs by normal rat and human prostate and prostate cancer cells. Prostate 24:204-211, 1994.

78. Nakamoto T, Chang CS, Li AK, Chodak GW. Basic fibroblast growth factor in human prostate cancer cells. Cancer Res 52:571-577, 1992.

79. Kondapaka SB, Fridman R, Reddy KB. Epidermal growth factor and amphiregulin up-regulate matrix metalloproteinase-9 (MMP-9) in human breast cancer cells. Int J Cancer 70:722-726, 1997.

80. Jeffers M, Rong S, Vande Woude GF. Enhanced tumorigenicity and invasion-metastasis by hepatocyte growth factor/scatter factor-met signalling in human cells concomitant with induction of the urokinase proteolysis network. Mol Cell Biol 16:1115-1125, 1996.

81. Hicks DG, Gokan T, O'Keefe RJ, Totterman SMS, Fultz PJ, Judkins AR, Myers SP, Rubens DJ, Sickel JZ, Rosier RN. Primary lymphoma of bone: Correlation of magnetic resonance image features with cytokine production by tumor cells. Cancer 75:973-980, 1995.

82. O'Keefe RJ, Hicks DG, Pollice P, Teot LA, Puzas JE, Rosier RN. Cytokine and growth factor expression in carcinomas with skeletal metastasis. J Bone Miner Res 11(Suppl I):180, 1996.

83. Clohisy DR, Ogilvie CM, Ramnaraine ML. Tumor osteolysis in osteopetrotic mice. J Orthop Res 13:892-897, 1995.

84. Wu G, Iwamura M, di Sant'Agnese PA, Deftos LJ, Cockett AT, Gershagen S. Characterization of the cell-specific expression of parathyroid hormone–related protein in normal and neoplastic prostate tissue. Urology 51(5ASuppl):110-120, 1998.

85. Kitazawa S, Maeda S. Development of skeletal metastases. Clin Orthop 312:45-50, 1995.

86. Luckman SP, Coxon FP, Ebetino FH, Russell RGG, Rogers MJ. Heterocycle-containing bisphosphonates cause apoptosis and inhibit bone resorption by preventing protein prenylation: Evidence from the structure-activity relationships in J774 macrophates. J Bone Miner Res 13:1668-1678, 1998.

87. Sasaki A, Boyce BF, Story B, Wright KR, Chapman M, Boyce R, Mundy GR, Yoneda T. Bisphosphonate risedronate reduces metastatic human breast cancer burden in bone in nude mice. Cancer Res 55:3551-3557, 1995.

88. Boissier S, Magnetto S, Frappart L, Cuzin B, Ebetino FH, Delmas PD, Clezardin P. Bisphosphonates inhibit prostate and breast carcinoma cell adhesion to unmineralized and mineralized bone extracellular matrices. Cancer Res 57:3890-3894, 1997.

89. Pelger RC, Hamdy NA, Zwinderman AH, Lycklama a Nijeholt AA, Papapoulos SE. Effects of the bisphosphonate olpadronate in patients with carcinoma of the prostate metastatic to the skeleton. Bone 22:403-408, 1998.

90. Diel IJ, Solomayer EF, Costa SD, Gollan C, Goerner R, Wallwiener D, Kaufmann M, Bastert G. Reduction in new metastases in breast cancer with adjuvant clodronate treatment. N Engl J Med 339:357-363, 1998.

91. Houston SJ, Rubens RD. The systemic treatment of bone metastases. Clin Orthop 312:95-104, 1995.

92. Conte PF, Giannessi PG, Latreille J, Mauriac L, Koliren L, Calabresi F, Ford JM. Delayed progression of bone metastases with pamidronate therapy in breast cancer patients: A randomized, multicenter phase III trial. Ann Oncol 5(Suppl 7):S41-S44, 1994.

93. Yoneda T, Sasaki A, Dunstan C, Williams PJ, Bauss F, De Clerck YA, Mundy GR. Inhibition of osteolytic bone metastasis of breast cancer by combined treatment with the bisphosphonate ibandronate and tissue inhibitor of the matrix metalloproteinase-2. J Clin Invest 99:2509-2517, 1997.

94. Pearson W, Batley J, O'Keefe RJ, Puzas JE, Reynolds PR, Hicks DG, Rosier RN. Suppression of metastatic potential by inhibition of matrix metalloproteinases. Trans Orthop Res Soc 21:184, 1996.

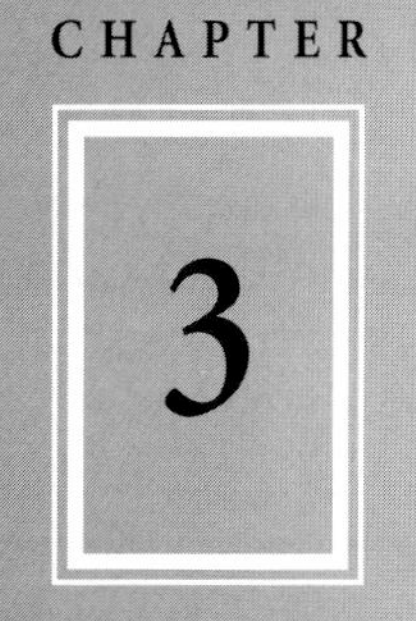

Pathology of Metastatic Disease

Fadi W. Abdul-Karim, M.D., and
Scott E. Kilpatrick, M.D.

Metastatic carcinoma, multiple or solitary, is the most common malignant tumor affecting the skeleton.[1] Large autopsy series have shown that, even with limited sampling, skeletal metastases can be found in 27% of patients who have died of carcinoma.[2] With extensive sampling or radiographic documentation, approximately 70% to 80% of patients with carcinoma have skeletal involvement.[3] Only 15% to 20% of these patients, however, have clinically evident or symptomatic disease.[3]

The majority of bone metastases in adults are from carcinomas of the breast, prostate, lung, kidney, and thyroid.[1-4] The complete list of primary tumors includes stomach, large intestine, and gynecologic malignancies and malignant melanoma.[5] Virtually every malignant neoplasm, even ones that rarely metastasize, have been observed in bone. In the pediatric age group, the most common metastatic lesion of marrow is neuroblastoma, followed by rhabdomyosarcoma and retinoblastoma.[6] However, in up to approximately 15% of patients with metastases to the skeleton, the primary site cannot be established, despite extensive examination.[1,2,7,8] Statistically, bone remains the second most common site after lymph nodes for metastasis of an unknown primary tumor.[8]

About 70% of bone metastases involve the axial skeleton, and the remaining affect the appendicular skeleton.[9-11] Although any bone may be involved, metastatic disease distal to the knee and the elbow is rare.[12] Such metastases may be accompanied by visceral involvement or may represent the only apparent site of dissemination.

The general surgical pathologist is far more likely to encounter a skeletal focus of metastatic cancer than a primary bone tumor.[13] The specimens may be submitted as those obtained by fine-needle aspirate biopsy (FNAB), needle core biopsy (NCB), open biopsy (with or without frozen section confirmation), or resection. The advantages and merits of these procedures in the diagnosis of metastatic disease have been well studied.

DIAGNOSTIC PROCEDURES

FNAB has been documented to be a safe, economical, and expedient method of evaluating skeletal lesions.[14] FNAB enables a significant volume of tumor, in particular the epicenter or areas of radiographic heterogeneity, to be sampled. It also allows for biopsy of regions such as the pelvis or vertebrae, which are not readily amenable to open biopsy, and of poorly vascularized bones such as the clavicle, which is prone to infection and slow healing.

The diagnosis of metastatic disease by FNAB is usually readily made because identification of epithelial cells generally indicates metastasis (Fig. 3-1). Immature marrow elements, megakaryocytes, and osteoclasts may mimic metastatic cells and should be recognized. Similarly, osteoblasts with epithelioid features and eccentric nuclei can mimic cells derived from poorly differentiated adenocarcinoma. The FNAB findings should always be correlated and interpreted in light of the clinical findings. Any potential discrepancy between the cytologic interpretation and the clinical presentation necessitates further investigation. NCB, on the other hand, has the advantage of providing the architectural details of a lesion and readily lends itself to the application of ancillary diagnostic tests (e.g., immunohistochemistry).

Considering the potential difficulties inherent in interpreting small amounts of tissue, a high degree of diagnostic accuracy, ranging from 67% to 97%, has been obtained with FNAB or NCB for both primary and metastatic bone tumors. Metastatic bone disease has been the most common indication for FNAB or NCB. The potential for synergy between these two techniques appears promising.[15,16] When FNAB sample adequacy is assessed immediately at the time of collection, the yield of adequate samples for both FNAB and NCB is improved.[15,16] Immediate interpretation also allows the radiologist to redirect the approach or technique, if necessary, and to obtain additional samples for ancillary studies (e.g., flow cytometry, cytogenetic analysis). This potentially obviates the need for the patient to return to the radiologic or operative suite for another biopsy. The pathologist interpreting FNAB and NCB has the advantage of combining cytologic with architectural detail to facilitate a specific diagnosis. A concomitantly obtained FNAB cell block may also provide histologic architecture for analysis.

PATHOLOGIST'S ROLE IN DIAGNOSIS

Irrespective of the biopsy modality, the pathologist's role in the diagnosis of metastatic bone dis-

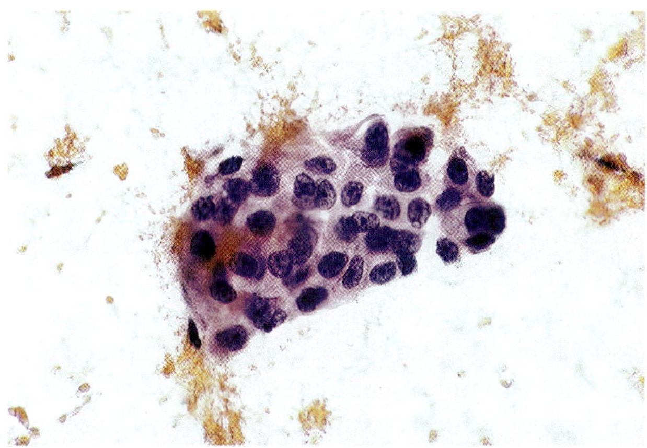

Fig. 3-1 Fine needle aspirate biopsy smear from metastatic squamous cell carcinoma. The cells are in a cohesive cluster, which is consistent with their epithelial nature. Eosinophilic cytoplasm and distinct cell borders are characteristic of squamous cell carcinoma.

ease can be defined in terms of five categories[1]:

1. The pathologist confirms bone metastasis in a patient with a solitary or (more commonly) multiple skeletal lesions and a known primary neoplasm. This decision is usually facilitated by review of the tissue sections from the previous primary disease.
2. The pathologist confirms bone metastasis in a patient with solitary or multiple bone lesions but no known history of a primary neoplasm. In this setting the pathologist may help guide the clinician in a search for the primary neoplasm. In most cases the primary neoplasm, with thorough investigation, will be readily apparent. Renal cell carcinoma is an example of a tumor that frequently presents as a skeletal (often solitary) metastasis from a clinically occult primary neoplasm.
3. The pathologist establishes whether the bone metastasis originated from a known primary or a secondary cancer. As the interval of time between treatment of the primary cancer and development of metastasis lengthens, the possibility increases that the metastasis may represent a second primary neoplasm. In one series of skeletal metastasis from breast cancer, 7% of the patients had a second malignancy.[17]
4. The pathologist excludes nonneoplastic conditions affecting bone, which simulate bone metastasis. Such mimickers include Paget's disease (especially monostotic lesions), osteomyelitis, metabolic bone disease, osteoporosis, irradiation osteitis, and fractures unrelated to metastatic disease.
5. Finally, the pathologist distinguishes between metastatic disease and a primary bone tumor. This distinction is readily apparent when certain bone tumors, such as hemangioma or enchondroma, do not share overlapping histopathologic features with metastatic disease. However, the distinction between a metastatic sarcomatoid variant of renal cell carcinoma and malignant fibrous histiocytoma of bone can be difficult and may necessitate further clinical and pathologic investigation.

Occasionally, metastatic carcinoma induces significant osseous (blastic) changes, mimicking a primary bone tumor. These changes will be addressed later in this chapter.

PATHOLOGIC FEATURES
Gross Findings

There are no gross diagnostic tests that allow distinction between metastatic and primary skeletal tumors (Figs. 3-2 and 3-3). Osteoblastic metastases tend to be firm and ill defined. Osteolytic metastases are usually soft or mushy, with a more sharply defined border.

Histopathologic Categories

The variation in the histopathologic features of metastatic bone disease is a reflection of the morphologic spectrum of the various primary tumors. This may be further compounded by the unique changes attributable to the host reaction to metastatic deposits. In general, the histopathologic findings of metastatic tumors can be divided into five categories.

Category 1: Indicative of Site of Origin

In the first histopathologic category, distinctive features are readily recognizable as indicative of the source of the primary tumors, such as metastatic well-differentiated follicular thyroid carcinoma, clear cell carcinoma of kidney, and metastatic pigmented malignant melanoma. The presence of colloid within follicles, organoid groups of clear cells with prominent delicate vascular arborization, and

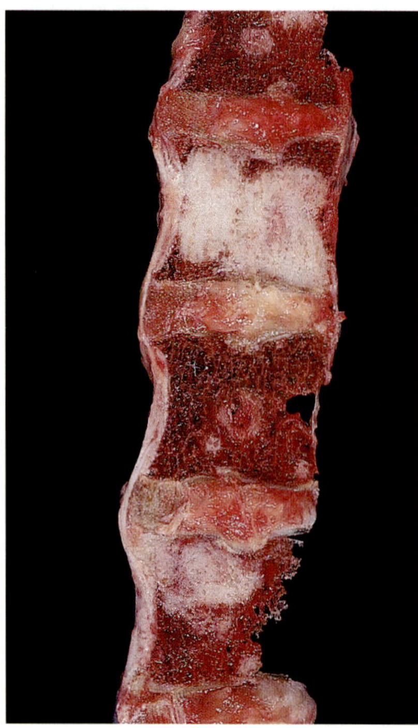

Fig. 3-2   Metastatic breast carcinoma to vertebrae. The lesion is grossly fibrotic and densely sclerotic; however, no specific gross features generally allow for determination of the primary site.

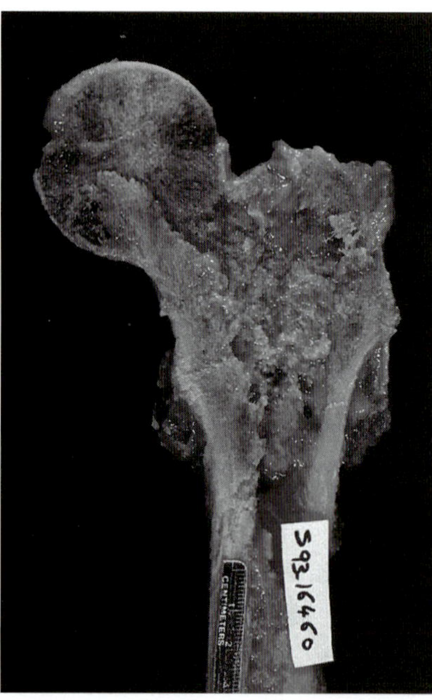

Fig. 3-3   Metastatic adenocarcinoma of lung, involving the femoral neck. Mottled areas of hemorrhage and necrosis related to prior radiation therapy are noted. No gross features, however, are characteristic of a metastatic lesion or the primary site of origin.

intracytoplasmic melanin are distinctive features of these tumors and allow for their identification (Figs. 3-4 and 3-5).

Category 2: Suggestive of Site of Origin

In the second category, relatively distinctive features strongly suggest the primary site. Included in this category are metastatic lesions of carcinomas of the breast and colon. Ductal structures with a comedolike pattern of necrosis or a linear arrangement of the tumor cells are strongly suggestive, in the proper clinical setting, of metastatic breast cancer. It is important to note that estrogen receptors are also shared by tumors other than breast carcinoma, including ovaries, endometrium, and stomach, and cannot be employed as a sole determinant of breast origin. Colonic carcinoma exhibits small glandular spaces lined by pseudostratified columnar cells with hyperchromatic elongated nuclei, luminal brush borders, and "dirty" central necrosis (Fig. 3-6).

Category 3: Nonspecific as to Site of Origin

In the third category, the histopathologic features allow for recognition of metastatic disease but are nonspecific in regard to primary site. For example, the diagnosis of metastatic squamous cell carcinoma is not difficult; however, primary squamous cell carcinomas of lung, head and neck, esophagus, cervix, and (less commonly) other sites share similar histopathologic features. Metastatic adenocarcinoma without any specific differentiating features is generally elusive as to the primary site of origin (Fig. 3-7). Occasionally, clear cell adenocarcinoma of ovary, endometrium, or lung may simulate clear cell renal cell carcinoma. Tumors in this category emphasize the hazards of attempting to identify an unknown primary site on the basis of the histopathologic findings alone.

Category 4: Not Readily Recognized as Metastatic

Fourth are the poorly differentiated neoplasms that lack specific histopathologic patterns and are not readily recognized as metastatic carcinoma. This category includes metastatic large cell carcinoma of the lung or pancreas, anaplastic carcinoma of the thyroid, and nonglandular solid components of poorly differentiated adenocarcinomas, irrespective of their primary site of origin (Fig. 3-8). One

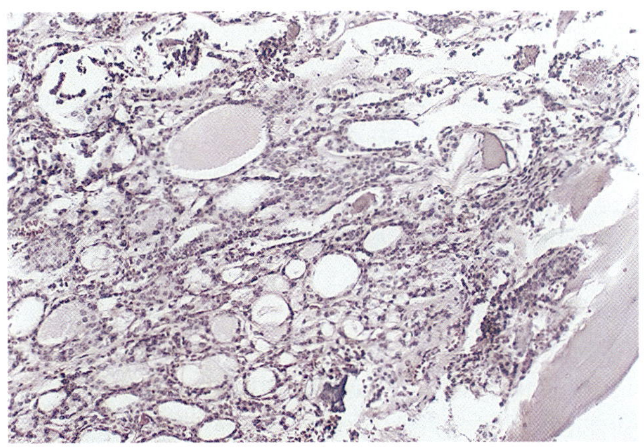

Fig. 3-4 Metastatic follicular carcinoma of thyroid. The presence of well-formed follicles and colloid allows for specification of the primary site.

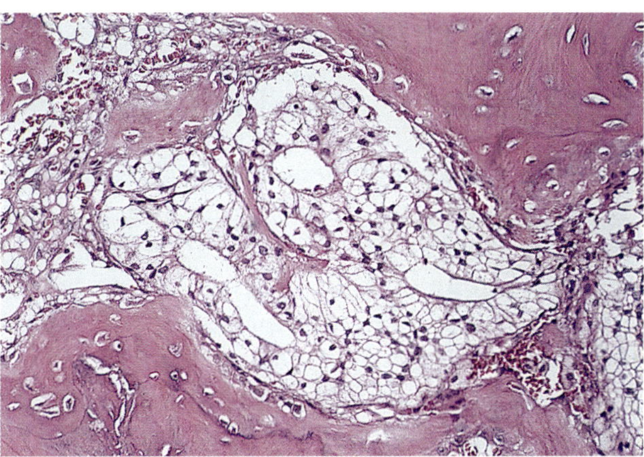

Fig. 3-5 Metastatic clear cell carcinoma of kidney. The tubules and nests of cells have abundant clear cytoplasm containing glycogen or lipid. Prominent vascular proliferation and hemorrhage are usually present.

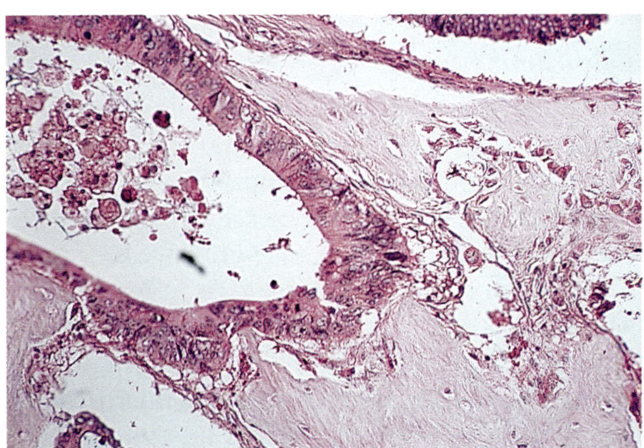

Fig. 3-6 Metastatic adenocarcinoma with tall columnar cells and a luminal brush border consistent with metastatic adenocarcinoma of colon.

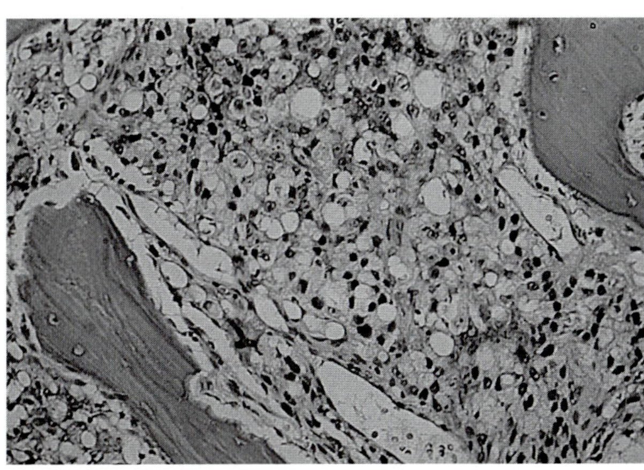

Fig. 3-7 Metastatic adenocarcinoma with no specific features characteristic of a certain primary site. Mucin stain was positive. The patient was subsequently found to have a primary tumor of the lung.

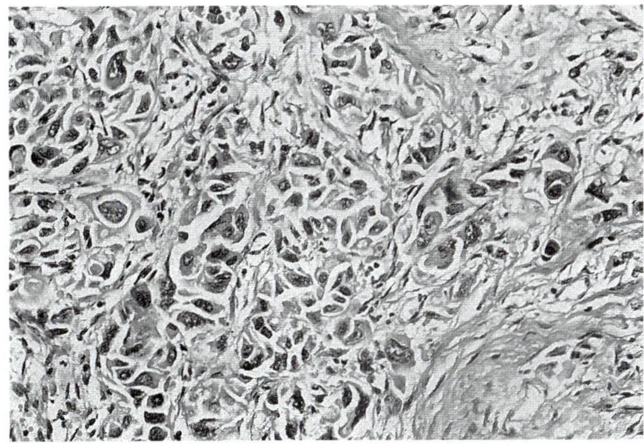

Fig. 3-8 Metastatic large cell carcinoma of lung. The histopathologic features resemble those of primary bone sarcoma. Knowledge of the presence of a primary lung tumor and positive staining for cytokeratin supported the diagnosis of metastatic carcinoma.

must also consider such nonepithelial tumors as anaplastic large cell (Ki-1+) lymphoma, poorly differentiated angiosarcoma, and, although rare, metastatic sarcoma. Without a history or known existence of a concomitant lesion, a specific diagnosis may be difficult to establish. Immunohistochemical stains for epithelial markers can readily identify the epithelial nature of some of these tumors but do not assist in suggesting a primary site.[18] Exceptions include positive staining for specific tumor markers such as prostatic acid phosphatase with prostate-specific antigen (Fig. 3-9) and the melanoma antigen HMB45.

Category 5: Overlapping With Primary Bone Tumors

Metastatic tumors exhibiting histopathologic features that are similar to or that considerably overlap those of primary bone sarcomas comprise the fifth category. This category represents a continuation of the previous one and includes tumors that fall under the general categories of spindle cell, clear cell, epithelioid cell, and small cell neoplasms.

Histopathologic Presentations
Spindle Cell Tumors

Spindle (sarcomatoid) squamous cell carcinomas are infrequently observed in the lung, head and neck, and esophagus. Metastatic skeletal lesions from these neoplasms can mimic primary bone sarcomas, such as fibrosarcoma. Sampling of the specimen often reveals at least focal obvious epithelial differentiation. However, a small biopsy sample, such as one obtained by FNAB or NCB, may show only the anaplastic spindle cell tumor component. Review of tissue sections from the suspected primary tumor and positive immunohistochemical staining for epithelial markers are essential for establishing a diagnosis. Similarly, metastasis from a sarcomatoid renal cell carcinoma can have features similar to those of malignant fibrous histiocytoma and thus can be misdiagnosed as primary fibrous histiocytoma of bone[19] (Fig. 3-10). The existence of disseminated bone involvement is a strong clue to the metastatic nature of the bone lesion. Immunohistochemical stains for epithelial markers may also assist in the differential diagnosis; however, some sarcomatoid carcinomas do not show epithelial differentiation. Furthermore, some

sarcomas may be focally positive for keratin. In all these cases, before definitive therapy it is important to rule out (clinically) the possibility of a sarcomatoid carcinoma in an adult patient. Metastatic sarcomas to bone, such as leiomyosarcoma, rarely occur but may be indistinguishable, morphologically, from primary bone sarcomas.[20,21]

Clear Cell Tumors

Metastatic clear cell neoplasms in bone, especially those of renal origin, can mimic primary bone tumors such as clear cell chondrosarcoma.[22] However, clear cell chondrosarcoma is extraordinarily rare and, in addition to cytoplasmic clearing, exhibits an admixture of osteoclast-like giant cells, heterogeneous osteoid matrix often resembling osteoblastoma, and angiectatic blood-filled spaces.[23] Unlike renal cell carcinoma, clear cell chondrosarcoma expresses S100 protein but not keratin.

Epithelioid Tumors

The differential diagnosis of epithelioid angiosarcoma of bone includes metastatic carcinoma and metastatic malignant melanoma. The latter tumor may also exhibit a variety of cellular patterns, including spindling, which may enhance its resemblance to primary bone sarcomas. In general, angiosarcomas exhibit endothelial cell specific markers such as factor VIII–related antigen, CD31, CD34, and ulex europaeus. Electron microscopy is an important diagnostic adjunct in separating epithelioid angiosarcoma from carcinoma and melanoma. Anaplastic or carcinoma-like epithelioid osteosarcoma may contain focal areas that are histopathologically indistinguishable from metastatic carcinoma (Fig. 3-11). Limited sampling may not demonstrate the presence of tumor osteoid, which is critical for the diagnosis of osteosarcoma. Knowledge of the clinical and radiographic presentation and ancillary studies are invaluable in this differential diagnosis.[24,25]

Small Cell Tumors

In pediatric patients, metastatic neuroblastoma and primitive alveolar rhabdomyosarcoma are considered in the differential diagnosis of primary round cell tumors of bone. These predominantly include Ewing's sarcoma and related primitive neuroectodermal tumors, lymphoma, small cell osteosarcoma, and mesenchymal chondrosarcoma. Clin-

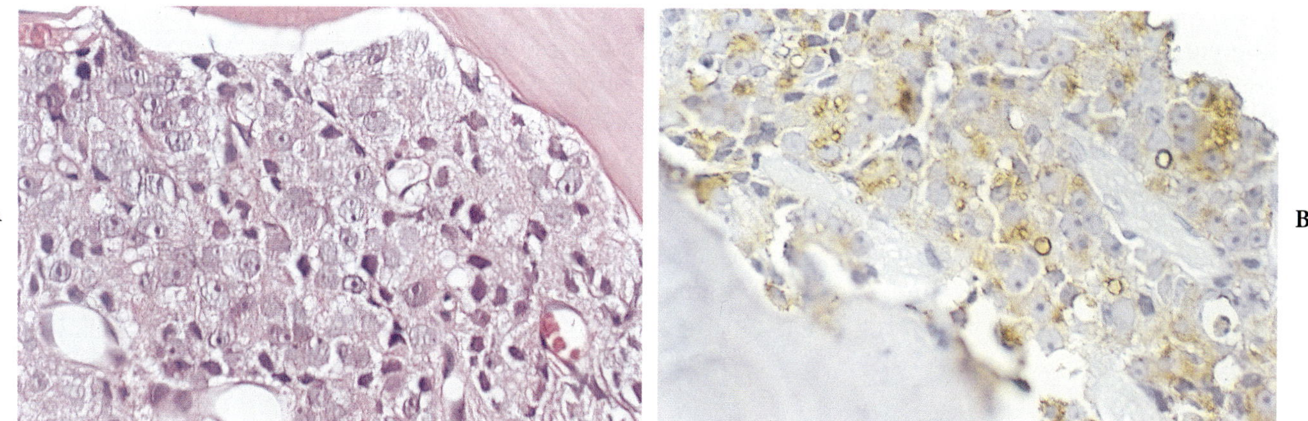

Fig. 3-9 Metastatic adenocarcinoma in a patient with lung and prostate adenocarcinomas. **A,** The poorly differentiated histopathologic features of this lesion do not allow for determination of the primary site. **B,** Immunohistochemical staining for prostatic acid phosphatase and prostate-specific antigen confirm the diagnosis of metastatic prostate carcinoma.

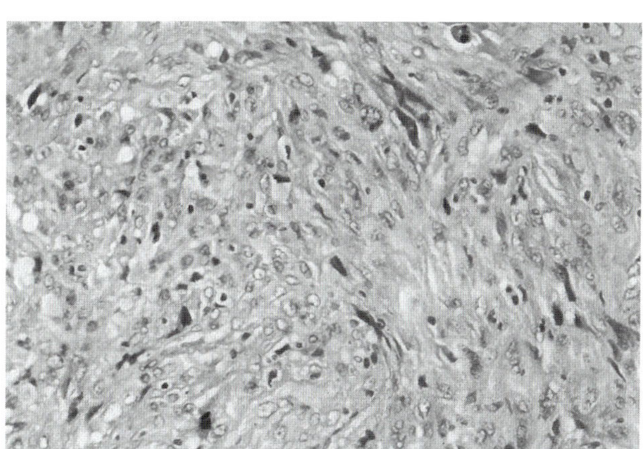

Fig. 3-10 Metastatic spindle cell or sarcomatoid renal cell carcinoma. The patient had a nephrectomy 2 years before the development of bony lesions. Purely on histopathologic grounds, the distinction between this tumor and a primary bone sarcoma such as malignant fibrous histiocytoma or fibrosarcoma may be difficult. In general, it may be advisable to exclude clinically a primary renal tumor whenever a spindle cell "sarcoma" of bone is diagnosed. Most patients will have a history of renal carcinoma.

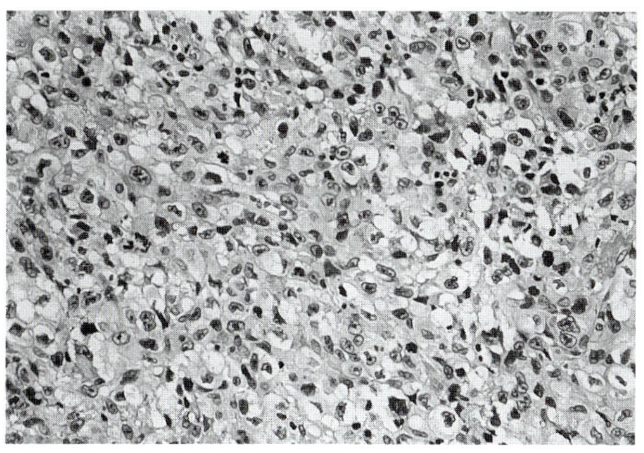

Fig. 3-11 Anaplastic or epithelioid (carcinoma-like) osteosarcoma. The histopathologic features are indistinguishable from those of metastatic carcinoma. Elsewhere in the sections, tumor osteoid was identified. The radiographic findings were characteristic of osteosarcoma, and the patient was not known to have a second primary tumor. It is essential to correlate the histopathologic and clinical features and to submit the entire biopsy tissue for histopathologic examination.

ically, neuroblastoma usually affects young children (<5 years of age), and pathologically, in its differentiated form, it often demonstrates pseudorosettes in a fibrillar background (Fig. 3-12). Metastatic alveolar rhabdomyosarcoma, which is far less common than neuroblastoma, almost never occurs in the absence of a known primary site. Nevertheless, primary Ewing's sarcoma and primitive neuroectodermal tumor of bone usually arise in patients between the ages of 5 and 25 years and are virtually never observed in African Americans. In the most primitive forms, small round cell tumors, whether primary or metastatic, may be indistinguishable by light microscopic analysis alone. A battery of ancillary studies, including immunostaining, electron microscopy, flow cytometry, and cytogenetic analysis, is helpful and often essential for proper identification.[9,26] Among adults, metastatic small cell carcinoma may simulate primary malignant lymphoma. However, the tumor cells of small cell carcinoma are generally more organoid and coherent than those of lymphoma and frequently exhibit nuclear molding, a "salt-and-pepper" chromatin pattern, and, occasionally, marked crush artifact (Fig. 3-13). Immunohistochemical staining for epithelial and neuroendocrine markers (chromogranin, synaptophysin, and neuron-specific enolase), as well as electron microscopy, can differentiate small cell carcinoma from lymphoma in the vast majority of difficult cases.

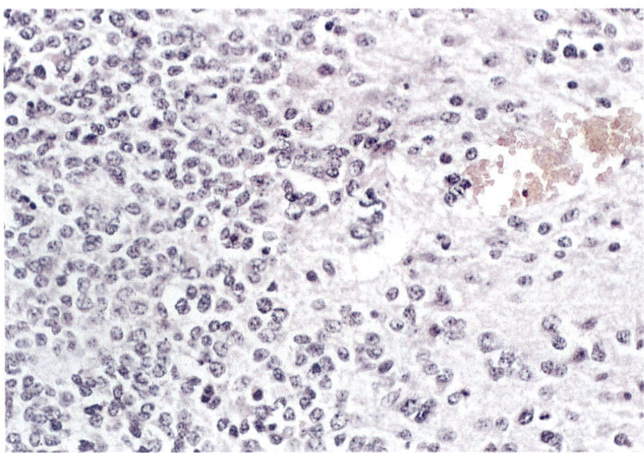

Fig. 3-12 Metastatic neuroblastoma. The tumor is characterized by the presence of small, round blue cells in a fibrillar (neuropil) background. Rosette arrangements may also be observed.

NONNEOPLASTIC SKELETAL RESPONSES TO METASTATIC DISEASE

Differentiating metastatic carcinoma from the associated osteoblastic or fibroblastic (desmoplastic response) proliferation is usually not a difficult task. However, an exuberant osteoblastic and fibroblastic proliferation, compounded by a periosteal reaction, fracture callus, hemorrhage or necrosis, or proliferation of osteoclasts, may occasionally obscure the metastatic deposit and sometimes simulate a primary bone tumor.[27]

Desmoplastic Response

Osteoblastic and fibroblastic proliferations typically accompany metastasis from breast and prostate cancer and may be so pronounced as to mask the underlying neoplasm.[28] Often in these cases the tumor cells are seen only as individual cells or arranged in small aggregates that may be easily missed. Similarly, fibrotic reactions may compress metastatic cells into barely visible cells. An unexplained intraosseous osteoblastic or fibroblastic proliferation should raise suspicion of a possible underlying lesion (Figs. 3-14 and 3-15). Multiple sections (levels) should be prepared and immunohistochemical stains for epithelial markers performed to help exclude the presence of malignant cells (Fig. 3-16). In cases of metastatic adenocarcinoma a mucin stain may suffice (Fig. 3-17).

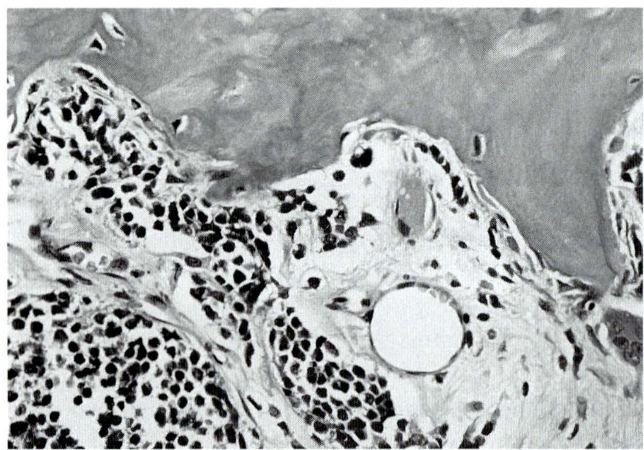

Fig. 3-13 Metastatic small cell undifferentiated carcinoma of lung. The cells are small and hyperchromatic, and they demonstrate clustering and nuclear molding. Ancillary studies can aid in the differential diagnosis with other small cell tumors including lymphoma.

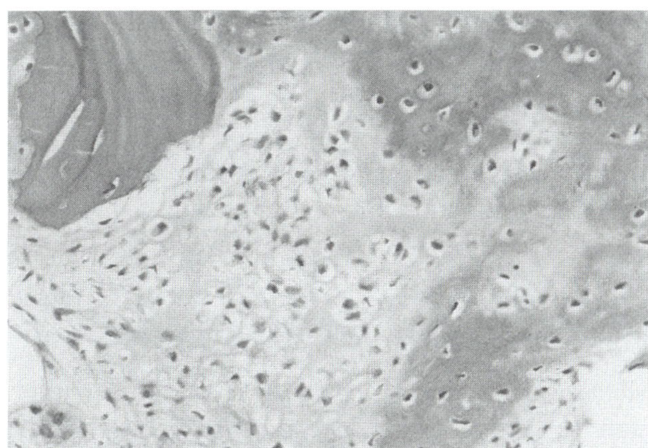

Fig. 3-14 Fulminant osteoblastic reaction at the periphery of metastatic carcinoma. This figure shows only the osteoblastic proliferation, osteoid and mineralized bone. Sampling of these areas without the carcinomatous component may result in interpretation of the lesion as a reactive or neoplastic osseous process.

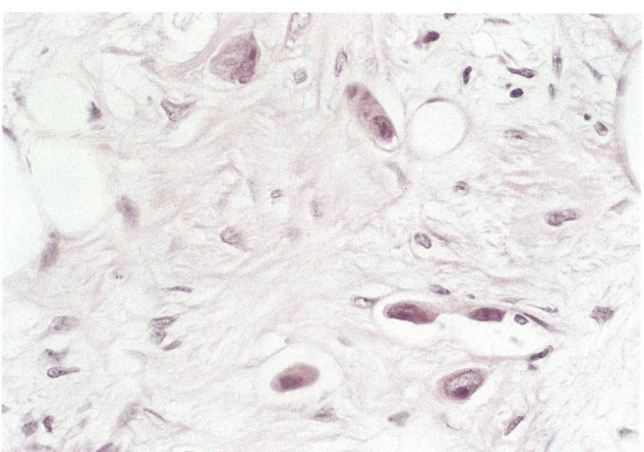

Fig. 3-15 Isolated cells forming metastatic breast carcinoma are entrapped in a prominent desmoplastic stromal response. These cells may be overlooked if examination is not thorough. Mucin stain or immunohistochemical stains for cytokeratin can highlight these cells.

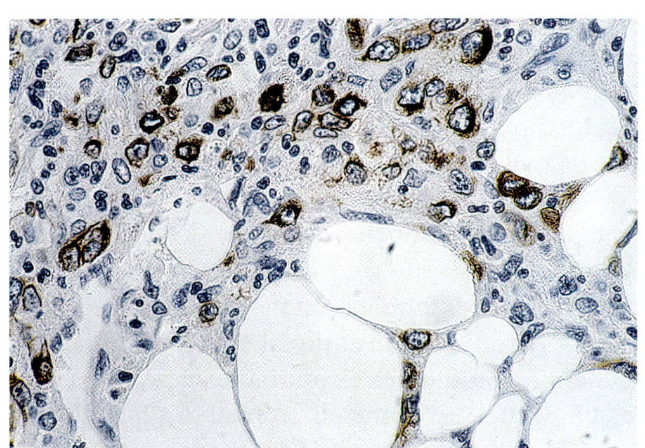

Fig. 3-16 Immunohistochemical stain for cytokeratin (AE 1/3) highlights individual metastatic cells from breast carcinoma. On routine staining these cells may be inconspicuous in a background of marrow fibrosis.

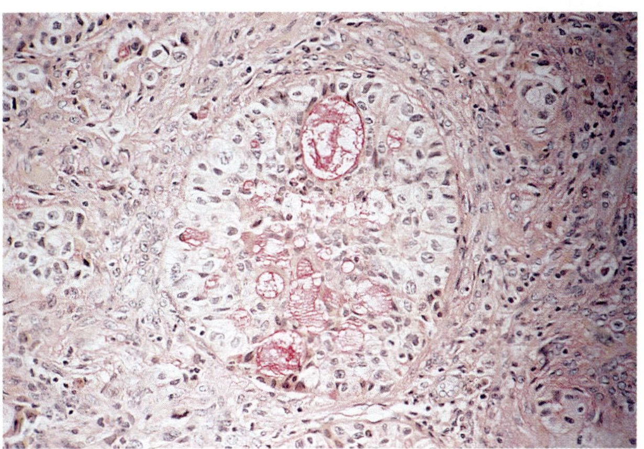

Fig. 3-17 A positive mucin stain (reddish pink), intracellular and in luminal secretions, is an inexpensive method of ascertaining whether a metastatic carcinoma is an adenocarcinoma. The presence of mucin, however, does not generally assist in determining the primary site. Exceptions include renal cell carcinoma and hepatocellular carcinomas, which are usually negative for mucin.

Periosteal Reaction

An exuberant periosteal reaction is rarely observed in metastatic disease but may accompany soft tissue extension, resulting in pathologic findings similar to those described earlier in this chapter.

Pathologic Fracture

Florid fracture callus with resultant fibroosseous, fibrocartilaginous, or cartilaginous proliferation may also mask metastatic disease. To the uninitiated, these changes may be confused with osteogenic sarcoma or chondrosarcoma. Unexplained clinical fracture always merits further investigation and requires meticulous gross inspection and, if necessary, judicious sampling.

Necrosis and Hemorrhage

Metastatic disease may cause necrosis and hemorrhage of bone marrow. Unexplained marrow necrosis is another indication for additional biopsies at adjacent clinically suspect sites[29] (Fig. 3-18).

Proliferation of Osteoclastic Giant Cells

Metastatic tumors can be accompanied by a prominent population of osteoclasts that focally and with limited sampling may occasionally resemble a giant cell tumor of bone. Examination of the "background stromal cells" is of critical importance in this situation.

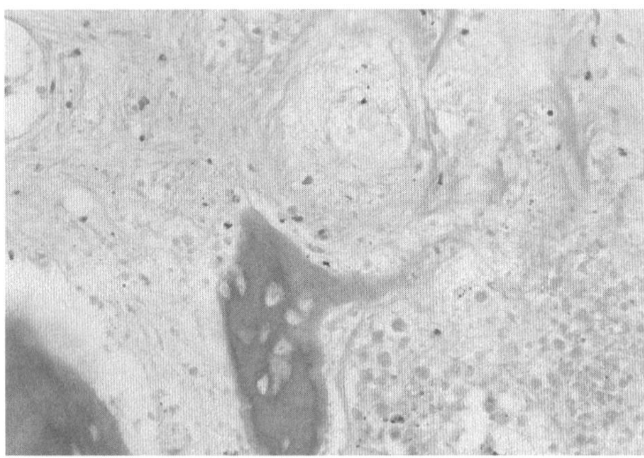

Fig. 3-18 Extensive necrosis of bone. Bone marrow has shadows of totally necrotic metastatic tumor cells, which are present in the right lower quadrant. Other areas demonstrated viable tumor cells derived from small cell carcinoma of lung. Biopsies of these lesions should avoid central necrotic areas, which may not yield diagnostic tissue.

Granulomatous Reaction

Rare metastatic tumors may be associated with a granulomatous response, suggesting an infectious origin. Meticulous attention to the presence of abnormal cells adjacent to the granulomas and the use of special stains for infectious organisms (e.g., acid-fast bacillus or silver stains) are helpful in excluding this diagnosis.

CONCLUSION

Metastatic carcinoma is the most common malignant tumor of bone. The primary malignancies that most commonly metastasize to bone are those of the breast, prostate, lung, and kidney. The sites of bone metastasis are usually the vertebral bodies, pelvic bones, proximal femur and humerus, and ribs. Metastasis distal to the elbows and knees is uncommon.

The correct diagnosis usually can be reached when the clinical history is considered. However, it should not be assumed that skeletal lesions in patients with known carcinomas are necessarily related to metastasis. The differential diagnosis of metastatic bone disease includes a primary bone tumor, Paget's disease, fracture, osteomyelitis, and hematopoietic malignancies.

Metastatic carcinoma is especially likely to be a diagnostic problem when only one skeletal lesion is found and no "primary" tumor is known. In difficult cases the pathologists may employ a variety of ancillary studies (conventional stains, immunohistochemical studies, electron microscopy, and cytogenetics) that aid in the differential diagnosis.

REFERENCES

1. Schwinn C. The pathologist and the diagnosis of bone metastasis. In Weiss L, Gilbert HA, eds. Bone Metastasis. Boston: GK Hall, 1981, pp 168-189.
2. Fechner RE, Mills SE. Tumors of the bones and joints. In Rosai J, Sobin LH, eds. Atlas of Tumor Pathology. Washington, DC: Armed Forces Institute of Pathology, 1993, pp 245-252.
3. Mirra JM, Picci P, Gold RH. Metastasis. In Mirra JM, ed. Bone Tumors: Clinical, Radiologic and Pathologic Correlations. Philadelphia: Lea & Febiger, 1989, pp 1495-1517.
4. Brunning RD. Bone marrow. In Rosai J, ed. Ackerman's Surgical Pathology, 8th ed. St. Louis: Mosby, 1996, pp 1797-1915.
5. Abdul-Karim FW, Masatoshi K, Wentz WB, Carter JR, Sorensen K, Macfee M, Zika J, Makley JT. Bone metastasis from gynecologic carcinomas: A clinicopathologic study. Gynecol Oncol 39:108-114, 1990.
6. Leeson MC, Makley JT, Carter JR. Metastatic skeletal disease in the pediatric population. J Pediatr Orthop 5:261-267, 1985.

7. Mackey B, Ordonez NG. Pathological evaluation of neoplasms with unknown primary tumor site. Semin Oncol 20: 206-228, 1993.

8. Bullough PG. Malignant non-matrix-producing bone tumors. In Bullough PG, ed. Bullough and Vigorita's Orthopaedic Pathology, 3rd ed. London: Mosby-Wolfe, 1997, pp 417-432.

9. Wold LE, McLeod RA, Sim FH, Unni KK. Metastatic carcinoma. In Zorab R, ed. Atlas of Orthopedic Pathology. Philadelphia: WB Saunders, 1990, pp 264-268.

10. Enneking WF. Malignant neoplasms of bone. In Enneking WF, ed. Clinical Musculoskeletal Pathology. Gainesville, Fla.: Storter Printing, 1977, pp 281-330.

11. Unni KK. Conditions that commonly stimulate primary neoplasms of bone. In Unni KK, Dahlin DC, eds. Dahlin's Bone Tumors: General Aspects and Data on 11,087 Cases, 5th ed. Philadelphia: Lippincott-Raven, 1996, pp 355-432.

12. Leeson MC, Makley JT, Carter JR. Metastatic skeletal disease distal to the elbow and knee. Clin Orthop 206:94-99, 1986.

13. Dorfman HD, Czerniak B. Metastatic tumors in bone. In Dorfman HD, Czerniak B, eds. Bone Tumors. St. Louis: Mosby, 1998, pp 1009-1040.

14. Agarwal PK, Goel MM, Chandra T, Agarwal S. Predictive value of fine needle aspiration cytology of bone lesions. Acta Cytol 41:659-665, 1997.

15. Schweitzer ME, Gannon FH, Deely DM, O'Hara BJ, Juneja V. Percutaneous skeletal aspiration and core biopsy: Complementary techniques. Am J Radiol 166:415-418, 1996.

16. Koscick RL, Petersilge CA, Makley JT, Abdul-Karim FW. CT guide fine needle aspiration and needle core biopsy of skeletal lesions: Complementary diagnostic techniques. Acta Cytol 42:697-702, 1998.

17. Miller F, Whitehill R. Carcinoma of the breast metastatic to the skeleton. Clin Orthop 184:121-127, 1984.

18. Athanasou NA, Quinn J, Heryet A, Woods CG, McGee JO. Effect of decalcification agents on immunoreactivity of cellular antigens. J Clin Pathol 40:874-878, 1987.

19. Ro JY, Ayala AG, Sella A, Samuels ML, Swanson DA. Sarcomatoid renal cell carcinoma: Clinicopathologic study of 42 cases. Cancer 59:516-526, 1987.

20. Fornaisier VL, Paley D. Leiomyosarcoma in bone: Primary or secondary? A case report and review of literature. Skeletal Radiol 10:147-153, 1983.

21. Antonescu CR, Erlandson RA, Huvos AG. Primary leiomyosarcoma of bone: A clinicopathologic, immunohistochemical and ultrastructural study of 33 patients and a literature review. Am J Surg Pathol 21:1281-1294, 1997.

22. Swanson PE. Clear cell tumors of bone. Semin Diagn Pathol 14:281-291, 1997.

23. Bjoernsson J, Beabout JW, Unni KK, Sim FH, Dahlin DC. Clear cell chondrosarcoma: Observations in 47 cases. Am J Surg Pathol 8:223-230, 1984.

24. Hasegawa T, Shibata T, Hirose T, Seki K, Hizawa K. Osteosarcoma with epithelioid features: An immunohistochemical study. Arch Pathol Lab Med 117:295-298, 1993.

25. Kramer K, Hicks DG, Palis J, Rosier RN, Oppenheimer J, Fallon MD, Cohen HJ. Epithelioid osteosarcoma of bone. Cancer 71:2977-2982, 1993.

26. Ilson DH, Motzer RJ, Rodriguez E, Chaganti RSK, Bosl GJ. Genetic analysis in the diagnosis of neoplasms of unknown primary tumor site. Semin Oncol 20:229-237, 1993.

27. Lipton A, Mundy G, Singer FR. Introduction to skeletal complications of malignancy. Am Cancer Soc 80:527-528, 1997.

28. Goltzman D. Mechanisms of the development of osteoblastic metastases. Cancer 80(Suppl):1581-1587, 1997.

29. Sun NCJ. Bone marrow. In Silverberg SG, DeLellis RA, Frable WJ, eds. Principles and Practice of Surgical Pathology and Cytopathology, 3rd ed. New York: Churchill Livingstone, 1997, pp 773-831.

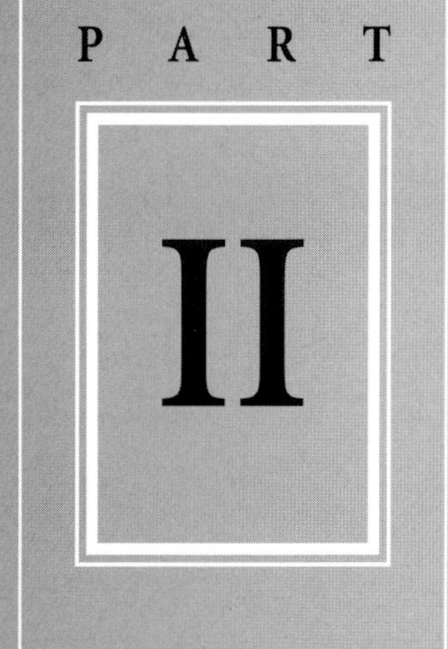

Clinical Presentation and Evaluation

Signs and Symptoms of Metastatic Disease and Serologic Markers

John P. Heiner, M.D., Mary M. Checovich, M.S., and James A. Stewart, M.D.

Metastatic disease to bone may be manifested by focal symptoms such as pain. It may also be asymptomatic and diagnosed during the staging of a primary tumor. This chapter will discuss the presenting signs and symptoms of metastatic disease and the serologic findings common to selected tumors.

SIGNS AND SYMPTOMS OF METASTATIC DISEASE

The most common presenting symptom of metastatic disease to the skeleton is pain. Galasko[1] found that although pain is the most common symptom, 30% to 50% of patients have asymptomatic bone metastases found during staging studies for primary tumors. In many patients the pain may represent only one of many metastatic lesions found on a technetium bone scan. In a review of 100 consecutive patients with pain, 80% had pain in more than one area and 34% had four or more areas of bone pain.[2] The clinician may assign pain to one of several categories: pain at rest, severe pain with motion or weightbearing, and mild-to-moderate pain with ambulation. A routine radiographic evaluation of the entire bone is necessary to evaluate the risk of pathologic fracture. Increasing pain or pain at rest may indicate an impending pathologic fracture. A palpable soft tissue mass may also accompany large lytic bone metastases. The patient usually can localize the pain in extremity lesions reasonably well, but pelvic and spine metastases may be manifested by severe but poorly localized pain.

Patients may also have a pathologic fracture at presentation. Such a fracture in the long bones of the lower limb is particularly devastating. If a patient has a history of minimal trauma with a subsequent fracture, the physician should suspect a neoplastic process that may not be clearly seen on the initial radiographic evaluation. Further studies, such as magnetic resonance imaging (MRI), may be beneficial.

Paraplegia is a less common initial symptom of metastatic disease, but the underlying cause needs to be recognized immediately. Typically a patient with a known malignancy has increasing leg weakness and back pain. The upper extremities are frequently spared, because thoracic and lumbar metastases are more common than cervical metastases. It is estimated that 5% of patients with cancer have metastases affecting the spinal cord.[3-5] In a study of men with prostate cancer, Rana et al.[6] showed a 2% incidence of paraplegia as the first sign of metastatic cancer. Breast, lung, and prostate cancer are the most common tumors to cause spinal cord compression. Fifteen percent of patients have no known primary tumor.[4,7] In the pediatric population, leukemia, osteosarcoma, Ewing's sarcoma, and rhabdomyosarcoma have all been reported to cause spinal cord compression.[5,8,9]

With the advent of MRI the diagnosis of cord compression from metastatic lesions has improved. Needle or open biopsy can quickly confirm the diagnosis. Radiation or surgical decompression with stabilization is usually performed on an emergent basis. If a patient has a complete spinal cord lesion with no function below the level of the compression, recovery of neurologic function may be limited.[10-13] Glucocorticoid treatment is also used to minimize edema and decrease compression of the spinal cord.[14] Survival of patients with spinal cord compression resulting from metastatic disease has been limited, but in certain tumors, such as lymphomas, longer survival periods, of several years, have been reported.[15,16]

Many patients have no symptoms of metastatic skeletal disease, and the first indication is found during a bone scan while the primary tumor is being staged.[17-19] Often the increased uptake on a bone scan is the first sign of metastatic disease and will often change the clinician's approach to the patient. The routine radiograph may or may not detect the underlying lesion.[20] MRI or biopsy is often necessary to confirm the findings of the technetium bone scan.

A painful soft tissue mass is one of the least common signs of metastatic disease to the musculoskeletal system. The mass may be due to hematogenous spread of the primary tumor to muscle, or the mass may have started as an intramedullary bone lesion and subsequently spread to the surrounding soft tissues. Routine radiographs and MRI will often differentiate between the true extraosseous metastases and those metastases arising from adjacent bones. Fatigue is also a symptom of widespread metastatic disease to bone. The fatigue is due to anemia caused by replacement of the normal marrow with tumor. This symptom usually occurs late in the disease. Confusion and other symptoms resulting from hypercalcemia and paraneoplastic symptoms are discussed elsewhere in this text.

One specific metastatic lesion warrants specific recommendations: an unknown primary malignancy. In a prospective study, Rougraff et al.[21] evaluated bone or soft tissue lesions in 40 patients with no known primary tumor. The evaluation was made before biopsy and included a complete history and physical examination; a complete blood cell count; determinations of the Westergren sedimentation rate, electrolyte levels, and liver enzyme and alkaline phosphatase levels; and serum protein electrophoresis. If the result of serum protein electrophoresis was positive for multiple myeloma, the patient was excluded from the study.

Radiographic evaluation included a radiograph of the chest and of the involved bone(s); technetium 99m phosphonate bone scan; and computed tomography (CT) scan of the chest, abdomen, and pelvis. With this evaluation the primary site was identified in 34 (85%) of 40 patients. In two patients the primary tumor was not apparent until the later stages of the disease. The single test that most frequently revealed the primary site was radiography of the chest. In 17 patients (43%) the diagnosis was revealed on chest x-ray film, with an additional 6 patients (15%) receiving a diagnosis based on CT scan of the chest. The history and physical examination correctly showed the diagnosis in only 3 (8%) of 40 patients. The most common primary tumor found was lung carcinoma, with 23 cases. Rougraff et al.[21] suggested that this strategy will help the clinician identify 85% of the primary tumor sites before biopsy of the metastatic lesion.

Metastatic disease to the musculoskeletal system may be manifested in any number of ways. The clinician must have a high index of suspicion. With the advent of multiple serum markers for various tumors, following the serologic changes has changed the clinician's ability to judge the activity of the disease. The following sections discuss various serum markers that are currently available for the assessment of malignant neoplasms.

MARKERS OF BONE METABOLISM

The dispersion of metastases to the skeleton is a complex process. Bone metastases usually arise from malignant cells in the bone marrow. They first develop in the trabecular bone and then involve the cortical bone. Once the malignant cells are established in the bone, the cells are attracted to the bone surface by collagen fragments and growth factors released from the bone surface. These malignant cells produce paracrine factors that stimulate osteoclasts to resorb bone. These cells also stimulate immune cells to produce osteoclast-activating factors.[22] These paracrine factors include prostaglandin, growth factors, cytokines, and parathyroid hormone–related protein.[23] The varied importance of each of these factors is still not understood nor clearly defined.

Skeletal metastases display a variety of physiologic abnormalities that can be detected by serologic studies. Biochemical markers of bone metabolism specifically reflect the metabolic activity of bone. Traditionally, alkaline phosphatase and hydroxyproline have been employed in the detection of bone metastases. Recently, new markers for the assessment of bone and collagen metabolism have been developed. Specific biochemical markers can reflect the entire skeletal turnover and may provide serial information for monitoring or predicting the response to therapy. It is possible that some markers of bone metabolism might even predict the appearance of bone metastases before bone scans will detect them. These biochemical markers could complement scanning techniques in monitoring the response to treatment.

DETECTION OF MARKERS OF BONE METABOLISM

Biochemical markers of bone metabolism specifically reflect the metabolic activity of the bone. The rate of formation and resorption of the bone matrix can be assessed either by measuring the enzymatic activity of the bone-forming or resorbing cells or by measuring components of the bone matrix that are released into circulation during the formation or resorption of bone. Markers of bone metabolism are generally divided into two categories: formation and resorption (Table 4-1). Most of these biochemical markers of bone metabolism

Table 4-1   Biochemical markers of metastatic disease activity

Measurement	Source	Changes in osteolytic bone disease
Bone formation		
Alkaline phosphatase	Liver/bone/gut	Increased
Skeletal alkaline phosphatase	Bone: osteoblasts	Increased
Osteocalcin	Bone: osteoblasts	Increased
Hydroxyproline	Posttranslational maturation of collagen	Increased
Extension peptides		
Carboxyterminal propeptide of type I procollagen	Procollagen type I	Increased
Aminoterminal propeptide of type I procollagen	Procollagen type I	Increased
Decarboxylated osteocalcin	Bone: osteoblasts	Increased
Bone resorption		
Dialyzable hydroxyproline	Collagen degradation	Increased
Glucosylgalactosyl/galactosyl hydroxylysine	Skin/bone collagen	Decreased
Acid phosphatase	Osteoclasts and other tissues	Increased
Tartrate-resistant acid phosphatase	Osteoclasts (platelets)	Increased
Deoxypyridinoline (Dpd) and pyridinoline (Pyd) (high-performance liquid chromatography)	Collagen cross-links	Increased
Pyridinoline (Pyrilink, Quidel Corporation, San Diego, Calif.)	Collagen cross-links	Increased
Deoxypyridinoline (D-pyrilink, Quidel Corporation, San Diego, Calif.)	Collagen cross-links	Increased
Aminoterminal telopeptide of type I collagen (Osteomark NTx, Ostex International, Seattle, Wash.)	Collagen and cross-links	Increased
Carboxyterminal telopeptide of type I collagen (Crosslaps, Osteometer A/S, Denmark)	Collagen and cross-links	Increased

are of unequal sensitivity and specificity; most have not been fully investigated. Many of these markers are not disease specific but may be more sensitive or specific in assessing the skeletal turnover in one disease state over another. Additionally, many of these markers exhibit physiologic changes that may be due to diurnal variation or aging or may be gender dependent.

MARKERS OF BONE FORMATION

Alkaline Phosphatase and the Bone-Specific Isoenzyme of Alkaline Phosphatase. Serum alkaline phosphatase is one of the most commonly used clinical markers of bone formation. Besides being produced by osteoblasts, alkaline phosphatase is derived from liver, kidney, and many other cells. Because only part of the circulating levels are normally derived from adult bone, alkaline phosphatase lacks sensitivity in conditions with a mild increase in bone turnover. Additionally, a moderate increase of serum alkaline phosphatase is ambiguous because it may reflect a mineralization effect or the effect of one of numerous medications shown to increase the hepatic isoenzyme of alkaline phosphatase. To overcome the lack of specificity of alkaline phosphatase, researchers developed techniques to differentiate bone and liver isoenzymes, which differ only by posttranslational modifications as they are coded by a single gene.[24] Bone-specific alkaline phosphatase reflects the phase of matrix development and maturation. Measurement of bone-specific alkaline phosphatase relies on techniques that use differentially effective activators and inhibitors (heat, phenylalanine, and urea), separation by electrophoresis, lectin precipitation, and the use of antibodies. In general, these assays have only slightly enhanced the sensitivity of this marker.

Serum Osteocalcin. Osteocalcin, or bone Gla protein, is a small noncollagenous protein that is specific for bone tissue and dentin. Next to collagen, it is the most abundant constituent of the bone matrix; 20% of noncollagenous matrix protein consists of osteocalcin. Osteocalcin is predominantly synthesized by the osteoblasts, and the majority of new bone Gla protein is incorporated into bone matrix, where it remains until the bone is resorbed.

The precise function of osteocalcin remains unknown; however, some researchers postulate that its main function is to retard mineralization of bone and dentin and to contribute to serum calcium homeostasis.[25] Enzyme-linked immunosorbent assay (ELISA), immunoradiometric assay (IRMA), or radioimmunoassay (RIA) techniques based on monoclonal or polyclonal antibodies against human or bovine osteocalcin determine the plasma osteocalcin concentration. Osteocalcin assay results are not standardized; comparisons between different assays are therefore possible only when the average serum concentration of osteocalcin in the abnormal population is compared with the average osteocalcin values of a normal population. Even after such a correction, interassay concordance is poor.

Carboxyterminal Propeptide of Type I Procollagen. This carboxyterminal propeptide is a 100,000 molecular-weight globular glycoprotein. Procollagen type I carboxyterminal propeptide (PICP) is released into the circulation during the conversion of procollagen into collagen outside of the cell. PICP is cleared from plasma by liver metabolism. A high PICP concentration may result from decreased liver clearance or end-stage liver disease and therefore must be interpreted with caution. PICP is related to the early proliferation phase

of bone formation and is considered to be a formation marker. Levels of PICP are usually measured in serum by the RIA technique.[26,27] The reason for the lack of sensitivity is not clear. Despite its potential value, this marker is not currently a valid clinical alternative to other markers of bone formation.[28]

Aminoterminal Propeptide of Type I Procollagen. During the extracellular processing of collagen I, there is cleavage of the aminoterminal propeptide of type I procollagen (PINP) and the carboxyterminal (PICP) before fibril formation. The aminoterminal propeptide (PINP) of the procollagen molecule is a 35,000 molecular-weight phosphorylated protein consisting of a helical and a globular domain. In contrast to PICP, the aminoterminal propeptide (PINP) is cleaved from the procollagen molecule in the later stages of bone formation. These peptides circulate in the blood, where they might be useful markers of bone formation because collagen is one of the most abundant organic components of the bone matrix.[29]

MARKERS OF BONE RESORPTION

Urinary Calcium. Fasting urinary calcium measured at the first morning void and corrected by creatinine excretion is an economical assay for bone resorption. It is useful for determining a marked increase in bone resorption but lacks sensitivity.

Hydroxyproline. Hydroxyproline (OH-Pro) is a traditional marker of bone resorption and, until recently, was the marker most widely used. Most of the measurable OH-Pro is derived from the degradation of various forms of collagen. Because only 50% of the human collagen is in bone, OH-Pro is not a specific marker. Additionally, OH-Pro is easily influenced by diet or by soft tissue destruction from tumors.[30,31] Assays based on colorimetric and high-performance liquid chromatography (HPLC) methods are used for the biochemical detection of OH-Pro in urine.

Isoenzyme of Tartrate-Resistant Acid Phosphatase. Acid phosphatase is another marker of bone resorption. The enzyme is also present in the prostate, thrombocytes, erythrocytes, and the spleen. The isoenzyme of osteoclastic origin is resistant to inhibition by L-tartrate. A bioassay is performed from the detection of acid phosphatase; the observed inhibition after incubation with L-tartrate is used for the assessment of activity by the isoenzyme of tartrate-resistant acid phosphatase (TRAP). The clinical use of TRAP as a marker of bone resorption is limited by a lack of specificity, instability, and the presence in plasma of enzyme inhibitors other than tartrate. However, the development of an immunoassay using monoclonal antibodies specifically directed against the bone isoenzyme of TRAP could prove to be valuable in assessing osteoclastic activity.[32]

Galactosyl Hydroxylysine. Galactosyl hydroxylysine is an amino acid unique to collagen and collagen-like proteins. After bone resorption, the kidneys excrete 50% to 100% of galactosyl hydroxylysine. Urinary galactosyl hydroxylysine is separated by HPLC, followed by fluorometric quantification. Unlike OH-Pro, urinary excretion of galactosyl hydroxylysine is not influenced by dietary-contributed collagen. The relative proportion and the total content of this amino acid vary between bone and soft tissue. Therefore it might be a more sensitive marker of bone resorption than OH-Pro.

Urinary Total Pyridinium Cross-links. Pyridinoline (Pyd) and deoxypyridinoline (Dpd) are nonreducible cross-links that stabilize the collagen chains within the extracellular matrix.[33] Although Pyd is found in both bone and cartilage, virtually all the Pyd in urine is from bone because bone mass is greater than cartilage and because of the higher turnover of bone. As expected, the ratio of Pyd to Dpd in urine is similar to that found in bone. Both Pyd and Dpd are released into the circulation with bone resorption as the collagen matrix degrades; therefore these cross-links are of potential use as markers of bone resorption. The measurement of the cross-linking compounds of collagen can overcome the relative lack of specificity exhibited by other markers of osteoclastic activity. After degradation of the bone matrix, Pyd cross-links are released into the circulation. The cross-links are excreted unchanged by the kidneys. Dpd and Pyd values have to be adjusted to urinary creatinine values to account for body size and urine dilution.

Carboxyterminal Telopeptide of Type I Collagen. The carboxyterminal telopeptide of type I collagen (ICTP), a compound molecule, consists of parts of the carboxyterminal telopeptide regions connected by pyridinium cross-links to helical segments of adjacent collagen fibrils. During bone resorption, this part is cleaved from the collagen molecule and released into the circulation. ICTP is not degraded metabolically. Instead, the molecule is excreted by filtration through the glomerular basal membrane. Levels of ICTP appear not to be influenced by renal function. An RIA for the determination of ICTP in serum is described by Risteli and Risteli.[24] An ELISA for ICTP in urine was evaluated by Bonde et al.[34]

Aminoterminal Telopeptide of Type I Collagen. The aminoterminal telopeptide of collagen I (INTP) is also a marker of bone resorption. Similar to ICTP, the INTP molecule is not readily metabolized and is removed by renal clearance. INTP is determined in urine by an enzyme-linked immunoassay. The probe used in the INTP (NTx) assay is directed against the aminoterminal telopeptide of the α_2-chain of collagen I, the collagen type predominant in bone matrix.[35] Specificity for bone-derived collagen fragments is further enhanced by assaying for the Dpd type of cross-links. Because the Dpd cross-link has a higher concentration in bone collagen than in collagen derived from other tissues, the INTP assay is considered to have a high specificity for collagen fragments released by bone resorption.

CLINICAL APPLICATION OF BIOCHEMICAL MARKERS OF BONE METABOLISM

Monoclonal antibodies to various tumor antigens have been developed. Tumor antigens and antibodies have been developed. Carcinoembryonic antigen (CEA; gastrointestinal tract),[36,37] cancer antigen 15-3 (CA 15-3; breast cancer),[38] and cancer antigen 125 (CA 125; ovarian cancer)[39] have been used in monitoring the response to treatment for many years. Several authors have hypothesized about the possibility of monitoring the response of bone metastases to therapy by a set of tumor markers. Some authors have found that the presence of CEA and CA 15-3 can predict bone metastases[40]; others have not.[41] When bone metastases were monitored, alkaline phosphatase and OH-Pro had a higher degree of sensitivity. In prostatic cancer, prostate-specific antigen (PSA) is used as a marker of disease activity. PSA is a specific marker for overall disease activity; however, its value for detection and monitoring of bone involvement is limited.[42,43] Overall, these markers have been useful in following the disease in general but have not been specific for the musculoskeletal metastases.

STUDIES IN PATIENTS WITH BREAST CANCER

In breast cancer, more bone metastases are osteolytic[44,45]; therefore bone resorption markers are more sensitive than bone formation markers in those patients. In the patient with osteoblastic metastatic disease, the bone formation markers will be more helpful (Table 4-2).

Alkaline Phosphatase. Although the alkaline phosphatase level is typically elevated in patients with bone metastases from breast cancer, it generally has low sensitivity for the detection of bone metastases.[40,46] Koizumi et al.[47] found that only 27 of 100 patients with skeletal metastases demonstrated elevated alkaline phosphatase levels. Alkaline phosphatase concentrations did not differ from those in patients without bone metastases.

Additionally, Nguyen et al.[48] reported that alkaline phosphatase could not discriminate between bone and liver metastases.

Bone-Specific Alkaline Phosphatase. In breast cancer, bone-specific alkaline phosphatase seems to be able to distinguish between bone metastases and soft tissue metastases. Nguyen et al.[48] reported elevated values in patients with bone metastases in comparison with nonbone metastases. Reale et al.[49] reported that elevated bone-specific alkaline phosphatase measurements were confirmed by a positive technetium bone scan approximately 100 days later.

Osteocalcin. Osteocalcin was found to have low sensitivity for bone metastases from breast cancer[50,51] and did not correlate with the degree of bone metastasis as determined by bone scintigra-

Table 4-2 Biochemical markers in patients with breast cancer

Marker	+ Metastases	− Metastases	Assay	% Sensitivity	% Specificity	Reference
Alkaline phosphatase	47	0	Colorimetric	66	NA	19
	32	28	Colorimetric	48	83	30
	100	167	Colorimetric	27	96	26
Bone-specific alkaline phosphatase	88	100	Electrophoresis	43	91	31
	23	74	RIA	79	86	28
	75	25	Electrophoresis	42	98	29
Osteocalcin	32	28	ELISA	30	78	30
	100	167	RIA	29	89	26
	75	252	RIA	34	77	29
Carboxyterminal propeptide of type I procollagen	100	167	RIA	29	89	26
	75	25	RIA	25	83	29
Tartrate-resistant acid phosphatase	80	111	Colorimetric	69	74	47
Hydroxyproline	88	70	Colorimetric	75	81	31
	48	0	Colorimetric	32	NA	19
	75	25	HPLC/fluorometry	74	30	29
Galactosyl hydroxylysine	24	40	HPLC/fluorometry	92	90	32
Pyridinoline/deoxypyridinoline	10	10	ELISA	95	92	33

NA, Not available; RIA, radioimmunoassay; ELISA, enzyme-linked immunosorbent assay; HPLC, high-performance liquid chromatography.

phy.[47] Patients with breast cancer who had a single metastatic bone lesion did not have altered osteocalcin levels; these levels were similar to those of subjects without any metastatic bone disease.

Carboxyterminal Propeptide of Type I Procollagen. Koizumi et al.[47] reported that PICP levels in patients with breast cancer who had bone metastases were higher than in patients without bone metastases. In this study, however, elevation of PICP values was a function of the extent of bone involvement rather than the ability of PICP to differentiate between the presence and absence of even a single bone metastasis.

Tartrate-Resistant Acid Phosphatase. Nguyen et al.[48] reported that TRAP could not differentiate patients with and without bone metastases.

Hydroxyproline. Frenay et al.[52] demonstrated that OH-Pro has good sensitivity and specificity for the presence or absence of bone metastases. During a follow-up study, 10 of the 20 patients with bone metastases had elevated OH-Pro levels 5.5 months before evidence with bone scintigraphy was demonstrated.

Galactosyl Hydroxylysine. Moro et al.[53] reported that galactosyl hydroxylysine might be an early marker of bone metastases. They based their report on findings in a group of patients with abnormalities on bone scans and with elevated galactosyl hydroxylysine levels.

Pyridinoline and Deoxypyridinoline. Checovich et al.[54] reported that cancer patients with and without evidence of bone metastases had significantly higher levels of Pyd. All patients with breast cancer had significantly higher Pyd and Dpd values than normal control subjects, although there was no significant difference between the breast cancer groups. However, retrospective follow-up 24 months after the initial collection of urine demonstrated that of the 20 patients with breast cancer who were initially assigned to a group without evidence of metastatic bone disease, four subsequently had neoplastic bone disease. Two patients had levels of pyridinium cross-links within the normal range, and the other two had elevated Pyd and Dpd levels. Statistical analyses designed to distinguish the diagnostic and prognostic values of the Pyd and Dpd assays—the log-rank test—demonstrated that Pyd was the best single predictor for development of metastatic bone disease.

STUDIES IN PATIENTS WITH PROSTATE CANCER

It is generally believed that bone metastases from prostate cancer are osteoblastic in origin. If so, formation markers would be better predictors of bone metastases than resorption markers in prostatic cancer (Table 4-3).

Alkaline Phosphatase. Many authors have reported elevated levels of alkaline phosphatase with metastatic bone disease in patients with prostate cancer. However, the ability of this assay to distinguish between patients with and without bone metastases is mixed, and the assay is generally insensitive.[55]

Skeletal Alkaline Phosphatase. Because metastatic spread to the liver is not common in prostate cancer, isolating the skeletal portion of alkaline phosphatase is generally not beneficial in these patients. Nonetheless, Morote et al.[56] demonstrated that normal skeletal alkaline phosphatase levels with PSA values less than 10 ng/ml was 100% predictive of the absence of bone metastasis.

Osteocalcin. Osteocalcin can be elevated in prostate cancer with bone metastasis. However, Koizumi et al.[47] could not find any difference in osteocalcin values in prostate cancer patients with or without bone metastases.

Carboxyterminal Propeptide of Type I Procollagen. Various authors have reported elevated levels in the majority of patients with bone metastases from prostate cancer. Koizumi et al.[47] could not find any difference in PICP values in prostate cancer patients with or without bone metastases.

Tartrate-Resistant Acid Phosphatase. Francini et al.[57] reported high sensitivity for the TRAP assay but low specificity in prostate cancer patients with or without bone metastases as determined radiographically.

Hydroxyproline. Miyamoto et al.[58] found no difference in urinary OH-Pro excretion in patients with benign prostatic hypertrophy, in those with primary prostate cancer, and in those with bone metastases from prostate cancer. These findings were confirmed by Francini et al.[57]

Pyridinoline and Deoxypyridinoline. Pyd and Dpd excretion is increased in patients with bone metastases from prostatic cancer. Yoshida et al.[59] reported that Dpd values could differentiate between benign prostatic hyperplasia and prostate cancer;

Table 4-3   Biochemical markers in prostate cancer

Marker	+ Metastases	− Metastases	Assay	% Sensitivity	% Specificity	Reference
Alkaline phosphatase	25	11	Colorimetric	96	64	35
	25	13	Colorimetric	32	100	26
Bone-specific alkaline phosphatase	68	72	RIA	99	85	34
Osteocalcin	25	13	RIA	24	92	26
	25	11	RIA	80	100	35
Carboxyterminal propeptide of type I procollagen	25	13	RIA	22	91	26
	10	0	RIA	70	NA	44
Tartrate-resistant acid phosphatase	40	40	Colorimetric	60	60	47
	25	11	Colorimetric	92	27	35
	10	0	Colorimetric	40	NA	44
Hydroxyproline	25	11	Colorimetric	92	27	35
	26	29	HPLC/fluorometry	31	97	36
Pyridinoline/deoxy-pyridinoline	26	29	HPLC/fluorometry	39	97	36
	25	13	ELISA	40	92	26
Carboxyterminal telopeptide of type I procollagen	25	13	RIA	35	100	26

NA, Not available; RIA, radioimmunoassay; ELISA, enzyme-linked immunosorbent assay; HPLC, high-performance liquid chromatography.

however, differences were not obvious between prostate cancer patients with and those without bone metastases.

Carboxyterminal Telopeptide of Type I Collagen. A twofold to threefold increase in ICTP (Crosslaps) was demonstrated in patients with bone metastases in comparison with control subjects.[60]

STUDIES IN PATIENTS WITH MISCELLANEOUS PRIMARY TUMORS

Alkaline Phosphatase. In several studies with patients who had miscellaneous primary tumors (Table 4-4), the radiographic appearance of the metastatic lesion, whether it was osteoblastic or osteolytic, had an effect on the ability of alkaline phosphatase to discriminate between those with and those without secondary bone metastases.[61-63] In general, alkaline phosphatase is not a sensitive marker for lytic bone lesions. A major limitation of this marker is its ability to distinguish between patients with bone metastases and those with liver metastases.

Skeletal Alkaline Phosphatase. In contrast to alkaline phosphatase, skeletal alkaline phosphatase is able to distinguish between patients with bone metastases and those with liver metastases. Berruti et al.[64] reported a positive correlation between skeletal alkaline phosphatase levels and the appearance of skeletal abnormalities on bone scintigraphy.

Osteocalcin. Francini et al.[65] reported on patients with osteoblastic or osteolytic metastases from various primary tumors. Osteocalcin levels were not elevated in patients with osteolytic metastases.

Carboxyterminal Propeptide of Type I Procollagen. In the study cited above, Francini et al.[65] also reported that PICP levels were increased in only a

Table 4-4 Biochemical markers in miscellaneous primary tumors

Marker	+ Metastases	− Metastases	Assay	% Sensitivity	% Specificity	Reference
Alkaline phosphatase	47	0	Colorimetric	66	NA	43
	44	21	Colorimetric	65	57	41
	37	0	Colorimetric	51	NA	44
	44	11	Colorimetric	65	57	39
	98	55	Colorimetric	47	78	40
Bone-specific alkaline phosphatase	7	96	Electrophoresis	33	97	48
	44	11	Electrophoresis	65	90	39
	44	21	Electrophoresis	65	91	41
Osteocalcin	44	11	RIA	55	81	39
	47	0	RIA	38	NA	43
	44	21	RIA	55	81	41
Carboxyterminal propeptide of type I procollagen	47	0	RIA	51	NA	43
	37	0	RIA	46	NA	44
Tartrate-resistant acid phosphatase	37	0	Colorimetric	30	NA	44
Hydroxyproline	47	0	Colorimetric	40	NA	43
Pyridinoline/deoxy-pyridinoline	41	56	HPLC/fluorometry	66/58	57/70	45
	98	55	HPLC/fluorometry	89/77	42/53	40
Carboxyterminal telopeptide of type I procollagen	30	64	ELISA	31	90	46

NA, Not available; RIA, radioimmunoassay; HPLC, high-performance liquid chromatography; ELISA, enzyme-linked immunosorbent assay.

small percentage of patients with osteolytic metastases and elevated in all patients with osteoblastic metastases. In addition, Berruti et al.[64] reported higher PICP levels in patients with osteoblastic-like metastases.

Tartrate-Resistant Acid Phosphatase. Santi et al.[66] demonstrated that in patients with radiographic evidence of bone metastases, no discernible difference could be observed when compared to healthy individuals.

Hydroxyproline. For OH-Pro, Santi et al.[66] demonstrated that in patients with radiographic evidence of bone metastases, no discernible difference from healthy individuals could be observed. Francini et al.[65] reported that only about 50% of

patients with osteolytic metastases had elevated OH-Pro levels, whereas only 25% of patients with osteoblastic metastases had increased levels.

Pyridinoline and Deoxypyridinoline. Pecherstorfer et al.[62] reported a higher sensitivity of Pyd and Dpd for bone metastases than was reported in a study by Lipton et al.[67] Demers et al.[68] demonstrated that Dpd was more discriminatory for bone metastases than Pyd and that both markers were better markers than alkaline phosphatase, skeletal alkaline phosphatase, and ICTP.

Aminoterminal Telopeptide of Type I Collagen. Berruti et al.[64] concluded that ICTP is not a reliable marker for bone metastases because of the variable results in patients without discernible bone metastases. In patients with positive findings for bone metastases, good correlation was observed with ICTP.

CONCLUSION

The markers of bone turnover—in particular, the more specific collagen cross-links—are increased in the majority of patients with metastatic bone disease. However, they still do not provide adequate accuracy to determine the presence or absence of bone metastases in an individual. Markers of bone metabolism reflect the uncoupling between bone resorption and formation, generally caused by bone metastases.

Among the resorption markers, Dpd is considered to be the most correlative with clinical findings of osteolytic bone disease (breast cancer). ICTP and probably INTP are promising markers for early bone involvement. In osteoblastic metastases (prostate cancer), markers of bone formation are most valuable for the detection of bone metastases.

REFERENCES

1. Galasko CSB. Diagnosis of skeletal metastases and assessment of response to treatment. Clin Orthop 312:64-75, 1995.
2. Hoskin PJ. Scientific and clinical aspects of radiotherapy in the relief of bone pain. Cancer Surv 7:69-86, 1998.
3. Bach F, Larsen BH, Rhode K, Borgesen SE, Gjerris F. Metastatic spinal cord compression: Occurrence, symptoms, clinical presentations and prognosis in 398 patients with spinal cord compression. Acta Neurochir (Wien) 107:37-43, 1990.
4. Byrne TN. Spinal cord compression from epidural metastases. N Engl J Med 327:614-619, 1992.
5. O'Connor MI, Currier BL. Metastatic bone disease: Metastatic disease of the spine. Orthopedics 15:611-620, 1992.
6. Rana A, Chisholm GD, Rashwan HM, Salim A, Merrick MV, Elton RA. Symptomatology of metastatic prostate cancer: Prognostic significance. Br J Urol 73:683-686, 1994.
7. Grant R, Papadopoulos SM, Greenberg HS. Metastatic epidural spinal cord compression. Neurol Clin 9:825-841, 1991.
8. Klein SL, Sanford RA, Muhlbauer MS. Pediatric spinal epidural metastases. J Neurosurg 74:70-75, 1991.
9. Perrin R. Metastatic tumors of the axial spine. Curr Opin Oncol 4:525-532, 1992.
10. Zelefsky JM, Scher HI, Krol G, Porteny RK, Leibel SA, Fuks ZY. Spinal epidural tumor in patients with prostate cancer. Cancer 70:2319-2325, 1992.
11. Hill ME, Richards MA, Gregory WM, Smith P, Rubens RD. Spinal cord compression in breast cancer: A review of 70 cases. Br J Cancer 68:969-973, 1993.
12. Leviov M, Dale J, Stein M, Ben-Shahar M, Ben-Arush M, Milstein D, Goldsher D, Kuten A. The management of metastatic spinal cord compression: A radiotherapeutic success ceiling. Int J Radiat Oncol Biol Phys 27:231-234, 1993.
13. Maranzano E, Latini P, Checcaglini F, Ricci S, Panizza BM, Aristei C, Perrucci E. Radiation therapy in metastatic spinal cord compression: A prospective analysis of 105 consecutive patients. Cancer 67:1311-1317, 1991.
14. Weissman DE. Glucocorticoid treatment for brain metastases and epidural spinal cord compression: A review. J Clin Oncol 6:543-551, 1998.
15. Lyons MK, O'Neill BP, Marsh WR, Kurtin PJ. Primary spinal epidural non-Hodgkin's lymphoma: Report of eight patients and review of the literature. Neurosurgery 30:675-680, 1992.
16. Rathmell AJ, Gospodarowicz MK, Sutcliffe SB, Clark RM. Localized epidural lymphoma: Survival relapse pattern and functional outcome. Radiother Oncol 24:14-20, 1992.
17. Front D, Schneck SO, Frankel A, Robinson E. Bone metastases and bone pain in breast cancer: Are they closely associated? JAMA 242:1747-1748, 1979.
18. Galasko CSB. Skeletal metastases and mammary cancer. Ann R Coll Surg Engl 50:3-28, 1972.
19. Galasko CS. The significance of occult skeletal metastases, detected by skeletal scintigraphy, in patients with otherwise apparently "early" mammary carcinoma. Br J Surg 62:694-696, 1975.
20. Galasko CSB, Doyle FH. The detection of skeletal metastases from mammary cancer: A regional comparison between radiology and scintigraphy. Clin Radiol 23:295-297, 1972.
21. Rougraff BT, Kneisl JS, Simon MA. Skeletal metastases of unknown origin: A prospective study of a diagnostic strategy. J Bone Joint Surg Am 75:1276-1281, 1993.
22. Yoneda T, Alsina MA, Chavez JB, Bonewald L, Nishimura R, Mundy GR. Evidence that tumor necrosis factor plays a pathogenetic role in the paraneoplastic syndromes of cachexia, hypercalcemia, and leukocytosis in a human tumor in nude mice. J Clin Invest 87:977-985, 1991.
23. Boyce BF. Normal bone remodelling and its disruption in metastatic bone disease. In Rubens RD, Fogelman I, eds. Bone Metastases: Diagnosis and Treatment. London: Springer-Verlag, 1991.
24. Risteli L, Risteli J. Biochemical markers of bone metabolism. Ann Med 25:385-393, 1993.
25. Price PA. Vitamin K–dependent formation of bone Gla protein (osteocalcin) and its function. Vitam Horm 42:65-108, 1985.
26. Melkko J, Niemi S, Risteli L, Risteli J. Radioimmunoassay of the carboxyterminal propeptide of type I procollagen. Clin Chem 36:1328-1332, 1990.
27. Taubman MB, Goldberg B, Scherr CJ. Radioimmunoassay for human procollagen. Science 186:1115-1117, 1974.
28. Parfitt AM, Simon LS, Villanueva AR, Krane SM. Procollagen type I carboxy-terminal extension peptide in serum as a marker of collagen biosynthesis in bone: Correlation with iliac bone formation rates and comparison with total alkaline phosphatase. J Bone Miner Res 2:427-436, 1987.
29. Simon LS, Krane SMK. Procollagen extension peptides as markers of collagen synthesis. In Frame B, Potts JT Jr, eds.

Clinical Disorders of Bone and Mineral Metabolism. Amsterdam: Excerpta Medica, 1983, pp 108-111.

30. Gasser A, Celada A, Courvoisier B, Depierre D, Hulme PM, Rinsler M, Williams D, Wootton R. The clinical measurement of urinary total hydroxyproline excretion. Clin Chim Acta 95:487-491, 1979.

31. Colwell A, Russell RGG, Eastell R. Factors affecting the assay of urinary 3-hydroxy pyridinium cross-links of collagen as markers of bone resorption. Eur J Clin Invest 23:341-349, 1993.

32. Kraenzlin ME, Lau KH, Liang L, Freeman TK, Singer FR, Stepan J, Baylink DJ. Development of an immunoassay for human serum osteoclastic tartrate-resistant acid phosphatase. J Clin Endocrinol Metab 71:442-451, 1990.

33. Eyre D. Collagen cross-linking amino acids. Methods Enzymol 144:115-139, 1987.

34. Bonde M, Qvist P, Fledelius C, Riis BJ, Christiansen C. Immunoassay for quantifying type I collagen degradation products in urine evaluated. Clin Chem 40:2022-2025, 1994.

35. Hanson DA, Weis MA, Bollen AM, Maslan SL, Singer FR, Eyre DR. A specific immunoassay for monitoring human bone resorption: Quantification of type I collagen crosslinked *N*-telopeptides in urine. J Bone Miner Res 7:1251-1258, 1992.

36. Sharkey RM, Goldenberg DM, Goldenberg H, Lee RE, Ballance C, Pawlyk D, Varga D, Hansen HJ. Murine monoclonal antibodies against carcinoembryonic antigen: Immunological, pharmacokinetic, and targeting properties in humans. Cancer Res 50:2823-2831, 1990.

37. Siccardi AG, Buraggi GL, Callegaro L, Colella AC, De Filippi PG, Galli G, Mariani G, Masi R, Palumbo R, Riva P. Immunoscintigraphy of adenocarcinomas by means of radiolabeled F(ab')₂ fragments of an anti-carcinoembryonic antigen monoclonal antibody: A multicenter study. Cancer Res 49:3095-3103, 1989.

38. Hayes DF, Zurawski VR Jr, Kufe DW. Comparison of circulating CA15-3 and carcinoembryonic antigen levels in patients with breast cancer. J Clin Oncol 4:1542-1550, 1986.

39. Zurawski VR Jr, Knapp RC, Einhorn N, Kenemans P, Mortel R, Ohmi K, Bast RC Jr, Ritts RE Jr, Malkasian G. An initial analysis of preoperative serum CA 125 levels in patients with early stage ovarian carcinoma. Gynecol Oncol 30(1):7-14, 1988.

40. Francini G, Montagnani M, Petrioli R, Paffetti P, Masili S, Leone V. Comparison between CEA, TPA, CA 15/3 and hydroxyproline, alkaline phosphatase, whole body retention of ⁹⁹ᵐTc MDP in the follow-up of bone metastases in breast cancer. Int J Biol Markers 5:65-72, 1990.

41. Suzuki S. Early diagnosis for bone metastasis of breast cancer based on bone metabolism. Fukushima J Med Sci 36(1):11-27, 1990.

42. Oesterling JE. Prostate specific antigen: A critical assessment of the most useful tumor marker for adenocarcinoma of the prostate. J Urol 145:907-923, 1991.

43. Andriole GL. Serum prostate-specific antigen: The most useful tumor marker. J Clin Oncol 10:1205-1207, 1992.

44. Kamby C, Vejbog I, Daugaard S, Guldhammer B, Dirksen H, Rossing N, Mouridesen HT. Clinical and radiologic characteristics of bone metastases in breast cancer. Cancer 60:2524-2531, 1987.

45. Stoll BA. Natural history, prognosis, and staging of bone metastases. In Stoll BA, Parbho S, eds. Bone Metastases Monitoring and Treatment. New York: Raven Press, 1983, pp 1-4.

46. Moro L, Gazzarrini C, Crivellari D, Galligioni E, Talamini R, de Bernard B. Biochemical markers for detecting bone metastases in patients with breast cancer. Clin Chem 39:131-134, 1993.

47. Koizumi M, Yamada Y, Takiguchi T, Nomura E, Furukawa M, Kitahara T, Yamashita T, Maeda H, Takahashi S, Aiba K, Ogata E. Bone metabolic markers in bone metastases. J Cancer Res Clin Oncol 121:542-548, 1995.

48. Nguyen M, Bonneterre J, Hecquet B, Desoize B, Demaille A. Plasma acid and alkaline phosphatase in patients with breast cancer. Anticancer Res 11:831-833, 1991.

49. Reale MF, Santini D, Marchei GG, Manna A, del Nero A, Bianco V, Marchei P, Frati L. Skeletal alkaline phosphatase as a serum marker of bone metastases in the follow-up of patients with breast cancer. Int J Biol Markers 10:42-46, 1995.

50. Berutti A, Torta M, Poivesan A, Raucci CA, Orlandi F, Panero A, Dogliotti L, Angeli A. Biochemical picture of bone metabolism in breast cancer patients with bone metastases. Anticancer Res 15:2871-2875, 1995.

51. Kamby C, Egsmose C, Soletormos G, Dombernowsky P. The diagnostic and prognostic value of serum bone Gla protein (osteocalcin) in patients with recurrent breast cancer. Scand J Clin Lab Invest 53:439-446, 1993.

52. Frenay M, Namer M, Boublil JL, Khater R, Viot M, Francois E, Milano G. Value of urinary hydroxyproline and bone isoenzyme of alkaline phosphatase in the early detection and follow-up of bone metastasis in breast cancer patients. Bull Cancer 75:533-539, 1988.

53. Moro L, Gazzarrini C, Modricky C, Rovis L, de Bernard B, Galligioni E, Criverllari D, Morassut S, Monfardini S. High predictivity of galactosyl-hydroxylysine in urine as an indicator of bone metastases from breast cancer. Clin Chem 36:772-774, 1990.

54. Checovich MM, Heiner JP, Heisey D, Kinsella T, Stewart J. Urinary pyridinoline and deoxypyridinoline in breast cancer patients with and without bone metastases. Trans Orthop Res Soc 43:553, 1997.

55. Van Hoof VO, van Oosterom AT, Leoutre LG, de Broe ME. Alkaline phosphatase isoenzyme patterns in malignant disease. Clin Chem 38:2546-2551, 1992.

56. Morote J, Lorente JA, Encabo G. Prostate carcinoma staging: Clinical utility of bone alkaline phosphatase in addition to prostate specific antigen. Cancer 78:2374-2378, 1996.

57. Francini G, Bigazzi S, Leone V, Gennari C. Serum osteocalcin concentration in patients with prostatic cancer. Am J Clin Oncol 11:83-87, 1988.

58. Miyamoto KK, McSherry SA, Robins SP, Besterman JM, Mohler JL. Collagen crosslink metabolites in urine as markers of bone metastases in prostatic carcinoma. J Urol 151:909-913, 1994.

59. Yoshida K, Hosoya U, Aria K, Sumi S, Honda M. Serum concentration of the pyridinoline crosslinked carboxyterminal

telopeptide of type I collagen and urinary concentration of deoxypyridinoline as markers of bone metastases in human prostate carcinoma. Clin Chim Acta 254:93-95, 1996.

60. Vinholes J, Guo CY, Purohit OP, Eastell R, Coleman RE. Evaluation of new bone resorption markers in a randomized comparison of pamidronate or clodronate for hypercalcemia of malignancy. J Clin Oncol 15(1):131-138, 1997.

61. Burlina A, Rubine D, Secchiero S, Sciacovelli L, Zaninotto M, Plebani M. Monitoring skeletal cancer metastases with the bone isoenzyme of tissue unspecific alkaline phosphatase. Clin Chim Acta 226:151-158, 1994.

62. Pecherstorfer M, Zimmer-Roth I, Schilling T, Woitge HW, Schmidt H, Baumgartner G, Thiebaud D, Ludwig H, Seibel MJ. The diagnostic value of urinary pyridinium cross-links of collagen, serum total alkaline phosphatase, and urinary calcium excretion in neoplastic bone disease. J Clin Endocrinol Metab 80:97-103, 1995.

63. Zaninotto M, Secchiero S, Rubin D, Sciacovelli L, Trovo M, Bortolus R, Plebani M. Serum bone alkaline phosphatase in the follow-up of skeletal metastases. Anticancer Res 15:2223-2228, 1995.

64. Berruti A, Piovesan A, Torta M, Raucci CA, Gorzegno G, Paccotti P, Dogliotti L, Angeli A. Biochemical evaluation of bone turnover in cancer patients with bone metastases: Relationship with radiograph appearances and disease extension. Br J Cancer 73:1581-1587, 1996.

65. Francini G, Gonnelli S, Petrioli R, Bruni S, Marsili S, Aquino A, Camporeale A. Procollagen type I carboxy-terminal propeptide as a marker of osteoblastic bone metastases. Cancer Epidemiol Biomarkers Prev 2:125-129, 1993.

66. Santi I, Monti M, Vaigano A, D'Aprile E, Rampoldi E, Castellani L, Accinni R, Cunietti E. Serum levels of procollagen type I carboxyterminal extension peptide in cancer patients with bone metastases. Int J Biol Markers 10:107-112, 1995.

67. Lipton A, Demers L, Daniloff Y, Curley E, Hamilton C, Harvey H, Witters L, Seaman J, van der Giessen R, Seyedin S. Increased urinary excretion of pyridinium crosslinks in cancer patients. Clin Chem 39:614-618, 1993.

68. Demers LM, Costa L, Chichilli VM, Gaydos L, Curley E, Lipton A. Biochemical markers of bone turnover in patients with metastatic bone disease. Clin Chem 41:1489-1494, 1995.

Radiologic Evaluation

Michael J. Tuite, M.D.

Despite the increasing use of newer imaging modalities such as magnetic resonance imaging (MRI), radiographs still play an important role in patients with suspected or known metastatic disease. Radiographs are easily available and relatively inexpensive but provide valuable information either about the status of the bones in cancer patients with focal skeletal complaints or about an abnormality on radionuclide bone scan or MRI scan. Radiographs can usually distinguish metastases from benign lesions or degenerative disease; more expensive imaging modalities, however, are often less informative.

The goal of this chapter is to present the variety of radiographic appearances of metastases and to discuss the role of radiography in the management of patients with musculoskeletal metastases.

COMMON SITES OF MUSCULOSKELETAL METASTASES

When one is considering whether a lesion on an x-ray film could be a metastasis, it is helpful to know a few facts about the usual behavior of metastases. Within the musculoskeletal system, metastases tend to deposit at sites that meet three criteria.[1] First, most tumors metastasize through the vascular system and therefore tend to deposit in areas with good blood flow. The increased blood flow to hematopoietic marrow relative to fatty marrow is one of the reasons that metastases are more common in the proximal than in the distal femur. Second, the local tissue environment must be able to sustain and nurture the growth of deposited tumor cells. Hematopoietic marrow, which provides an excellent substrate for tumor growth, is a more common site for metastases than is skeletal muscle, even though both have a comparably rich blood supply. Finally, there should be sluggish blood flow through a rich capillary network to allow tumor cells time to gain a foothold, a situation that is optimally present in thoracolumbar vertebral bodies.

The most common route of tumor metastasis to the musculoskeletal system is via the venous circulation.[2] The thin walls of veins are more vulnerable to tumor invasion than are arteries, which is the reason that many malignancies also metastasize to the lungs. In the case of metastases to the musculoskeletal system, two of the most common sites are the thoracolumbar spine and the posterior ribs, both of which not only have hematopoietic marrow but, depending on intra-abdominal pressure, can receive blood flow via Batson's venous plexus.[3] Prostate carcinoma is one of several tumors that often metastasize to the spine and ribs by shedding cells into veins that drain into Batson's plexus.

Metastases via the systemic arterial system are uncommon but, when seen, are usually from lung

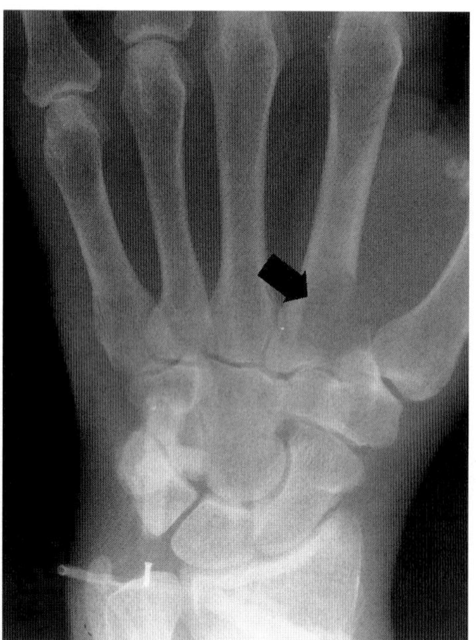

Fig. 5-1 Posteroanterior view of the hand in a 59-year-old man with lung carcinoma. There is a lytic metastasis *(arrow)* at the base of the second metacarpal bone with cortical destruction.

carcinomas.[2] Tumors in the lung can invade through the thin-walled pulmonary veins and thus shed tumor emboli into the peripheral skeleton, including the hands and feet (Fig. 5-1).

There are other routes that tumors can take to metastasize to bones. Skeletal metastases via the lymphatic vessels are typically from osseous invasion by a tumor-involved lymph node. This is most common in the mediastinum but also occurs in the lumbosacral spine, particularly on the left, where the lymph nodes are located close to the spine.[2] Although not what we usually consider a metastasis, direct tumor invasion into an adjacent bone is another skeletal manifestation of nonlocalized malignancy. This is particularly common for malignancies in the mediastinum or retroperitoneum (Fig. 5-2). Finally, some "drop metastases" within the central nervous system, which deposit adjacent to the dura, can enlarge and invade into an adjacent vertebra.

With this background, it is not surprising that the most common sites of skeletal metastases are, in decreasing order of frequency, the thoracolumbar spine and sacrum, proximal femur, pelvis, ribs, sternum, proximal humerus, and skull.[2-4] When one is evaluating a patient for metastases, these are the sites that should be looked at most carefully and are the bones typically included in a radiologic skeletal survey.

Appendicular Skeleton

Most metastases to the appendicular skeleton deposit within the medullary portion of the pelvis or the proximal diaphysis of the femur or humerus. When small, these metastases are difficult to see radiographically because they tend to infiltrate between the bone trabeculae. Even as the metastasis enlarges and begins to destroy trabeculae, studies have shown that 30% to 50% of the cancellous bone has to be destroyed before appearing as a lytic lesion on plain film.[5] Medullary bone metastases are usually visible on nuclear medicine bone scan or MRI scan before they can be seen on radiographs (Fig. 5-3).

Metastases to cortical bone do occur but are less common than metastases to cancellous bone.[6] Cortical bone lacks the fertile substrate of hematopoietic marrow and the rich capillary network and anastomosing veins that are present in the medullary cavity. Because the blood supply is mainly arterial, cortical metastases are most often from lung malignancies, where tumor cells can enter the arterial system via the pulmonary veins. Cortical metastases, when they do occur, are easier to identify on radiographs than are medullary lesions because of the superior contrast between the dense bone and the lesion. The risk of pathologic fracture is greater, however, for cortical metastases. Subperiosteal metastases are also usually from lung carci-

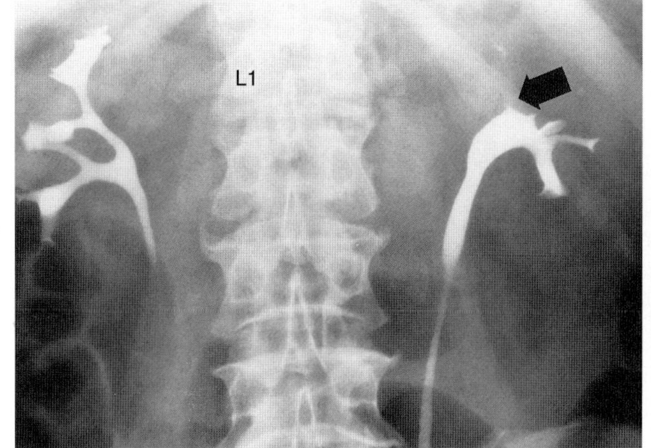
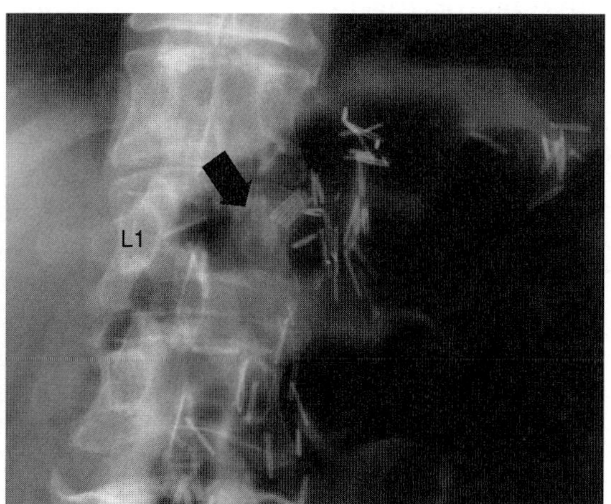

Fig. 5-2   A, Anteroposterior view of the abdomen during bilateral retrograde urethrography demonstrates amputation of the left upper pole renal calix *(arrow)* by a transitional cell carcinoma. **B,** One year later, after resection, anteroposterior view of the thoracolumbar junction shows destruction of the left L1 pedicle *(arrow)* by recurrent tumor.

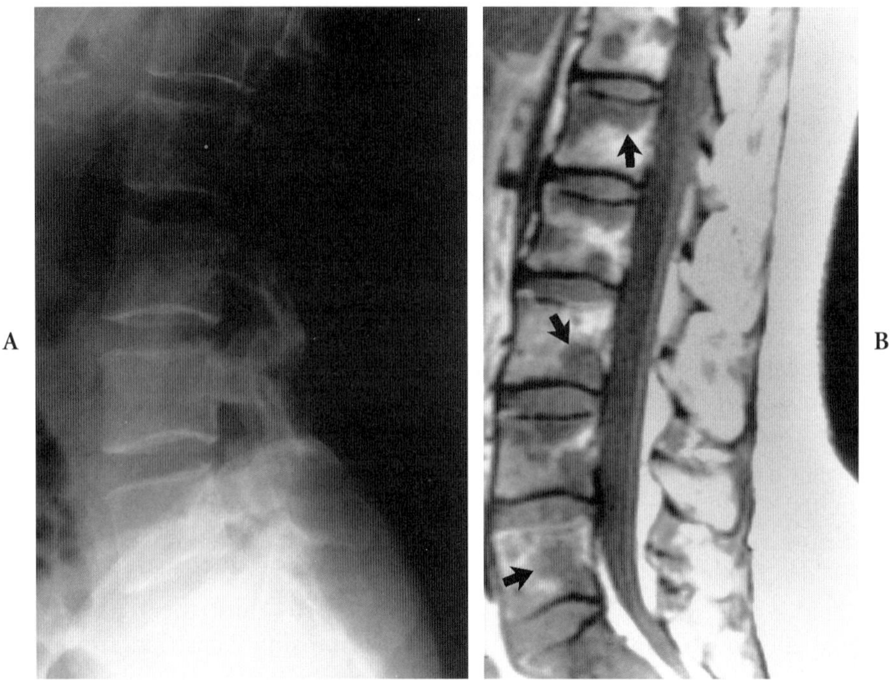

Fig. 5-3   Lateral radiograph (**A**) and sagittal T1-weighted MRI image (**B**) of the lumbar spine in a 37-year-old woman with breast carcinoma. Note that the multiple vertebral-body metastases *(arrows)* are seen much better on the MRI than on the x-ray film.

nomas and result in a "cookie bite" lesion of the external cortex on radiographs (Fig. 5-4).[2]

Metastases are also more common in areas that have additional reasons for increased blood flow.[2,7] These areas include sites of healing fractures, internal fixation, or Paget's disease (Fig. 5-5), all of which should be carefully evaluated in patients with suspected metastatic disease.

Axial Skeleton

Because the axial skeleton contains hematopoietic marrow, metastases are common to all the bones of the axial skeleton, including the ribs, skull, and sternum. The most common location of metastases to the axial skeleton, however, is within the medullary portion of the thoracolumbar vertebral bodies.[2] Most of the hematopoietic marrow in older individuals is located here. The main vessels that anastomose with Batson's plexus are the basivertebral vein and the anterior venous channels of the vertebral bodies.

Although the radiology literature often emphasizes the importance of evaluating the pedicles for

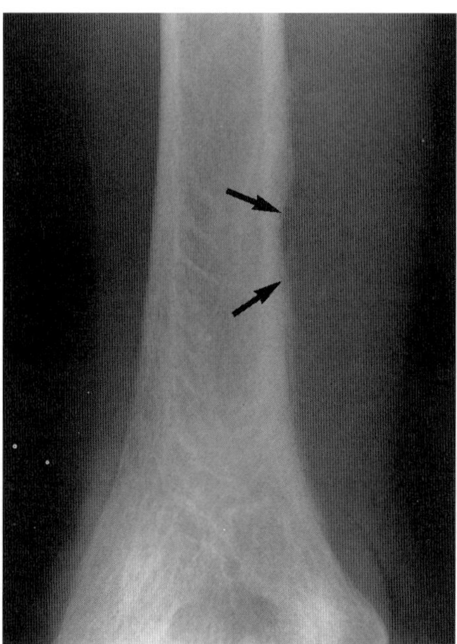

Fig. 5-4   Anteroposterior view of the humerus in a 62-year-old man with lung carcinoma and a subperiosteal metastasis causing a "cookie bite" lesion *(arrows)*.

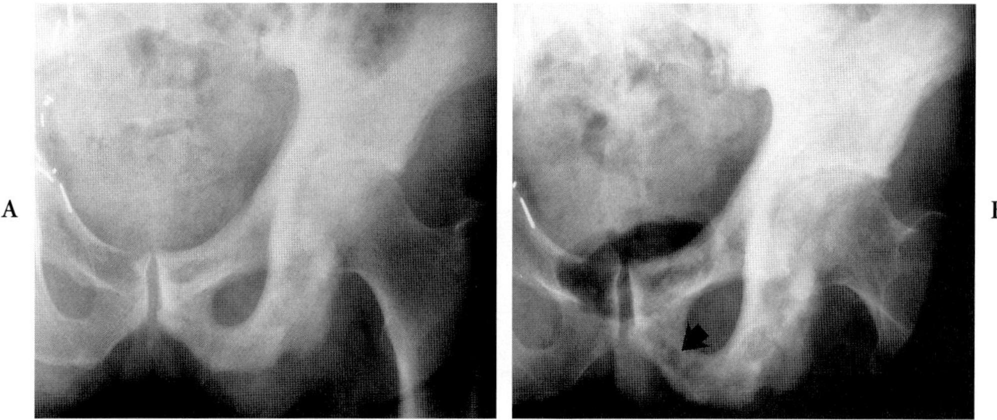

Fig. 5-5 **A,** Anteroposterior view of the pelvis in a 77-year-old man with Paget's disease of the left innominate bone and with prostate carcinoma. **B,** Three years later, there is a superimposed lytic metastasis *(arrow)* in the left inferior pubic ramus.

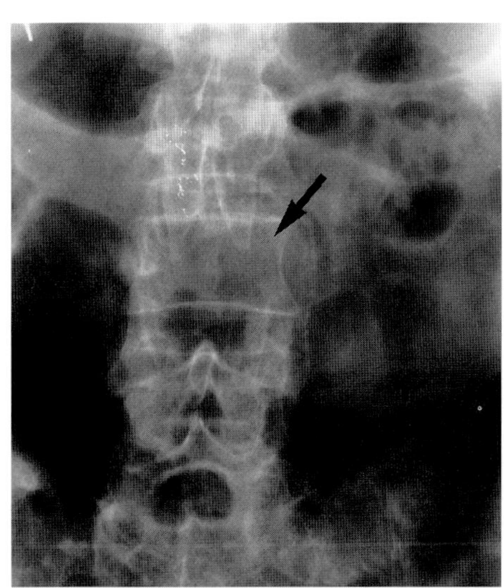

Fig. 5-6 View of diffuse lung carcinoma metastases to the lumbar spine in a 74-year-old man. Anteroposterior radiograph demonstrates only destruction of the left L3 pedicle *(arrow).*

metastatic disease, metastases occur to the vertebral bodies more often than to the posterior elements.[2] What is true is that lytic lesions of the pedicle are rare in multiple myeloma and therefore, when seen, are much more likely to represent metastatic disease. In addition, it is not uncommon to identify metastatic involvement of a pedicle on an x-ray film before the larger, more extensive disease in the vertebral body is seen (Fig. 5-6).

Soft Tissue

Although metastases to parts of the musculoskeletal system other than the bones are uncommon, they occasionally do occur to muscle or other soft tissue. With the superior soft tissue detail of computed tomography (CT) and MRI, the role of radiography in imaging these lesions is limited. Radiography may be useful in some tumors, such as adenocarcinomas of the gastrointestinal tract, which calcify and therefore are visible on radiographs (Fig. 5-7). Knowing that a region of tumor is calcified is helpful if an MRI scan is obtained for presurgical or radiation planning, because the MRI appearance of calcification can be confusing. The differential diagnosis of a calcified soft tissue mass in an extremity of a patient with a suspected metastasis also includes chondrosarcoma, osteosarcoma, and myositis ossificans.

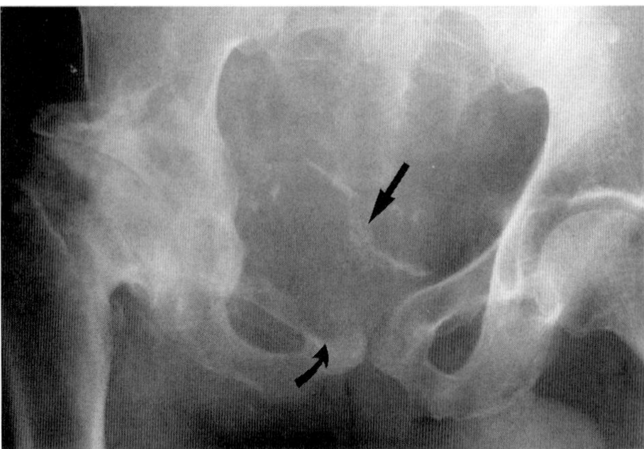

Fig. 5-7 Anteroposterior view of the pelvis in a 58-year-old man with mucinous adenocarcinoma. Note the tumor calcification *(straight arrow)* and right superior pubic ramus bone destruction *(curved arrow)*. Patient also has developmental dysplasia of the right hip.

Radiography also may be useful in patients with soft tissue metastases to determine whether there is extrinsic erosion or invasion of the adjacent bone. Bronchogenic carcinoma, which can metastasize to muscle via the arteries, is the most common malignancy to cause extrinsic bone cortical invasion.[8]

RADIOGRAPHIC EVALUATION

Most radiographs of patients with suspected metastatic disease are for evaluation of an abnormality identified on a screening bone scan. Because of the low specificity of bone scintigraphy, radiography is required of any abnormality that is detected. Osteoarthritis and degenerative disc disease are common in older patients and often have a similar appearance to metastases on bone scan. Fractures, bone infarcts, Paget's disease, and benign tumors also can be confused with metastases on scintigraphy but are distinguishable on radiographs (Fig. 5-8).

New bone or joint pain in patients with cancer should also be first evaluated with radiographs. Radiographs are less expensive than a bone scan, and many benign conditions, such as osteoarthritis and degenerative disc disease, are readily diagnosed on the basis of plain films. If a metastasis is identified, radiographs provide valuable information on the integrity of the underlying bone and often obviate the need for additional expensive imaging tests.

Table 5-1 Skeletal survey for metastases: Radiographic views

Location	View
Skull	Lateral
Cervical spine	Lateral
Thoracic spine	Anteroposterior and lateral
Lumbar spine	Anteroposterior and lateral
Pelvis	Anteroposterior
Femurs	Anteroposterior
Humeri	Anteroposterior

Chest x-ray film to evaluate ribs and sternum.

Skeletal Survey

Most authors recommend a nuclear medicine bone scan in patients with newly diagnosed malignancies that have a predilection for metastasizing to the skeleton.[9,10] Compared with a skeletal survey, a bone scan is 40% to 70% more sensitive for detecting metastatic lesions, especially those with the typical intramedullary location.[3] Skeletal surveys are also limited to only the visualized bones and involve a higher radiation dose to the patient. Recent articles have reported that whole-body MRI scanning with fast spin-echo inversion recovery may be a more sensitive and specific alternative than bone scanning.[11]

Traditionally the skeletal survey has been used mainly in patients with multiple myeloma, in which the bone scan finding is falsely negative in up to 50% of lesions.[12] A skeletal survey is also sometimes performed in patients with highly anaplastic tumors, such as neuroblastoma, renal cell carcinoma, and thyroid carcinoma, in which no abnormality is shown on the bone scan.[13] Although at least some of a patient's metastatic lesions are usually seen on a bone scan, 5% of radiographically evident metastases are not visualized with scintigraphy, either because of insufficient osteoblastic activity or obscuration by bladder activity.[7] Metastases may also be difficult to identify on bone scan if they are diffuse and extensive (Fig. 5-9).

If a skeletal survey is performed, radiographs of the bones should be obtained where skeletal metastases occur most commonly. These sites include the

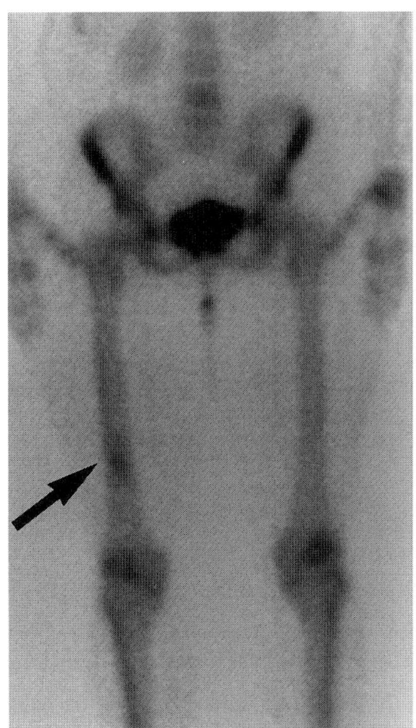 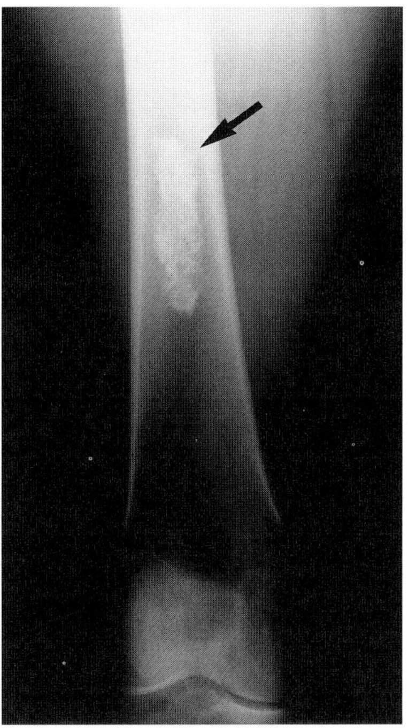

A **B**

Fig. 5-8 **A,** Bone scan of a 56-year-old woman with newly diagnosed breast carcinoma shows an abnormality in the mid right femur *(arrow).* **B,** Anteroposterior radiograph of the right femur demonstrates the well-defined matrix calcification of a benign enchondroma or bone infarct *(arrow).*

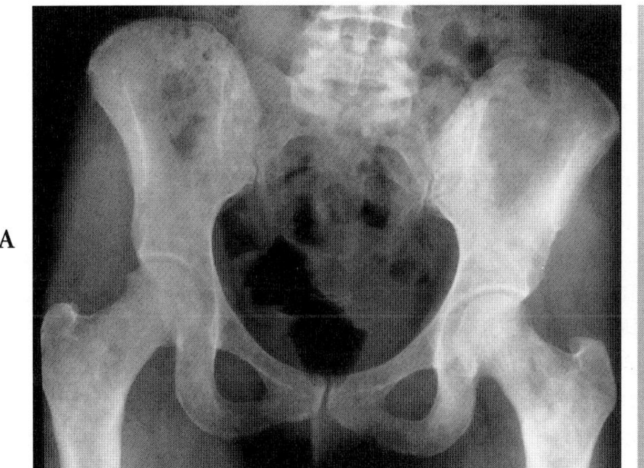

A

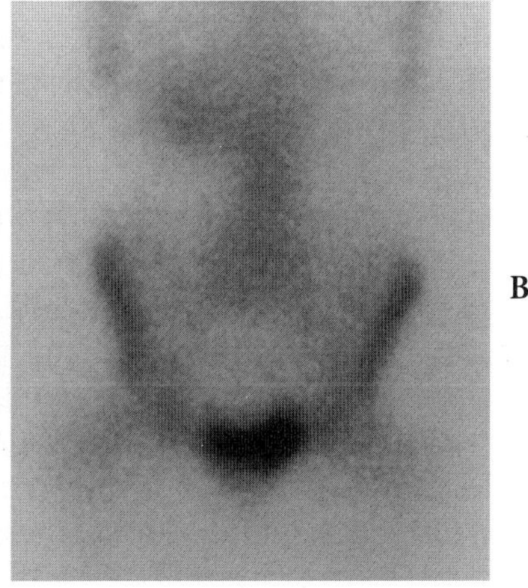

B

Fig. 5-9 **A,** Anteroposterior radiograph of a 47-year-old woman with extensive metastases to the skeleton from breast carcinoma. Multiple areas of sclerosis and lucency are seen throughout the pelvis and femurs from diffuse, mixed-density metastases. **B,** Bone scan with normal findings.

axial skeleton, the pelvis, and the proximal long bones. Radiographic views for a skeletal survey are listed in Table 5-1.

For patients with treated malignancies, the role of a skeletal survey is also limited. If a patient's original metastases were seen on plain film and not on scintigraphy, it is usually preferable to follow up with a skeletal survey. In addition, metastases in patients undergoing treatment often appear worse on bone scan for several months because of increased radiopharmaceutical uptake at sites of healing metastases, known as the "flare phenomenon."[13] Radiographs are often more accurate for distinguishing healing from recurrence during this period.

Detection of Metastases

Because metastases can be difficult to see on plain films, it is important that certain radiographic technical factors be optimal. For conventional film-screen cassettes, fine- or medium-screen extremity film provides higher spatial resolution than fast-speed film. For computed or digital radiography, contrast can be improved with later processing, and lesions often can be made more conspicuous despite lower spatial resolution.

The choice of x-ray beam voltage is also important in the radiography of skeletal metastases. A peak voltage of 50 to 60 kV should be selected for optimal contrast between normal bone and skeletal metastases. The electrical current required to expose film adequately at these peak kilovoltage settings is easily obtained in a dedicated radiography room but may be unavailable for a portable x-ray machine. Metastases that are small or located within the medullary bone are often missed on portable radiographs.

Although plain-film tomography was often used in the past to assess skeletal metastases, it has largely been replaced by CT. Both techniques demonstrate well the amount of cortical destruction, which is useful in diagnosing an impending pathologic fracture, but CT provides superior transaxial images. There are currently very few indications for plain film tomograms of skeletal metastases.

It is difficult to give a precise value for the sensitivity of radiographs for detecting skeletal metastases. The ability to see a metastasis depends on a number of factors, such as its location and size, whether the lesion is osteoblastic or osteolytic, and the quality of the radiograph. Most authors estimate that a skeletal survey has a false-negative rate of about 50% for metastases.[13]

When one is considering whether a lesion on a radiograph may represent a metastasis, it is helpful to know whether a patient's primary malignancy tends to metastasize to the musculoskeletal system. Although any tumor can result in skeletal metastases, the malignancies that do so most frequently are, in decreasing order of frequency, prostate, breast, kidney, lung, thyroid, and bladder.[2-4] The first four of these primary malignancies account for more than 75% of bone metastases in adults.[14] Based on the incidence of the primary malignancy, carcinomas of the breast, lung, and uterus are common tumors causing skeletal metastases in women, and carcinomas of the prostate, lung, and bladder commonly cause metastases in men.[14]

Patients with skeletal metastases typically have multiple lesions at presentation, although 10% of metastases are first seen as a solitary lesion on x-ray film.[3] Because metastases can be difficult to see on radiographs, however, only a single lesion may be seen on a skeletal survey in patients with multiple metastases demonstrated on bone scan or MRI.

If a solitary lesion is seen on bone scan in a patient with a known malignancy, the lesion will be benign in one third of cases.[12] Solitary bone scan abnormalities are more likely to be due to a metastasis if they are located in the thoracolumbar spine, where 80% are malignant, than in the ribs, where only 17% are due to metastatic disease. Radiographic correlation can be difficult because only 35% of the solitary lesions found on bone scan to be metastases could be seen on x-ray films.

DIAGNOSTIC RADIOGRAPHY

Skeletal metastases are often categorized radiographically by their density. The three main categories are osteoblastic, osteolytic, and a mixed appearance of osteolysis with areas of sclerosis (Table 5-2).

Osteoblastic Metastases

Osteoblastic metastases are most commonly seen in men with metastatic prostate carcinoma. The bone formation in osteoblastic metastasis is a result of two processes.[1] First, metastases stimulate osteoblasts to form woven bone, similar to that seen adjacent to fractures and osteomyelitis. The woven bone is eventually remodeled to lamellar bone, although remodeling may not have a chance to occur in a rapidly enlarging metastasis. Second, metastases that are osteoblastic almost always produce a fibrous stroma, which then undergoes intramembranous ossification (Fig. 5-10). Prostate carcinoma metastases are the classic tumors that synthesize significant amounts of fibrous stroma, but some breast carcinoma metastases also produce abundant stroma.

Osteolytic Metastases

Purely osteolytic metastases occur either when there is extremely rapid growth that does not allow time for the host bone to respond or in very cellular tumors.[5] As in mixed-density metastases, tumor-secreted lytic enzymes and osteoclast stimulation also contribute to this appearance. Purely osteolytic metastases can have permeative margins, as in aggressive melanoma lesions, or can be well defined, as commonly seen in renal cell carcinoma (Fig. 5-11).[2]

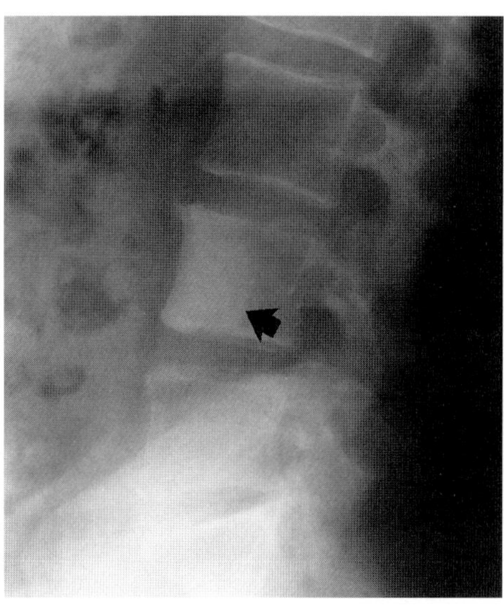

Fig. 5-10 Radiograph of a 52-year-old man with cholangiocarcinoma and an osteoblastic metastasis to the L4 vertebral body *(arrow).*

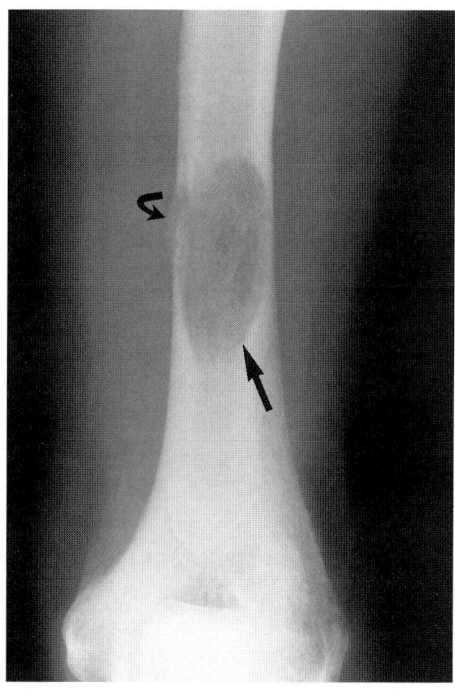

Fig. 5-11 Radiograph of a 54-year-old man with renal cell carcinoma. Note the well-defined margins of this osteolytic metastasis *(straight arrow)* in the humerus, as well as the periostitis *(curved arrow)* from a healing pathologic fracture.

Table 5-2 Radiographic appearance of metastases

Osteoblastic*	Purely osteolytic	Mixed (mainly lytic)
Breast	Kidneys	Lung
Bronchial carcinoid	Thyroid gland	Breast
Bowel (stomach)	Adrenal glands	Cervix
Bladder (with prostate invasion)	Gastrointestinal tract	Ovary
Brain (medulloblastoma)	Melanoma	Testicles
Bone (osteosarcoma)	Head and neck	Neuroblastoma
Lymphoma	Chordoma	Chondrosarcoma
Prostate	Mesothelioma	
	Fibrosarcoma	
	Malignant fibrous histiocytoma	
	Ewing's sarcoma	
	Hepatoma	
	Pheochromocytoma	

*Mnemonic: Six "bees" lick pollen.

Mixed Metastases

One of the most common radiographic appearances of metastases, particularly for breast carcinoma in women, is the mixed or mainly osteolytic lesion. These lesions typically have an ill-defined region of bone lucency with varying amounts of adjacent sclerosis (Fig. 5-12). Osteolysis results mainly from tumor-secreted lytic enzymes and the stimulation of osteoclasts, and the enlarging tumor also causes osteoblasts to produce reactive new bone.[2] The margins of the metastases often have a permeative appearance: a wide zone of transition from abnormal to normal bone. There is usually little or no periostitis and no soft tissue mass, both of which are useful features distinguishing metastases from primary bone malignancies.[3,6] If a periosteal reaction is seen, it often indicates an accompanying pathologic fracture.

Although Table 5-2 lists metastases by their usual radiographic appearance, many malignancies have a variable appearance even within the same patient.[2] For example, some breast metastases are purely osteolytic, whereas others are densely osteoblastic. Prostate metastases can also be predominantly osteolytic, particularly in the cervical spine and in elderly men.[2]

In patients with an unknown primary malignancy and a radiographic lesion that is a suspected metastasis, some x-ray features are more common in certain tumors. For example, a lytic lesion of the skull with a central region of sclerosis, a "button sequestrum," is suggestive of a breast carcinoma me-

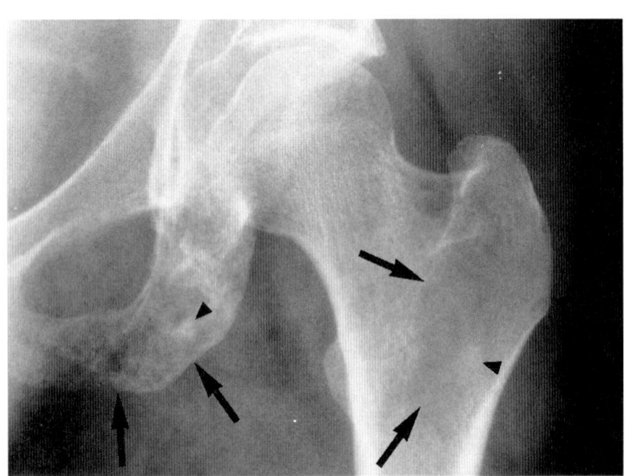

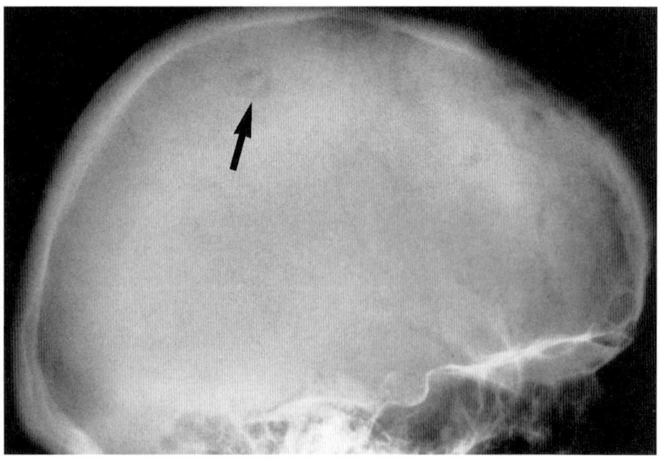

Fig. 5-12 Radiograph of a 37-year-old woman with breast carcinoma metastases to the left ischium and proximal femur (same patient as in Fig. 5-3). Metastases are mixed osteolytic lesions *(arrows)* with areas of sclerosis *(arrowheads)*.

Fig. 5-13 Radiograph of a 50-year-old woman with breast carcinoma metastases to the skull, including one with a "button sequestrum" appearance *(arrow)*.

tastasis (Fig. 5-13).[15] Other distinctive appearances of metastases are included in Table 5-3.

Differential Diagnosis

There are several other conditions to consider when a suspected metastasis is identified on radiographs. In older individuals the most common lesion that is similar in appearance is multiple myeloma. Useful distinguishing characteristics of multiple myeloma are its well-defined rather than permeative margins, endosteal scalloping, and lesion size uniformity.[2] Multiple myeloma also may involve the mandible, shoulder, and elbow, especially the olecranon process, all of which are unusual for metastases. As previously mentioned, both metastases and multiple myeloma occur in vertebral bodies, but metastases are much more likely to involve the pedicle.

Within the spine, another common differential is between a metastatic pathologic fracture and an osteoporotic compression fracture. Metastases are more likely to show trabecular or posterior cortical

---

Table 5-3 Distinctive radiographic appearances

Feature	Malignancy
General	
Common osteoblastic	Male: prostate; female: breast
Common osteolytic, adult	Male: lung; female: breast
Common osteolytic, child	Neuroblastoma
Location	
Foot	Lung, colon, and kidney
Hand	Lung
T12 vertebra	Lung
L2 vertebra	Breast, prostate
Lytic in cervical spine	Also prostate
Sclerotic in thoracolumbar spine	Also pancreatic carcinoma
Characteristic	
Lytic, expansile	Kidney, thyroid (vs. multiple myeloma)
Soap-bubble lytic	Kidney
Blastic, expansile	Prostate
Solitary	Lung, kidney, thyroid
Cortical	Bronchogenic carcinoma
"Cookie bite" subperiosteal	Bronchogenic carcinoma
Metaphyseal lucent band, child	Neuroblastoma (vs. leukemia)
Cross joints, small calcifications	Thyroid
Ivory vertebral body	Prostate (vs. lymphoma, Paget's disease)
Skull, button sequestrum	Breast (vs. eosinophilic granulomatosis, osteomyelitis)
Soft tissue	
Pelvic metastasis with soft tissue mass	Colon
Sunburst periostitis	Prostate, gastrointestinal tract, retinoblastoma, neuroblastoma
Muscle ossification	Stomach carcinoma

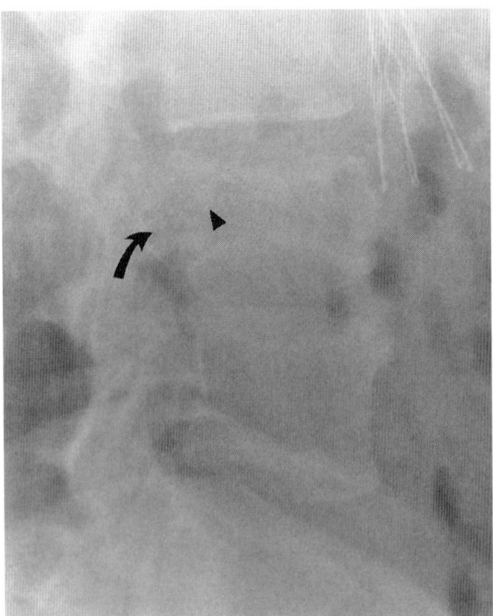

Fig. 5-14 Lateral radiograph of the lumbar spine in a 55-year-old man with a poorly differentiated carcinoma of unknown primary origin and pain after minimal trauma. There is a pathologic compression fracture of L3 with posterior vertebral body cortical destruction *(arrow)* and ill-defined patchy areas of sclerosis *(arrowhead)*. There is also a filter in the inferior vena cava.

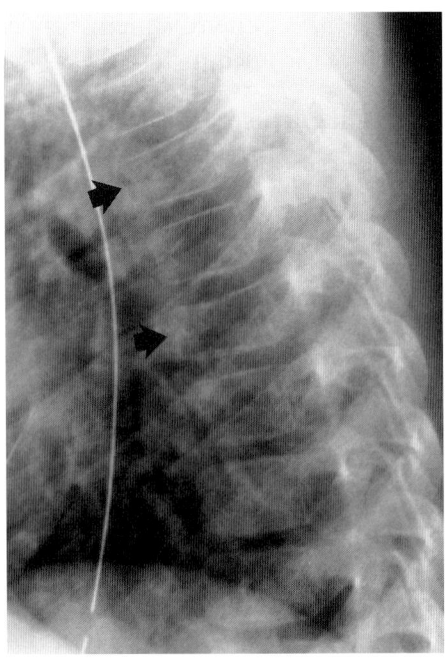

Fig. 5-15 Lateral view of the thoracic spine in a 3-year-old child with neuroblastoma and back pain. Two mildly wedged pathologic vertebral body compression fractures are seen *(arrows)*.

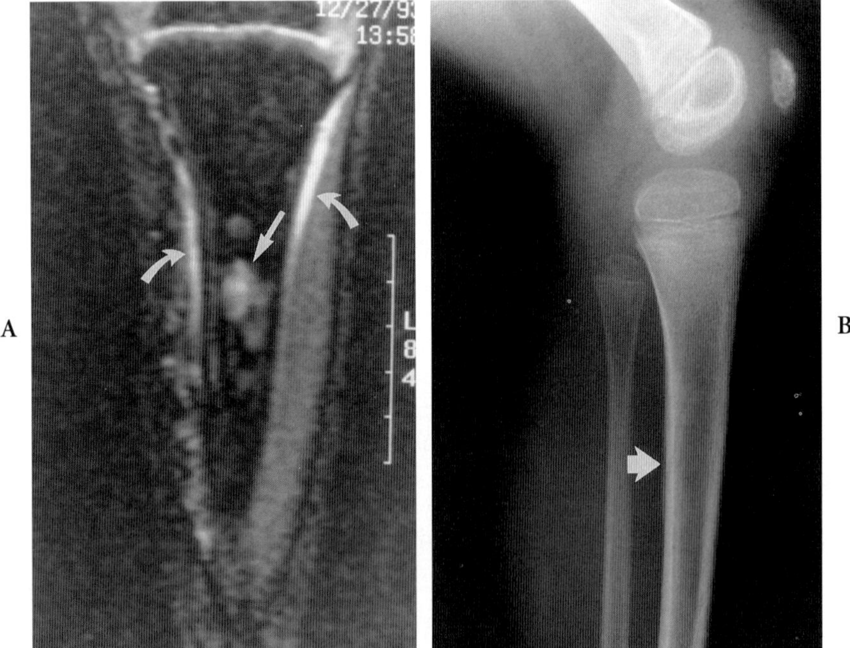

Fig. 5-16 A 7-year-old boy with neuroblastoma treated with whole-body radiation and a bone marrow transplant now has leg pain after resuming activity. **A,** Coronal T2-weighted MRI image of the tibia shows high signal within the medullary canal *(straight arrow)* and adjacent to the cortex *(curved arrows)* from periostitis. **B,** Lateral radiograph 2 weeks later shows an uninterrupted single layer of periostitis *(arrow)*, consistent with a stress fracture.

destruction, significant compression, and a focal paravertebral soft tissue mass (Fig. 5-14).[16] Metastases also may involve noncontiguous vertebral bodies, whereas osteoporotic fractures commonly appear as several contiguous vertebrae with mild anterior wedging.[2] In addition, osteoporotic fractures rarely occur within the upper thoracic spine. Despite these differences in imaging features, MRI, CT, or even biopsy is sometimes required to distinguish between these two entities.

Osteomyelitis is also occasionally considered in evaluations for suspected metastases. Osteomyelitis usually has a greater periosteal reaction and more soft tissue edema than metastases and will often extend into and destroy the disc or joint space. Joint cartilage and disc are usually preserved until late in metastatic disease.[7]

Pediatric Metastases

In children the tumor that most commonly metastasizes to the skeleton is neuroblastoma.[17] These metastases are usually osteolytic and are often multiple and bilateral. A pathologic compression fracture of a vertebral body with cord compression is also common (Fig. 5-15). Other malignancies in children that commonly metastasize include medulloblastoma, which is more likely to metastasize in children than in adults and is occasionally osteoblastic; retinoblastoma; and a type of Wilms' tumor that has been called "bone-metastasizing renal tumor of childhood."[2] With current therapeutic regimens, patients with Ewing's tumor and osteosarcoma are living longer and also may have metastases at presentation of a recurrence. Ewing's metastases are usually osteolytic, whereas those of osteosarcoma are osteoblastic.

Radiographs can be helpful in identifying some additional features of metastases in children. One example is a metastasis adjacent to a physis, which may be difficult to identify on bone scintigraphy because of the normal increased activity at the physis. Another characteristic of metastases in children is that children are more likely than adults to have periostitis and a soft tissue mass. Finally, some children who receive whole-body radiation, followed by a bone marrow transplant for metastases, develop leg pain and undergo MRI. Abnormal regions within the femur or tibia suspected as metastases are often identified on the MRI images but

actually represent stress fractures. Radiographs of these areas are helpful because stress fractures have a distinctive appearance on x-ray film, which can obviate the need for a bone biopsy (Fig. 5-16).[18]

IDENTIFYING COMPLICATIONS

There are multiple complications from skeletal metastases that can be seen on radiographs, including such metabolic abnormalities as hypercalcemia and oncogenic osteomalacia.[2] Radiography is most useful for pathologic fractures, however, in making the diagnosis and in identifying impending fractures.

For the appendicular skeleton, the risk that a metastasis will progress to a pathologic fracture depends on several factors, although this topic is somewhat controversial. The most commonly cited risk factors in the radiology literature are (1) destruction of 50% or more of the cortex and (2) a painful femoral metastasis that measures at least 2.5 cm in diameter, even if confined to the medullary portion of the femur (Fig. 5-17).[2,19] Accurately deciding whether a metastasis satisfies these criteria on radiographs can be difficult, however. CT is preferable for determining the degree of cortical destruction, and MRI may be required to measure accurately the size of a femoral metastasis with ill-defined margins.

Mirels[20] has pointed out, however, that the studies evaluating these two risk factors involved relatively few patients. He proposed a more objective scoring system to determine the likelihood of having a pathologic fracture based on the grading of four factors: (1) site (upper vs. lower limb), (2) pain, (3) radiographic appearance (lytic vs. blastic), and (4) size (relative to the width of the bone, not cortical destruction).[20] Although his scoring system reasonably separates out those patients at higher risk of having a pathologic fracture, equal emphasis is given to the site and to the size of the metastasis, even though his own data show that size is a much more important risk factor.[20]

Radiography is also useful in determining whether a metastasis is the cause of an extremity fracture after minimal trauma. In many older patients with osteoporosis, radiographs can reveal a focal lesion of bone that is easily distinguished from a benign insufficiency fracture. The fracture pattern is often helpful for this purpose, because transverse and isolated lesser trochanteric fractures

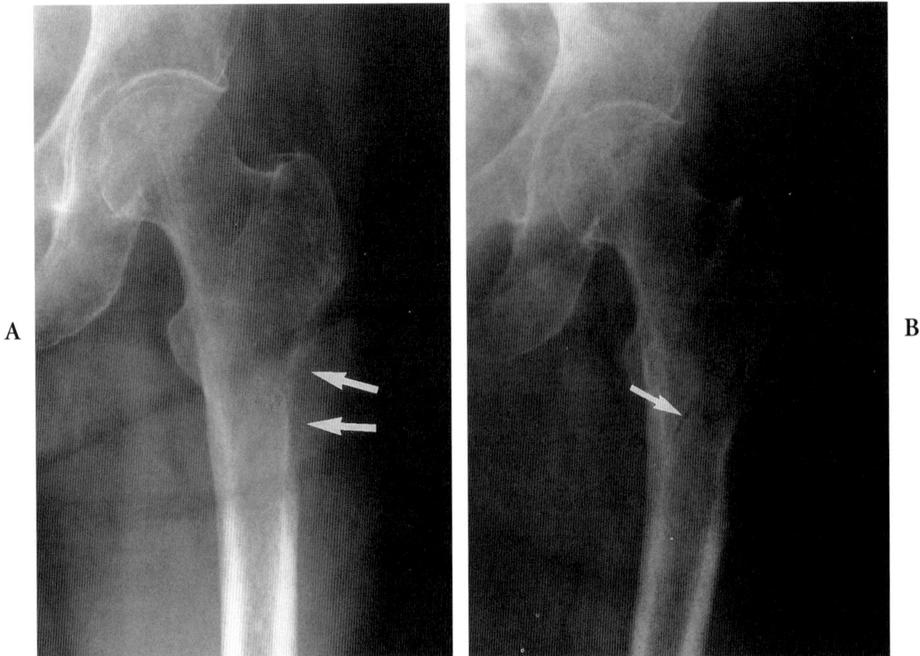

Fig. 5-17   **A,** Anteroposterior view of the femur of a 68-year-old woman with lung carcinoma demonstrates a large lytic metastasis with cortical destruction *(arrows).* **B,** Radiograph obtained 4 days later shows a pathologic fracture *(arrow).*

in adults are usually pathologic.[2] Radiographs are also useful in planning the treatment of fractures and impending pathologic fractures.

For the spine, we have already discussed radiographic characteristics helpful in distinguishing metastatic from osteoporotic fractures. It is useful to remember that one third of patients with systemic malignancy and vertebral compression have a nonmalignant cause for the collapse.[21] Vertebral body metastases often initially are seen with a compression fracture, however, and 5% of patients with skeletal metastases will have resultant extradural cord or nerve root compression.[22] Radiographs are also useful for planning radiation therapy in these patients.

ROLE IN FOLLOW-UP

Radiographs of metastases are frequently obtained after chemotherapy, radiation, or surgical treatment. In this section we will discuss the radiographic appearance of metastases in patients who undergo chemotherapy, the general bone changes that occur with radiation therapy, and the role of radiographs in orthopedic fixation.

The radiographic appearance of treated metastases depends mainly on the density of the original lesion. In patients with lytic or mixed metastases, the earliest healing response is a peripheral rim of sclerosis.[23,24] Treated metastases will then slowly fill in with sclerosis before fading as normal bone remodeling occurs. A common scenario in treated metastatic breast carcinoma is the development of sclerotic lesions in previously normal-appearing bone. The most common cause of this finding is not the development of new osteoblastic metastases but, rather, the sclerotic healing of radiographically occult metastases involving less than 30% destruction of the cancellous bone (Fig. 5-18).[23,24]

Radiographic evidence of recurrence includes the development of an area of osteolysis either that is larger than the original lesion or that develops faster than would be expected with simple fading as a result of bone remodeling.[3] Recurrence should also be suspected if the lesion becomes radiolucent relative to the surrounding normal bone.

For osteoblastic metastases that have been treated, the lesions may remain radiographically unchanged, a finding that is particularly common in

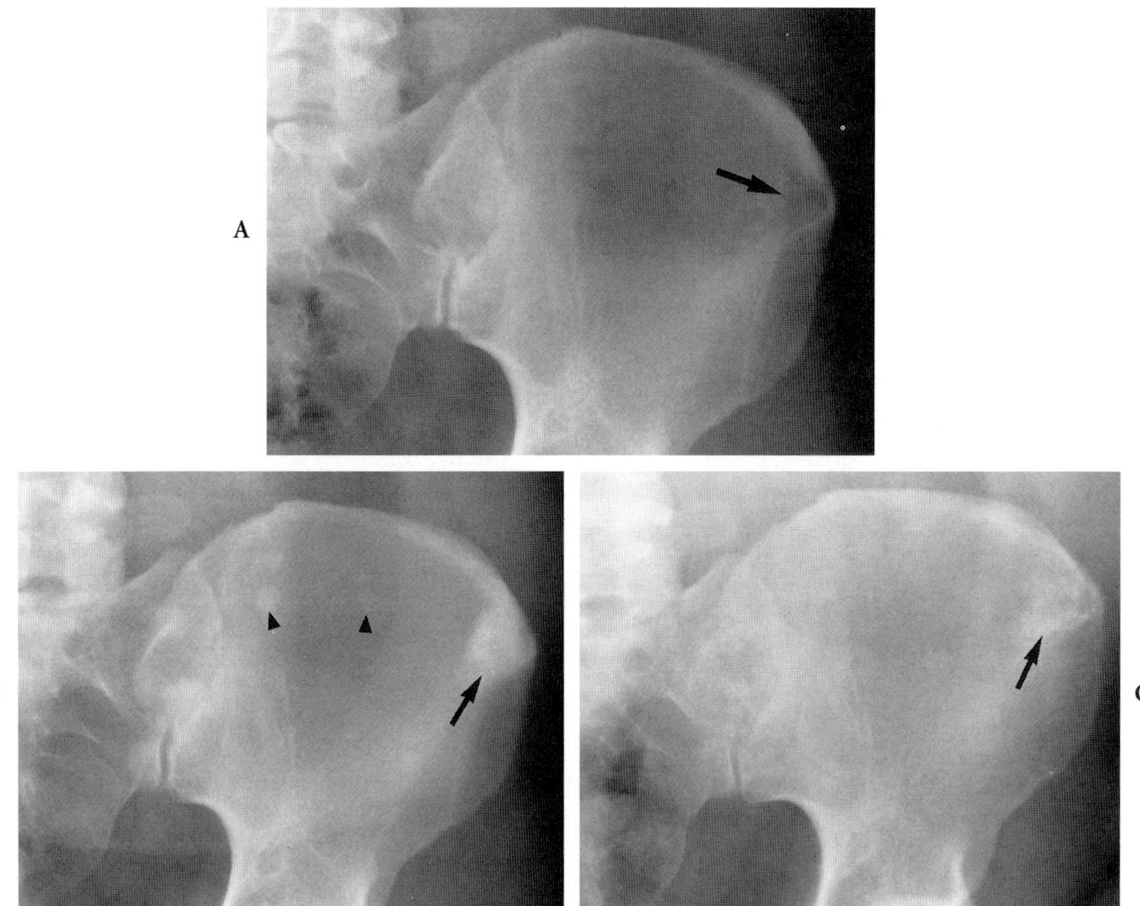

Fig. 5-18   **A,** Anteroposterior view of the left ilium of a 38-year-old woman with breast carcinoma shows a predominantly lytic metastasis *(arrow)*. **B,** Six months later, after chemotherapy, the metastasis *(arrow)* has filled in with sclerosis, consistent with healing. Several new osteoblastic lesions have appeared *(arrowheads)* in previously normal bone, representing sclerotic healing of occult metastases. **C,** Twenty-one months after radiograph **B** was obtained, there is new lytic destruction of the healed metastases *(arrow)* from tumor recurrence. The patient died 1 year later.

healing prostate carcinoma metastases.[25] Other types of blastic metastases may initially increase in density before decreasing in diameter and eventually fading to normal.[2] New sclerotic foci in patients with osteoblastic metastases who are undergoing treatment can be difficult to sort out because they may represent either new lesions or healing of previously radiographically occult lesions. Tumor recurrence will usually be seen initially as an increase in the size of the sclerotic lesion. The development of new osteolytic areas within a sclerotic focus may also represent recurrence, although such a recurrence can be difficult to distinguish from the normal fading of a treated lesion.

In patients who receive radiation therapy for a metastatic lesion, the healing response of the metastasis is similar to that seen with chemotherapy. The adjacent bone will often become abnormal, however, with the development of patchy lytic areas that may appear similar to tumor recurrence. Several clues can be used to help differentiate radiation changes from tumor recurrence. Radiated bone typically has coarse, thickened trabeculae and unnaturally straight margins that correlate with the radiation field.[2] Radiation changes to bone will usually peak in 2 to 3 years, so the development of a new bone abnormality within the radiation field after this time limit should be further evaluated.[3]

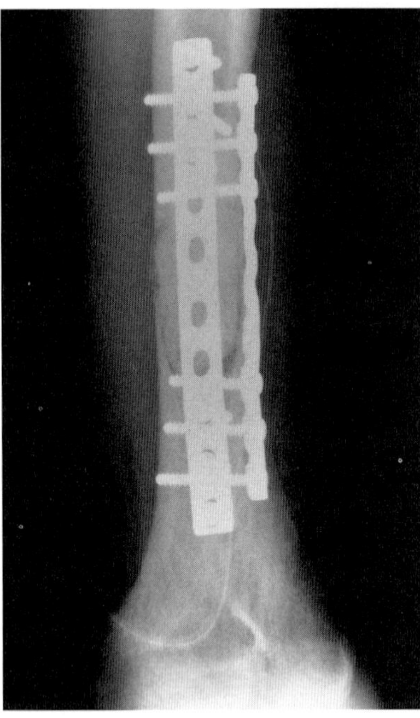

Fig. 5-19   Anteroposterior view of the humerus of a 54-year-old man with a painful pathologic fracture resulting from a renal cell carcinoma metastasis (same patient as in Fig. 5-11). There has been curettage, cementing, and placement of reconstruction plates across the metastasis.

Surgical resection and fixation of metastases are occasionally performed either for pathologic or impending pathologic fracture or for severe pain.[19] Radiographs are obtained after surgery to check for proper placement of the hardware or for alignment across a pathologic fracture (Fig. 5-19). Subsequent radiographs may be obtained if the patient has recurrent pain, either to identify hardware failure or new bone destruction from local recurrence.

REFERENCES

1. Galasko CSB. The anatomy and pathways of skeletal metastasis. In Weiss L, Gilbert HA, eds. Bone Metastasis. Boston: GK Hall, 1981, pp 49-83.
2. Resnick D, Niwayama G. Skeletal metastases. In Resnick D, Niwayama G, eds. Diagnosis of Bone and Joint Disorders, 2nd ed. Philadelphia: WB Saunders, 1988, pp 3944-4010.
3. Pagani JJ, Libshitz HI. Imaging bone metastases. Radiol Clin North Am 20:545-560, 1982.
4. Krane SM, Schiller AL. Hyperostosis, neoplasms, and other disorders of bone and cartilage. In Petersdorf RG, Adams RD, Braunwald E, Isselbacher KJ, Martin JB, Wilson JD, eds. Principles of Internal Medicine, 10th ed. New York: McGraw-Hill, 1983, p 1967.
5. Rankin S. Radiology. In Rubens RD, Fogelman I, eds. Bone Metastases: Diagnosis and Treatment. London: Springer-Verlag, 1991, pp 63-81.
6. Hendrix RW, Rogers LF, Davis TM. Cortical bone metastases. Radiology 181:409-413, 1991.
7. Greenfield GB. Radiology of Bone Diseases, 4th ed. Philadelphia: JB Lippincott, 1986, p 437.
8. Resnick D, Niwayama G. Soft tissues. In Resnick D, Niwayama G, eds. Diagnosis of Bone and Joint Disorders. Philadelphia: WB Saunders, 1988, p 4230.
9. Olson P, Everson LI, Griffiths HJ. Staging of musculoskeletal tumors. Radiol Clin North Am 32:151-162, 1994.
10. Gold RI, Seeger LL, Bassett LW, Steckel RJ. An integrated approach to the evaluation of metastatic disease. Radiol Clin North Am 28:471-483, 1990.
11. Eustace S, Tello R, DeCarvalho V, Carey J, Wroblicka JT, Melhem ER, Yucel EK. A comparison of whole-body turboSTIR MR imaging and planar 99mTc-methylene diphosphonate scintigraphy in the examination of patients with suspected skeletal metastases. AJR Am J Roentgenol 169:1655-1661, 1997.
12. Corcoran RJ, Thrall JH, Kyle RW, Kaminski RJ, Johnson MC. Solitary abnormalities in bone scans of patients with extraosseous malignancies. Radiology 121:663-667, 1976.
13. Mettler FA, Guiberteau MJ. Essentials of Nuclear Medicine Imaging, 2nd ed. Philadelphia: WB Saunders, 1985, pp 253-259.
14. Wilner D. Radiology of Bone Tumors and Allied Disorders. Philadelphia: WB Saunders, 1982, p 364.
15. Rosen IW, Nadel HI. Button sequestrum of the skull. Radiology 92:969, 1969.
16. Laredo JD, Lakhdari K, Bellaiche L, Hamze B, Janklewicz P, Tubiana JM. Acute vertebral collapse: CT findings in benign and malignant nontraumatic cases. Radiology 194:41-48, 1995.
17. Azouz EM. Tumors. In Reed MH, ed. Pediatric Skeletal Radiology. Philadelphia: Williams & Wilkins, 1992, pp 506-566.
18. Tuite MJ, DeSmet AA, Gaynon PS. Tibial stress fracture mimicking neuroblastoma metastasis in two young children. Skeletal Radiol 24:287-290, 1995.
19. Springfield D, Jennings C. Pathologic fractures. In Rockwood CA, Green DP, Bucholz RW, eds. Fractures in Adults, 3rd ed. Philadelphia: JB Lippincott, 1991, pp 417-425.
20. Mirels H. Metastatic disease in long bones. Clin Orthop 249:256-264, 1989.
21. Fornasier VL, Czitrom AA. Collapsed vertebrae: A review of 659 autopsies. Clin Orthop 131:261-265, 1978.
22. Barron KD, Hirano A, Araki S, Ferry RD. Experience with metastatic neoplasms involving the spinal cord. Neurology 9:91, 1959.
23. Libshitz HI, Hortobagyi GN. Radiographic evaluation of therapeutic response in bony metastases of breast cancer. Skeletal Radiol 7:159-165, 1981.
24. Barry WF, Wells SA, Cox CE, Haagensen DE. Clinical and radiographic correlations in breast cancer patients with osseous metastases. Skeletal Radiol 6:27-32, 1981.
25. Pollen JJ, Shlaer WJ. Osteoblastic response to successful treatment of metastatic cancer of the prostate. AJR Am J Roentgenol 132:927-931, 1979.

Computed Tomography and Magnetic Resonance Imaging

Murali Sundaram, M.D., F.R.C.R., *and*
Douglas J. McDonald, M.D.

Metastasis is the single most common malignant tumor of bone. However, metastasis to soft tissue that requires imaging ranks among the rarest of soft tissue malignancies. Not every known or suspected metastasis to bone requires further evaluation with either computed tomography (CT) or magnetic resonance imaging (MRI), but every soft tissue mass requiring biopsy, irrespective of the clinician's level of diagnostic certainty, merits further imaging by MRI.[1] The difference in approach is because of the frequency with which skeletal metastases to bone can be documented and characterized by radiography. Soft tissue metastasis, like other soft tissue masses, can be reliably depicted and characterized only by MRI. This chapter will be devoted largely to discussing the rationale for CT or MRI in the evaluation of suspected skeletal metastases. It also will briefly address our experience with soft tissue metastases.

RATIONALE

Metastasis to soft tissues presenting as an indeterminate mass and mimicking a sarcoma is a relatively rare occurrence.[2] Solitary metastasis to bone is far more frequently encountered than sarcoma of bone. On the basis of the age of the individual and the location of the lesion, metastasis to bone can frequently be identified by radiographic appearance alone. CT and MRI usually further characterize the lesion and also influence treatment. For example, in flat bones such as the ilium, even large metastases can be difficult to characterize by radiography alone. In these circumstances, CT, MRI, or both can help determine the diagnosis and extent of tumor. The modalities are also useful in the follow-up of treated metastasis. Recognition of a benign lesion mimicking metastasis in an elderly person could prevent unnecessary imaging, biopsies, or both. These lesions would include insufficiency fractures of the sacrum and pubis, monostotic Paget's disease of the sacrum, and benign vertebral compression fractures. Intravenous injection of gadolinium is usually reserved for lesions in vertebrae and is rarely used elsewhere in the skeleton.

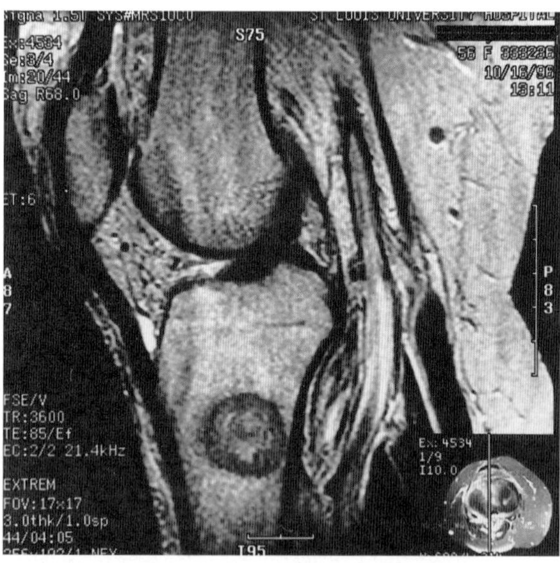

Fig. 6-1 Metastasis to proximal tibia. The patient had pain and a normal radiograph at presentation. Technetium bone scan showed increased radiotracer accumulation. The configuration of the abnormality on the MRI is that of a tumor. This appearance, together with normal radiographic findings, favors metastasis over sarcoma.

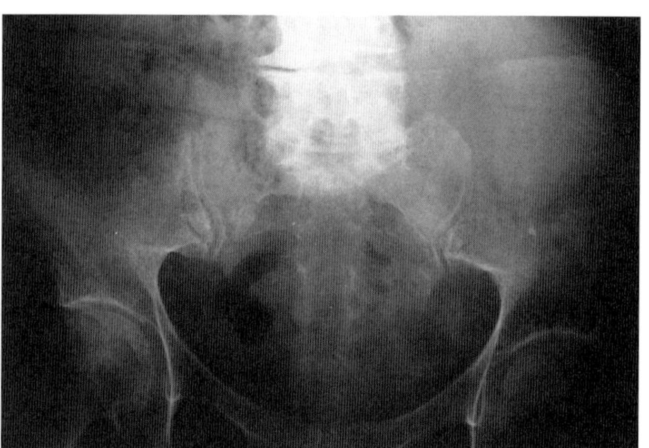
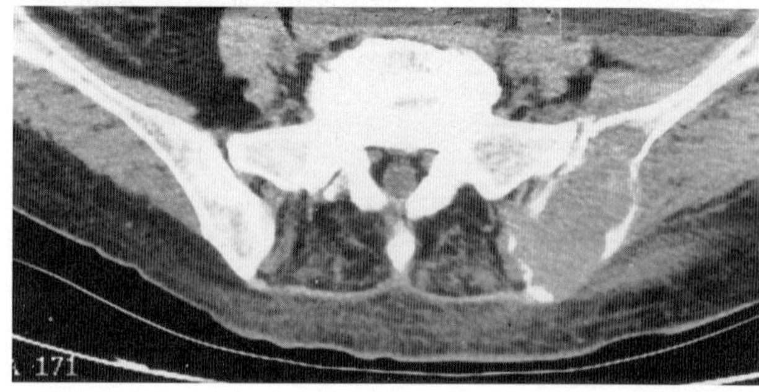

Fig. 6-2 Large left ilial metastasis. Radiograph (**A**) shows an ill-defined soft tissue density, which on the CT scan (**B**) demonstrates unequivocally an expanding, osteolytic lesion that on other sections had clearly breached the cortex and produced a large extraosseous mass.

GUIDELINES

Because of the seeming ubiquity of suspected metastases, it might appear too restrictive to adhere to guidelines for evaluation. Yet guidelines are required so that all lesions of bone can be approached in a consistent and logical fashion, with the opportunity for modifications and refinement as technology and experience evolve. Broadly, three categories of suspected metastatic disease merit further imaging by either CT or MRI.

Further imaging is necessary to confirm a lesion in patients with normal radiographic findings but abnormalities on bone scan (Fig. 6-1) or equivocal radiographic findings (i.e., flat bones, distal femur, proximal humerus) (Fig. 6-2). CT or MRI is also indicated for further characterization of the matrix of a lesion not well seen on a radiograph, usually in the pelvis, vertebra, sternum, or scapula (see Figs. 6-2 and 6-3). Finally, further CT or MRI is needed to depict for the surgeon, radiotherapist, or medical oncologist the extent and dimensions of a lesion that, although evident on the radiograph, needs to be further staged locally before surgery or radiation therapy and to serve as a baseline before chemotherapy (Fig. 6-3).

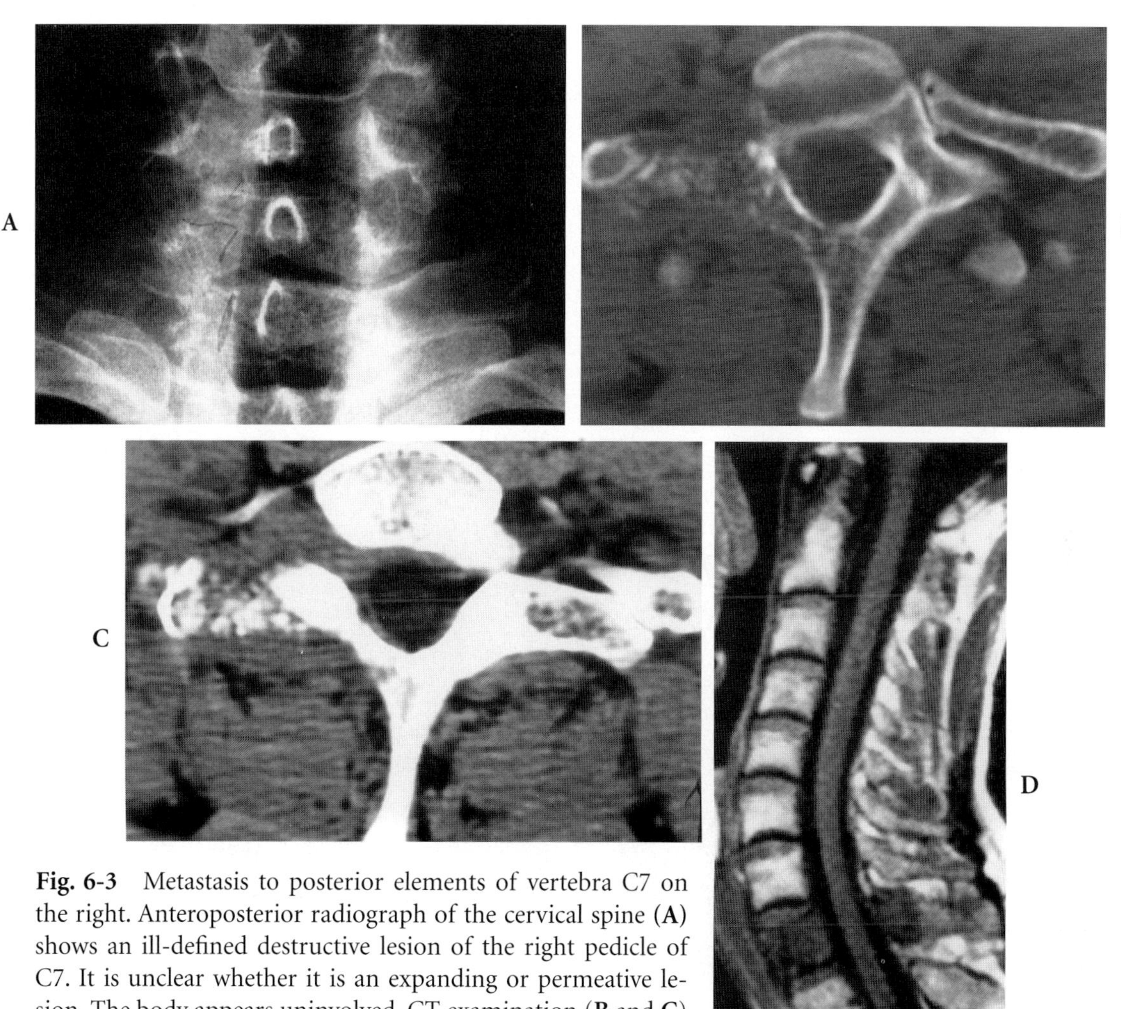

Fig. 6-3 Metastasis to posterior elements of vertebra C7 on the right. Anteroposterior radiograph of the cervical spine (**A**) shows an ill-defined destructive lesion of the right pedicle of C7. It is unclear whether it is an expanding or permeative lesion. The body appears uninvolved. CT examination (**B** and **C**) shows a permeative, destructive lesion of the pedicle of C7 that is predominantly osteolytic. Scattered bone fragments are seen amidst this destructive lesion. Sagittal T1-weighted MRI (**D**) shows that the body of C7 has retained its normal morphologic configuration but with complete replacement of normal fatty marrow, indicating tumor infiltration of the body as well.

COMPUTED TOMOGRAPHY VS. MAGNETIC RESONANCE IMAGING

Unlike CT, in which the major determinants of the scanning technique are thickness of slice and reformatting, MRI, in its evolution over the past decade, has spawned a plethora of pulse sequences permitting imaging in coronal, axial, sagittal, and oblique planes, which can be further augmented by intravenously administered gadolinium. The mainstay of our sequences was, is, and has remained the spin-echo pulsing sequence with, more recently, fast spin echo replacing conventional spin echo for both T1- and T2-weighted sequences. Fat-suppressed T2-weighted sequences are included for pelvic lesions, vertebral lesions, and occasional appendicular lesions (if radiographic appearances are equivocal) primarily to increase conspicuity of lesion rather than to stage. The use of intravenously administered gadolinium to visualize the pelvis and appendicular skeleton is the exception rather than the rule.[3] Gadolinium is routinely used for vertebral lesions to aid in differentiating postmenopausal vertebral collapse from metastatic disease. MRI is carried out invariably in two planes, with the axial plane always included and augmented by either coronal or sagittal imaging, depending on the anatomic structure being imaged.

The need to use both imaging modalities should be exceptional. MRI, because of its superior sensitivity to lesions in marrow, exquisite soft tissue detail, and ease of direct multidirectional imaging, is the preferred modality. In the search for metastases involving the vertebral column, MRI affords a highly sensitive and quick technique for scanning the entire spinal column in the sagittal plane (Fig. 6-4) and for providing further detail with axial images of sites of interest. We tend to reserve CT as the preferred modality when the matrix of a lesion (i.e., osteolytic, calcified, ossified) is not clearly evident on a radiograph and when that information could influence further investigation and the possible mode of biopsy.

DIAGNOSIS

Multiple skeletal metastases rarely pose a diagnostic dilemma; their presence initiates a search for a primary neoplasm by CT of the thorax, abdomen, and pelvis. Diagnosis is usually established by biopsy of the most accessible lesion by the least invasive method. Thus CT-guided percutaneous biopsies are a commonplace and efficacious technique for determining diagnosis. CT-guided biopsies also have a similar role in the solitary lesion that is suggestive of metastasis (Fig. 6-5). Solitary aggressive

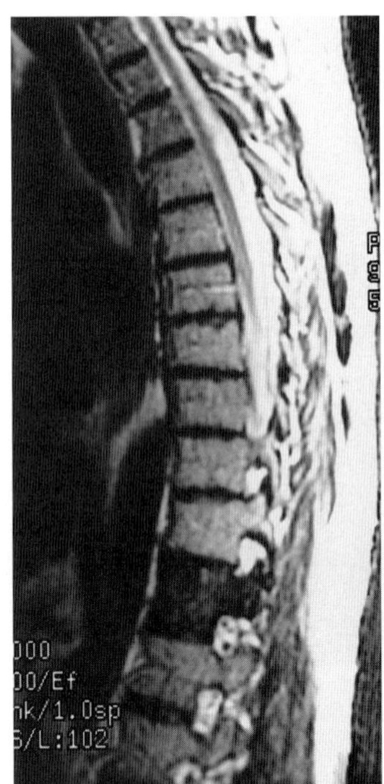
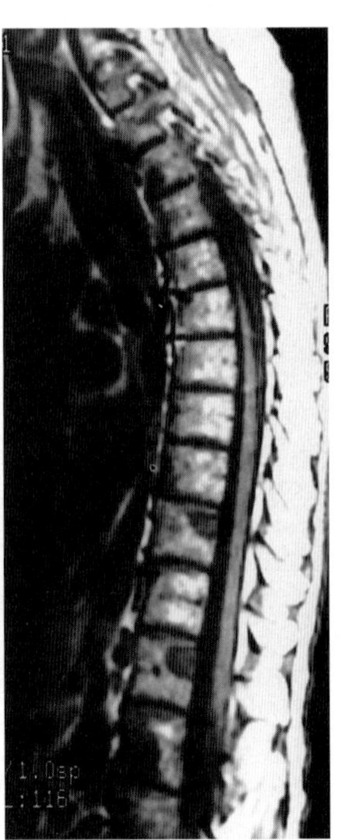

Fig. 6-4 Sagittal T1-weighted MRI scans of two patients. **A,** Solitary marrow-replacing lesion of T12. **B,** Multiple marrow-replacing lesions. For both patients, radiographic findings were normal. In a patient with a known malignancy, the favored diagnosis is metastasis. In a patient without a known primary malignancy a common differential diagnosis to be considered with metastases is multiple myeloma. Note presentation of normal vertebral height and configuration of involved vertebrae.

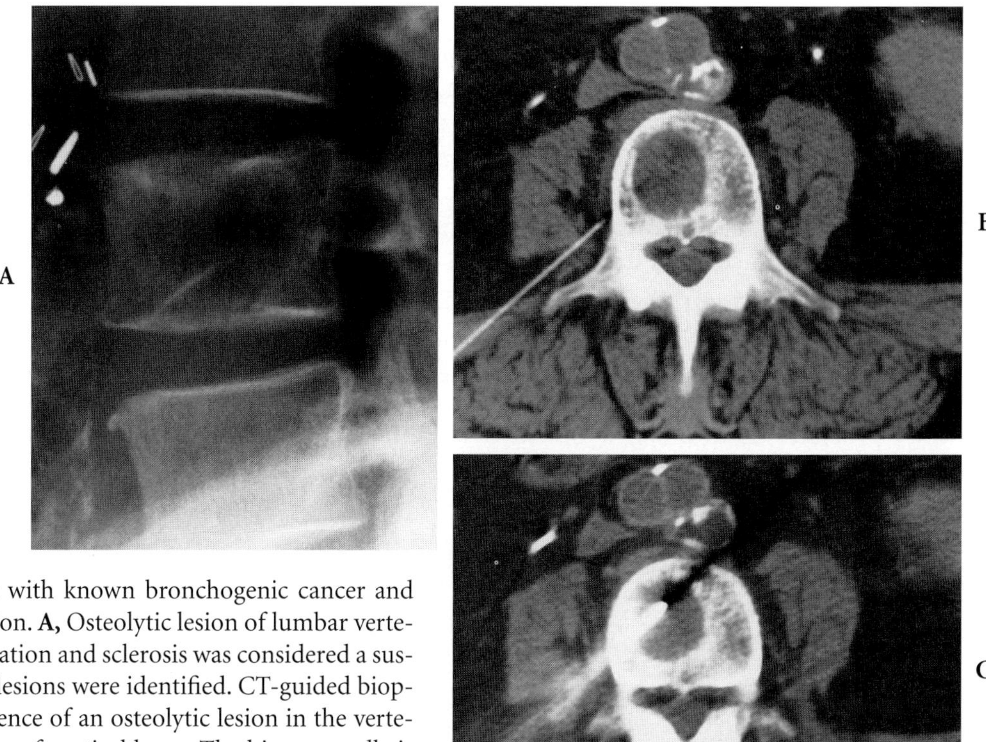

Fig. 6-5 Images of patient with known bronchogenic cancer and solitary lumbar vertebral lesion. **A,** Osteolytic lesion of lumbar vertebral body with slight deformation and sclerosis was considered a suspected metastasis. No other lesions were identified. CT-guided biopsy (**B** and **C**) shows the presence of an osteolytic lesion in the vertebral body within the confines of cortical bone. The biopsy needle is passed through cortical bone into the lesion. Cytologic confirmation of adequate tissue and diagnosis was provided instantly in the CT suite, confirming metastasis from the lung.

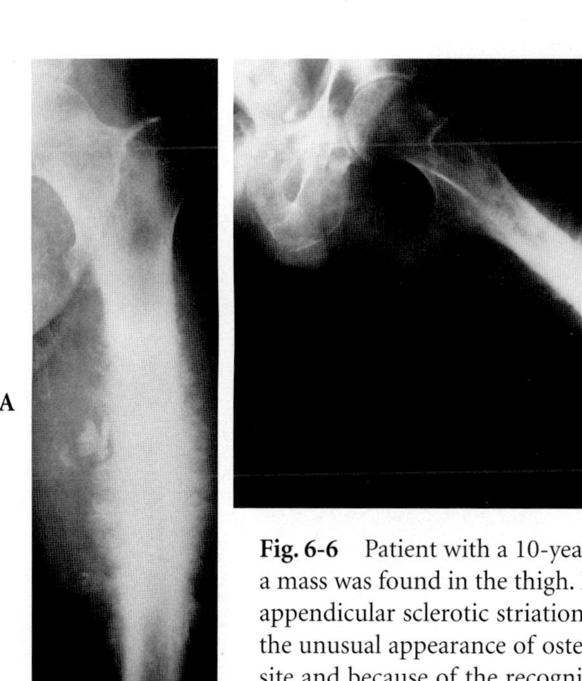

Fig. 6-6 Patient with a 10-year history of prostatic cancer was thought to be doing well until a mass was found in the thigh. Radiographs (**A** and **B**) show a diaphyseal, sclerotic lesion with appendicular sclerotic striations of bone indistinguishable from an osteosarcoma. Because of the unusual appearance of osteosarcoma in an elderly man who had not had radiation at this site and because of the recognition that prostatic metastasis could be manifested by this pattern, biopsy was performed without any further imaging. The surgeon, however, took care in the biopsy approach so that, if the lesion was found to be an osteosarcoma, a limb salvage procedure would not be compromised by the biopsy technique.

lesions of bone occurring in patients at ages when metastases abound pose management problems. Metastatic disease to the skeleton, even when solitary, is a far more frequent occurrence than a sarcoma of bone. However, when a sarcoma cannot be excluded (usually in patients with a solitary tumor of bone and no known primary malignancy), we would image and stage as we would for a sarcoma (i.e., stage before biopsy). An open biopsy rather than a CT-guided percutaneous biopsy is performed in such circumstances. However, in patients with a known primary malignancy (e.g., breast, lung, prostate, or kidney), a destructive solitary lesion of bone is presumed to be metastatic and is approached as such even if at times it might mimic a sarcoma of bone. A well-known mimic is prostatic metastasis to the appendicular skeleton, which may radiographically suggest an osteosarcoma (Fig. 6-6).[4]

Benign Lesions Mimicking Metastases

In practice, a solitary aggressive, destructive lesion will come to biopsy. What one wishes to avoid is the biopsy of those benign lesions that mimic metastases on any one of several imaging studies. In adults, three such lesions are postmenopausal in-

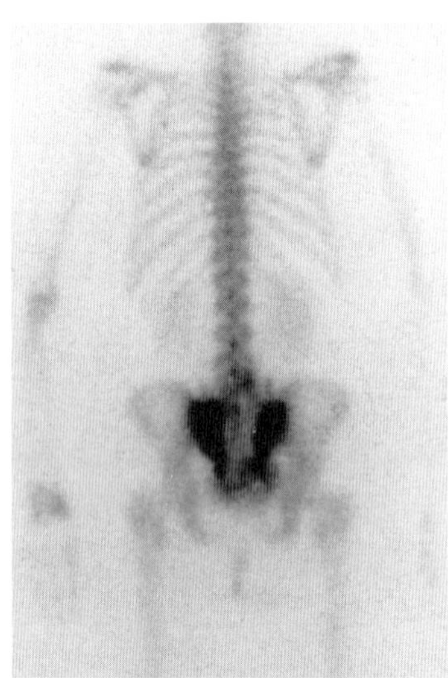

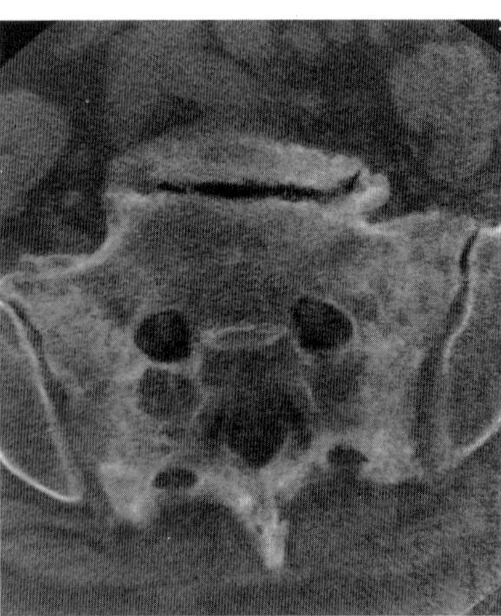

A   B

Fig. 6-7 Elderly woman with known breast cancer had low back pain. Radiographs showed no abnormalities, apart from osteopenia. Technetium bone scan (**A**) showed increased radiotracer accumulation in a linear orientation. CT (**B**) demonstrated the characteristic linear orientation with sclerosis bilaterally, characteristic of insufficiency fractures. There is no soft tissue mass.

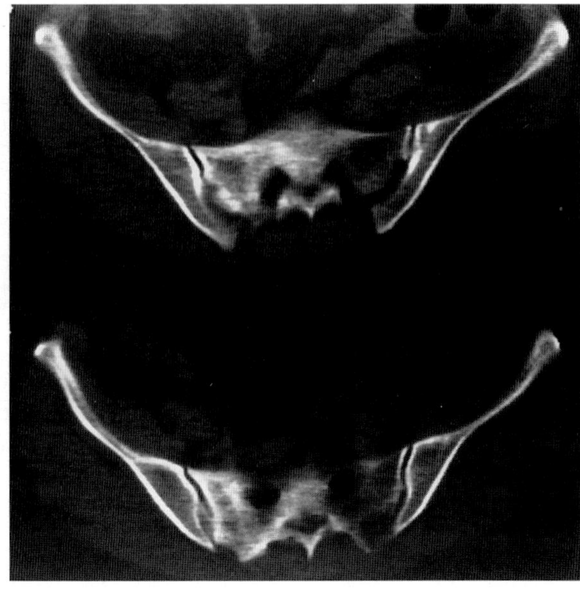

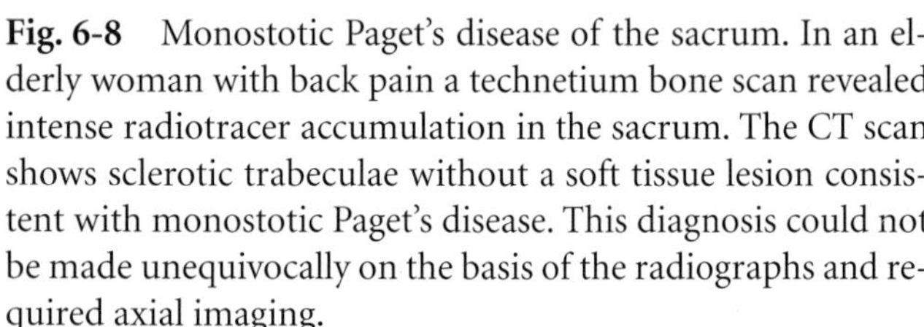

Fig. 6-8 Monostotic Paget's disease of the sacrum. In an elderly woman with back pain a technetium bone scan revealed intense radiotracer accumulation in the sacrum. The CT scan shows sclerotic trabeculae without a soft tissue lesion consistent with monostotic Paget's disease. This diagnosis could not be made unequivocally on the basis of the radiographs and required axial imaging.

sufficiency fractures of the sacrum[5,6] (Fig. 6-7) and pubis,[6] monostotic Paget's disease of the sacrum (Fig. 6-8), and postmenopausal vertebral collapse. Analogous mimics in children are less of a problem because of familiarity with vertebra plana in eosinophilic granuloma, with femoral and tibial stress fractures from increased activity on scintigraphy, and with the bone edema pattern on MRI.

Metastases Mimicking Benign Lesions

Usually metastases are rapidly growing and do not behave in an indolent manner. However, a common metastasis that is an exception to that rule is prostatic metastasis, which can show radiographic abnormalities and remain relatively dormant even when untreated (Fig. 6-9). Neither CT nor MRI is required to suggest the correct diagnosis.

Soft Tissue Metastases

During the past 10 years we have encountered five soft tissue metastases (all from lung) manifested by a growing soft tissue mass (Fig. 6-10). In each of these instances, radiographs and CT scans of the thorax, performed for staging a presumed sarcoma, identified a pulmonary or hilar mass. Three of these patients were surprisingly young (in their

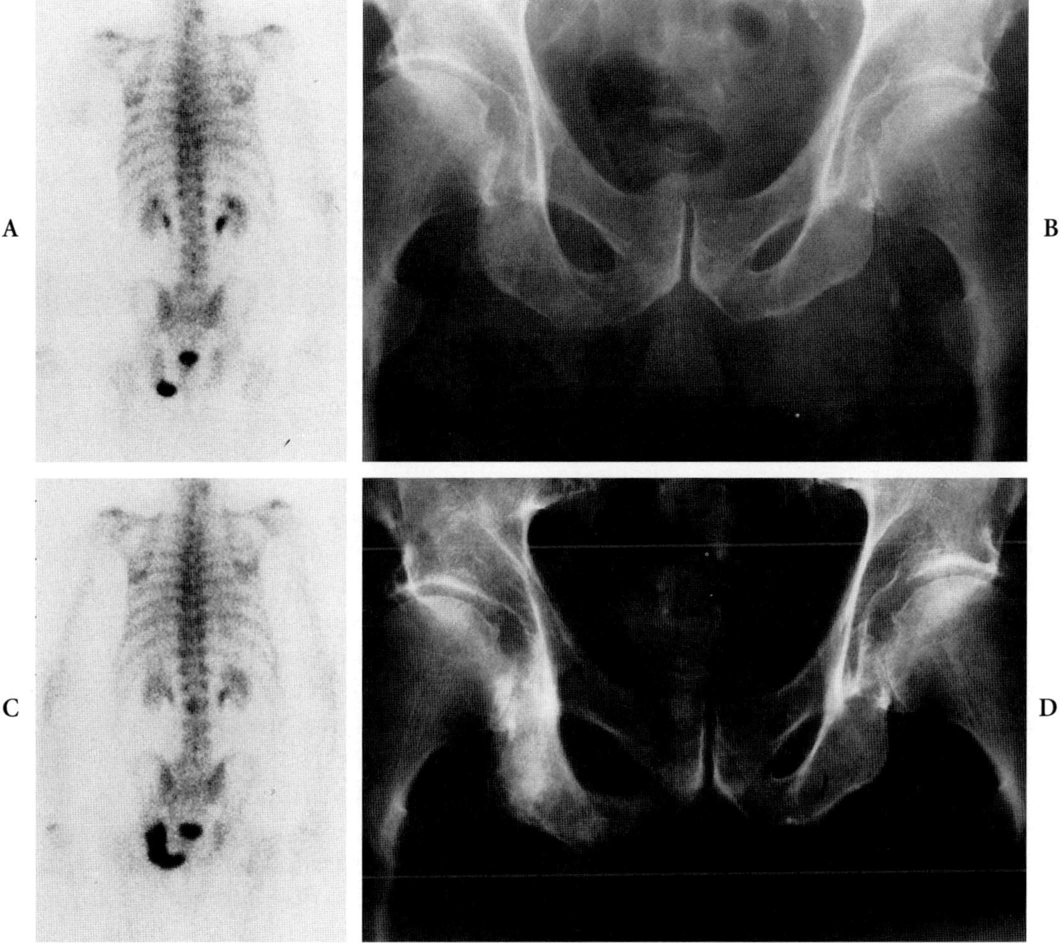

Fig. 6-9 Patient was seen in 1992 with pain in the hip. **A,** Technetium bone scan shows localized, intense radiotracer accumulation in the ischium. **B,** Radiograph shows faint sclerosis in the ischium, and the combination of findings was erroneously interpreted as early Paget's disease. The patient was seen again 5 years later. **C,** Technetium bone scan shows more extensive radiotracer accumulation in the ischium as the only finding. **D,** Radiograph shows sclerosis of the ischium and inferior pubis on the right, without coarsened trabeculae or bone expansion. Biopsy confirmed prostatic metastasis.

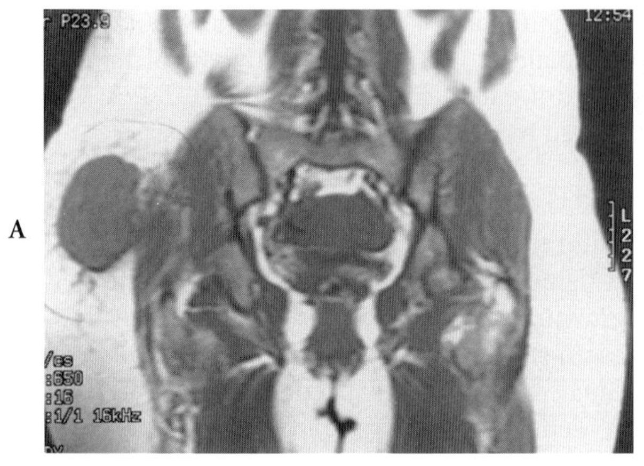

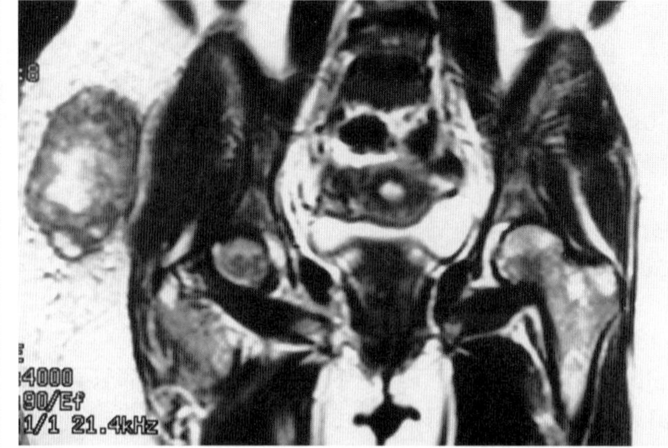

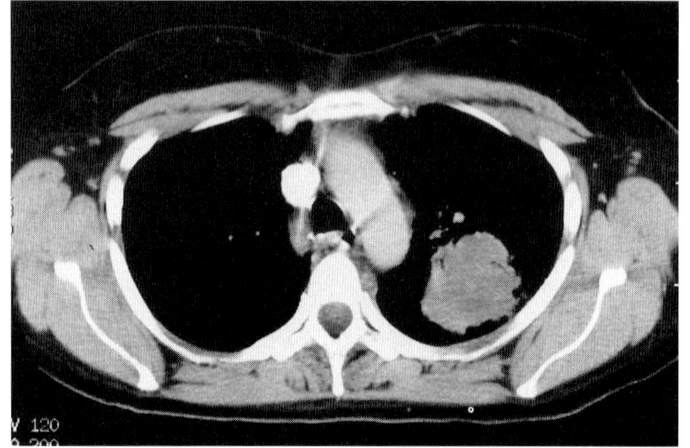

Fig. 6-10 A 42-year-old woman had a mass in the right buttock. Coronal T1 (**A**) and T2 (**B**) MRI scans confirm a large necrotic mass in the gluteus, which, because of size and depth, suggested a soft tissue sarcoma. As part of the staging of this soft tissue mass, the patient underwent radiography of the chest and CT scanning (**C**), which revealed a large mass in the left lung that proved to be a peripheral bronchogenic carcinoma. The mass in the buttock was a metastasis from a lung cancer.

forties) and female. The combination of a solitary appendicular soft tissue mass and a solitary mass in the lung or a nodal mediastinal mass should suggest a bronchogenic cancer that has spread to the soft tissues, rather than vice versa.[2] The logical imaging approach to the indeterminate soft tissue mass includes imaging not only of the mass but also of the thorax and abdomen. When a lung mass is found in addition to a soft tissue mass, the latter is likely a metastasis rather than a sarcoma.

TREATMENT
Pathologic Fracture

Accurate imaging is the basis on which many treatment decisions are made. In the extremities, the primary goals of treatment for metastatic carcinoma are to relieve pain and improve function. Achieving these goals requires effective management of the pathologic fracture or impending pathologic fracture.

Adequate imaging of a pathologic fracture generally can be done with good-quality radiographs, which should show the entire length of the involved bone. Managing the impending fracture is more difficult because it requires the ability to predict the risk of fracture. This risk is directly related to the load on the bone. Ideally, assessment of the load requires knowledge of defect geometry, including size, shape, and anatomic site; remaining bone properties; and the type of load supplied. Practically, the risk is estimated on the basis of defect geometry and anatomic site.

Defect geometry is assessed in long bones by means of standard anteroposterior and lateral radiographs. Cortical destruction is measured relative to the overall bone diameter, with lesions involving greater than 50% of the cortical diameter or lesions greater than 2.5 cm in length thought to have a greater incidence of impending fracture. Assessment is particularly significant in high stress areas such as the subtrochanteric part of the femur.

Permeative destruction of bone can also lead to increased risk of pathologic fracture but is much harder to assess. In such circumstances, CT may

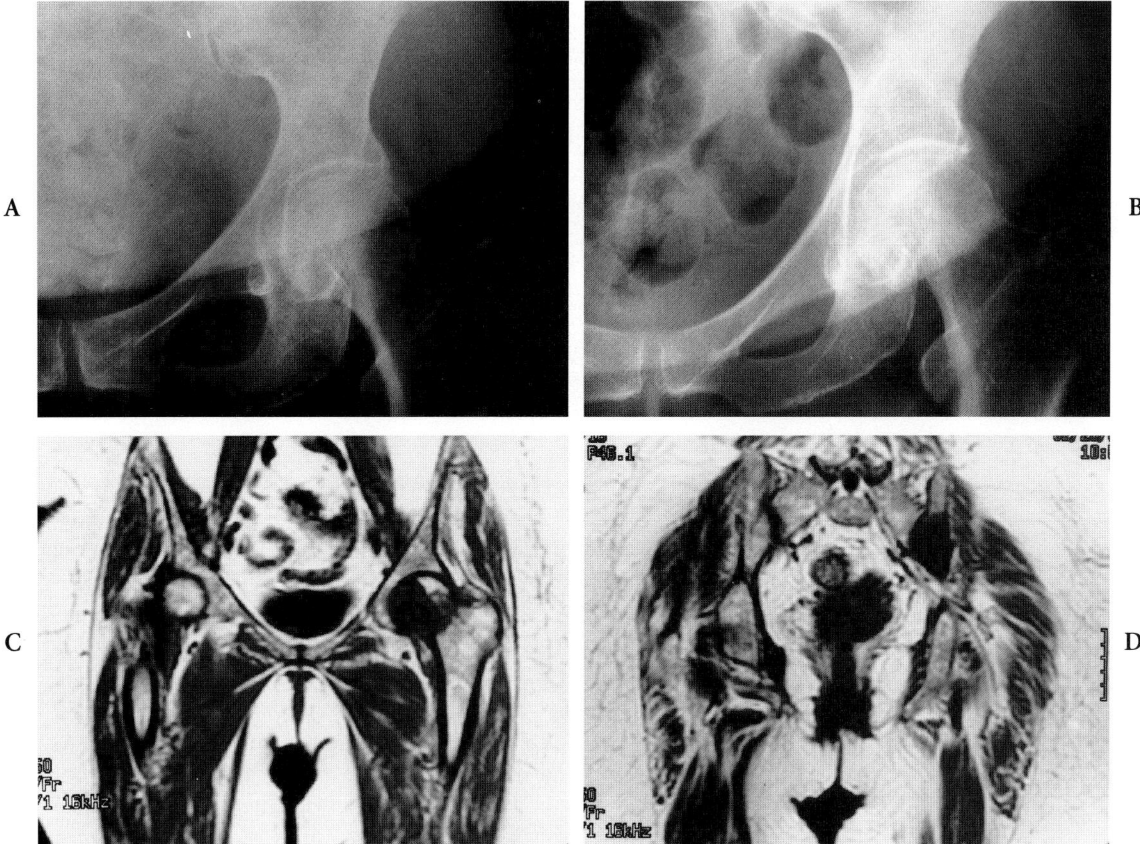

Fig. 6-11   **A,** Anteroposterior radiograph of the hip of a 63-year-old woman with hip pain and a history of soft tissue sarcoma. Other than some diffuse osteopenia, no obvious lesion was noted. **B,** Anteroposterior radiograph of the same patient 1 month later. A clear subcapital impacted femoral neck fracture is seen. **C,** T1-weighted coronal MRI scan clearly shows the marrow-replacing lesion within the left femoral head and neck. This is not the appearance that one would expect from a fracture and fits best with a neoplastic process. **D,** T1-weighted coronal MRI scan further posterior in the pelvis shows a second lesion within the posterior ilium, also consistent with neoplasm.

give a much clearer view of the amount of bone destruction present. In addition, MRI is also beneficial because it gives a much clearer extent of intramedullary bone involvement (Fig. 6-11). Once the decision has been made to treat a fracture or impending fracture surgically, it is important to have adequate radiographs of the entire bone involved or, if the lesion involves a joint surface, an accurate assessment of both sides of the joint. Most lesions are internally fixed with an intramedullary implant, with or without cement augmentation. It is important to instrument all areas of involvement to prevent subsequent fractures.

Pelvic Reconstruction

In the pelvis, imaging of lesions with CT or MRI, in addition to the use of radiographs, is often required to determine the appropriate treatment. In the pelvis, functionally significant lesions generally occur around the acetabulum (Fig. 6-12, *A*). Total hip replacement with acetabular reconstruction, although a demanding surgery, can be of great benefit for the patient. Accurate assessment of the extent of bone destruction of the pelvis does generally require CT imaging (Fig. 6-12, *B*). If adequate bone stock remains, reconstruction can generally be done with conventional hip arthroplasty. If ex-

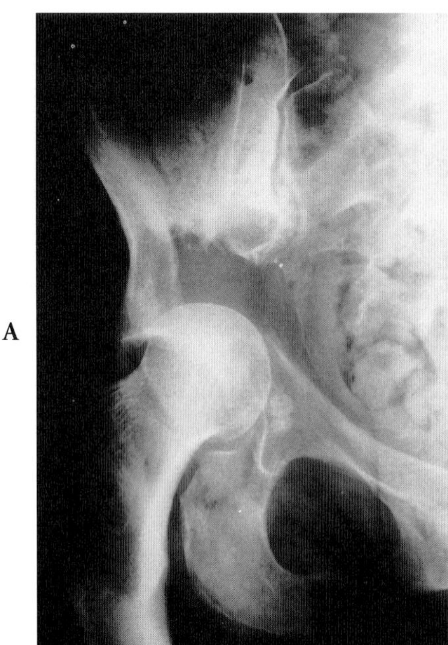

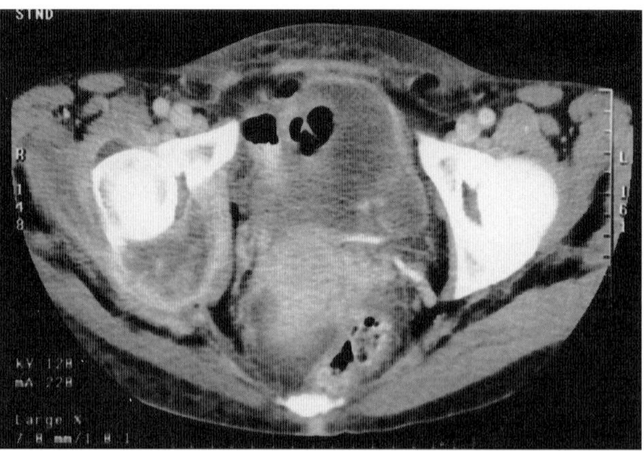

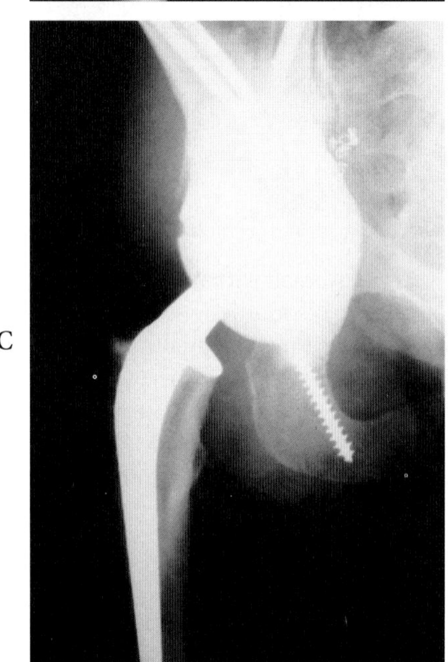

Fig. 6-12 A, Anteroposterior radiograph of a 44-year-old woman with known metastatic renal cell carcinoma to bone. An obvious lesion in the ilium has resulted in almost complete destruction of the supra-acetabular bone. The femoral head has protruded into the pelvis as well. **B,** CT scan through the pelvis in the same patient. Although the CT scan is not needed for diagnosis, it is extremely helpful in treatment planning because it allows the surgeon to define more clearly the extent of disease and remaining bone. **C,** Anteroposterior radiograph of the same hip after surgical reconstruction. A total hip arthroplasty was done, with reconstruction of the pelvic defect primarily with bone cement. Large, threaded Steinmann pins were used to anchor the cement into the remaining bone, particularly superiorly. Note the embolization coils in the internal iliac system. Preoperative arterial embolization is extremely helpful in minimizing blood loss in patients with metastatic renal cell carcinoma of the pelvis who require surgical intervention.

tensive bone is involved, major acetabular reconstruction is necessary, or a nonconventional prosthesis, such as the saddle prosthesis, may be needed (Fig. 6-12, *C*). MRI of the pelvis may also be helpful in determining treatment options, because the extent of marrow involvement may alter one's choice of reconstruction.

Spine Surgery

In the spine, the important therapeutic decisions are based on assessment of the mechanical integrity of the spine and the neurologic status of the patient. CT and MRI are invaluable to the spine surgeon in this regard because they are generally more accurate than radiographs in assessing the extent of bone involvement and the integrity of the remaining bone. In patients for whom surgery is indicated, the decisions regarding surgical approach, be it anterior, posterior, or both, are generally made on the basis of the location and extent of the lesion as visualized by CT scan. When spinal fusion is contemplated, the MRI is valuable in determining the status of the vertebrae above and below the site of main involvement. This gives the surgeon information that will influence the length of fusion and the sites and type of fixation that will be required.

CONCLUSION

There is a fine line between appropriate use and overuse of the multiple imaging modalities now available. If the dominant question of how further imaging will affect management by providing a specific diagnosis or by influencing the mode of biopsy or treatment is satisfactorily answered, inappropriate imaging can be limited. If the radiologist works on the surmise that common things happen commonly, has a working knowledge of therapeutic options, and is familiar with the strengths and limitations of CT and MRI, then a balanced, logical, and consistent approach to the imaging of musculoskeletal metastases can be achieved.

ACKNOWLEDGMENT

We gratefully acknowledge the assistance provided by Mrs. Lois Hebel in preparing this chapter.

REFERENCES

1. Sharafuddin MJA, Sundaram M. The role of magnetic resonance imaging in the diagnosis of soft tissue lesions. CRC Crit Rev Diagn Imaging 35:379-483, 1994.
2. Glockner JF, White LM, Sundaram M, McDonald DJ. Unsuspected metastases presenting as solitary soft tissue lesions: A fourteen-year review. Skeletal Radiol 29:270-274, 2000.
3. Sundaram M, Glockner J. The use of gadolinium in the MR imaging of bone tumors. Semin Ultrasound CT MR 18:307-311, 1997.
4. Igou D, Sundaram M, McDonald DJ, Janney C. Appendicular metastatic prostate cancer simulating osteosarcoma, Paget's disease, and Paget's sarcoma. Skeletal Radiol 24:447-449, 1995.
5. Cooper KL, Beabout JW, Swee RG. Insufficiency fractures of the sacrum. Radiology 156:15-20, 1995.
6. Davies AM, Evans NS, Struthers GR. Parasymphyseal and associated insufficiency fractures of the pelvis and sacrum. Br J Radiol 61:103-108, 1988.

Radiopharmaceutical Imaging

Scott B. Perlman, M.D.

Skeletal Scintigraphy
Positron Emission Tomography
Gallium Scintigraphy
Lymphoscintigraphy
Thyroid Cancer Imaging
Antibody and Peptide Imaging
    Scintigraphy for Staging Cases of Prostate Cancer
    Somatostatin Receptor Scintigraphy
    Metaiodobenzylguanidine

Many of the imaging modalities and techniques that identify metastatic disease rely on the direct identification of a tumor or of anatomic changes that occur in adjacent tissue as a result of metastasis. Radiopharmaceutical imaging identifies the metastasis or the physiologic response that occurs as a result of the metastatic disease. These radiopharmaceutical techniques are unique in that they identify the increased blood flow, increased metabolism, tumor receptor sites, or other physiologic characteristics of the tumor. This chapter will discuss the various physiologic imaging methods available in clinical nuclear medicine for the identification of metastatic disease.

SKELETAL SCINTIGRAPHY

Skeletal scintigraphy uses diphosphonates, such as methylene diphosphonate, labeled with technetium 99m. These radiopharmaceuticals are rapidly incorporated into the newly developed hydroxyapatite crystal matrix. This technique identifies new bone formation and thus is a sensitive method of identifying metastatic disease to the skeleton.

The technique is sensitive, and small metastases can be detected if there is an active skeletal remodeling response, because it is this osteoblastic response, not the actual tumor, that is usually identified on the scan. A patient with a purely osteolytic skeletal response to a bone metastasis may have normal bone scan findings if no active osteoblastic healing response to the metastasis is present. A photopenic "cold" skeletal defect can sometimes be seen, representing bone destruction, although this is often difficult to appreciate.

The technique is straightforward. The patient is given the radiopharmaceutical intravenously and is asked to drink extra fluids (approximately four 8-ounce glasses) within the next few hours to help clear the soft tissues and urinary system of the radiopharmaceutical. Approximately 3 hours after injection, imaging is performed. A whole body planar bone scan is acquired, including anterior and posterior views of the skeleton, with approximately 20 to 30 minutes of imaging time needed to complete the process.

The planar images are relatively quick to acquire, but determining the depth and exact location of a lesion may be difficult and can only be estimated from these images. In some circumstances the exact location of a lesion will help determine whether an area of increased uptake is due to a benign finding, such as degenerative disease or metastatic disease. Furthermore, if one wishes to correlate the bone scan with an anatomic imaging modality such as computed tomography (CT), then more precise location of an abnormal bone scan finding is necessary. In these circumstances, additional imaging using single-photon emission computed tomography (SPECT) will allow better localization of the radioactivity signal. The addition of the SPECT technique does not require a second dose of radiopharmaceutical and involves acquiring an additional set of images with a rotating gamma camera. These SPECT images can then be viewed in any plane, typically the coronal, sagittal, and transaxial planes. Even-Sapir et al.[1] demonstrated that 83% of lesions showing uptake in the body and pedicle were metastatic disease, whereas benign disease was usually present if uptake was abnormal in the vertebral body and posterior elements but was normal in the pedicle (Figs. 7-1 and 7-2).

The high sensitivity of the bone scan for the detection of areas of increased bone turnover leads to the identification of many benign processes, such as common degenerative disease, that also demonstrate increased uptake of the radiopharmaceutical, although usually to a mild degree. Image interpretation therefore requires the use of pattern recognition, intensity of lesion uptake, and location to determine whether the finding may be due to metastatic disease. The typical appearance of metastatic disease consists of multiple focal areas of significantly increased radiopharmaceutical uptake scattered throughout the skeleton (see Fig. 7-2). The distribution of the metastatic lesions often follows the red marrow in the bone, because of the increased blood flow to this region. This fact can be of great help when determining the etiology of a "superscan," which indicates extensive widespread increased radiopharmaceutical uptake throughout the skeleton and an increased ratio of bone to soft tissue (Fig. 7-3). If the entire axial and appendicular skeleton demonstrates this pattern, then metabolic bone disease, which may occur in disorders such as hyperthyroidism, hyperparathyroidism, and systemic mastocytosis, should be considered. If the increased uptake predominantly involves the

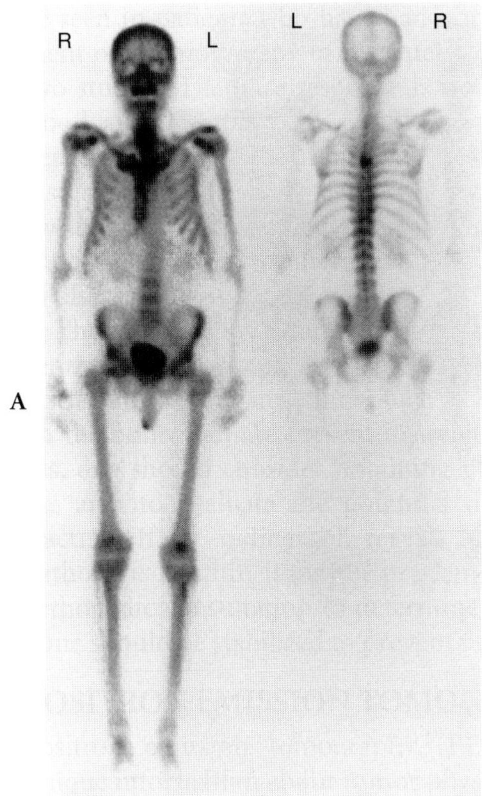

Fig. 7-1   **A,** Whole-body bone scan of elderly man with prostate cancer. The examination is performed to rule out metastatic disease. A solitary focal abnormality is present at the T5 level, which may be due to metastatic disease, trauma, or degenerative changes. **B,** Four transaxial planes of the thoracic spine at the level of T5 from the SPECT bone scan of the patient shown in **A.** The SPECT scan demonstrates that the abnormal area initially identified on the planar images involves the left side of the vertebral body and the left pedicle. Thus the bone scan finding is likely due to metastatic disease.

axial skeleton, then metastatic disease is the most likely explanation.

These general imaging principles are important to the proper interpretation of the scan. Thus a small area of mildly abnormal uptake in the medial plateau of the tibia in an elderly patient is almost certainly due to degenerative disease, whereas a few focal areas of highly increased radiotracer accumulation in the vertebral bodies and humeral and femoral diaphyses in a young woman with breast cancer is most likely due to metastatic disease. Furthermore, a finding of three ribs with contiguous, small focal areas of abnormal radiotracer accumulation is common in rib trauma, but a single rib with a long linear area of involvement should make one suspect that a metastatic lesion or local invasion by tumor is present (Fig. 7-4).

Correlation with plain radiographs is often helpful. The radiographs may demonstrate arthritic changes in a joint in the same location as the finding on the bone scan, reinforcing the diagnosis of arthritis. However, radiographs with normal findings in the location of abnormalities on a bone scan

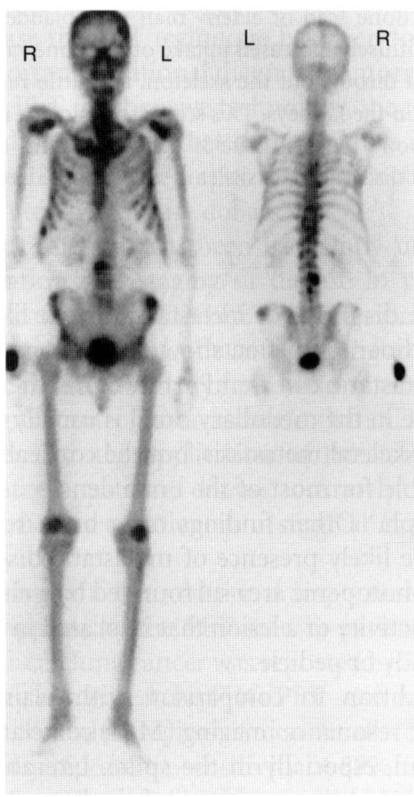

Fig. 7-2   Follow-up bone scan of patient shown in Fig. 7-1. The scan now demonstrates multiple skeletal metastases.

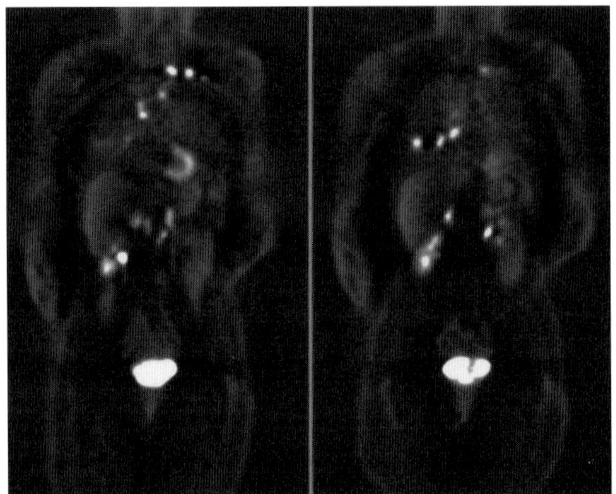

Fig. 7-5   FDG PET scan of patient with non-small-cell lung cancer. The two coronal images of the chest, abdomen, and pelvis demonstrate multiple areas of increased FDG uptake consistent with metastatic disease in the chest and abdomen. The heart, kidneys, and bladder are also seen, consistent with normal myocardial uptake and normal renal excretion of the radiopharmaceutical.

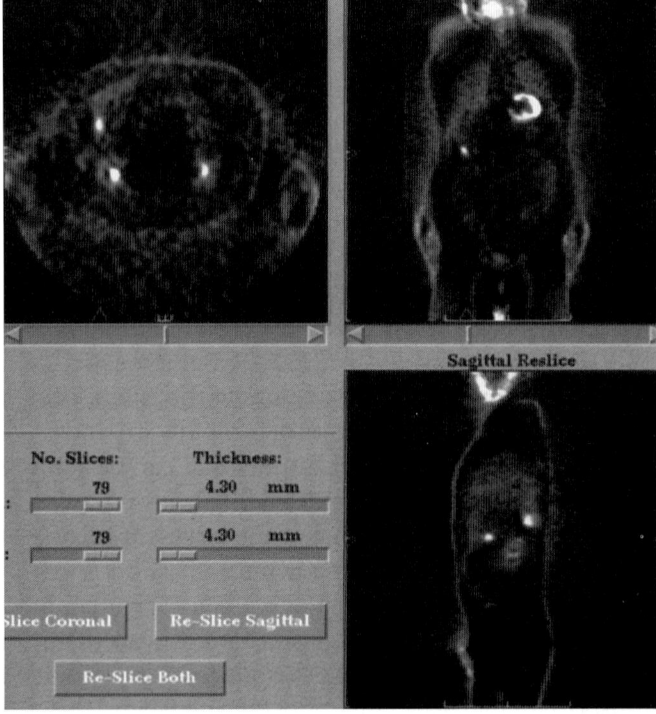

Fig. 7-6   FDG PET scan of patient with colon cancer. Transaxial, coronal, and sagittal planes are shown, demonstrating the small hypermetabolic metastasis in the inferior aspect of the liver anterior to the right renal pelvis. Normal myocardial uptake and normal FDG excretion into the renal pelvis are also present.

ings have been reported by others using PET imaging to stage cases of lung cancer.[9-12]

PET imaging has also been found to be useful for patients with colorectal carcinoma. The PET technique is often able to identify unsuspected metastatic disease,[13] which is important in the selection of patients who may benefit from hepatic resection or cryosurgery of the liver metastases (Fig. 7-6). In a series of 24 patients with suspected colorectal cancer recurrence in the liver, Vitola et al.[14] demonstrated that the FDG PET scan had a higher accuracy (93%) than either CT or CT portography (both 76%) in the identification of metastatic disease to the liver. The PET scan also altered the surgical plans in 6 (25%) of 24 patients.[14] The PET scan has also been reported to be an accurate way of staging disease in patients with colorectal carcinoma.[15]

A large benefit the PET scan offers is the ability to image the entire body. This is especially important when one is evaluating patients with a malig-

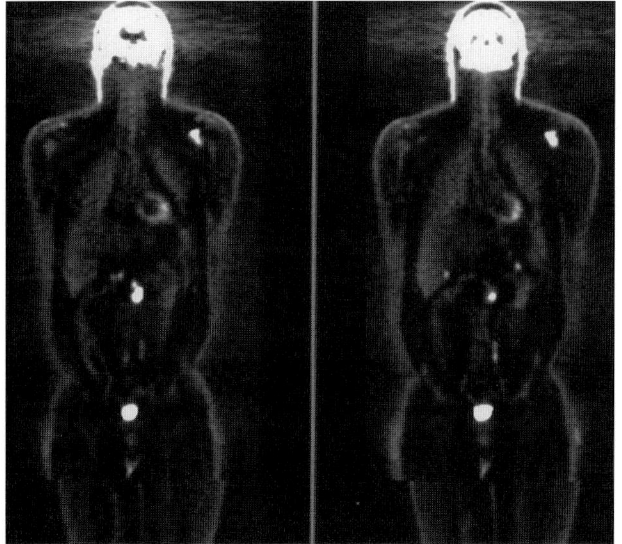

Fig. 7-7   FDG PET scan of patient with a melanoma. Hypermetabolic metastases are present in the left shoulder and abdomen. Normal FDG uptake is present in the brain, and normal urinary excretion is noted in the bladder.

nant melanoma (Fig. 7-7). FDG PET imaging is an accurate method of staging disease in these patients and can accurately identify metastatic disease in lymph nodes.[16,17]

Other PET radiopharmaceuticals used for the evaluation of metastatic disease include the evaluation of the use of the amino acid analog C-11-methionine and the evaluation of tumor hypoxia by using F-18-fluoromisonidazole.[18-20] Radiopharmaceuticals such as these show much promise but at this time are still used mainly for investigational purposes.

A current limitation of positron tomography is that the PET system is relatively expensive, and most of the PET scanners are located in large hospitals and medical centers. An exciting development that will make the PET technology available to smaller hospitals is the recent development of gamma cameras, which can also perform coincidence imaging with the PET radiopharmaceuticals. These cameras do not have the high degree of sensitivity and resolution of dedicated PET systems,[21] but they are significantly less expensive and have the ability to perform general nuclear medicine imaging, including SPECT imaging and coincidence PET imaging. Thus the imaging departments that cannot afford dedicated PET systems can still have access to this technology. Investigations and comparisons currently under way have demonstrated that these gamma camera systems can reliably image sites of metabolic primary tumor and metastatic disease, although it is still not clear which patients should be examined with a dedicated PET system vs. the gamma camera hybrid system.

GALLIUM SCINTIGRAPHY

The mechanism of gallium uptake into tumor cells is not well understood. Gallium 67 binds to transferrin in the blood and is transported into the cell, where it binds to iron-binding proteins such as lactoferrin and ferritin, found in increased concentration in tumors. Intracellular localization of the radiotracer is in the lysosomes of tumor cells.[22]

Gallium-67 imaging has been used for a number of years to stage Hodgkin's and non-Hodgkin's lymphoma (Fig. 7-8). One of the most frequent indications is whether a mass present after therapy represents active disease vs. scar tissue. A mass present on palpation or CT examination that had gallium uptake before treatment and is now absent from the gallium scan is likely scar tissue. A recent review lists a sensitivity of gallium imaging of 76% to 100% and a specificity of 75% to 96% for the determination of residual cancer vs. fibrosis and necrosis.[23] Gallium has also been used to evaluate a patient's treatment response early in the course of chemotherapy. A positive finding that becomes negative early in the course of therapy predicts a favorable treatment response. Front et al.[24] reported

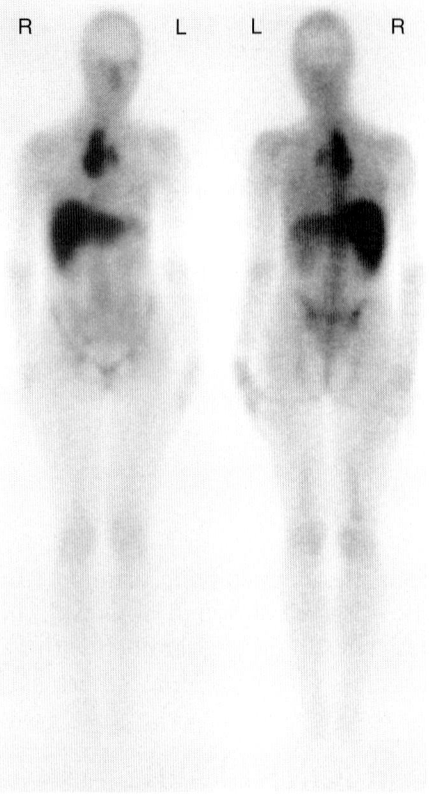

Fig. 7-8 Gallium scan of 29-year-old patient with Hodgkin's disease. The examination was performed 72 hours after injection of the gallium. Note the increased gallium uptake into the known anterior mediastinal mass, consistent with active tumor.

that, in patients with Hodgkin's disease and non-Hodgkin's lymphoma, positive results on a gallium scan, followed by negative results after treatment, accurately predicted disease-free survival, whereas positive gallium scan findings that continued after treatment predicted disease recurrence or failure to achieve remission.

LYMPHOSCINTIGRAPHY

Lymphoscintigraphy is used for the identification of the sentinel lymph node to determine whether a malignant tumor has spread via the lymphatic channels. The procedure is based on the idea that the nearest lymph node that drains the area of the primary malignancy is likely to have tumor in it if there has been lymphatic spread of the tumor. Thus the lymph node that is the closest to the primary tumor, the sentinel lymph node, holds important information about tumor spread. The development of small hand-held probes is a great help to the surgeon, who can search for the area of radioactivity while at surgery to identify the sentinel lymph node. It is best used as an addition to the gamma camera technique, which can readily determine whether there is an unusual pattern of lymph node drainage that would be difficult to identify with a hand-held probe. However, after the gamma camera has located the sentinel lymph node, the probe can serve as an excellent method of locating the lymph node during surgery.

The procedure is used most commonly for patients with breast cancer or a melanoma to determine the lymph node drainage pattern. However, this technique can be used whenever the lymph node drainage pattern is questioned.

This procedure involves the administration of a form of Tc-99m–labeled sulfur colloid, which is fil-

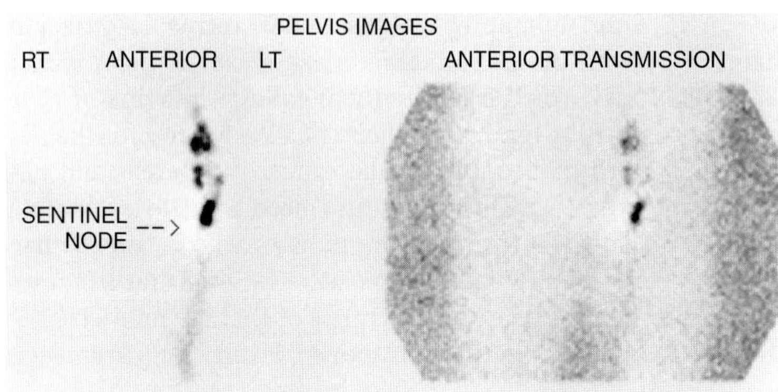

Fig. 7-9 Radionuclide lymphoscintigram of patient with a Merkel's cell tumor of the left calf. The examination identified the lymph channels draining the area. There appear to be two lymph nodes identified in the groin, each of which may represent a sentinel lymph node.

tered to allow the administration of smaller-sized radiopharmaceutical particles. Injections are made around the periphery of the lesion (intradermal in the case of a melanoma), and gamma camera imaging is performed for a period of up to 2 to 3 hours. The location of the sentinel lymph node is marked on the skin with ink before surgery. The excised sentinel lymph node can then be carefully examined by a pathologist to determine whether metastatic disease is present (Fig. 7-9).

THYROID CANCER IMAGING

Well-differentiated thyroid cancers will often organify iodine, similar to normal thyroid tissue. Therefore the administration of radioactive iodine 131 can be helpful in staging a differentiated thy-

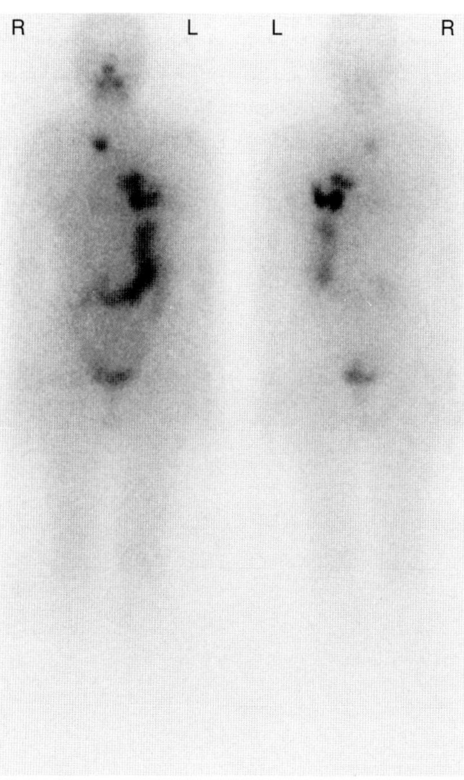

Fig. 7-10   Metastatic survey of elderly woman with a papillary thyroid cancer. The anterior and posterior planar images demonstrate iodine-131 uptake into metastases in the right clavicle and in multiple areas of the left lung. The metastases take up and organify the radioactive iodine. Therefore this patient can be treated with a higher dose of radioactive ^{131}I than the dose used for the diagnostic scan. Note normal uptake into the nasopharyngeal area and normal excretion into the bowel and bladder.

roid cancer. The typical protocol involves cessation of replacement thyroid hormone after thyroidectomy. The thyrotropin level is allowed to rise, and after it is significantly elevated, radioactive iodine 131 is administered orally. Imaging is performed 2 to 3 days later to look for evidence of residual thyroid activity in the thyroid bed and evidence of metastatic disease. Identification of abnormal activity may indicate surgery for removal of metastatic tumor, such as tumor in a lymph node. It may also indicate administration of a therapeutic dose of radioactive iodine 131 in many cases. The metastatic survey is also an important part of the follow-up of these patients and should be performed at regular intervals or as part of the search for metastatic disease in a patient with an elevated serum thyroglobulin level (Fig. 7-10).

ANTIBODY AND PEPTIDE IMAGING
Scintigraphy for Staging Cases of Prostate Cancer

In-111-capromab pendetide is a murine monoclonal antibody that is targeted against prostate-specific membrane antigen (PSA). In patients with prostate cancer, this radiolabeled monoclonal antibody imaging procedure is performed before local therapy to determine whether metastatic disease is present and to evaluate those patients who are thought, because of indicators such as a rising PSA level after prostatectomy, to have metastatic disease. It has been suggested that the scan is best used in patients with a moderate to high probability of extraprostatic disease, as determined by an elevated serum PSA level, high Gleason grade, or advanced clinical stage[25] (Fig. 7-11).

Hinkle et al.[26] reported that the In-111-capromab pendetide scan had an accuracy of 81% for the detection of extraprostatic disease in patients with prostate cancer, compared with CT, MRI, and ultrasonography, which had a combined accuracy of 48% for extraprostatic disease detection. The scan detected occult disease in more than 50% of patients with prostate carcinoma who were studied and provided important information about lymph node involvement with metastatic disease.[26]

The scan has also been shown to have important predictive ability in patients in whom radical prostatectomy has failed. Kahn et al.[27] demonstrated that men with prostate cancer, radical prostatectomy failure, and negative findings on In-111-capro-

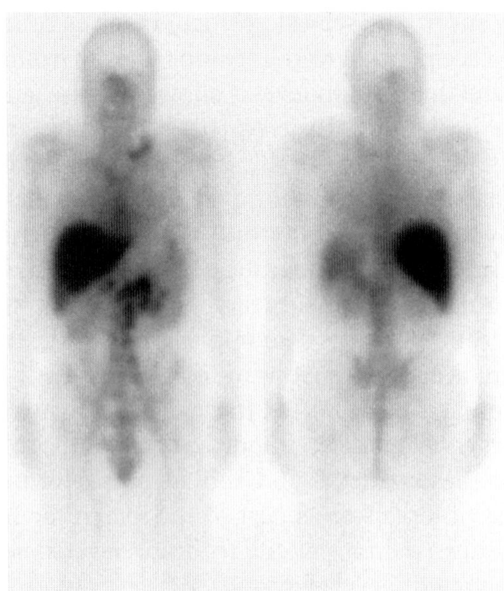

Fig. 7-11 Scintigraphic examination of patient with prostate cancer, after prostatectomy (prostate-specific antigen, a PSA 0.3). Anterior and posterior planar images demonstrate involvement of multiple lymph nodes in the abdomen and uptake into lymph nodes in the left supraclavicular region.

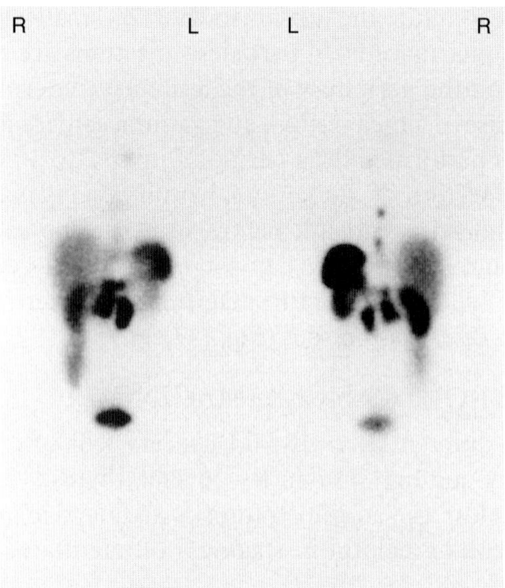

Fig. 7-12 Anterior and posterior planar images of an indium 111 octreotide scan of patient with a gastrinoma and an increased serum gastrin level. Note abnormal uptake in the thoracic spine and in the midline of the abdomen, consistent with metastatic disease. Normal liver, spleen, colon, renal, and bladder activity are seen.

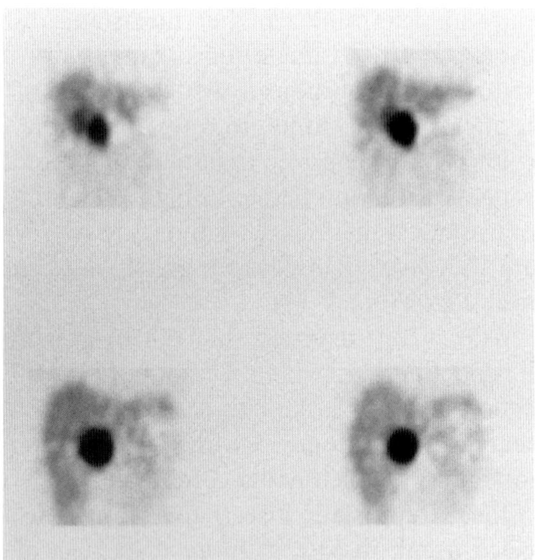

Fig. 7-13 Indium 111 octreotide scan of woman with a pancreatic mass. Coronal images of the SPECT examination demonstrate significant uptake into the mass and no evidence of metastatic disease. At surgery, a neuroendocrine tumor of the pancreas was found, consistent with an islet cell tumor. No tumor was found in the lymph nodes at surgery.

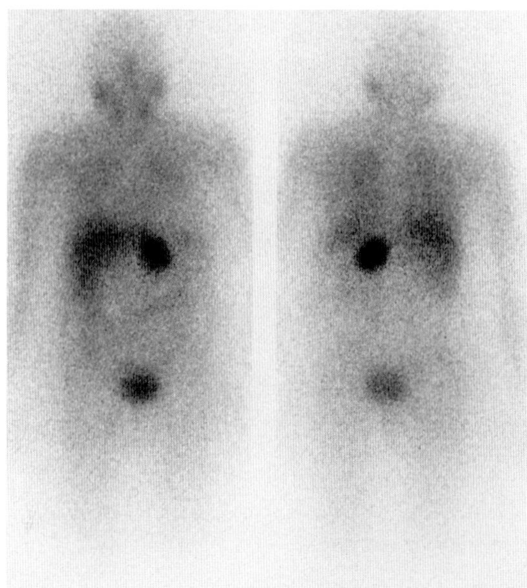

Fig. 7-14 Patient with long-standing hypertension and a left adrenal mass. The patient also has an increase in catecholamine and metabolite levels. The MIBG scan (anterior and posterior planar images) demonstrates highly increased uptake into the left adrenal mass. At surgery the tumor was found to be a pheochromocytoma. Normal uptake in many areas, including the liver, colon, and bladder, is present.

mab scan outside the pelvis were more likely to have a complete durable PSA response after salvage radiotherapy than men with positive findings on a scan outside the pelvis.

Somatostatin Receptor Scintigraphy

Octreotide, an eight-amino-acid fragment of somatostatin, can readily be labeled with indium 111. This radiopharmaceutical identifies somatostatin receptors and has proved to be accurate in imaging various tumors of neuroendocrine origin including carcinoid tumors, pheochromocytomas, gastrinomas, insulinomas, medullary carcinomas of the thyroid, and patients with small-cell lung cancer (Figs. 7-12 and 7-13).

A major advantage of this imaging technique is that the entire body can be imaged for evidence of metastatic disease. This was shown to be important in imaging patients with neuroendocrine tumors, and 50% of patients in one investigation had previously unexpected lesions detected.[28] In a European multicenter trial, the octreotide scan often was also found to demonstrate more tumor sites than conventional imaging. Furthermore, the octreotide scan often affected patient management, including surgical decisions, and provided important information about therapy with octreotide.[29] Although the radiopharmaceutical is expensive, the procedure is cost-effective if used appropriately.[30]

Metaiodobenzylguanidine

Radiopharmaceutical imaging using metaiodobenzylguanidine (MIBG) labeled with iodine 131 is useful for the identification of the primary tumor and metastatic disease in patients with pheochromocytoma,[31] neuroblastoma,[31] or functioning paraganglioma.[32] MIBG is concentrated in the sympathomedullary system present in the adrenal medulla, neurons, and other neuroendocrine tissues. The radiopharmaceutical is sequestered in neurosecretory granules[31] (Fig. 7-14).

In addition to the imaging procedures described, a number of new and promising antibodies, antibody fragments, and peptides have either recently been approved or are under investigation for the evaluation of metastatic disease. The U.S. Food and Drug Administration (FDA) recently has approved arcitumomab, a Fab′ antibody fragment labeled with technetium 99m. This radiopharmaceutical targets the colorectal cancer tumor marker carci-

noembryonic antigen and has shown good results in identifying metastatic disease in patients with colorectal cancer.[33] Another Fab antibody fragment labeled with technetium 99m, nofetumomab merpentan (Verluma, NeoRx Corp., Seattle, Wash.), has recently been approved by the FDA. This agent has been shown to stage disease accurately in patients with small-cell and non-small-cell lung cancer.[33,34] These new radiopharmaceuticals will certainly play an increasing role in the diagnostic evaluation of patients with cancer.

In summary, radiopharmaceutical imaging of metastatic disease has become an important part of the initial evaluation and follow-up of patients with malignancy. The standard procedures described and the exciting new techniques will help physicians and their patients make important therapeutic decisions.

REFERENCES

1. Even-Sapir E, Martin RH, Barnes DC, Pringle CR, Iles SE, Mitchell MJ. Role of SPECT in differentiating malignant from benign lesions in the lower thoracic and lumbar vertebrae. Radiology 187:193-198, 1993.
2. Jacobsen AF, Stomper PC, Cronin EB, Kaplan WD. Bone scans with one or two new abnormalities in cancer patients with no known metastases: Reliability of interpretation on initial correlative radiographs. Radiology 174:503-507, 1990.
3. Gold RI, Seeger LL, Bassett LW, Steckel RJ. An integrated approach to the evaluation of metastatic bone disease. Radiol Clin North Am 28:471-483, 1990.
4. Frank JA, Ling A, Patronas NJ, Carrasquillo JA, Horvath K, Hickey AM, Dwyer AJ. Detection of malignant bone tumors: MR imaging vs scintigraphy. AJR Am J Roentgenol 155:1043-1048, 1990.
5. Gosfield E III, Alavi A, Kneeland B. Comparison of radionuclide bone scans and magnetic resonance imaging in detecting spinal metastases. J Nucl Med 34:2191-2198, 1993.
6. Coleman RE, Mashiter G, Whitaker KB, Moss DW, Rubens RD, Fogelman I. Bone scan flare predicts successful systemic therapy for bone metastases. J Nucl Med 29:1354-1359, 1988.
7. Huang S, Phelps ME. Principles of tracer kinetic modeling in positron emission tomography and autoradiography. In Phelps ME, Mazziotta JC, Schelbert HR, eds. Positron Emission Tomography and Autoradiography. New York: Raven Press, 1986, p 300.
8. Steinert HC, Hauser M, Allemann F, Engel H, Berthold T, von Schulthess GK, Weder W. Non-small cell lung cancer: Nodal staging with FDG PET versus CT with correlative lymph node mapping and sampling. Radiology 202:441-446, 1997.
9. Sazon DAD, Santiago SM, Hoo GWS, Khonsary A, Brown C, Mandelkern M, Blahd W, Williams AJ. Fluorodeoxyglucose–positron emission tomography in the detection and staging of lung cancer. Am J Respir Crit Care Med 153:417-421, 1996.

10. Valk PE, Pounds TR, Hopkins DM, Haseman MK, Hofer GA, Greiss HB, Myers RW, Lutrin CL. Staging non-small cell lung cancer by whole-body positron emission tomography imaging. Ann Thorac Surg 60:1573-1582, 1995.

11. Sasaki M, Ichiya Y, Kuwabara Y, Akashi Y, Yoshida T, Fukumura T, Murayama S, Ishida T, Sugio K, Masuda K. The usefulness of FDG positron emission tomography for the detection of mediastinal lymph node metastases in patients with non-small cell lung cancer: A comparative study with x-ray computed tomography. Eur J Nucl Med 23:741-747, 1996.

12. Patz EF Jr, Lowe VJ, Goodman PC, Herndon J. Thoracic nodal staging with PET imaging with 18FDG in patients with bronchogenic carcinoma. Chest 108:1617-1621, 1995.

13. Lai DT, Fulham M, Stephen MS, Chu KM, Solomon M, Thompson JF, Sheldon DM, Storey DW. The role of whole-body positron emission tomography with [18F]fluorodeoxyglucose in identifying operable colorectal cancer metastases to the liver. Arch Surg 131:703-707, 1996.

14. Vitola JV, Delbeke D, Sandler MP, Campbell MG, Powers TA, Wright K, Chapman WC, Pinson CW. Positron emission tomography to stage suspected metastatic colorectal carcinoma to the liver. Am J Surg 171:21-26, 1996.

15. Abdel-Nabi H, Doerr RJ, Lamonica DM, Cronin VR, Galantowicz PJ, Carbone GM, Spaulding MB. Staging of primary colorectal carcinomas with fluorine-18 fluorodeoxyglucose whole-body PET: Correlation with histopathologic and CT findings. Radiology 206:755-760, 1998.

16. Steinert HC, Huch Boni RA, Buck A, Boni R, Berthold T, Marincek B, Burg G, von Schulthess GK. Malignant melanoma: Staging with whole-body positron emission tomography and 2-[F-18]-fluoro-2-deoxy-D-glucose. Radiology 195:705-709, 1995.

17. Wagner JD, Schauwecker D, Hutchins G, Coleman JJ III. Initial assessment of positron emission tomography for detection of nonpalpable regional lymphatic metastases in melanoma. J Surg Oncol 64:181-189, 1997.

18. Nettelbladt OS, Sundin AE, Valind SO, Gustafsson GR, Lamberg K, Langstrom B, Bjornsson EH. Combined fluorine-18-FDG and carbon-11-methionine PET for diagnosis of tumors in lung and mediastinum. J Nucl Med 39:640-647, 1998.

19. Leskinen-Kallio S, Huovinen R, Nagren K, Lehikoinen P, Ruotsalainen U, Teras M, Joensuu H. [C-11]Methionine quantitation in cancer PET studies. J Comput Assist Tomogr 16:468-474, 1992.

20. Valk PE, Mathis CA, Prados MD, Gilbert JC, Budinger TF. Hypoxia in human gliomas: Demonstration by PET with fluorine-18-fluoromisonidazole. J Nucl Med 33:2133-2137, 1992.

21. Coleman RE, Laymon CM, Turkington TG. FDG imaging of lung nodules: A phantom study comparing SPECT, camera-based PET, and dedicated PET. Radiology 210:823-828, 1999.

22. Thrall JH, Ziessman HA. Tumors. In Thrall JH, Ziessman HA, eds. Nuclear Medicine: The Requisites. St. Louis: Mosby, 1995, p 173.

23. Front D, Bar-Shalom R, Israel O. The continuing clinical role of gallium-67 scintigraphy in the age of receptor imaging. Semin Nucl Med 27(1):68-74, 1997.

24. Front D, Ben-Haim S, Israel O, Epelbaum R, Haim N, Even-Sapir E, Kolodny G, Robinson E. Lymphoma: Predictive value of Ga-67 scintigraphy after treatment. Radiology 182:359-363, 1992.

25. Polascik TJ, Manyak MJ, Haseman MK, Gurganus RT, Rogers B, Maguire RT, Partin AW. Comparison of clinical staging algorithms and 111indium-capromab pendetide immunoscintigraphy in the prediction of lymph node involvement in high-risk prostate carcinoma patients. Cancer 85:1586-1592, 1999.

26. Hinkle GH, Burgers JK, Neal CE, Texter JH, Kahn D, Williams RD, Maguire R, Rogers B, Olsen JO, Badalament RA. Multicenter radioimmunoscintigraphic evaluation of patients with prostate carcinoma using indium-111 capromab pendetide. Cancer 83:739-747, 1998.

27. Kahn D, Williams RD, Haseman MK, Reed NL, Miller SJ, Gerstbrein J. Radioimmunoscintigraphy with In-111-labeled capromab pendetide predicts prostate cancer response to salvage radiotherapy after failed radical prostatectomy. J Clin Oncol 16(1):284-289, 1998.

28. Shi W, Johnston CF, Buchanan KD, Ferguson WR, Laird JD, Crothers JG, McIlrath EM. Localization of neuroendocrine tumours with [111In]DTPA-octreotide scintigraphy (Octreoscan): A comparative study with CT and MR imaging. QJM 91:295-301, 1998.

29. Krenning EP, Kooij PP, Pauwels S, Breeman WA, Postema PT, DeHerder WW, Valkema R, Kwekkeboom DJ. Somatostatin receptor: Scintigraphy and radionuclide therapy. Digestion 57(Suppl 1):57-61, 1996.

30. Kwekkeboom DJ, Lamberts SW, Habbema JD, Krenning EP. Cost-effectiveness analysis of somatostatin receptor scintigraphy. J Nucl Med 37:886-892, 1996.

31. Freitas JE. Adrenal cortical and medullary imaging. Semin Nucl Med 25:235-250, 1995.

32. Maurea S, Cuocolo A, Reynolds JC, Tumeh SS, Begley MG, Linehan WM, Norton JA, Walther MM, Keiser HR, Neumann RD. Iodine-131—metaiodobenzylguanidine scintigraphy in preoperative and postoperative evaluation of paragangliomas: Comparison with CT and MRI. J Nucl Med 34:173-179, 1993.

33. Zuckier LS, DeNardo GL. Trials and tribulations: Oncological antibody imaging comes to the fore. Semin Nucl Med 27:10-29, 1997.

34. Breitz HB, Sullivan K, Nelp WB. Imaging lung cancer with radiolabeled antibodies. Semin Nucl Med 28:127-132, 1993.

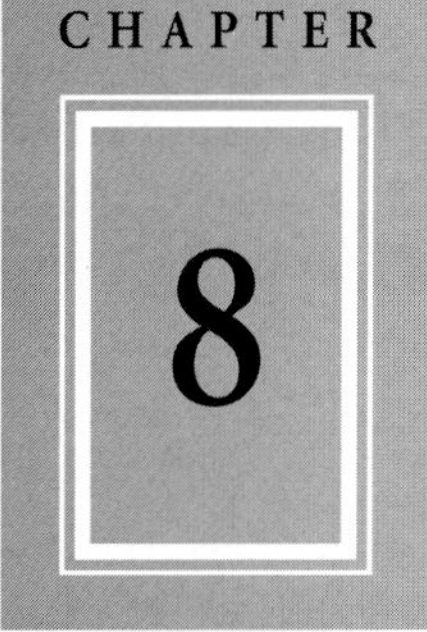

Interventional Radiology

John C. McDermott, M.D.

The interventional radiologist can assist the clinician and orthopedic surgeon in performing image-guided biopsy of various skeletal lesions to arrive at a diagnosis of a primary bone tumor or metastatic disease. The interventionist can also assist in performing embolization of vascular osseous metastatic lesions before orthopedic fixation with the hope of reducing perioperative blood loss. Finally, he or she can inject alcohol percutaneously to reduce the pain associated with osseous metastases or inject methylmethacrylate to stabilize lesions and thus lessen pain or prevent collapse.

PERCUTANEOUS SKELETAL BIOPSY
Historical Perspectives

Martin and Ellis,[1] in 1930, reported the first series of technically successful percutaneous bone biopsies. In their series, percutaneous aspiration biopsy was performed on eight musculoskeletal lesions. In this study an 18-gauge needle was employed for biopsy of both primary bone tumors and bone metastases. In 1945 the same group published their series of 567 skeletal aspiration biopsies with an accuracy rate of 82%.[1,2] In the ensuing 50 years, there has been marked improvement in fluoroscopic systems and the arrival of computed tomography (CT). These sophisticated advances in imaging guidance have increased the number of osseous lesions that can be safely approached.

In tandem with the revolution in imaging, there have been technical improvements in the biopsy needles. A prototype drill for bone biopsy that provided a larger sample was introduced by Martin and Ellis.[1] This prototype subsequently led to a commercially available biopsy drill that can be used in obtaining an osseous core for diagnosis or employed for percutaneous removal and ablation of an osteoid osteoma. Ackerman[3] developed a trephinated needle for cutting through lesions with intact cortex. This needle was later improved on by Craig,[4] who increased the inner diameter of the trephine and thus increased the diameter of obtainable osseous material from 1.5 to 3.5 mm.[5]

Open Surgical Biopsy vs. Percutaneous Imaging-Guided Biopsy

Percutaneous imaging-guided biopsy of skeletal lesions offers certain advantages over surgical biopsy.

The trauma to both normal and neoplastic tissue is reduced. The damage to the structural integrity of the bone is reduced. The risk of tumor cell dissemination may be decreased. The cost of percutaneous biopsy is less, and general anesthesia is not needed (with the exception of a biopsy in the pediatric population). If an insufficient amount of tissue is obtained, an open surgical biopsy can still be performed.

Yet the enthusiasm for percutaneous imaging-guided skeletal biopsy must be balanced in the context of diagnosis. The value of closed needle biopsy in the diagnosis of skeletal metastases is the well-accepted standard. However, the use of percutaneous biopsy in the diagnosis of primary bone tumors, with the exception of a solitary plasmacytoma, is controversial at best. In fact, a consensus of many surgical pathologists is that the diagnosis of a primary bone tumor is best obtained by the performance of an open biopsy, with a sizable amount of tissue provided for histologic examination. In primary bone tumors the degree of biologic aggressiveness and cell type can vary across the lesion, thus making diagnosis of a primary bone tumor on the basis of a percutaneous sample subject to error. Furthermore, because most primary bone tumors are treated surgically, the diagnosis is optimally made at the time of surgery by providing a copious amount of tissue for the surgical pathologist. Finally, cartilaginous tumors cannot be graded from the small samples provided by the use of closed biopsy, nor can a definitive subclassification of sarcomatous neoplasms be accomplished with the small amount of tissue provided by the use of percutaneous biopsy.[6]

Indications

The overwhelming use of percutaneous skeletal biopsy is to determine the presence of metastatic disease in the presence of a known primary tumor. Another common indication for biopsy is a lesion suggestive of metastatic disease but without a known primary tumor. The third indication is a vertebral compression fracture when the patient has not taken steroids and has not had a diagnosis of a primary tumor. Here the clinical concern is an occult tumor that has metastasized to the spine. Before undertaking an imaging-guided skeletal biopsy, one should review the pertinent films and discuss the imaging approach with the clinician and pathologist.

Lesion Location and Analysis, With Technical Considerations

Metastatic disease from breast, prostate, kidney, lung, and thyroid account for 80% of metastatic disease to the skeleton. In a recent review of 153 percutaneous bone biopsy specimens by Mink,[7] 138 of 153 lesions were located in the spine, ribs, humeri, femurs, or pelvic bones. Of these sites, 61 were in either the thoracic or lumbar spine.

When a patient is referred to the angiography interventional section for possible biopsy, the relevant imaging studies are reviewed. These include plain films, nuclear medicine bone scans, CT, and magnetic resonance imaging. The lesion is analyzed by anatomic location (i.e., spine, long bones, flat bones) and underlying pathologic change. With respect to pathologic change, the lesion is characterized as lytic or blastic, intact cortex or destroyed cortex, presence or absence of soft tissue extension, and finally, with respect to spinal column lesions, vertebral collapse or not.

The location of the osseous abnormality guides the interventionist in the appropriate choice of imaging guidance. All our percutaneous skeletal biopsies are done either in an angiography suite, which is equipped with a ceiling-mounted C arm that can rotate 180 degrees as well as provide cephalad or caudal angulation, or under CT guidance. Biopsy specimens of lesions located in the extremities and well delineated on plain films are nearly universally obtained under fluoroscopic guidance. Lesions in the spine are approached under either fluoroscopic or CT guidance, depending on the proximity of the lesion to the cord and the presence or absence of cord compression symptoms. Lesions in the pelvis are nearly always approached with CT guidance.

If the lesion is blastic and with an intact cortex, a trephinated needle or Jamshidi needle (produced by Baxter) is used to obtain a satisfactory aliquot of tissue. If the lesion is lytic and with an intact cortex, similarly a trephine or Jamshidi needle is used to gain access to the lytic focus. At this point the stylet is removed and the trephine is advanced through the lytic focus to obtain tissue. Alternatively, a cutting needle such as a Tru-cut or monopty device

can be advanced coaxially through the trephine to obtain tissue from the focus.[8] In situations in which the pathologic process has violated the cortex and extended into the surrounding soft tissue, either a cutting needle or a 21-gauge skinny needle can be used. In the former case a histologic sample is obtained, whereas in the latter an aspiration sample is acquired for cytopathologic examination. In most instances a cytopathologist is on site to make a "touch" preparation for immediate analysis. Some interventionists believe that the use of the beveled nonserrated cutting edge of the Jamshidi needle minimizes damage to the surrounding soft tissue on entry. It is also thought that the beveled and tapered tip limits or reduces the degree of crush artifact on the sample.[9]

Patient Preparation

Before percutaneous biopsy the coagulation factors and platelet count are checked. Bleeding diathesis is considered an absolute contraindication to percutaneous biopsy. Patient cooperation and pain control are the hallmarks of a technically successful procedure. The risks and benefits are discussed in depth with the patient and family. Specific to spinal column biopsy, the potential risks of pneumothorax and paraplegia are discussed. All patients have an intravenous line in place and are monitored by pulse oximetry and blood pressure measurements. Usually the patient receives midazolam and fentanyl as conscious sedation. A copious amount of 1% lidocaine is instilled into the soft tissues before advancement of the biopsy needle; it is imperative that a copious amount of lidocaine or an admixture of lidocaine and bupivacaine be infused into the periosteum before an attempt is made to pierce the cortex. General anesthesia is not routinely employed except in pediatric skeletal biopsies. The patient is monitored for 2 to 4 hours after the procedure and discharged if a complication does not intervene.

Technical Points in Biopsy of the Spine

Percutaneous biopsy of the spine is best discussed in some detail, because the most serious complications (paraplegia, quadriplegia) have occurred after biopsy of the spine. Currently, spinal biopsy is performed under either CT or fluoroscopic guidance (Figs. 8-1 through 8-4). If fluoroscopy is the

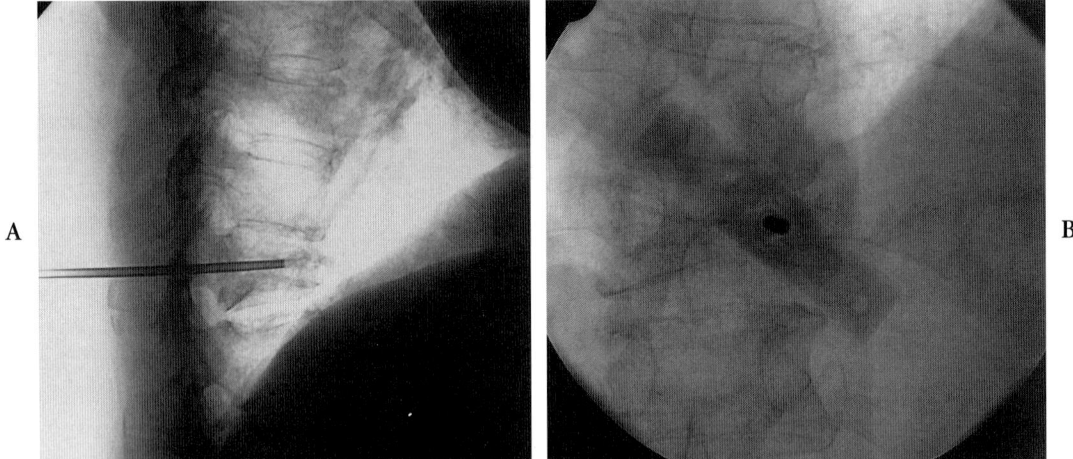

Fig. 8-1   A 71-year-old woman after bilateral mastectomy for adenocarcinoma of both breasts 15 years ago. She has new onset of back pain and a new compression fracture of the T11 vertebra. The clinical concern was metastatic breast cancer versus osteoporotic compression fracture. The patient was placed on the angiography table in the prone position. An 11-gauge Jamshidi biopsy needle was fluoroscopically advanced through the right pedicle of T11 to obtain tissue for histology. **A,** Lateral view; **B,** frontal view. The final pathology report noted normal marrow without metastatic adenocarcinoma.

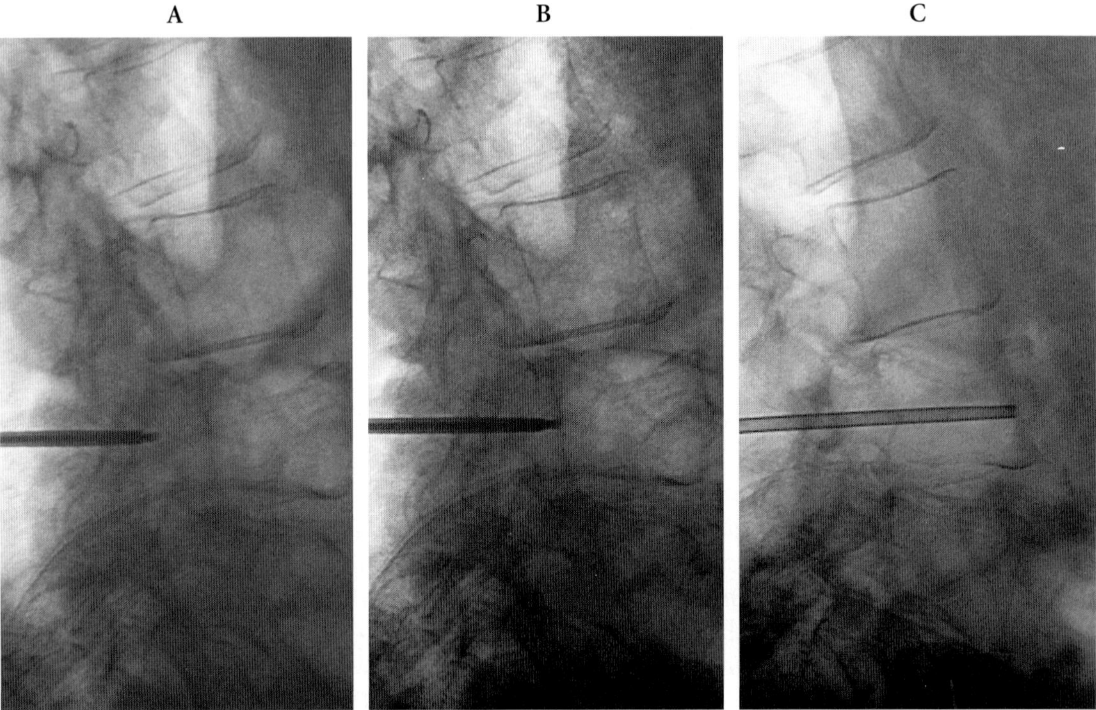

Fig. 8-2   A 66-year-old woman with severe back pain. Plain films of the spine showed a compression fracture of the L4 vertebra. A fluoroscopically guided biopsy of the L4 body was performed with the patient in the prone position. A Jamshidi needle was used. **A,** Needle is advanced to the edge of the cortex. **B,** Needle is advanced through the cortex. **C,** Bone biopsy specimen is obtained with needle. Biopsy result revealed plasmacytoma.

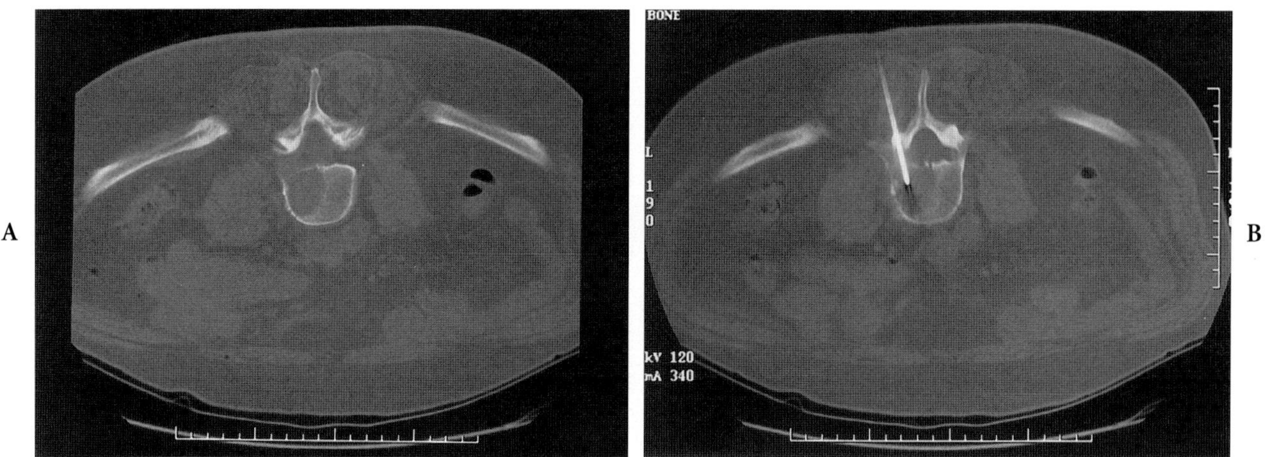

Fig. 8-3 A 75-year-old man with a history of prostate cancer and (**A**) new onset of lower back pain with L4 radiculopathy. **B,** CT-guided biopsy of the lytic lesion in the L4 vertebral body was performed with the patient in the prone position. Again, a Jamshidi needle was used.

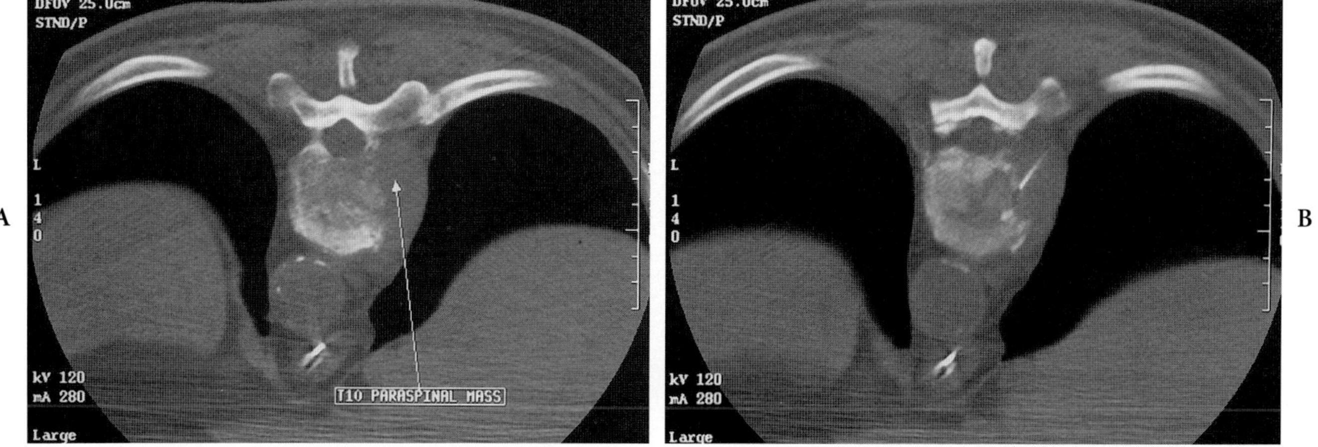

Fig. 8-4 A 66-year-old man with upper back pain. **A,** CT scan demonstrated a destructive lesion with associated paraspinal mass at T10 vertebra. **B,** Fine-needle aspiration biopsy was done with a 22-gauge needle. Cytopathologic results were positive for large cell carcinoma.

imaging method, the patient is placed in the prone oblique position on the angiography table. A spot is measured approximately 5 cm from the midline for a thoracic spine biopsy and 8 cm for biopsy of the lumbar spine. The thoracic spine and disc space can be reached through a "window" created by the heads of the ribs, the lateral margin of the articular processes, and the lateral edge of the vertebral body or disc.[10] Fluoroscopic guidance in both the antero-posterior and lateral projections is necessary for safe entry into the target without broaching the pleural reflection. Alternatively a thoracic spine biopsy can be performed under CT guidance with the patient in the prone position. In this situation a spot 5 cm from the midline is marked and the trephine or Jamshidi needle is advanced through the costovertebral joint and into the vertebral body or disc.[11] Similarly, a transpedicular approach will also allow safe passage into the vertebral body. At our institution, most biopsies of the spine, whether thoracic or lumbar, are performed with CT guidance. In performing thoracic spine biopsies, we routinely administer a copious amount of lidocaine. This not only reduces procedural pain but also increases the thickness of the paravertebral soft tissue, thereby reducing the incidence of pneumothorax during thoracic spine biopsy.[12] At other institutions a pneumothorax on the side of the biopsy is induced to create a larger window to facilitate the biopsy. Before this the results of the patient's pulmonary function tests should be checked to ensure a pneumothorax can be tolerated during the procedure.

Handling of the Specimen

Once the aliquot of tissue has been obtained from the biopsy site, an immediate "touch" preparation of the sample can be performed and analyzed by an on-site cytopathologist for malignant cells. This preparation guides the interventionist in determining the adequacy of the sample and the need for a second or third sample for histopathologic review. It is also important to submit any blood clot for histologic review. The osseous lesion is immediately placed in formalin after the touch preparation. Decalcification of the bone sample is done before histologic study. There is controversy over whether less crush artifact results from a trephinated needle or a Jamshidi needle. If there is clinical concern regarding the presence of osteomyelitis or discitis, or both, a portion of the sample is sent for appropriate stains and culture (e.g., Gram stain; anaerobic, aerobic, and fungal cultures).

Complications

The classic article that best analyzed the complication rate from percutaneous osseous biopsy was by Murphy et al.[5] The overall rate of complication reported in this article was approximately 0.2%. The complications are best segregated into minor and major groups. The minor group includes pain that is often a result of an inadequate amount of lidocaine administration and bleeding that is self-limited. The major complications in most cases result from vertebral column biopsy, particularly in reference to thoracic spine biopsy. The reported major complications after closed spine biopsy include quadriplegia, paraplegia, paraparesis, foot drop because of neural injury, and death. There have been two reported deaths from spinal cord injury during percutaneous spine biopsy. The reported incidence of serious neurologic injury stemming from biopsy was 0.08%. The reported death rate is 0.02%.[5] At our institution we routinely obtain a CT scan, with thin sections through the proposed site of biopsy in the spine, and look for incipient cord compression before biopsy. Another reported major complication has been severe bleeding after closed biopsy of a vascular metastasis to the skeletal system. Such a complication can be managed with either open surgery or embolotherapy. Finally, tumor tract seeding along the chosen approach is a much discussed complication but in our experience exceedingly rare.

Results

An accurate biopsy will answer the clinical question, does the lesion represent a primary bone malignancy, a metastatic focus, or a site of infection? To answer these questions, one must obtain a sufficient amount of material for histologic examination, touch preparation, and culture, depending on clinical context. More tissue is better than less. The on-site availability of a cytopathologist can facilitate the process and reduce the need for additional biopsies. Lesions that are primarily cystic or necrotic may not provide sufficient material for analysis. In this situation a repeated biopsy from the edge of the lesion, where there is solid tissue, will often provide a diagnostic yield. Where osteomyelitis is a concern, antibiotic therapy should be stopped at least 48 hours before the biopsy.

EMBOLOTHERAPY

Metastatic neoplasms tend to possess the same degree of vascularity as the primary tumor. It is well known that renal cell carcinoma, carcinoid, melanoma, and hepatoma are richly vascular neoplasms. Likewise, their metastatic foci are vascular. When such neoplasms metastasize to the skeleton, the interventional radiologist may be called on to embolize the site of osseous metastasis to prevent impending fracture, control pain refractory to radiation therapy and systemic opiates, and reduce blood loss during intraoperative fixation and stabilization[13] (Figs. 8-5 and 8-6).

At our institution we commonly receive referrals for metastatic renal cell carcinoma to the spine, pelvis, femur, and humerus for embolization. Before embolotherapy, the pertinent films are reviewed and the patient is screened for underlying comorbid risk factors (e.g., cardiac or renal disease). The patient's renal function and coagulation profile are checked. A detailed discussion occurs between the patient and the interventional radiologist regarding the procedure and its inherent risks and potential complications. After this discussion, an informed consent is obtained. It is imperative that diagnostic arteriography be performed to detail the major and minor feeders to the metastatic focus. If the patient has compromised renal function, then it is best not to combine both the staging diagnostic arteriogram and embolization in the same setting. The goal of embolization is selectively to engage the feeding vessels to the metastasis and occlude them with a permanent agent such as polyvinyl alcohol. This embolic agent is a particulate agent that comes in a range of particle sizes. Routinely we use polyvinyl alcohol ranging from 300 to 1000 μm. The goal is to obliterate the tumor stains as completely as possible without causing nontarget embolization. To this end, we often use a coaxi-

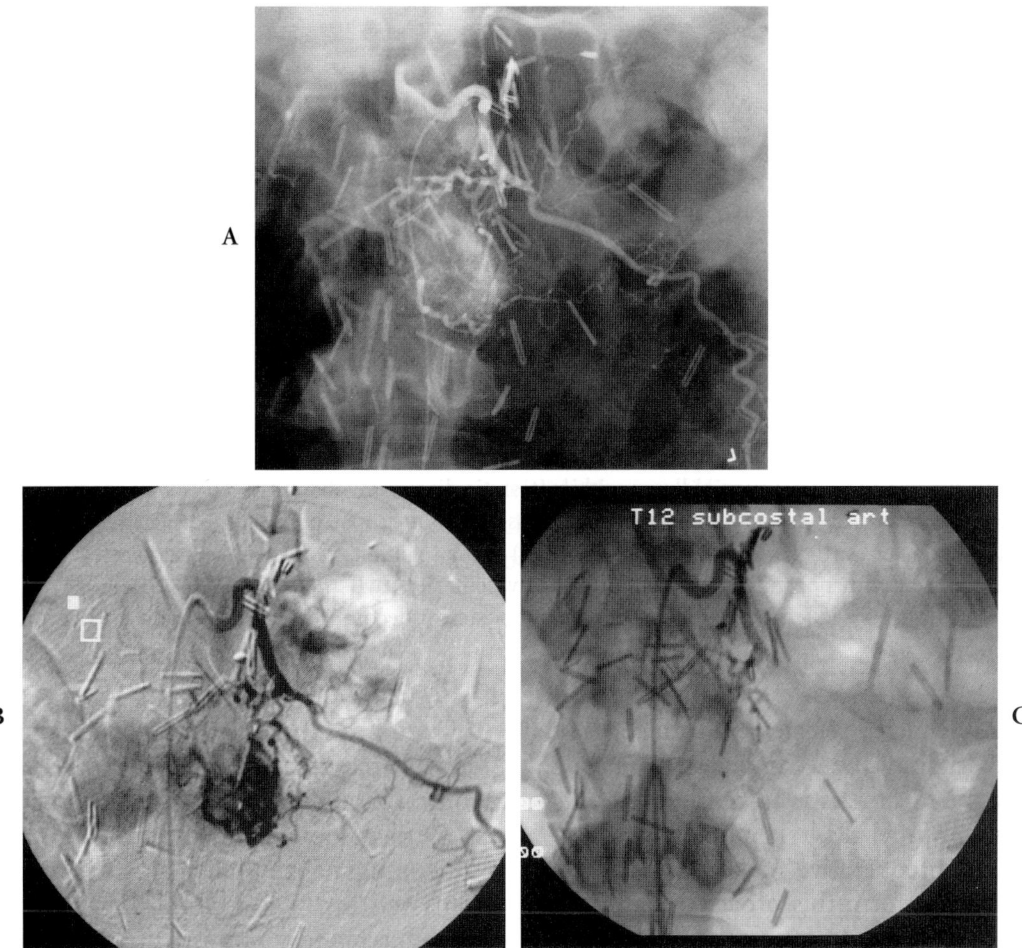

Fig. 8-5   A 59-year-old man with destruction of the left L1 pedicle. Several years ago, a radical nephrectomy for renal cell carcinoma was performed. Note the destroyed left L1 pedicle (**A**) and the hypervascular nature of this lesion in (**B**). This lesion was supplied by the left T-12 intercostal artery (the L1 lumbar artery had been tied off at the time of the radical nephrectomy). **C,** Postembolization film obtained after the lytic lesion was devascularized with microcoils and polyvinyl alcohol before surgical corpectomy.

7. Mink J. Percutaneous bone biopsy in the patient with known or suspected osseous metastases. Radiology 161:191-194, 1986.

8. Cohen MA, Zornoza J, Finkelstein JB. Percutaneous needle biopsy of long bone lesions facilitated by the use of a hand drill. Radiology 139:750-751, 1981.

9. Stoker DJ, Kissin C. Percutaneous vertebral biopsy: A review of 135 cases. Clin Radiol 36:569-577, 1985.

10. Laredo JD, Bard M. Thoracic spine: Percutaneous trephine biopsy. Radiology 160:485-489, 1986.

11. Brugieres PB, Gaston A, Heran F, Voisin MC, Marsault C. Percutaneous biopsies of the thoracic spine under CT guidance: Transcostovertebral approach. J Comput Assist Tomogr 14: 446-448, 1990.

12. Carlson P, Crummy AB, Wojtowycz M, McDermott JC. A safe route for deep pelvic biopsy with distention of the iliac muscle. J Vasc Interv Radiol 2:277-278, 1991.

13. Roscoe MW, McBroon RJ, St Louis E, Grossman H, Perrin R. Preoperative embolization in the treatment of osseous metastases from renal cell carcinoma. Clin Orthop 238:302-307, 1989.

14. Sun S, Lang EV. Bone metastases from renal cell carcinoma: Preoperative embolization. J Vasc Interv Radiol 9:263-269, 1998.

15. Smith TP, Gray L, Weinstein JN, Richardson WJ, Payne CS. Preoperative transarterial embolization of spinal column neoplasms. J Vasc Interv Radiol 6:863-869, 1995.

16. Gangi A, Kastler B, Klinert A, Dietmann JL. Injection of alcohol into bone metastases under CT guidance. J Comput Assist Tomogr 18: 932-935, 1994.

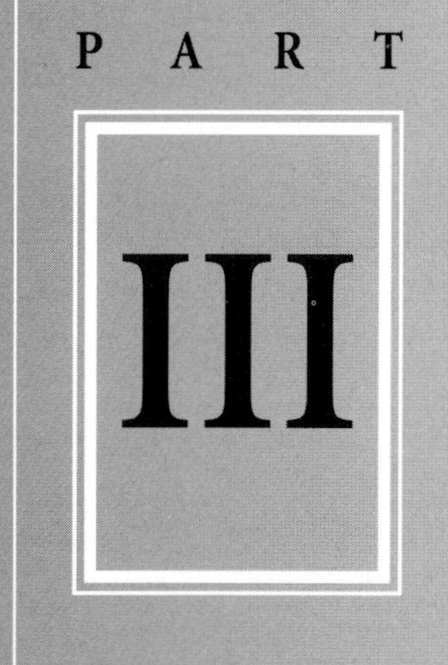

Therapeutic Approaches

Therapy Affecting Bone Resorption and Deposition

Theresa A. Guise, M.D.

Cancer is associated with significant morbidity in the skeleton. This was evident in 1889, when Stephen Paget observed that "in a cancer of the breast the bones suffer in a special way, which cannot be explained by any theory of embolism alone . . . the same thing is seen much more clearly in those cases of cancer of the thyroid body where secondary deposition occurs in the bones with astonishing frequency."[1] He also noted that "a general degradation of the bones sometimes occurs in carcinoma of the breast, yet without any distinct deposition of cancer in them." These early observations were profound, as it is now clear that cancer can involve bone through both metastatic and humoral mechanisms.

Cancer affects bone in several ways: (1) indirectly through elaboration of factors that act systemically on target organs of bone and kidney to disrupt normal calcium homeostasis, (2) locally and directly via secondary spread of tumor to bone, and (3) via direct involvement by primary bone tumors. This chapter focuses on pathophysiology of local involvement of metastatic tumor to bone and current nonsurgical therapy available, other than radiation, that may affect bone resorption and deposition.

The three most common neoplasms in humans—breast, prostate, and lung cancer—frequently affect the skeleton. Since most patients dying of cancer have bone involvement due either to metastatic spread or to the systemic effects of tumor-produced factors on bone and kidney, this is not a trivial problem. To improve therapy and prevention, one must understand the pathophysiology of the effects of cancer on bone, as it will continue to be a source of morbidity for years to come.

NORMAL BONE REMODELING

Bone is unique among target tissues affected by cancer because it is being continually remodeled by systemic hormones and local bone-derived growth factors. Bone consists of two physically and biologically distinctive structures. The outer cortical bone is hard, mineralized matrix in which cellular and metabolic activities are relatively low. Cortical bone makes up 85% of the total bone in the body and is most abundant in the long bones of the appendicular skeleton. The volume of cortical bone is regulated by the formation of periosteal bone, by remodeling within Haversian systems, and by endosteal bone resorption. Cancellous or trabecular bone, which constitutes the remaining 15% of the skeleton, is most abundant in the vertebral bodies. The adult skeleton is in a dynamic state, as the coordinated actions of osteoclasts and osteoblasts on trabecular surfaces and in Haversian systems effect continual bone resorption and formation. The normal mineralization of bone matrix is contingent upon adequate amounts of vitamin D, calcium, and phosphate. The mineralized bone matrix contains abundant amounts of growth factors, chiefly transforming growth factor (TGF)-β and insulinlike growth factor (IGF)-II.[2,3] Such growth factors are released from the bone matrix as a result of osteoclastic bone resorption,[4] a step in the normal remodeling process necessary to maintain the structural integrity of bone. The inner portion of bone consists of multicellular bone marrow in which hematopoietic stem cells, stromal cells, and immune cells reside. The hematopoietic stem cells have the potential to differentiate into the blood-forming elements and bone-resorbing osteoclasts, whereas the stromal cells support the differentiation of the hematopoietic cells and form bone-producing osteoblasts. Cells in the bone marrow, stromal and immune cells in particular, produce cytokines and growth factors that mediate cell-to-cell interactions in autocrine, paracrine, or juxtacrine fashions. Once cancer cells reach bone, the high concentrations of growth factors and cytokines in the bone microenvironment provide a fertile soil in which the cells can grow. Furthermore, when the tumor cells stimulate osteoclastic bone resorption, this bone microenvironment is even more enriched with bone-derived growth factors that enhance survival of the cancer and similarly disrupt normal bone remodeling, leading to bone destruction.

PATHOPHYSIOLOGY OF BONE METASTASIS AND RATIONALE FOR THERAPY DIRECTED AGAINST BONE RESORPTION AND BONE FORMATION

Both solid tumors and hematologic malignancies frequently affect the most vascular areas of the skeleton, specifically the red bone marrow of the axial skeleton in the proximal ends of the long bones, the ribs, and the vertebral bodies. The most common way in which cancer affects the skeleton is directly through local tumor-mediated stimulation of osteoclastic bone resorption. Such osteolytic bone lesions are typical of breast and lung carcinoma and hematologic malignancies such as multiple myeloma. Although breast cancer cells have been shown to resorb bone directly in vitro,[5] most evidence (scanning electron microscopic examination of adjacent bone surfaces[6] and response to osteoclast inhibitors) is consistent with the notion that factors secreted by cancer cells can activate osteoclasts locally. The resulting osteolytic bone destruction can lead to pain, pathologic fractures, nerve compression syndromes, and hypercalcemia.

Tumor in bone may stimulate new bone formation, which causes osteoblastic bone metastasis. This metastasis is most often associated with prostate cancer, although it less frequently occurs in breast cancer and rarely in a sclerotic variant of myeloma[7] and in other malignancies. Osteoblastic metastases are also associated with bone pain and nerve compression syndromes, but unlike osteolytic metastases, this type of bone involvement can cause hypocalcemia.[8,9] Pathologic fractures as well can occur with osteoblastic metastases because of the intrinsic weakness of the new woven bone or the concomitant osteolysis. In general, common sites of pathologic fractures are the vertebral bodies and the proximal ends of the long bones. Spinal cord compression is a catastrophic event often associated with metastatic bone disease and can be due to tumor directly impinging on the spinal cord, fracture of vertebral body consumed by destructive osteolytic lesions, or bone overgrowth of osteoblastic lesions.

Pathophysiologic Mechanisms of Bone Metastases

Breast and prostate cancer are the most common malignancies in which bone metastases occur. Breast cancer is most often associated with osteolytic metastasis, whereas osteoblastic metastases are more often manifest in prostate cancer. Mixed osteolytic and osteoblastic lesions are often evident in both breast and prostate cancer. The remainder of the chapter focuses on general principles of metastasis to bone and on mechanisms specific to osteolytic and osteoblastic metastasis, citing examples

from current research in breast and prostate cancer, respectively. The reader should understand that breast and prostate cancer, although predominantly lytic and blastic respectively, often have components of both osteolysis and osteosclerosis. In this chapter, delineation of osteolytic and osteoblastic mechanisms of bone metastasis from breast and prostate cancer, respectively, is by no means meant to be exclusive. It is likely that both mechanisms are often operative in the same patient.

General Mechanisms of Bone Metastases

Anatomic Factors. Tumor metastasis to bone is not a random event but rather a result of anatomic factors, tumor cell phenotype, and suitability of the metastatic site for tumor growth. Blood flow from the primary site is a significant determinant of the site of metastasis. Studies by Batson describe in detail a low-pressure, high-volume system of valveless vertebral veins that communicate between the spine and intercostal veins independent of the pulmonary, caval, or portal systems.[10] This plexus may serve as a major channel by which certain malignancies, such as prostate and breast cancer, metastasize to bone.

This concept that the vertebral system of veins acts as a direct conduit in the spread of prostatic carcinoma to the skeletal system was refuted by Dodds et al., who found that the distribution of metastases was virtually identical in patients with prostatic and nonprostatic tumors.[11] Of the patients with prostatic carcinoma, 25% had bone scan lesions exclusively outside the region of the sacrum, pelvis, and lumbar spine. The distribution of skeletal metastases from prostatic carcinoma did not support the concept that the vertebral veins have a substantial role in the dissemination of this tumor.

Seed and Soil. Regardless of whether blood flow or anatomic considerations are important determinants of the site of metastasis, they are not the only ones. The distribution of metastases to various organs is not predicted by anatomic considerations alone in approximately 40% of tumors.[12] Thus other determinants of the site of metastasis such as properties of both the tumor cell and the metastatic site are important. Metastasis is an extremely complex event that involves a cascade of linked sequential events that must be completed before a tumor cell successfully establishes a secondary tumor in bone. Specifically, a tumor cell must (1) detach from the primary site, (2) enter tumor vasculature to reach the circulation, (3) survive host immune response and physical forces in the circulation, (4) arrest in a distant capillary bed, (5) escape the capillary bed, and (6) proliferate in the metastatic site. The events involved in entering the tumor vasculature are similar to those involved with exiting the vasculature in the bone marrow cavity. These include (1) attachment of tumor cells to the basement membrane, (2) tumor cell secretion of proteolytic enzymes to disrupt the basement membrane, and (3) migration of tumor cells through the basement membrane. Attachment of tumor cells to basement membranes and to other cells are mediated through cell adhesion molecules such as laminin and *E*-cadherin. Tumor cell secretion of substances such as metalloproteinases facilitates disruption of the basement membranes and enhances invasion. Inherent tumor cell motility and motility in response to chemotactic stimuli are also important factors for tumor cell invasion to the secondary site.

Breast cancer is one of a limited number of primary neoplasms that display osteotropism, an extraordinary affinity to grow in bone. Greater than 70% of women dying from breast cancer have bone metastasis.[13-16] The mechanisms underlying this osteotropism are complex and involve unique characteristics of both the breast cancer cells and the bone to which these tumors metastasize.

Why is breast cancer one of the limited primary tumors to display osteotropism? Paget, during his observations of breast cancer in 1889, proposed the "seed and soil" hypothesis to explain this phenomenon: "When a plant goes to seed, its seeds are carried in all directions; but they can only grow if they fall on congenial soil."[1] In essence, the microenvironment of the organ to which the cancer cells metastasize may serve as a fertile soil in which the cancer cells (or seeds) may grow. Although this concept was proposed over a century ago, it remains a basic principle in the field of cancer metastasis at the present time. Thus breast cancer cells possess certain properties that enable them to grow in bone, and the bone microenvironment provides a fertile soil on which to grow.

Animal Models of Bone Metastases

Gaining an understanding of the pathophysiology of bone metastasis has been a slow process scientifically, as there are few useful animal models of spontaneous bone metastasis. Thus various techniques of experimental bone metastasis have been utilized throughout the years, including injection of tumor cells directly into the (1) intramedullary cavity,[17,18] (2) abdominal aorta,[19] (3) tail vein with inferior vena cava occlusion,[20] (4) left upper thigh muscle,[21] (5) left thoracic artery with renal artery occlusion, and (6) left cardiac ventricle.[22] A complete review of the advantages and disadvantages of these models has been made by Orr et al.[23] Most recently a mouse mammary carcinoma cell line has been demonstrated to spontaneously metastasize to bone after subcutaneous or mammary fat pad inoculation.[24]

Osteolytic Metastases

Cancer metastatic to bone often causes bone destruction or osteolysis. Although several tumor types, such as prostate, lung, renal cell, and thyroid, are associated with osteolytic lesions, breast cancer is the most common. A comprehensive review of over 500 patients dying of breast cancer revealed that 69% had bone metastasis, and bone was the most common site of first distant relapse.[25] In those patients with disease confined to the skeleton the median survival was 24 months compared with 3 months in those patients whose first relapse occurred in the liver. For these reasons the following discussion on the pathophysiology of cancer-mediated osteolysis will focus on breast cancer.

Breast Cancer Cells as the "Seed"

Various common characteristics are necessary for tumor cells to possess the metastatic phenotype. Such properties include (1) the production of proteolytic enzymes necessary for detachment from the primary site, invasion into surrounding soft tissues, intravasation, extravasation, and bone matrix degradation; (2) expression or loss of cell adhesion molecules essential for detachment from the primary site and arrest at a metastatic site; (3) migratory activity to travel in the circulation; (4) escape from the host immune surveillance to survive; and (5) capacity to respond to a chemoattractant. Although these properties are common to tumor cells metastasizing to any organ, they are insufficient to explain the propensity of breast cancer to metastasize to bone. Therefore it is likely that breast cancer cells have additional characteristics that are specifically required for causing metastases in bone.

Because bone is mainly composed of a hard, mineralized tissue, it is more resistant to destruction than other soft tissues are. Thus for cancer cells to grow in bone, they must be able to destroy bone. Histologic review of breast cancer metastatic to bone reveals that tumor cells are adjacent to osteoclasts resorbing bones,[6,26,27] indicating that breast cancer cells can stimulate osteoclastic bone resorption. Breast cancer cells may induce osteoclastic differentiation of hematopoietic stem cells, activate mature osteoclasts already present in bone, or do both, by releasing soluble mediators or by cell-to-cell contact. There is considerable evidence that tumor-produced parathyroid hormone–related protein (PTHrP) is a mediator of osteoclastic bone resorption at sites of breast cancer metastases to bone.

Parathyroid Hormone–Related Protein

Parathyroid hormone–related protein was purified from human lung cancer,[28] breast cancer,[29] and renal cell carcinoma[30] simultaneously by several independent groups and was cloned shortly thereafter.[31] PTHrP is a major mediator of humoral hypercalcemia of malignancy,[32] although rare cases of authentic tumor-produced PTH have been reported.[33-36] PTHrP has 70% homology to the first 13 amino acids of the *N*-terminal portion of PTH,[37] binds to PTH receptors,[38] and has biologic activity similar to that of PTH.[39] Specifically, it stimulates adenylate cyclase in renal and bone systems,[29,30,39-41] increases renal tubular reabsorption of calcium and osteoclastic bone resorption,[40,41] decreases renal phosphate uptake,[39,40] and stimulates 1α-hydroxylase.[39] PTHrP has been found in a variety of tumor types including squamous cell, breast, and renal carcinoma.[42] The regulation of PTHrP is complex, and factors such as prolactin,[43] epidermal growth factor (EGF),[44] insulin,[44] IGF-I[44] and IGF-II,[44] TGF-α,[46,47] TGF-β,[45,48,49] angiotensin II,[50] stretch,[51] and the src proto-oncogene[52] have been shown to increase expression, whereas glucocorticoids[44,46,53,54]

and $1,25(OH)_2D_3$ (1,25 dihydroxycholecalciferol)[44] decrease it. Estrogen has been shown to increase PTHrP expression in uterine tissue, and in vitro studies suggest that an estrogen response element is present in the *PTHrP* gene.[55,56] Mutations in codons 248 and 273 of the *p53* tumor suppressor gene repress *PTHrP* gene expression in some squamous cell carcinomas.[57] The cell death inhibitor Bcl-2 is downstream in a signaling pathway that is required for normal skeletal development.[58]

The human *PTHrP* gene is much larger and more complex than the human *PTH* gene. It spans approximately 15 kilobases of genomic DNA and has 9 exons and 3 promoters. There are three PTHrP isoforms of 139, 141, and 173 amino acids as well as multiple PTHrP messenger RNA species.[45] There is considerable sequence homology across species up to amino acid 111.[59] Like PTH and other endocrine peptides, PTHrP undergoes endoproteolytic, posttranslational processing that results in several secretory forms: (1) an amino-terminal PTHrP-(1-36), (2) a midregion species that begins at amino acid 38 and has an undefined carboxyl terminus,[60,61] and (3) a carboxylterminal species that is recognized by an antibody directed against the 109-138 region.[61-63]

PTHrP has been detected in a variety of tumor types as well as in normal tissue.[42] The widespread expression of PTHrP in normal tissue was the first evidence that the hormone had a role in normal physiology. Emerging work testifies to the fact that PTHrP has an important role in normal physiology in addition to its PTH-like effects. PTHrP appears to be important in

1. The regulation of cartilage differentiation and bone formation through endochondral ossification[64-66]
2. Growth and differentiation of skin,[67] mammary gland,[37,68-71] and pancreatic islets[72]
3. Cardiovascular function[73]
4. Transepithelial calcium transport in the distal nephron, mammary epithelia, and the placenta[74,75]
5. Relaxation of smooth muscle in the uterus, bladder, arteries, stomach, and ileum[50,75-77]
6. Host immune function[78-80]

Bone perichondrial cell production of PTHrP regulates cartilage cell differentiation and has been linked to expression of the *Indian hedgehog* gene.[81] Indian hedgehog protein expressed by prehypertrophic cartilage cells inhibited cartilage differentiation, and this inhibitory effect was mediated by PTHrP. The normal physiologic functions of PTHrP have been extensively reviewed elsewhere.[82,83]

The role of PTHrP in normal breast physiology sheds light on its potential importance in the pathophysiology of hypercalcemia and bone metastasis associated with breast cancer. PTHrP is expressed in lactating mammary tissue[84] and secreted into milk at concentrations 10,000 to 100,000 times greater than its plasma concentrations in humans with malignancy-associated hypercalcemia.[85-89] Elevated plasma PTHrP concentrations have been documented in at least two patients with the rare syndrome of lactational hypercalcemia[90-92] and in some breast-feeding mothers.[93]

Clinical and experimental evidence indicates that tumor-produced PTHrP is a major candidate for being the factor responsible for the osteoclastic bone resorption present at sites of breast cancer metastatic to bone.[94-96] PTHrP has been detected by immunohistochemistry[94] and in situ hybridization[95] in 92% of breast cancer metastases in bone but in only 17% of similar metastases to nonbone sites, an observation that prompted speculation that production of PTHrP as a bone-resorbing agent may contribute to the ability of breast cancers to grow as bone metastases. Bundred and colleagues found immunohistochemical staining positive for PTHrP in 56% of 155 primary breast tumors from normocalcemic women, and PTHrP expression was positively correlated to the development of bone metastases and hypercalcemic episodes.[97] PTHrP expression was detected by reverse transcriptase polymerase chain reaction (PCR) in 37 of 38 primary breast cancers, and subsequent development of bone metastases was associated with elevated PTHrP expression.[96] Finally, PTHrP was detected by immunohistochemistry in 83% of patients who developed bone metastases but in only 38% of those who developed lung metastases and 38% of those without recurrence.[98] There have been no consistent correlations between PTHrP expression in the primary breast tumor and standard prognostic factors, recurrence, or survival. The only significant and consistent correlations have

been between PTHrP positivity and the development of bone metastases and hypercalcemia.

These clinical observations have been extended by experimental studies using a mouse model of bone metastases[99] in which inoculation of a human breast cancer cell line, MDA-MB-231,[100] into the left cardiac ventricle reliably causes osteolytic metastases, usually in the absence of hypercalcemia or elevated plasma PTHrP concentrations. MDA-MB-231 cells produce low amounts of PTHrP in vitro, and when the cells were engineered to overexpress PTHrP, an increase in the number of osteolytic metastases was observed.[101] Specifically, MDA-MB-231 cells were transfected with (1) the cDNA for human preproPTHrP driven by a cytomegalovirus (CMV) promoter to produce PTHrP-overexpressing clones and (2) the PTHrP cDNA in the antisense orientation to depress PTHrP secretion. Stable clones expressing high and low concentrations of PTHrP were selected for study in vivo. Mice that had been inoculated in the left ventricle with the high-expressing clone MDA/PTHrP-1 had threefold more osteolytic bone lesions radiographically at 3 weeks than did mice inoculated with the low-expressing antisense clone MDA/PTHrP-AS or with the untransfected MDA-MB-231 cells. Mice in the MDA/PTHrP-1 group became mildly hypercalcemic compared with mice in the MDA/PTHrP-AS group and the parental MDA-MB-231 group, but neither of the latter two groups had detectable plasma PTHrP concentrations. Survival was significantly poorer in the mice bearing the MDA/PTHrP-1 cells than in either the antisense or parental group. These data demonstrate that osteolytic lesions were significantly enhanced by PTHrP overexpression in MDA-MB-231 cells and that the effects were local, as plasma PTHrP concentrations were undetectable.

In contrast, when mice were treated with monoclonal antibodies directed against the 1-34 region of PTHrP prior to inoculation with parental MDA-MB-231 cells, the number and size of observed osteolytic lesions were dramatically less than in similar animals treated with control IgG or that received no treatment. Histomorphometric analysis of long bones from tumor-bearing mice revealed significantly fewer osteoclasts per millimeter of the tumor-bone interface in mice treated with the

PTHrP antibody than in the controls. This is predictable, since neutralizing the effects of PTHrP should decrease osteoclastic bone resorption. The intriguing aspect of this, however, was that tumor burden in bone, assessed histomorphometrically, was significantly less in the PTHrP antibody–treated mice inoculated with MDA-MB-231 tumor cells than in similar tumor-bearing mice treated as controls. Thus neutralizing the effects of PTHrP decreases not only osteoclastic bone resorption but also tumor burden in bone. In a separate experiment in mice with established osteolytic metastases due to MDA-MB-231, the rate of progression of metastases slowed more in the mice treated with the PTHrP antibody than in the mice that received a control injection.[102,103] Similar findings have been demonstrated in this model using a human lung squamous cell carcinoma.[104]

Since neutralizing the effects of PTHrP had a significant impact on reducing tumor burden in bone, one would predict that decreasing the production of PTHrP by tumor cells would have similar effects. Glucocorticoids inhibit PTHrP secretion in vitro, but whether this can prevent bone metastases mediated by PTHrP is unknown. To determine if glucocorticoid treatment would reduce tumor-produced PTHrP and bone metastasis, the effect of dexamethasone on PTHrP production and the development and progression of bone metastasis caused by MDA-MB-231 was studied.[105] Dexamethasone, in a dose-dependent manner, significantly decreased the amount of PTHrP mRNA and protein produced by MDA-MB-231 cells. Placebo-treated mice inoculated in the left cardiac ventricle with MDA-MB-231 developed significantly more and larger bone metastases, as assessed by computerized image analysis of radiographs, than similarly inoculated mice treated with slow-release dexamethasone pellets (2.7 mg/kg/d). Histomorphometric analysis confirmed these data. In contrast, dexamethasone had no effect on tumor size when MDA-MB-231 cells were inoculated intramuscularly. PTHrP concentrations in bone marrow plasma from femora with osteolytic lesions were significantly higher in placebo mice compared with dexamethasone-treated mice. These data suggest that dexamethasone in large doses can effectively reduce tumor burden in bone by inhibiting PTHrP

expression. The adverse metabolic, immunologic, and musculoskeletal effects of high dose glucocorticoids unfortunately preclude their use for the treatment of bone metastases in humans. These data, however, serve as proof of concept to support the local role of PTHrP in mediating breast cancer–induced osteolysis. Taken together, these data strongly suggest that PTHrP expression by breast cancer cells is important for the development and progression of breast cancer metastases in bone. It stands to reason, then, that production of other osteoclast-stimulating factors should potentiate the development of bone metastases as well.

PTHrP stimulates osteoclastic bone resorption only indirectly, and the exact molecular mechanism is unclear. Thomas et al. have provided evidence that a recently identified osteoclast differentiation factor may mediate the effects of PTHrP on osteoclastic bone resorption.[106] Recently the stromal cell–derived RANK (receptor activator of NF-kappaB) ligand—also known as osteoclast differentiation factor (ODF), osteoprotegerin ligand (OPGL), and TRANCE—has been identified, and a soluble form of the molecule in combination with macrophage colony-stimulating factor (M-CSF) can generate osteoclasts from hematopoietic cells in the absence of osteoblastic stromal cells.[107-110] It was also identified by its ability to induce NF-kappaB and apoptosis of T cells as RANKL and TRANCE, respectively.[111-113] For simplicity, the nomenclature of RANK ligand as indicated by a recent review and consensus[114] will be used. RANK ligand is a member of the tumor necrosis factor (TNF) family and is a membrane-bound molecule. Two receptors for RANK ligand have been proposed. The first, which aided the identification of RANK ligand, was osteoprotegerin (OPG), also reported as osteoclastogenesis inhibitory factor (OCIF).[115,116] OPG, a secreted TNF receptor family member, has a relatively wide distribution. Overexpression of OPG in mice resulted in osteopetrosis.[115] Conversely, mice deficient in OPG demonstrate osteoporosis and calcification of the aorta. In agreement with the phenotypes of mice with altered OPG production, recombinant OPG inhibited osteoclast formation in cocultures of mouse osteoblastic cells and hematopoietic cells.[108,109] The ability of OPG to bind to RANK ligand and limit the biologic actions of

RANK ligand suggested that OPG may function as a decoy receptor.[108,109,116] The putative receptor responsible for signaling RANK ligand biologic actions appears to be RANK,[111] although other hitherto unrecognized receptors of the TNF-receptor family may have similar capabilities.

Thomas et al.[106] determined that the breast cancer cell lines MDA-MB-231, MCF-7, and T47D and primary breast cancers do not express ODF but express OPG and RANK. MCF-7, MDA-MB-231, and T47D cells did not act as surrogate osteoblasts to support osteoclast formation in coculture experiments, a result consistent with the fact that they do not express ODF. When MCF-7 cells overexpressing PTHrP were added to cocultures of murine osteoblasts and hematopoietic cells, osteoclast formation resulted without the addition of any osteotropic agents; cocultures with MCF-7 cells or MCF-7 cells transfected with pcDNAIneo required exogenous agents for osteoclast formation. When MCF-7 cells overexpressing PTHrP were cultured with murine osteoblasts, osteoblastic ODF mRNA levels were enhanced and osteoblastic OPG mRNA levels diminished; MCF-7 parental cells had no effect on ODF or OPG mRNA levels when cultured with osteoblastic cells. Using a murine model of breast cancer metastasis to bone, we established that MCF-7 cells that overexpress PTHrP cause significantly more bone metastases associated with increased osteoclast formation, plasma PTHrP concentrations, and hypercalcemia than parental or empty vector controls cause.[106]

Other Potential Breast Cancer Products Involved in Bone Metastases

Just as production of bone-resorbing factors by breast cancer cells enhances bone metastases, production of other factors may render the breast cancer cell ineffective as a seed and thus diminish metastases to bone or other sites. Using the same mouse model of breast cancer metastases to bone, we demonstrated that nude mice inoculated with MDA-MB-231 cells transfected to overexpress either the cell adhesion molecule *E*-cadherin or the tissue inhibitor of metalloproteinase-2 (TIMP-2) had fewer osteolytic metastases than mice inoculated with nontransfected MDA-MB-231 cells.[117]

Cancer cell expression of factors affecting motility are important in the general metastatic process[118] as well as in those processes specific to bone metastasis. Once tumor cells arrive in the bone marrow sinusoids, they must be able to move through those sinusoids to the bone tissue. Autocrine motility factor,[119,120] thymosin β15, and possibly the small heat shock protein 27 (Hsp27) have emerged as potential factors controlling cell motility. Thymosin β15 increases cell motility, and when its production was inhibited by expression of antisense constructs, as recently reported by Bao et al.,[121] metastases were prevented in the Dunning rat prostate adenocarcinoma model. Similarly, overexpression of Hsp27 in MDA-MB-231 cells reduced cell motility in vitro and bone metastasis in mice.[122]

Another important property of the breast cancer seed that enables it to establish growth in bone resides in the adhesion molecules. Experimental evidence supports the notion that tumor cell surface expression of adhesion molecules mediates targeting to bone and the resultant bone metastasis. For example, bone marrow stromal cells express the vascular cell adhesion molecule-1 (VCAM-1), a ligand for $\alpha_4\beta_1$ integrin.[123] Tumor cells expressing $\alpha_4\beta_1$ integrin may preferentially adhere to bone marrow stromal cells to establish bone metastasis. CHO cells transfected with $\alpha_4\beta_1$ integrin caused bone and lung metastases when inoculated intravenously into nude mice, whereas only lung metastases developed in mice similarly inoculated with untransfected CHO cells.[124] In that report, bone metastases were inhibited by antibodies against $\alpha_4\beta_1$ integrin or VCAM-1. Similar expression of $\alpha_3\beta_1$, $\alpha_6\beta_1$, or $\alpha_v\beta_1$ integrin did not induce bone metastases.[124] Although many breast cancer cells express the $\alpha_v\beta_3$ integrin receptor that binds the bone matrix protein osteopontin, a potential avenue for the development of bone metastasis, MDA-MB-231 cell populations with high-level expression of the $\alpha_v\beta_3$ integrin, were less likely to cause bone metastasis than those cells expressing low amounts of $\alpha_v\beta_3$ integrin in the mouse model of bone metastasis.[125] Bone sialoprotein peptides containing RGD sequences have been shown to decrease MDA-MB-231 cell adhesion to extracellular bone matrix in vitro.[126] Finally, tumor cell expression of CD44 may mediate binding to osteopontin via RGD-independent mechanisms.[127] Such observations illustrate the complex and multifactorial nature of the mechanisms underlying the metastatic process.

Bone Microenvironment as the "Soil"

Bone is unique among metastatic target tissues because it undergoes continual remodeling under the influence of systemic hormones and local bone-derived growth factors. Mineralized bone matrix is a repository for growth factors, chiefly TGF-β and IGF-II.[2] These growth factors are released from the bone matrix as a result of normal osteoclastic bone resorption,[4] a part of the normal remodeling process necessary for maintenance of the structural integrity of bone. The hematopoietic stem cells in the bone marrow can differentiate into bone-resorbing osteoclasts. Other cells in the bone marrow, stromal and immune cells in particular, produce cytokines and growth factors that may potentiate tumor cell growth or expression of osteolytic factors. Thus, once breast cancer cells arrest in bone, the high concentrations of growth factors and cytokines in the bone microenvironment provide a fertile soil on which the cells can grow. Such host cytokines may also enhance osteoclastic bone resorption stimulated by tumor-produced factors such as PTHrP. Furthermore, when the tumor cells stimulate osteoclastic bone resorption, this bone microenvironment is even more enriched with bone-derived growth factors that enhance survival of the cancer. Finally, bone-derived TGF-β may have an important role as a chemoattractant for breast cancer cells.

A large body of indirect evidence to support the concept that bone is a fertile soil, further enriched by the process of osteoclastic bone resorption, has accumulated in studies using bisphosphonates in the treatment of bone metastases. It is already clear from clinical studies that bisphosphonates—potent inhibitors of bone resorption—significantly reduce skeletal morbidity in advanced breast cancer.[128-134] In a recent multicenter trial that consisted of over 700 patients with stage IV breast cancer with two or more predominantly lytic lesions, with at least one lesion that was 1 cm or greater in diameter, patients treated with pamidronate 90 mg intravenously every 3 to 4 weeks for 12 months in conjunction with chemotherapy or hormonal therapy had significantly fewer skeletal complications and less bone pain than the control group had.[132] Bisphosphonates have also been shown to reduce the number of bone metastases and the tumor burden in animal models. Thus, decreasing osteoclastic bone resorption makes the bone microenvironment a less fertile soil for the growth of tumor.

TGF-β, which is present in high concentrations in the bone microenvironment and is expressed by some breast cancers and cancer-associated stromal cells,[135] has been shown to enhance secretion of and to stabilize the mRNA for PTHrP in a renal cell carcinoma, a squamous cell carcinoma,[48,49] and a human breast adenocarcinoma from the MDA-MB-231 cell line.[136] In fact, of the known growth factors present in the mineralized bone matrix (e.g., TGF-β, IGF-I and -II, fibroblast growth factor [FGF] 1 and 2, bone morphogenetic proteins [BMPs], and platelet-derived growth factor [PDGF]), only TGF-β has been shown to significantly stimulate PTHrP secretion from the human breast cancer cell line MDA-MB-231.[136] The fact that TGF-β is abundant in bone[2] and can enhance PTHrP expression by cancer cells makes it an important candidate factor in the establishment and progression of breast cancer metastases to bone. TGF-β is a member of a large superfamily of proteins that are important regulators of bone cell activity.[137] Multiple isoforms of TGF-β exist in mammals and appear to control cell proliferation and differentiation in many human cell types.[138] The prototype of these isoforms, TGF-β1, is highly expressed by differentiated osteoblasts and osteoclasts and is stored in bone matrix and released in active form during osteoclastic bone resorption.[4] The effects of TGF-β include stimulation of mesenchymal cell proliferation, inhibition of epithelial cell proliferation, synthesis of extracellular matrix proteins, and enhancement of cell adhesion. These effects of TGF-β are mediated through complex receptor interactions.[138-141] TGF-β binds to the type II receptor, and this complex recruits and phosphorylates the type I receptor, which in turn initiates signal transduction mediated by the recently identified Smad protein family.[138,139] The effects of TGF-β on cancer cells are complex and variable.[142] In some cancer cells, TGF-β inhibits growth, whereas in others it stimulates growth or enhances metastases.[143]

Further evidence for the role of bone-derived TGF-β in the development and progression of breast cancer metastasis to bone has been demonstrated in the same in vivo mouse model of osteolysis described above. Since TGF-β increases PTHrP expression by MDA-MB-231 cells in vitro, this cell line was transfected with a cDNA encoding a TGF-β-II receptor lacking a cytoplasmic domain (TβRIIΔcyt).[144] This receptor binds TGF-β, but since it cannot phosphorylate the type I receptor, signal transduction is not initiated, and it acts in a dominant-negative fashion to block the biologic effects of TGF-β.[145] Stable clones expressing TβRIIΔcyt did not increase PTHrP secretion in response to TGF-β stimulation, whereas controls of untransfected MDA-MB-231 cells or cells transfected with the empty vector did increase secretion. Mice in which the left cardiac ventricle was inoculated with MDA-MB-231 cells expressing TβRIIΔcyt had fewer osteolytic lesions and a smaller area of osteolytic lesions determined by radiography and histomorphometry than the controls inoculated with the parental cells or with cells transfected with the empty vector had.[136] Reversal of the dominant-negative blockade by a constitutively active TGF-β type I receptor expressed in the breast cancer cells markedly enhanced osteolytic bone metastasis, increased PTHrP production and hypercalcemia, and decreased survival. These data indicate that responsiveness of this human breast cancer cell line to TGF-β is important for the expression of PTHrP in bone and the development of osteolytic bone metastasis in vivo. Figure 9-1 illustrates one proposed mechanism for osteolytic bone metastases.

In the mouse model of bone metastasis in which human tumor cells inoculated into the left cardiac ventricle cause bone metastasis, metastasis to the calvaria is rare because of the relatively low rate of bone turnover at this site compared with that in other bones. To increase the rate of bone turnover in the calvaria, Sasaki et al.[146] injected recombinant interleukin (IL)-1α subcutaneously over the calvariae of nude mice for 3 days. Upon completion of these treatments, MDA-MB-231 cells were inoculated into the left cardiac ventricle of female nude mice. Four weeks after tumor cell inoculation, IL-1 treated mice had obvious metastatic tumor deposits in the calvaria compared with none in the control-treated mice. Further experiments demonstrated that pretreatment of the mice injected with IL-1 with the bisphosphonate risedronate pro-

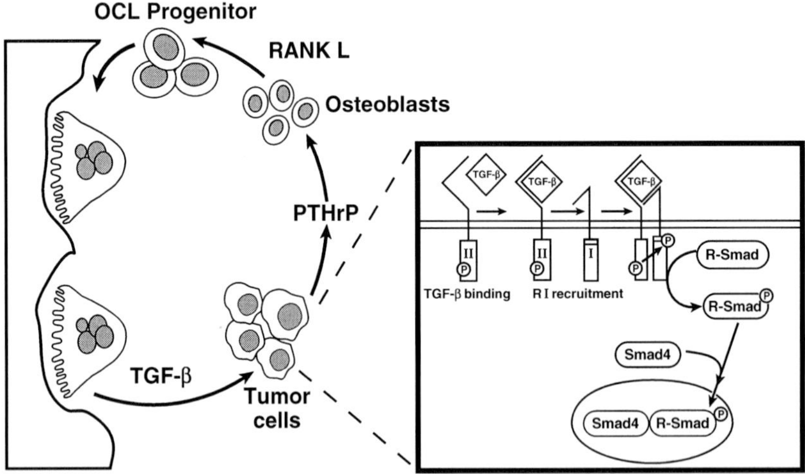

Fig. 9-1 Model for the establishment and progression of osteolytic bone metastases. Tumor-produced parathyroid hormone–related protein (PTHrP) stimulates osteoclastic bone resorption by increasing the production of receptor activator of NF-kappaB (RANK) ligand by the osteoblast. Transforming growth factor beta (TGF-β), released from the bone matrix as a consequence of osteoclastic bone resorption, further increases the production of PTHrP by the breast cancer cells via the TGF-β receptor–Smad signaling pathway. Such a cycle would enhance the osteolytic potential of tumors once established in bone. (RI, receptor I; OCL, osteoclast.)

foundly inhibited the development of metastatic tumor deposits in the calvaria.[146] These data suggest that growth factors released from bone matrix may potentiate tumor cell growth in bone metastases. These findings, however, do not exclude some other alteration in the bone matrix or microenvironment that may be enhanced by increased bone turnover.

Growth factors released from resorbing bone likely have significant effects on tumor cell growth as well. Experimental evidence suggests that IGFs may be important in this regard. Culture supernatants from resorbing neonatal mouse calvariae strongly increased the proliferation of MDA-MB-231 breast cancer cells in culture.[147] Inhibition of bone resorption by risedronate added to the calvarial organ cultures blocked the subsequent breast cancer cell proliferation. Additionally, neutralizing antibodies to the IGF-I receptor markedly impaired the growth-stimulating effects of the resorbing bone culture supernatants on the tumor cells.[147] These results strongly suggest that IGFs are released from bone during bone resorption and promote breast cancer cell proliferation.

Another property of bone that may explain the predilection of certain tumor types to grow in bone is the chemotactic attraction of circulating cancer cells. Culture supernatants of resorbing bone stimulate chemotactic movement of breast cancer cells in a Boyden chamber assay.[148] Bone matrix factors such as TGF-β, type I collagen and its fragments, osteocalcin, and IGFs have been shown to stimulate chemotaxis of breast cancer cells.[149] Most recently, IGF-I was shown to stimulate $\alpha_v\beta_5$ integrin-mediated chemotactic migration of human breast cancer cell lines.[150]

Tumor Cell–Bone Interactions

In addition to the properties of breast cancer as a seed and the bone microenvironment as a soil, there are likely complex interactions between the bone microenvironment and the tumor cell as well as between and within tumor cells that influence osteoclast activation. Both bone-derived and tumor-associated factors have been shown to increase PTHrP expression by tumor cells and to modulate the end-organ effects of PTHrP. Thus such factors may enhance the ability of tumor cells to activate osteoclasts and promote bone destruction.

Other tumor-associated factors in addition to bone-derived growth factors may be important regulators of PTHrP expression in breast cancer metastatic to bone. Many tumor-associated factors, such as epidermal growth factor (EGF),[44] TGF-α,[151] IL-6,[152] TNF, IGF-I and IGF-II,[44] have the potential not only to enhance tumor production of PTHrP but also to modulate its end organ effects on bone as well.

There is accumulating evidence that solid tumors may produce other factors, alone or in combination with PTHrP, that have the capacity to stimulate osteoclastic bone resorption and cause hypercalcemia.[153] These factors include IL-1, IL-6, TGF-α, and TNF. IL-1 injections in mice produced mild hypercalcemia[154]; this IL-1-induced hypercalcemia has been effectively blocked by the IL-1 receptor antagonist.[155] Mice bearing a renal carcinoma that cosecreted IL-6 and PTHrP developed hypercalcemia.[156] Human TGF-α and TNF-α have stimulated osteoclastic bone resorption in vitro and hypercalcemia in vivo.[157-161] TNF-α also caused hypercalciuria, without an increase in nephrogenous cyclic adenosine monophosphate (cAMP), and increased osteoclastic bone resorption in vivo in a mouse model.[162] In addition, some of these factors have been shown to modulate the end organ effects of PTHrP on bone and kidney.

There is clear evidence that other tumor-produced factors can modulate the end-organ effects of PTHrP as well as its secretion from tumors. Using an in vivo model of PTH- and PTHrP-mediated hypercalcemia, Uy demonstrated that both proteins, when produced by tumors in which the corresponding genes were transfected and then inoculated into nude mice, caused similar hypercalcemia as well as increases in osteoclastic bone resorption, more committed marrow mononuclear osteoclast precursors, and mature osteoclasts.[163,164] No stimulatory effects were seen on the multipotent osteoclast precursors, the granulocyte-macrophage colony-forming unit. In a similar model system, IL-6 potentiated the hypercalcemia and bone resorption mediated by PTHrP in vivo by stimulating production of early osteoclast precursors.[152] Likewise, TGF-α has been shown to enhance the hypercalcemic effects of PTHrP in an animal model of malignancy-associated hypercalcemia[151] and to modulate the renal and bone effects of PTHrP.[165,166] Sato

by human prostate cancer coupled with its profound effects on bone formation have obvious implications in the pathophysiology of prostate cancer–mediated osteoblastic metastasis.

Insulinlike Growth Factor–I and –II (IGF). The IGF system is fairly complex, consisting of two ligands, IGF-I and IGF-II; two receptors; and six binding proteins. The topic of IGFs, their binding proteins, and their biologic actions have been extensively reviewed by Jones and Clemmons.[204] Most of the cellular effects of the IGFs are mediated by binding of the peptides to the IGF-I receptor. The affinity of the IGF-I receptor for IGF-II is 2- to 15-fold less than for IGF-I. The IGF-II–cation-independent mannose 6-phosphate receptor has a 500-fold greater affinity for binding IGF-II than for binding IGF-I. IGFs mediate their biologic effects via interaction with their respective receptors, and these receptor interactions are affected by the presence of IGF binding proteins. Six IGF binding proteins (IGFBPs) have been identified, and binding of these proteins to IGFs can enhance or inhibit the biologic effects of IGFs. IGF-I and -II are weak bone cell mitogens but have clear and potent stimulatory effects on the differentiated function of the osteoblast, as evidenced by an increase in osteocalcin and type I collagen synthesis in osteoblasts. As a result, IGFs increase bone matrix apposition rates and bone formation. IGFs also decrease collagen degradation and the expression of interstitial collagenase, functions that suggest a role in the preservation of bone matrix. IGFs enhance bone formation in vivo, and mice with null mutation of IGF-I receptor have delayed skeletal development and ossification.[205] The anabolic properties of IGF-I and -II, their inhibitory actions on matrix degradation, and their abundance in bone tissue suggest that these factors play a central role in the maintenance of bone mass.[206]

Regulation of IGF-I in bone is further complicated by the production of IGFBPs by osteoblasts, which express all six IGFBPs. Binding of IGF to one of these binding proteins can inhibit or potentiate the biologic effect of IGF. Binding to IGFBP-1, for example, decreases the biologic activity of IGF-I. Conversely, IGFBP-5 has been shown to increase bone formation and thus appears to enhance the effect of IGF-I.[207] This system is further complicated by the observation that growth factors such as TGF-β, PDGF, FGF, and BMP-2 inhibit synthesis of IGFBP-5 in bone cell cultures, whereas IGF-I and retinoic acid increase it.[208] Thus it appears that the effect of IGFs on bone is anabolic and that local regulation of IGFs in bone is highly complex.

IGFs are potent mitogens for the growth of human prostate cancer cells, and primary cultures of prostate epithelial cells have been demonstrated to express all aspects of a functional IGF system: IGFs, IGF receptors, and IGFBPs.[209] Human seminal fluid contains IGF-I and -II, IGFBP-2 and -4, IGFBP-3 fragments, and IGFBP-3 protease activity.[210] This IGFBP-3 protease activity in seminal fluid has been attributed to prostate-specific antigen (PSA),[211] and production of other proteases such as urokinase receptor and cathepsin D have been demonstrated in prostate cancer.[212,213] IGFBP-2 appears to be the main binding protein produced by prostate cancer cells, and accordingly, clinical studies have demonstrated serum concentrations of IGFBP-2 to be increased and IGFBP-3 to be diminished in patients with prostate cancer.[214,215] Furthermore, significant positive correlations between serum concentrations of IGFBP-2 and PSA as well as between IGFBP-2 and tumor stage have been observed in men with prostate cancer.[214,215] Although at least one of these studies included patients with bone metastases, neither report comments on whether there was a significant correlation between IGFBP-2, PSA, and the bone metastases. Immunohistochemistry and in situ hybridization in prostate tissue containing benign epithelium, high-grade prostate intraepithelial neoplasia, and adenocarcinoma indicate that mRNA and immunostaining intensity for IGFBP-2 progressively increased from benign prostate tissue to malignant adenocarcinoma, whereas the immunostaining intensity for IGFBP-3 was greater in prostate intraepithelial neoplasia than in normal tissue, but was decreased in malignant cells.[216] These authors conclude that the decreased expression of IGFBP-3 in malignant prostate tissue may be due to pretranslational or posttranslational mechanisms, or both, including proteolysis and that these observations correlate with serum changes of IGFBPs described in men with prostate cancer.

There is accumulating evidence that prostate cancers produce a variety of proteases such as PSA, urokinase type plasminogen activator (uPA), and cathepsin D, which may be responsible for dissociating IGF-I and IGF-II from their respective binding proteins, thus enhancing their effects not only on tumor growth but also, in the case of prostate cancer metastatic to bone, on the mitogenic effects on osteoblasts. PA III cell–conditioned media has been shown to contain a 35 kDa proteinase capable of digesting IGFBPs, which may serve to increase the bioavailability of osteoblast-derived IGFs.[217] In addition to their proteolytic effects that activate growth factors, these proteases may be mitogenic for tumor cells as well.

On the basis of the preceding observations of the presence of an intact IGF system (including IGFBP proteases) in prostate cancer, the mitogenic effect of IGFs on prostate cancer and on osteoblasts, and the positive correlations between serum IGFBP-2 and PSA, it is conceivable that local production of IGFs by prostate cancer in bone may mediate the osteoblastic response so characteristic of prostate cancer metastatic to bone. Unfortunately the data described are associations at best, and a direct causal role has yet to be proven.

Proteases. *Prostate-specific antigen (PSA)* is a serine protease, single-chain glycoprotein that has trypsinlike and chymotrypsinlike enzymatic activity.[218] As PSA initially was believed to be produced exclusively by prostate epithelial cells, it has been used extensively as a marker for prostate cancer.[219] The three clinical diseases associated with an increased serum PSA concentration are prostate cancer, benign prostatic hypertrophy, and acute bacterial prostatitis.[220] In patients with prostate cancer the serum PSA concentration is a valuable biologic marker for diagnosis, prognosis, and management. The pretreatment serum PSA concentration has been shown to be a significant predictor of disease outcome after radiation therapy for local and regional prostate cancer.[221] Androgenic hormones increase the production of PSA via transcriptional regulation.[222] Radionuclide scanning has shown that serum PSA concentrations correlate significantly with the presence of bone metastases.[223] In a large clinical study of 521 men with newly diagnosed and untreated prostate cancer, only 1 of 306 patients with a serum PSA concentration of less than 20 ng/ml had a positive bone scan.[224] Serum PSA concentration proved to be a better predictor of bone scan findings than tumor grade, local clinical stage, acid phosphatase, or prostatic acid phosphatase.[224,225] Thus in a patient newly diagnosed with prostate cancer a serum PSA concentration of

less than 10 ng/ml and no skeletal symptoms, a bone scan may not be necessary,[223] although others recommend measurement of PSA in conjunction with bone-specific alkaline phosphatase.[226] Immunoreactive PSA recently has been demonstrated in 27% of 174 primary breast cancers,[227] even though it was once believed to be an exclusive product of prostate epithelium. Breast-derived PSA was identical to PSA derived from prostate,[228] and PSA has been shown to be produced at the ovarian metastatic site of a breast cancer.[229] Furthermore, in a larger study of breast tumor cytosols from women and men, a positive correlation between immunoreactive PSA and progesterone receptor was observed.[228,230]

The function of PSA in prostate cancer is unclear, but its proteolytic activity may prove to be important in the genesis of osteoblastic response to prostate tumor in bone. Fielder et al. have shown that IGFBP-3 proteolyzes into at least seven fragments with molecular weights of 13 to 26 kDa and that this binding protein has at least five different proteolytic recognition sites for PSA.[231] Three of the five proteolytic sites were consistent with a kallikreinlike enzymatic activity, and two of the sites were consistent with a chymotrypticlike enzymatic activity. Furthermore, some of the IGFBP-3 fragments retained the ability to bind IGF.[231] PSA has been shown to stimulate osteoblast proliferation at concentrations of 2.5 ng/ml, possibly through activation of latent TGF-β.[232] Thus it is tempting to speculate that PSA-induced proteolytic cleavage of the IGFBP-IGF complex results in locally active IGF at the site of prostate cancer metastatic to bone to stimulate the osteoblastic response. Furthermore, recent evidence demonstrates that PSA also cleaves PTHrP-(1-141) at the carboxylterminal phenylalanine-23 and inactivates the biologic effects of PTHrP, thus allowing stimulation of cAMP production in an osteoblast cell line.[233] This may have important implications for the predominantly osteoblastic phenotype observed in prostate cancer. The fact that breast cancers also express PSA is equally interesting; metastatic breast cancer to bone is one of the few other carcinomas associated with osteoblastic metastases, albeit at a much lower frequency than observed with prostate cancer.

Urokinase-type plasminogen activator (uPA) is a member of the serine protease family that also includes tissue-type plasminogen activator (tPA). These proteins are expressed in normal cells. The major function of tPA is related to intravascular thrombolysis, and uPA is involved in proteolysis during cell migration and tissue remodeling. Although both tPA and uPA have been identified in malignant tissue, uPA appears to play a more prominent role in malignancy because it promotes tumor cell migration and invasion by activating plasminogen to plasmin, which in turn cleaves extracellular matrix components of laminin, fibronectin, and collagen.

uPA has been isolated from several prostate cancer cell lines that promote new bone formation in vivo. The rat prostate PA III tumor line causes new bone formation when inoculated over the scapula of rats and athymic nude mice.[234] Conditioned media from PA III cells stimulated proliferation of osteoblasts in vitro. uPa expression by human PC-3 prostate cancer cells is increased by EGF and *trans*-retinoic acid and decreased by dexamethasone.[235] In an experiment to demonstrate the influence of uPA on prostate cancer metastasis, Achbarou et al. used gene transfer techniques to increase the expression of uPA in the rat prostate cancer cell line Mat LyLu to five times that of the same cells expressing empty vector. In a separate Mat LyLu cell line, which expressed uPA mRNA in the antisense orientation, the uPA mRNA was three times less than in the empty vector cells. The uPA-overexpressing, uPA-underexpressing, and parental cell lines were compared in a rat model of bone metastases in which tumor cells inoculated into the left cardiac ventricle of inbred male Copenhagen rats caused bone metastasis. Rats inoculated with the uPA-overexpressing cell line developed hind limb paralysis sooner than rats inoculated with empty vector Mat LyLu cells. Similarly, rats inoculated with the uPA antisense-expressing Mat LyLu cells developed hind limb paralysis later that rats inoculated with parental or uPA-overexpressing Mat LyLu cells.[183] Histologic assessment of the sites of tumor metastasis indicated that more metastatic tumor was present sooner in both skeletal and nonskeletal sites of the rats inoculated with the uPA-overexpressing Mat LyLu cell line than in those inoculated with the empty vector or antisense cell line. Furthermore, histologic analysis of bone indicated that although both osteolytic and os-

teoblastic lesions were present in both control and experimental rats, the osteoblastic response was the predominant feature in rats bearing the uPA-overexpressing Mat LyLu cells.

Fibroblast Growth Factors. Both acidic and basic FGFs, now known as FGF-1 and -2, respectively, are present in mineralized bone matrix and stimulate the replication of cells in the skeletal system but do not increase the differentiated function of the osteoblast. Therefore they may play an important role in bone repair in which bone cell mitogenesis may be necessary. FGFs enhance TGF-β expression in cells with the osteoblast phenotype and have powerful stimulatory effects on bone formation in vivo. When injected locally over the calvariae of mice, FGF increases bone thickness 50%. When administered to ovariectomized rats, FGF blocked the associated bone loss and increased trabecular connectivity and bone microarchitecture.[236]

Prostate cancer cells express large amounts of both FGF-1 and -2.[237,238] Various prostate cancer cell lines have been demonstrated to produce not only FGF-1 and -2[239-241] and FGF receptor but also FGF-like polypeptides.[241] An extended aminoterminal form of FGF-2 was purified from a human amnion tumor as a result of its ability to stimulate proliferation of the osteoblast cell line MG-63.[242] This tumor has been reported to cause bone formation in vivo when inoculated into nude mice. Other data suggest that FGF-2 inhibits osteoclast formation via stromal cells and osteoblasts.[243] Although this evidence supports the notion that FGFs may mediate the predominantly osteoblastic phenotype of metastasis in patients with prostate cancer, like TGF-β, there are presently no direct associations between tumor-produced FGFs and osteoblastic metastasis.

Bone Morphogenetic Proteins. BMPs are bone-derived polypeptides and, with the exception of BMP-1, are members of the extended TGF-β superfamily. At least 15 members are currently recognized, and the list is growing. BMP-2 through BMP-8 share some TGF-β-related gene sequences. BMPs are synthesized by bone cells locally and stimulate the formation of ectopic bone when injected intramuscularly or subcutaneously into rodents.[244] BMPs stimulate the replication and differentiation of normal cells of the osteoblast lineage and, in contrast to TGF-β, enhance the expression of the differentiated osteoblastic phenotype.[245] BMP-1, -2, -3, -4, and -6 are temporally expressed in primary cultures of fetal rat calvarial cells. BMP-2, -4, and -7 have been shown to induce differentiation of primitive mesenchymal cells into bone when implanted into subcutaneous tissue.[246] BMP-2 accelerates differentiation in primary cultures of fetal rat calvarial cells as demonstrated by an increase in expression of alkaline phosphatase and osteocalcin.[246] BMP-3 decreases osteoclastic bone resorption and is chemotactic for monocytes. BMP-7 (osteogenic protein-1) suppresses cell proliferation and stimulates the expression of markers characteristic of the osteoblast phenotype in rat osteosarcoma cells but stimulates growth and differentiation in rat calvarial cultures.[247] In vivo, human BMP-7 was capable of inducing new bone formation in the rat subcutaneous bone, induction model.[248] Recently, overexpression of BMP-4 in lymphocytes was described in association with the disabling ectopic osteogenesis of fibrodysplasia ossificans progressiva.[249]

Normal and neoplastic prostate tissues express BMP-2, -3, -4, and -6 mRNA. The predominant form in normal human prostate tissue was shown to be BMP-4. Although this pattern was observed in human prostate cancer cell lines PC-3 and DU-145, PC-3 also expressed BMP-2 and -3 in large amounts. The rat prostate cancer PA III cell expressed predominately BMP-3 mRNA.[250] PA III is a cell line derived from a strain of rats, Lobund-Wistar, that has a 10% incidence of spontaneous prostate adenocarcinoma.[251] PA III stimulates new bone formation in this strain of rats, as well as in nude mice, when inoculated over the scapula. Rat BMP-3 was isolated from PA III cells,[252] and transfection of the PA III tumor cells with a BMP-3 antisense construct somewhat reduced the osteoblastic response.[253] Thus biologically active BMPs expressed by prostate tumor in bone may contribute to the new bone formation at metastatic tumor sites in bone.

Endothelin-1. Endothelin-1 (ET-1) is the most recent factor implicated in the genesis of osteoblastic metastases. It is a potent vasoconstrictor and originally was purified from endothelial cells.[254] Prostatic epithelium produces ET-1, and receptors with high-affinity for ET-1 are present throughout the prostate gland.[255] ET-1 concentrations in semi-

nal fluid are 500 times greater than those in plasma. ET-1 stimulates mitogenesis in osteoblasts, and osteoblasts have high-affinity receptors for ET-1.[256,257] Osteoclastic bone resorption and osteoclast motility also are decreased by ET-1.[258] Moreover, mean plasma ET-1 concentrations in men with advanced, hormone-refractory prostate cancer with bone metastases were significantly higher than mean plasma ET-1 concentrations in men with organ-confined prostate cancer or in normal controls.[259] These endothelin measurements, however, were not correlated to tumor burden in bone and did not correlate with serum prostate-specific antigen concentrations. Human prostate cancer cell lines—DU-145, LNCaP, PC-3, PPC-1, and TSU—have been shown to express ET-1 by RT-PCR. Finally, in vivo, ET-1 stimulated BMP-induced bone formation as assessed by alkaline phosphatase activity in a rat model of matrix-induced bone formation.[259] Additionally, IL-6, but not estrogen, tamoxifen, TGF-β, TNF, γ-interferon, or IL-1, stimulated ET-1 production from human breast cancer cells MCF-7 and ZR-75-1.[260] This is of interest since breast cancer is occasionally associated with osteoblastic metastasis.

Recently, Yin et al. reported that the human breast cancer cell line ZR-75-1, which produces ET-1, causes osteoblastic metastases in nude mice.[261] Conditioned media from ZR-75-1 and synthetic ET-1 stimulated osteoblast proliferation and new bone formation in organ cultures of neonatal mouse calvariae, the effects of which were inhibited by the endothelin receptor antagonist BQ-123. In contrast, conditioned media from the human breast cancer cell line MDA-MB-231, which causes osteolytic metastases in the same mouse model and does not produce ET-1, did not stimulate new bone formation. To determine if ET-1 is a general mediator of osteoblastic metastases, other breast and prostate cancer cell lines were screened for ET-1 production in vitro and for the capacity to cause bone metastases in vivo. In addition to ZR-75-1, two other breast cancer cell lines, MCF-7 and T47D, produced significant amounts of ET-1 in vitro and caused osteoblastic bone metastases when inoculated into the left cardiac ventricle of female nude mice. In contrast, three other breast cancer lines and two prostate cancer lines that caused osteolytic metastases in vivo did not produce detectable ET-1 but did produce PTHrP. Conditioned media from MCF-7 and T47D stimulated osteoblast proliferation and new bone formation in neonatal mouse calvariae, and this effect was inhibited by BQ-123, as it was in ZR-75-1. To determine the relative roles of the ET_A and ET_B receptors in mediating the new bone formation induced by these cancer lines, the effects of selective ET_A and ET_B and of nonselective ET antagonists were tested on new bone formation stimulated by ET-1- and ZR-75-1-conditioned media in neonatal mouse calvariae. Both nonselective and selective ET_A antagonists completely inhibited ET-1- and ZR-75-1-mediated new bone formation. Treatment with ET_B antagonist produced a slight increase in ET-1-mediated new bone formation but had no effect, stimulatory or inhibitory, on ZR-75-1-mediated new bone formation. Neither ET_A antagonist (BQ-123 or ABT627) inhibited new bone formation simulated by the positive control FGF-2. In summary, the data demonstrate the following: (1) Breast cancer cell lines that cause osteoblastic metastases in vivo universally produce ET-1; (2) these effects of tumor-produced ET-1 are mediated via ET_A receptors; and (3) ET_B receptor may function as a clearance receptor. These results identify the ET_A receptor as a potential target for the treatment of osteoblastic bone metastases.

Thus the mechanisms responsible for the predominantly osteoblastic phenotype of prostate cancer metastatic to bone are complex and likely are the result of multiple tumor-produced factors affecting normal bone remodeling. Figure 9-2 is a schematic model based on available data from the literature that identify potential tumor-bone interactions.

Bone Microenvironment as the "Soil" for Prostate Cancer

As bone matrix is an abundant source of growth factors, some of which are released as a consequence of osteoclastic bone resorption, it is likely a fertile soil for prostate cancer cells as well as breast cancer cells. For example, human prostate cancer cell lines proliferate in response to conditioned media from human, rat, or bovine bone marrow.[262] Conditioned media from osteoblastlike cells enhance growth of LNCaP, PC-3, and DU-145.[263] Other in vitro studies indicate that TGF-β stimulated adhesion of the human prostate cancer cell line PC-3 to bone matrix and that this adhesion appears to be mediated via $\alpha_2\beta_1$ integrins.[264] TGF-β

Osteoblastic Metastasis

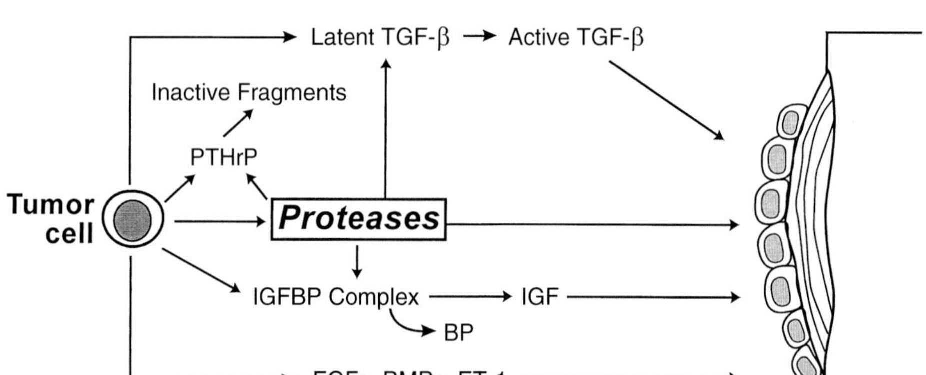

Fig. 9-2 Model for the formation of osteoblastic bone metastases from prostate cancer. Tumor production of factors such as transforming growth factor beta (TGF-β), fibroblast growth factors (FGFs), bone morphogenetic proteins (BMPs), and endothelin-1 (ET-1) may directly stimulate osteoblastic activity and subsequent bone formation. Proteases such as prostate-specific antigen, urokinase type plasminogen activator, and cathepsin D may activate latent TGF-β, release insulinlike growth factors (IGFs) from inhibitory binding proteins (BP) and inactivate parathyroid hormone–related protein (PTHrP).

has also been shown to stimulate cell motility of the Mat LyLu, an in vitro observation that suggests that bone-derived TGF-β may be an important chemotactic factor in prostate cancer.[265]

THERAPY FOR TUMOR IN BONE

Most patients with bone metastasis are normocalcemic. In a majority of breast cancer patients with bone metastases, local osteolysis occurs without hypercalcemia[25] or increases in nephrogenous cAMP[266] or PTHrP.[267] Osteolytic bone lesions occur most frequently in patients with carcinoma of the breast, carcinoma of the lung, and myeloma, the same malignancies that are associated with hypercalcemia. There are also, however, other solid tumors in which hypercalcemia is rare but in which osteolytic bone lesions occur relatively frequently. Among these is carcinoma of the thyroid. Patients with thyroid carcinoma suffer considerably because of their bone lesions, which cause intractable pain, pathologic fracture after trivial injury, and nerve compression syndrome such as spinal cord compression. Hypercalcemia also is likely to develop in these patients. Until recently, therapy for tumor in bone was directed against tumor cells for breast and prostate cancer, myeloma, and other malignancies. This usually involved chemotherapy or hormonal therapy, local field irradiation, radionuclide therapy, or surgery.[13,268,269] The advent of bisphosphonates has changed this perspective somewhat in that it has added therapy directed against the osteoclast to our current armamentarium of anticancer drugs.

Because metastatic bone disease is mediated by osteoclastic bone resorption and because factors that stimulate osteoclastic bone resorption, such as PTHrP, enhance bone destruction by tumor, it is logical to consider therapy with inhibitors of bone resorption to prevent the development of bone metastases or to delay their progression. Other mechanisms by which bisphosphonates decrease bone metastases may involve tumor cell adhesion to bone. In vitro studies demonstrate that a number of bisphosphonates decrease attachment of MDA-MB-231 breast cancer cells to extracellular bone matrix. Of interest is that the decrease in tumor adhesion effected by these bisphosphonates positively correlates to their antiresorptive potency.[270] Finally, there is evidence to suggest that bisphosphonates may induce tumor cell apoptosis.[271,272]

Several prospective, double-blind placebo-controlled trials have been published documenting the efficacy of the bisphosphonate pamidronate in decreasing the skeletal complications associated with breast cancer[131,273-275] and myeloma.[276] Bisphosphonates, analogues of pyrophosphate, have become the most useful antiresorptive agents among the drugs currently available for the treatment of hypercalcemia associated with malignancy. They have a high affinity for hydroxyapatite in bone and concentrate in areas of high bone turnover. The mechanisms by which bisphosphonates inhibit bone resorption are not clearly understood but potentially include induction of osteoclast apoptosis, inhibition of osteoclast formation and recruitment, and stimulation of osteoblasts to produce an inhibitor of osteoclast formation.[277,278] Bisphosphonates also might affect bone resorption by inhibiting the osteoclast's ability to attach and form a ruffled border.[277] Recent in vitro findings using rodent marrow cultures suggest that tyrosine phosphatase activity is important in osteoclast formation and function and is a potential molecular target of bisphosphonate action.[279] Bisphosphonates also inhibit axenic growth of amebas of the slime mold *Dictyostelium discoideum,* and the potency of this growth inhibition paralleled the potency of bone resorption inhibition.[280] These findings indicate that bisphosphonates may have a mechanism of action that is similar in both the osteoclast and *Dictyostelium discoideum.* On the basis of these studies, bisphosphonates can be classified into at least two groups with different modes of action. Bisphosphonates that closely resemble pyrophosphate (such as clodronate and etidronate) can be metabolically incorporated into nonhydrolysable analogues of ATP that may inhibit ATP-dependent intracellular enzymes. The more potent, nitrogen-containing bisphosphonates (such as pamidronate, alendronate, risedronate, and ibandronate) are not metabolized in this way but can inhibit enzymes of the mevalonate pathway, thereby preventing the biosynthesis of isoprenoid compounds that are essential for the posttranslational modification of small GTPases. The inhibition of protein prenylation and the disruption of the function of these key regulatory proteins explains the loss of osteoclast activity and induction of apoptosis. The nitrogen-containing bisphosphonates also have proinflammatory properties. These different modes of action might account for subtle differences between compounds in terms of their clinical effects.[281,282]

Bisphosphonates vary in potency but, in general, are poorly absorbed and are most effective in treating hypercalcemia when given intravenously. Bisphosphonates are concentrated in bone and remain there until the bone is resorbed. Etidronate, the first available bisphosphonate in the United States, is the least potent. Pamidronate is a potent amino-bisphosphonate available for the treatment of hypercalcemia of malignancy. The drug combines high efficacy with a low toxicity profile and thus has become the current bisphosphonate of choice for the treatment of hypercalcemia of malignancy and metastatic bone disease due to breast cancer. It is highly effective in normalizing serum calcium concentrations, and when used in dosages recommended for hypercalcemia of malignancy, pamidronate is not associated with bone mineralization defects. Because of its propensity to cause mouth ulcers, oral pamidronate, although effective, is not likely to be approved for such use in the United States. Clodronate has been used in Europe and Canada for treatment of metastatic bone disease. The potent oral bisphosphonate alendronate is Food and Drug Administration (FDA) approved for use in the United States for postmenopausal osteoporosis and Paget's disease of bone, and tiludronate is approved for Paget's disease of bone.

The FDA has approved pamidronate for use in patients with myeloma and osteolytic lesions but who are not hypercalcemic. This approval is based on a finding that intravenous pamidronate given every 4 weeks for 9 cycles in almost 400 patients with myeloma significantly reduced skeletal complications (defined as pathologic fracture, requirement for radiation to bone or surgery, or spinal cord compression) and prevented hypercalcemia.[276] In addition, this treatment alleviated bone pain and improved quality of life. There was also a suggestion in these patients that overall survival was improved. Pamidronate is now being used widely early in the course of myeloma because it is a relatively nontoxic drug and may have a beneficial effect on more than just bone complications. There are now indications that pamidronate treatment of stage III myeloma patients on salvage therapy is associated with prolonged survival.[283]

Clinical studies have been ongoing for 20 years in normocalcemic patients with solid tumors and osteolytic bone metastases. All the available evidence from these studies suggests that drugs that decrease bone resorption such as the potent bisphosphonates have a beneficial effect on skeletal complications, including pain and pathologic fracture, prevention of hypercalcemia, and improved quality of life. In a recent multicenter trial, over 380 patients with stage IV breast cancer with one or more predominantly lytic lesions, with at least one lesion that was 1 cm or greater in diameter, were treated with pamidronate 90 mg intravenously every 3 to 4 weeks for 12 months in conjunction with chemotherapy; these patients had significantly fewer skeletal complications and less bone pain than the control group had.[132] There was continued benefit after 24 months of treatment, and no adverse effects of pamidronate were noted.[273] In an equivalent study of 372 stage IV patients treated with hormonal therapy, those treated simultaneously with pamidronate had significantly less skeletal morbidity[274] than those given placebo. High-dose pamidronate (120 mg 2-hour intravenous infusion) or placebo was given to 86 patients with heavily pretreated progressive bone metastases (52 with breast cancer, 17 with prostate cancer, and 17 others); those given pamidronate had significantly less morbidity than those given placebo. In this study, no other systemic anticancer treatment or radiotherapy was administered. Symptomatic improvement corresponded with changes in the rate of biochemical markers of bone resorption. In patients with the highest rates of bone resorption, however, clinical response or normalization of the rate of bone resorption was rarely observed.[284] Except for the study by Theirault et al.,[274] which demonstrated a significant survival benefit in women less than 50 years of age treated with hormonal therapy, no difference in overall survival has been observed in breast cancer patients treated with pamidronate.

Recently in patients with newly diagnosed breast cancer and tumor cells in the bone marrow, adjuvant clodronate therapy reduced skeletal and soft tissue metastases and increased overall survival. This was the first time such benefits have been demonstrated.[275] Although other studies using oral clodronate have shown a reduction in skeletal morbidity,[285] the effect on survival and soft tissue metastases demonstrated by Diel et al.[275] has yet to be duplicated by other investigators in clinical trials.

In experimental studies in which human breast cancer cells are inoculated into the left ventricle of the nude mouse, Sasaki et al.[286] have shown that bisphosphonates such as risedronate and ibandronate not only prevent the development of skeletal complications and bone metastases but also reduce tumor burden in bone. This likely occurs because the bisphosphonates make bone a less favorable environment for the growth of tumor cells by reducing bone turnover and decreasing the supply of local bone-derived growth factors that also act as tumor growth factors in the bone microenvironment. It is apparent from clinical studies that bisphosphonates reduce significant skeletal morbidity in advanced breast cancer. These data suggest that drugs that inhibit bone resorption prevent the growth of tumor cells in the skeleton and thus may be useful adjuvant therapy in patients with malignant disease. Other agents that inhibit osteoclastic bone resorption, such as gallium nitrate, are currently in clinical trials for the treatment of bone metastases.[287]

Studies using bisphosphonates in the treatment of prostate cancer metastatic to bone are fewer, and the results are less impressive. Clodronate treatment of men with advanced prostate cancer resulted not only in decreased osteoclastic bone resorption, as assessed histomorphometrically, but also in osteomalacia. The authors attributed the transient relief of bone pain in the clodronate group to this resultant osteomalacia.[288] In a small study of breast and prostate cancer patients with osteosclerotic lesions, pamidronate decreased bone pain. This response was predicted chiefly by a decrease in the urinary marker of bone resorption, deoxypyridinoline.[289] It has been suggested that the patients who have the best symptomatic responses to bisphosphonates are those with coexistent lytic bone metastases or elevated indexes of osteoclastic bone resorption, although this has been disputed by some.[290]

Another potential therapeutic target for osteoblastic metastases to bone are antagonists to the endothelin receptors. Since the animal models of osteoblastic bone metastases described in this chapter suggest that tumor-produced ET-1 produces its effects on osteoblast activity via the ETA receptor, ETA receptor antagonists should be a useful addition to the drugs treating prostate cancer bone metastases. Such agents are currently in clinical trials for diseases such as hypertension.[291]

Several important questions remain regarding the use of bisphosphonates for treatment of tumor in bone:

1. Will bisphosphonates be useful as adjuvant therapy in tumor types other than breast cancer and myeloma?
2. Will bisphosphonate treatment in cancer improve survival?
3. Will bisphosphonates be beneficial in prevention of bone metastasis if therapy is initiated before the development of bone metastasis in patients with limited disease?
4. Will bisphosphonate therapy in cancer prove to be cost effective?
5. Is there a role for bisphosphonate therapy in osteoblastic metastasis?

Although animal studies suggest that the answers to these questions may already be obvious, only prospective trials in humans will provide us with the definitive answers.

REFERENCES

1. Paget S. The distribution of secondary growths in cancer of the breast. Lancet 1:571-572, 1889.
2. Hauschka PV, Mavrakos AE, Iafrati MD, Doleman SE, Klagsbrun M. Growth factors in bone matrix. Isolation of multiple types by affinity chromatography on heparin-sepharose. J Biol Chem 261:12665-12674, 1986.
3. Mohan S, Baylink DJ. Bone growth factors. Clin Orthop 263:30-48, 1991.
4. Pfeilschifter J, Mundy GR. Modulation of type β transforming growth factor activity in bone cultures by osteotropic hormones. Proc Natl Acad Sci USA 84:2024-2028, 1987.
5. Eilon G, Mundy GR. Direct resorption of bone by human breast cancer cells in vitro. Nature 276:726-728, 1978.
6. Boyde A, Maconnachie E, Reid SA, Delling G, Mundy GR. Scanning electron microscopy in bone pathology: Review of methods. Potential and applications. Scanning Electron Microscopy 4:1537-1554, 1986.
7. Case Records of the Massachusetts General Hospital (case 29-1972). N Engl J Med 287:138-143, 1972.
8. Szentirmai M, Constantinou C, Rainey JM, Loewenstein JE. Hypocalcemia due to avid calcium uptake by osteoblastic metastases of prostate cancer. West J Med 163:577-578, 1995.

9. Weigand MC, Burshell A, Jaspan J, Odugbesan AO. Case report: Clinical hypocalcemia. The endocrine conference of the Alton Ochsner Medical Institutions and Tulane University Medical Center. Am J Med Sci 19:194-196, 1994.

10. Batson OV. The function of the vertebral veins and their role in the spread of metastases. Ann Surg 112:138-149, 1940.

11. Dodds PR, Caride VJ, Lytton B. The role of vertebral veins in the dissemination of prostatic carcinoma. J Urol 126:753-755, 1981.

12. Liotta LA, Kohn E. Cancer invasion and metastases. JAMA 263:1123-1126, 1990.

13. Aaron AD. The management of cancer metastatic to bone. JAMA 272:1206-1209, 1994.

14. Walther HE. Krebsmetastasen. Basel: Bens Schwabe Verlag, 1948.

15. Weiss L. Comments on hematogenous metastatic patterns in humans as revealed by autopsy. Clin Exp Metastasis 10:191-199, 1992.

16. Cifuentes N, Pickren JW. Metastases from carcinoma of mammary gland: An autopsy study. J Surg Oncol 11:193-205, 1979.

17. Galasko CS, Bennett A. Relationship of bone destruction in skeletal metastases to osteoclast activation and prostaglandins. Nature 263:508-510, 1976.

18. Wu T, Sikes RA, Cui Q, Thalmann GN, Kao C, Murphy CF, Yang H, Zhau HE, Balian G, Chung LWK. Establishing human prostate cancer cell xenografts in bone: Induction of osteoblastic reaction by prostate-specific antigen-producing tumors in athymic and SCID/bh mice using LNCaP and lineage-derived metastatic sublines. Int J Cancer 77:887-894, 1998.

19. Powles TJ, Clark SA, Easty DM, Easty GC, Neville AM. The inhibition by aspirin and indomethacin of osteolytic tumor deposits and hypercalcaemia in rats with Walker tumour and its possible application to human breast cancer. Br J Cancer 28:316-321, 1973.

20. Shevrin D, Kukreja SC, Ghosh L, Lad TE. Development of skeletal metastasis by human prostate cancer in athymic nude mice. Clin Exp Metastasis 6:401-409, 1988.

21. Kostenuik PJ, Singh G, Suyama KL, Orr FW. A quantitative model for spontaneous bone metastasis: Evidence for a mitogenic effect of bone on Walker 256 cancer cells. Clin Exp Metastasis 10:403-410, 1992.

22. Arguello F, Baggs RB, Frantz CN. A murine model of experimental metastasis to bone and bone marrow. Cancer Res 48:6876-6881, 1988.

23. Orr FW, Sanchez-Seatman OH, Kostenuik P, Singh G. Tumor-bone interactions in skeletal metastasis. Clin Orthop 312:19-33, 1995.

24. Lelekakis M, Moseley JM, Martin TJ, Hards D, Williams E, Ho P, Lowen D, Javni J, Miller FR, Slavin J, Anderson RL. A novel orthotopic model of breast cancer metastasis to bone. Clin Exp Metastasis 17:163-170, 1999.

25. Coleman RE, Rubens RD. The clinical course of bone metastases from breast cancer. Br J Cancer 55:61-66, 1987.

26. Taube T, Elomaa I, Blomqvist C, Beneton MNC, Kanis JA. Histomorphometric evidence for osteoclast-mediated bone resorption in metastatic breast cancer. Bone 15:161-166, 1994.

27. Francini G, Petrioloi R, Maioli E, Gonnelli S, Marsili S, Aquino A, Bruni S. Hypercalcemia in breast cancer. Clin Exp Metastasis 11:359-367, 1993.

28. Moseley JM, Kubota M, Diefenbach-Jagger H, Wettenhall REH, Kemp BE, Suva LJ, Rodda CP, Ebeling PR, Hudson PJ, Zajac JD, Martin TJ. Parathyroid hormone–related protein purified from a human lung cancer cell line. Proc Natl Acad Sci USA 84:5048-5052, 1987.

29. Burtis WJ, Wu T, Bunch C, Wysolmerski JJ, Insogna KL, Weir EC, Broadus AE, Stewart AF. Identification of a novel 17,000-dalton parathyroid hormone–like adenylate cyclase-stimulating protein from a tumor associated with humoral hypercalcemia of malignancy. J Biol Chem 262:7151-7156, 1987.

30. Strewler GJ, Stern PH, Jacobs JW, Eveloff J, Klein RF, Leung SC, Rosenblatt M, Nissenson R. Parathyroid hormone–like protein from human renal carcinoma cells. Structural and functional homology with parathyroid hormone. J Clin Invest 80:1803-1807, 1987.

31. Suva LJ, Winslow GA, Wettenhall REH, Hammonds RG, Moseley JM, Dieffenbach-Jagger H, Rodda C, Kemp BE, Rodriguez H, Chen EY, Hudson PJ, Martin TJ, Wood W. A parathyroid hormone–related protein implicated in malignant hypercalcemia: Cloning and expression. Science 237:893-896, 1987.

32. Wysolmerski JJ, Broadus AE. Hypercalcemia of malignancy: The central role of parathyroid hormone–related protein. Annu Rev Med 45:189-200, 1994.

33. Strewler GJ, Budayr AA, Clark OH, Nissenson RA. Production of parathyroid hormone by a malignant nonparathyroid tumor in a hypercalcemic patient. J Clin Endocrinol Metab 76:1373-1375, 1993.

34. Nussbaum SR, Gaz RD, Arnold A. Hypercalcemia and ectopic secretion of parathyroid hormone by an ovarian carcinoma with rearrangement of the gene for parathyroid hormone. N Engl J Med 323:1324-1328, 1990.

35. Yoshimoto K, Yamasaki R, Sakai H, Tezuka U, Takahashi M, Iizuka M, Sekiya T, Saito S. Ectopic production of parathyroid hormone by small cell lung cancer in a patient with hypercalcemia. J Clin Endocrinol Metab 68:976-981, 1989.

36. Rizzoli R, Pache JC, Didierjean L, Burger A, Bonjour JP. A thymoma as a cause of true ectopic hyperparathyroidism. J Clin Endocrinol Metab 79:912-915, 1994.

37. Wysolmerski JJ, Philbrick WM, Dunbar ME, Lanske B, Kronenberg H, Broadus AE. Rescue of the parathyroid hormone–related protein knockout mouse demonstrates that parathyroid hormone–related protein is essential for mammary gland development. Development 125(7):1285-1294, 1998.

38. Abou-Samra AB, Jüppner H, Force T, Freeman MW, Kong XF, Schipani E, Urena P, Richards J, Bonventre JV, Potts JT Jr, Kronenberg HM, Segre GV. Expression cloning of a common receptor for parathyroid hormone and parathyroid hormone–related peptide from rat osteoblast-like cells: A single receptor stimulates intracellular accumulation of both cAMP and inositol triphosphates and increases intra-

cellular free calcium. Proc Natl Acad Sci USA 89:2732-2736, 1992.

39. Horiuchi N, Caulfield MP, Fisher JE, Goldman ME, McKee RL, Reagan JE, Levy JJ, Nutt RF, Rodan SB, Schoefield TL, Clemens T, Rosenblatt M. Similarity of synthetic peptide from human tumor to parathyroid hormone in vivo and in vitro. Science 238:1566-1568, 1987 (published erratum appears in Science 239:128, 1988).

40. Kemp BE, Moseley JM, Rodda CP, Ebeling PR, Wettenhall REH, Stapleton D, Dieffenbach-Jagger H, Ure F, Michelangeli VP, Simmons HA, Raisz LG, Martin TJ. Parathyroid hormone–related protein of malignancy: Active synthetic fragments. Science 238:1568-1570, 1987.

41. Yates AJP, Gutierrez GE, Smolens P, Travis PS, Katz MS, Aufdemorte TB, Boyce BF, Hymer TK, Poser JW, Mundy GR. Effects of a synthetic peptide of a parathyroid hormone–related protein on calcium homeostasis, renal tubular calcium reabsorption, and bone metabolism in vivo and in vitro in rodents. J Clin Invest 81:932-938, 1988.

42. Danks JA, Ebeling PR, Hayman J, Chou ST, Moseley JM, Dunlop J, Kemp BE, Martin TJ. Parathyroid hormone–related protein: Immunohistochemical localization in cancers and in normal skin. J Bone Miner Res 4:273-278, 1989.

43. Thiede MA. The mRNA encoding a parathyroid hormone–like peptide is produced in mammary tissue in response to elevations in serum prolactin. Mol Endocrinol 3:1443-1447, 1989.

44. Sebag M, Henderson J, Goltzman D, Kremer R. Regulation of parathyroid hormone–related peptide production in normal human mammary epithelial cells in vitro. Am J Physiol 267:C723-C730, 1994.

45. Southby J, Murphy LM, Martin TJ, Gillespie MT. Cell-specific and regulator-induced promoter usage and messenger ribonucleic acid splicing for parathyroid hormone–related protein. Endocrinology 137:1349-1357, 1996.

46. Rizzoli R, Feyen JHM, Grau G, Wohlwend A, Sappino AP, Bonjour J-P. Regulation of parathyroid hormone–related protein production in a human lung squamous cell carcinoma line. J Endocrinol 143:333-341, 1994.

47. Burton PBJ, Knight DE. Parathyroid hormone–related peptide can regulate growth of human lung cancer cells. FEBS Lett 305:228-232, 1992.

48. Merryman JI, DeWille JW, Werkmeister JR, Capen CC, Rosol TJ. Effects of transforming growth factor-β on parathyroid hormone–related protein production and ribonucleic acid expression by a squamous carcinoma cell line in vitro. Endocrinology 134:2424-2430, 1994.

49. Kiriyama T, Gillespie MT, Glatz JA, Fukumoto S, Moseley JM, Martin TJ. Transforming growth factor-β stimulation of parathyroid hormone–related protein (PTHrP): A paracrine regulator? Mol Cell Endocrinol 92:55-62, 1993 (published erratum appears in Mol Cell Endocrinol 94:145, 1993).

50. Pirola CJ, Wang H-M, Kamyar A, Wu S, Enomoto H, Sharifi B, Forrester JS, Clemens TL, Fagin JA. Angiotensin II regulates parathyroid hormone–related protein expression in cultured rat aortic smooth muscle cells through both transcriptional and posttranscriptional mechanisms. J Biol Chem 268:1987-1994, 1993.

51. Daifotis AG, Weir EC, Dreyer BE, Broadus AE. Stretch-induced parathyroid hormone–related protein gene expression in the rat uterus. J Biol Chem 267:23455-23458, 1992.

52. Li X, Drucker DJ. Parathyroid hormone–related peptide is a downstream target for *ras* and *src* activation. J Biol Chem 269:6263-6266, 1994.

53. Glatz JA, Heath JK, Southby J, O'Keeffe LM, Kiriyama T, Moseley JM, Martin TJ, Gillespie MT. Dexamethasone regulation of parathyroid hormone–related protein (PTHrP) expression in a squamous cancer cell line. Mol Cell Endocrinol 101:295-306, 1994.

54. Lu C, Ikeda K, Deftos LJ, Gazdar AF, Mangin M, Broadus AE. Glucocorticoid regulation of parathyroid hormone–related peptide gene transcription in a human neuroendocrine cell line. Mol Endocrinol 3:2034-2040, 1989.

55. Thiede MA, Harm SC, Hasson DM, Gardner RM. In vivo regulation of parathyroid hormone–related peptide messenger ribonucleic acid in the rat uterus by 17 β-estradiol. Endocrinology 128:2317-2323, 1991.

56. Paspaliaris V, Petersen DN, Thiede MA. Steroid regulation of parathyroid hormone–related protein expression and action in the rat uterus. J Steroid Biochem Mol Biol 53:259-265, 1995.

57. Foley J, Wysolmerski JJ, Broadus AE, Philbrick WM. Parathyroid hormone–related protein gene expression in human squamous carcinoma cells is repressed by mutant isoforms of p53. Cancer Res 56:4056-4062, 1996.

58. Amling M, Neff L, Tanaka S, Inoue D, Kuida K, Weir E, Philbrick WM, Broadus AE, Baron R. Bcl-2 lies downstream of parathyroid hormone–related peptide in a signaling pathway that regulates chondrocyte maturation during skeletal development. J Cell Biol 136:205-213, 1997.

59. Martin TJ, Moseley JM, Gillespie MT. Parathyroid hormone–related protein: Biochemistry and molecular biology. Crit Rev Biochem Mol Biol 26:377-395, 1991.

60. Soifer NE, Dee KE, Insogna KL, Burtis WJ, Matovcik LM, Wu TL, Milstone LM, Broadus AE, Philbrick WM, Stewart AF. Parathyroid hormone–related protein. Evidence for secretion of a novel mid-region fragment by three different cell types. J Biol Chem 267:18236-18243, 1992.

61. Burtis WJ, Fodero JP, Gaich G, Debeyssey M, Stewart AF. Preliminary characterization of circulating amino- and carboxyl-terminal fragments of parathyroid hormone–related peptide in humoral hypercalcemia of malignancy. J Clin Endocrinol Metab 75:1110-1114, 1992.

62. Burtis WJ, Brady TG, Orloff JJ, Ersbak JB, Warrell RP Jr, Olson BR, Wu TL, Mitnick ME, Broadus AE, Stewart AF. Immunochemical characterization of circulating parathyroid hormone–related protein in patients with humoral hypercalcemia of cancer. N Engl J Med 322:1106-1112, 1990.

63. Orloff JJ, Soifer NE, Fodero JP, Dann P, Burtis WJ. Accumulation of carboxyl-terminal fragments of parathyroid hormone–related protein in renal failure. Kidney Int 43:1371-1376, 1993.

64. Karaplis AC, Luz A, Glowacki J, Bronson RT, Tybulewicz VL, Kronenberg HM, Mulligan RC. Lethal skeletal dysplasia from targeted disruption of the parathyroid hormone–related peptide gene. Genes Dev 8:277-289, 1994.

116. Yasuda H, Shima N, Nakagawa N, Mochizuki SI, Yano K, Fujise N, Sato Y, Goto M, Yamaguchi K, Kuriyama M, Kanno T, Murakami A, Tsuda E, Morinaga T, Higashio K. Identity of osteoclastogenesis inhibitory factor (OCIF) and osteoprotegerin (OPG): A mechanism by which OPG/OCIF inhibits osteoclastogenesis in vitro. Endocrinology 139:1329-1337, 1998.

117. Mbalaviele G, Dunstan CR, Sasaki A, Williams PJ, Mundy GR, Yoneda T. E-cadherin expression in human breast cancer cells suppresses the development of osteolytic bone metastases in an experimental metastasis model. Cancer Res 56:4063-4070, 1996.

118. Coffey DS. Prostate cancer metastasis: Talking the walk. Nature Med 2:1305-1306, 1996.

119. Watanabe H, Carmi P, Hogan V, Raz T, Silletti S, Nabi IR, Raz A. Purification of human tumor cell autocrine motility factor and molecular cloning of its receptor. J Biol Chem 266:13442-13448, 1991.

120. Watanabe H, Takehana K, Date M, Shinozaki T, Raz A. Tumor cell autocrine motility factor is the neuroleukin/phosphohexose isomerase polypeptide. Cancer Res 56:2960-2963, 1996.

121. Bao L, Loda M, Janmey PA, Stewart R, Anand-Apte B, Zetter BR. Thymosin β15: A novel regulator of cell tumor motility upregulated in metastatic prostate cancer. Nature Med 2:1322-1328, 1996.

122. Lemieux PM, Guise TA, Dallas M, Oesterreich S, Yin JJ, Selander K, Fuqua SAW. Low cell motility induced by Hsp27 overexpression decreases osteolytic metastases of human breast cancer cells in vivo. J Bone Miner Res 14(9):1570-1575, 1999.

123. Kikuchi T, Takeuchi Y, Matsumoto T, Fujita T, Ogata E. Direct interaction of melanoma cells with bone marrow stromal cells via $\alpha_4\beta_1$ integrin/VCAM-1 inhibits osteoblastic differentiation. J Bone Miner Res 11(Suppl 1): S117, 90 (abstract), 1996.

124. Matsuura N, Puzon-McLaughlin W, Irie A, Morikawa Y, Kakudo K, Takada Y. Induction of experimental bone metastasis in mice by transfection of integrin $\alpha_4\beta_1$ into tumor cells. Am J Pathol 148:55-61, 1996.

125. Tondravi M, Quiroz M, Wang M, Teitelbaum SL. Increased rate of skeletal metastases by human breast cancer cells expressing low levels of $\alpha_1\beta_1$ integrin. J Bone Miner Res 11(Suppl 1):S98, 15 (abstract), 1996.

126. van der Pluijm G, Vloedgraven HJM, Ivanov B, Robey FA, Grzesik WJ, Robey PG, Papapoulos SE, Löwik CWGM. Bone sialoprotein peptides are potent inhibitors of breast cancer cell adhesion to bone. Cancer Res 56:1948-1955, 1996.

127. Weber GF, Ashkar S, Glimcher MJ, Cantor H. Receptor-ligand interaction between CD44 and osteopontin (Eta-1). Science 271:509-512, 1996.

128. Glover D, Lipton A, Keller A, Miller AA, Browning S, Fram RJ, George S, Zelenakas K, Macerata RS, Seaman JJ. Intravenous pamidronate disodium treatment of bone metastases in patients with breast cancer. A dose-seeking study. Cancer 74:2949-2955, 1994.

129. van Holten-Verzantvoort AT, Bijvoet OL, Cleton FJ, Hermans J, Kroon HM, Harinck HIJ, Vermes P, Elte JW, Neijt JP, Beex LV, Blijham G. Reduced morbidity from skeletal metastases in breast cancer patients during long-term bisphosphonate (APD) treatment. Lancet 2:983-985, 1987.

130. Morton AR, Cantrill JA, Pilliai GV, McMahon A, Anderson DC, Howell A. Sclerosis of lytic bone metastases after disodium aminohydroxypropylidene bisphosphonate (APD) in patients with breast carcinoma. BMJ 297:772-773, 1988.

131. Paterson AH, Powles TJ, Kanis JA, McCloskey E, Hanson J, Ashley S. Double-blind controlled trial of oral clodronate in patients with bone metastases from breast cancer. J Clin Oncol 11:59-65, 1993.

132. Hortobagyi GN, Theriault RL, Porter L, Blayney D, Lipton A, Sinoff C, Wheeler H, Simeone JF, Seaman J, Knight RD. Efficacy of pamidronate in reducing skeletal complications in patients with breast cancer and lytic bone metastases. Protocol 19 Aredia Breast Cancer Study Group. N Engl J Med 335:1785-1791, 1996.

133. Delmas PD. Bisphosphonates in the treatment of bone diseases. N Engl J Med 335:1836-1837, 1996.

134. Delmas PD, Balena R, Confravreaux E, Hardouin C, Hardy P, Bremond A. Bisphosphonate risedronate prevents bone loss in women with artificial menopause due to chemotherapy of breast cancer: A double blind placebo-controlled trial. J Clin Oncol 15:955-962, 1997.

135. van Roozendaal CEP, Klijn JGM, van Ooijen B, Claassen C, Eggermont AMM, Henzen-Logmans SC, Foekens JA. Transforming growth factor beta secretion from primary breast cancer fibroblasts. Mol Cell Endocrinol 111:1-6, 1993.

136. Yin JJ, Selander K, Chirgwin JM, Dallas M, Grubbs BG, Wieser R, Massagué J, Mundy GR, Guise TA. Blockade of TGF-beta signaling blockade inhibits PTHrP secretion by breast cancer cells and bone metastases development. J Clin Invest 103(2):197-206, 1999.

137. Centrella M, Horowitz MC, Wozney JM, McCarthy TL. Transforming growth factor β gene family members and bone. Endocr Rev 15:27-39, 1994.

138. Massagué J. TGF-β signal transduction. Ann Rev Biochem 67:753-791, 1998.

139. Christian JL, Nakayama T. Can't get no SMADisfaction: Smad proteins as positive and negative regulators of TGF-β family signals. Bioessays 21:382-390, 1999.

140. Massagué J, Hata A, Liu F. TGF-β signalling through the Smad pathway. Trends Cell Biol 7:187-192, 1997.

141. Zhang Y, Derynck R. Regulation of Smad signalling by protein associations and signalling crosstalk. Trends Cell Biol 9:274-279, 1999.

142. Arteaga CL, Dugger TC, Hurd SD. The multifunctional role of transforming growth factor (TGF)-β on mammary epithelial cell biology. Breast Cancer Res Treat 38:49-56, 1996.

143. Oft M, Heider KH, Beug H. TGF-β signaling is necessary for carcinoma cell invasiveness and metastasis. Curr Biol 8(23):1243-1252, 1998.

144. Wieser R, Attisano L, Wrana JL, Massagué J. Signaling activity of transforming growth factor β type II receptors lacking specific domains in the cytoplasmic region. Mol Cell Biol 13:7239-7247, 1993.

145. Wrana JL, Attisano L, Wieser R, Ventura F, Massagué J. Mechanism of activation of the TGF-β receptor. Nature 370:341-347, 1994.

146. Sasaki A, Williams P, Mundy GR, Yoneda T. Osteolysis and tumor growth are enhanced in sites of increased bone turnover in vivo. J Bone Miner Res 9(Suppl 1):S294, B257 (abstract), 1994.

147. Yoneda T, Williams P, Dunstan C, Chavez J, Niewolna M, Mundy GR. Growth of metastatic cancer cells in bone is enhanced by bone-derived insulin-like growth factors (IGFs). J Bone Miner Res 10(Suppl 1):P269 [abstract], 1995.

148. Orr W, Varani J, Gondex MK, Ward PA, Mundy GR. Chemotactic responses of tumor cells to products of resorbing bone. Science 203:176-179, 1979.

149. Mundy GR, DeMartino S, Rowe DW. Collagen and collagen fragments are chemotactic for tumor cells. J Clin Invest 68:1102-1105, 1981.

150. Doerr ME, Jones JI. The role of integrins and extracellular matrix proteins in the insulin-like growth factor I–stimulated chemotaxis of human breast cancer cells. J Biol Chem 271:2443-2447, 1996.

151. Guise TA, Yoneda T, Yates AJP, Mundy GR. The combined effect of tumor-produced parathyroid hormone–related peptide and transforming growth factor-α enhance hypercalcemia in vivo and bone resorption in vitro. J Clin Endocrinol Metab 77:40-45, 1993.

152. delaMata J, Uy HL, Guise TA, Story B, Boyce BF, Mundy GR, Roodman GD. IL-6 enhances hypercalcemia and bone resorption mediated by PTHrP in vivo. J Clin Invest 95:2846-2852, 1995.

153. Mori H, Aoki K, Katayama I, Nishioka K, Umeda T. Humoral hypercalcemia with elevated plasma PTHrP, TNF alpha and IL-6 in cutaneous squamous cell carcinoma. J Dermatol 23:460-462, 1986.

154. Sabatini M, Boyce B, Aufdemorte T, Bonewald L, Mundy GR. Infusions of recombinant human interleukins 1α and 1β cause hypercalcemia in normal mice. Proc Natl Acad Sci USA 85:5235-5239, 1988.

155. Guise TA, Garrett IR, Bonewald LF, Mundy GR. The interleukin-1 receptor antagonist inhibits hypercalcemia mediated by interleukin-1. J Bone Miner Res 8:583-587, 1993.

156. Weissglas M, Schamhart D, Lowik C, Papapoulos S, Vos P, Kurth KH. Hypercalcemia and cosecretion of interleukin-6 and parathyroid hormone-related peptide by a human renal cell carcinoma implanted into nude mice. J Urol 153:854-857, 1995.

157. Stern PH, Krieger NS, Nissenson RA, Williams RD, Winkler ME, Derynck R, Strewler GJ. Human transforming growth factor-alpha stimulates bone resorption in vitro. J Clin Invest 76:2016-2019, 1985.

158. Ibbotson KJ, Twardzik DR, D'Souza SM, Hargreaves WR, Todaro GJ, Mundy GR. Stimulation of bone resorption in vitro by synthetic transforming growth factor-alpha. Science 228:1007-1009, 1985.

159. Tashjian AH Jr, Voelkel EF, Lloyd W, Derynck R, Winkler ME, Levine L. Actions of growth factors on plasma calcium. Epidermal growth factor and human transforming growth factor-alpha cause elevation of plasma calcium in mice. J Clin Invest 78:1405-1409, 1986.

160. Yates AJ, Boyce BF, Favarato G, Aufdemorte TB, Marcelli C, Kester MB, Walker R, Langton BC, Bonewald LF, Mundy GR.

161. Bertolini DR, Nedwin GE, Bringman TS, Smith DD, Mundy GR. Stimulation of bone resorption and inhibition of bone formation in vitro by human tumour necrosis factors. Nature 319:516-518, 1986.

162. Johnson RA, Boyce B, Mundy GR, Roodman GD. Tumors producing human tumor necrosis factor induce hypercalcemia and osteoclastic bone resorption in nude mice. Endocrinology 124:1424-1427, 1989.

163. Uy HL, Dallas M, Calland JW, Boyce BF, Mundy GR, Roodman GD. Use of an in vivo model to determine the effects of interleukin-1 on cells at different stages in the osteoclast lineage. J Bone Miner Res 10:295-301, 1995.

164. Uy HL, Guise TA, DeLaMata J, Taylor SD, Story BM, Dallas MR, Boyce BF, Mundy GR, Roodman GD. Effects of parathyroid hormone (PTH)–related protein and PTH on osteoclasts and osteoclast precursors in vivo. Endocrinology 136:3207-3212, 1995.

165. Pizurki L, Rizzoli R, Caverzasio J, Bonjour JP. Effect of transforming growth factor α and parathyroid hormone–related protein on phosphate transport in renal cells. Am J Physiol 259:F929-F935, 1990.

166. Pizurki L, Rizzoli R, Caverzasio J, Bonjour JP. Stimulation by parathyroid hormone–related protein and transforming growth factor α of phosphate transport in osteoblast-like cells. J Bone Miner Res 6:1235-1241, 1991.

167. Sato K, Fujii Y, Kasono K, Ozawa M, Imamura H, Kanaji Y, Kurosawa H, Tsushima T, Shizume K. Parathyroid hormone–related protein and interleukin-1 alpha synergistically stimulate bone resorption in vitro and increase the serum calcium concentration in mice in vivo. Endocrinology 124:2172-2178, 1989.

168. Torring O, Turner RT, Carter WB, Firek AF, Jacobs CA, Heath H. Inhibition by human interleukin-1 of parathyroid hormone–related peptide effects on renal calcium and phosphorus metabolism in the rat. Endocrinol 131:5-13, 1992.

169. Uy HL, Mundy GR, Boyce BF, Story BM, Dunstan CR, Yin JJ, Roodman GD, Guise TA. Tumor necrosis factor enhances parathyroid hormone–related protein (PTHrP)–induced hypercalcemia and bone resorption without inhibiting bone formation in vivo. Cancer Res 57:3194-3199, 1997.

170. Burton PB, Moniz C, Knight DE. Parathyroid hormone–related peptide can function as an autocrine growth factor in human renal cell carcinoma. Biochem Biophys Res Commun 167:1134-1138, 1990.

171. Paling MR, Pope TL. Computed tomography of isolated osteoblastic colon metastases in the bony pelvis. J Comput Tomogr 12:203-207, 1988.

172. Kingston JE, Plowman PN, Smith BF, Garvan NJ. Differentiated astrocytoma with osteoblastic skeletal metastases in a child. Childs Nervous System 2:219-221, 1986.

173. Gamis AS, Egelhoff J, Roloson G, Young J, Woods GM, Newman R, Freeman AI. Diffuse bony metastases at presentation in a child with glioblastoma multiforme. A case report. Cancer 66:180-184, 1980.

174. McLennan MK. Case report 657: Malignant epithelial thymoma with osteoblastic metastases. Skeletal Radiol 20:141-144, 1991.

175. Giordano N, Nardi P, Vigni P, Palumbo F, Battisti E, Gennari C. Osteoblastic metastases from carcinoid tumor [letter]. Clin Exp Rheumatol 12:228-229, 1994.

176. Liaw CC, Ho YS, Koon-Kwan NG, Chen TL, Tzann WC. Nasopharyngeal carcinoma with brain metastasis: A case report. J Neurooncol 22:227-230, 1994.

177. Pingi A, Trasimeni G, Di Biasi C, Gualdi G, Piazza G, Corsi F, Chiappetta F. Diffuse leptomeningeal gliomatosis with osteoblastic metastases and no evidence of intraaxial lesions. Am J Neuroradiol 16:1018-1020, 1995.

178. Pederson RT, Haidak DJ, Ferris RA, Macdonald JS, Schein PS. Osteoblastic bone metastasis in Zollinger-Ellison syndrome. Radiology 118:63-64, 1976.

179. George J, Lai FM. Metastatic cervical carcinoma presenting as psoas abscess and osteoblastic and lytic bony metastases. Singapore Med J 36:224-227, 1995.

180. Thalmann GN, Anezinis PE, Chang S, Zhau H, Kim EE, Hopwood VL, Pathak S, von Eschenbach AC, Chung LWK. Androgen-independent cancer progression and bone metastasis in the LNCaP model of human prostate cancer. Cancer Res 54:2577-2581, 1994.

181. Greenberg NM, DeMayo F, Finegold MJ, Medina D, Tilley WD, Aspinall JO, Cunha GR, Donjacour AA, Matusik RJ, Rosen JM. Prostate cancer in a transgenic mouse. Proc Natl Acad Sci USA 92:3439-3443, 1995.

182. Gingrich JR, Barrios RJ, Morton RA, Boyce BF, DeMayo FJ, Finegold JJ, Angelopoulou R, Rosen JM, Greenberg NM. Metastatic prostate cancer in a transgenic mouse. Cancer Res 56:4096-4102, 1996.

183. Achbarou A, Kaiser S, Tremblay G, Ste-Marie L-G, Brodt P, Goltzman D, Rabbani SA. Urokinase overproduction results in increased skeletal metastasis by prostate cancer cells in vivo. Cancer Res 54:2372-2377, 1994.

184. Charhon SA, Chapuy MC, Delvin EE, Valentin-Opran A, Edouard CM, Meunier PJ. Histomorphometric analysis of sclerotic bone metastases from prostatic carcinoma special reference to osteomalacia. Cancer 51:918-924, 1983.

185. Simpson E, Harrod J, Eilon G, Jacobs JW, Mundy GR. Identification of a messenger ribonucleic acid fraction in human prostatic cancer cells coding for a novel osteoblast-stimulating factor. Endocrinology 117:1615-1620, 1985.

186. Martínez J, Silva S, Sántibañez JF. Prostate-derived soluble factors block osteoblast differentiation in culture. J Cell Biochem 61:18-25, 1996.

187. Koutsilieris M, Rabbani SA, Bennett HP, Goltzman D. Characteristics of prostate-derived growth factors for cells of the osteoblast phenotype. J Clin Invest 80:941-946, 1987.

188. Robey PG, Young MF, Flanders KC, Roche NS, Kondaiah P, Reddi AH, Termine JD, Sporn MB, Roberts AB. Osteoblasts synthesize and respond to transforming growth factor-type-β in vitro. J Cell Biol 105:457-463, 1987.

189. Lyons RM, Keski-Oja J, Moses HL. Proteolytic activation of latent transforming growth factor-β from fibroblast-conditioned medium. J Cell Biol 106:1659-1665, 1988.

190. Miyazano K, Hellman U, Wernstedt C. Latent high molecular weight complex of transforming growth factor β1. Purification from human platelets and structural characterization. J Biol Chem 263:6407-6415, 1988.

191. Noda M, Rodan GA. Type beta transforming growth factor (TGF beta) regulation of alkaline phosphatase expression and other phenotype-related mRNAs in osteoblastic rat osteosarcoma cells. J Cell Physiol 133:426-437, 1987.

192. Noda M, Yoon K, Prince CW, Butler WT, Rodan GA. Transcriptional regulation of osteopontin production in rat osteosarcoma cells by type β transforming growth factor. J Biol Chem 263:13916-13921, 1988.

193. Noda M. Transcriptional regulation of osteocalcin production by transforming growth factor-β in rat osteoblast-like cells. Endocrinology 124:612-617, 1989.

194. Ignotz RA, Massagué J. Transforming growth factor-beta stimulates the expression of fibronectin and collagen and their incorporation into the extracellular matrix. J Biol Chem 261:4337-4345, 1986.

195. Ignotz R, Endo T, Massagué J. Regulation of fibronectin and type 1 collagen mRNA levels by transforming growth factor-beta. J Biol Chem 262:6443-6446, 1987.

196. Sporn MB, Roberts AB, Wakefield LM, deCrombrugghe B. Some recent advances in the chemistry and biology of transforming growth factor-β. J Cell Biol 105:1039-1045, 1987.

197. Marcelli C, Yates AJP, Mundy GR. In vivo effects of human recombinant transforming growth factor beta on bone turnover in normal mice. J Bone Miner Res 5:1087-1096, 1990.

198. Erlebacher A, Derynck R. Increased expression of TGF-β2 in osteoblasts results in an osteoporosis-like phenotype. J Cell Biology 132:195-210, 1996.

199. Marquardt H, Lioubin MN, Ikeda T. Complete amino acid sequence of human transforming growth factor type beta 2. J Biol Chem 262:12127-12130, 1987.

200. Muir GH, Butta A, Shearer RJ, Fisher C, Dearnaley DP, Flanders KC, Sporn MB, Colletta AA. Induction of transforming growth factor beta in hormonally treated human prostate cancer. Br J Cancer 69:130-134, 1994.

201. Steiner MS, Zhou Z-Z, Tonb DC, Barrack ER. Expression of transforming growth factor-β1 in prostate cancer. Endocrinology 135:2240-2247, 1994.

202. Eklov S, Funa K, Nodgren H, Olofsson A, Kanzaki T, Miyazono K, Nilsson S. Lack of the latent transforming growth factor beta binding protein in malignant, but not benign prostatic tissue. Cancer Res 53:3193-3197, 1993.

203. Steiner MS, Barrack ER. Transforming growth factor-beta 1 overproduction in prostate cancer: Effects on growth in vivo and in vitro. Mol Endocrinol 6:15-25, 1992.

204. Jones JI, Clemmons DR. Insulin-like growth factors and their binding proteins: Biological actions. Endocr Rev 16:3-34, 1995.

205. Liu JP, Baker J, Perkins AS, Robertson EJ, Efstratiadis A. Mice carrying null mutations of the genes encoding insulin-like growth factor I and type 1 IGF receptor. Cell 75:59-72, 1993.

206. Canalis E. Editorial: Skeletal growth factors and aging. J Clin Endocrinol Metab 78:1009-1010, 1994.

207. Canalis E, Gabbitas B. Skeletal growth factors regulate the synthesis of insulin-like growth factor binding protein-5 in bone cell cultures. J Biol Chem 270:10771-10776, 1995.

208. Dong Y, Canalis E. Insulin-like growth factor I and retinoic acid induce the synthesis of IGF-binding protein 5 in rat osteoblastic cells. Endocrinology 136:2000-2006, 1995.

209. Cohen P, Peehl DM, Lamson G, Rosenfeld RG. Insulin-like growth factors (IGFs), IGF receptors and IGF binding proteins in primary cultures of prostate epithelial cells. J Clin Endocrinol Metab 73:401-407, 1991.

210. Cohen P, Peehl DM, Rosenfeld RG. The IGF axis in the prostate. Horm Metab Res 26:81-84, 1994.

211. Cohen P, Graves HC, Peehl DM, Kamarei M, Giudice LC, Rosenfeld RG. Prostate specific antigen (PSA) is an insulin-like growth factor binding protein-3 (IGFBP-3) protease found in seminal plasma. J Clin Endocrinol Metab 75:1046-1053, 1992.

212. Conover CA, Perry JE, Tindall DJ. Endogenous cathepsin D-mediated hydrolysis of insulin-like growth factor–binding proteins in cultured human prostatic carcinoma cells. J Clin Endocrinol Metab 80:987-993, 1995.

213. Koutsilieris M, Frenette G, Lazure C, Lehoux JG, Govindan MV, Polychronakos C. Urokinase-type plasminogen activator: A paracrine factor regulating the bioavailability of IGFs in PA-III cell-induced osteoblastic metastases. Anticancer Res 13:481-486, 1993.

214. Cohen P, Peehl DM, Stamey TA, Wilson KF, Clemmons DR, Rosenfeld RG. Elevated levels of insulin-like growth factor–binding protein-2 in the serum of prostate cancer patients. J Clin Endocrinol Metab 76:1031-1035, 1993.

215. Kanety H, Madjar Y, Dagan Y, Levi J, Papa MZ, Pariente C, Goldwasser B, Karasik A. Serum insulin-like growth factor–binding protein-2 (IGFBP-2) is increased and IGFBP-3 is decreased in patients with prostate cancer: Correlation with serum prostate-specific antigen. J Clin Endocrinol Metab 77:229-233, 1993.

216. Tennant MK, Thrasher JB, Twomey PA, Birnbaum RS, Plymate SR. Insulin-like growth factor–binding protein-2 and -3 expression in benign human prostate epithelium, prostate intraepithelial neoplasia, and adenocarcinoma of the prostate. J Clin Endocrinol Metab 81:411-420, 1996.

217. Koutsilieris M, Polychronakos C. Proteinolytic activity against IGF-binding proteins involved in the paracrine interactions between prostate adenocarcinoma cells and osteoblasts. Anticancer Res 12:905-910, 1992.

218. Watt KW, Lee P-J, M'Timkulu T, Chan WP, Loor R. Human prostate-specific antigen: Structural and functional similarity with serine proteases. Proc Natl Acad Sci USA 83:3166-3170, 1986.

219. Stamey TA, Yang N, Hay AR, McNeal JE, Frieha FS, Redwine E. Prostate-specific antigen as a serum marker for adenocarcinoma of the prostate. N Engl J Med 317:909-916, 1987.

220. Murphy GP. The second Stanford conference on international standardization of prostate specific antigen assays. Cancer 75:122-128, 1995.

221. Zagars GK, von Eschenbach AC. Prostate-specific antigen. An important marker for prostate cancer treated by external beam radiation therapy. Cancer 72:538-548, 1993.

222. Henttu P, Liao S, Vihko P. Androgens up-regulate the human prostate-specific antigen messenger ribonucleic acid (mRNA), but down-regulate the prostatic acid phosphatase mRNA in the LNCaP cell line. Endocrinology 130:766-772, 1992.

223. Oesterling JE. Prostate specific antigen: A critical assessment of the most useful tumor marker for adenocarcinoma of the prostate. J Urol 145:907-923, 1991.

224. Chybowski FM, Keller JJ, Bergstralh EJ, Oesterling JE. Predicting radionuclide bone scan findings in patients with newly diagnosed, untreated prostate cancer: Prostate specific antigen is superior to all other clinical parameters. J Urol 145:313-318, 1991.

225. Oesterling JE. Using prostate-specific antigen to eliminate unnecessary diagnostic tests: Significant worldwide economic implications. Urology 46(3 Suppl A):26-33, 1995.

226. Lorente JA, Morote J, Raventos C, Encabo G, Valenzuela H. Clinical efficacy of bone alkaline phosphatase and prostate specific antigen in the diagnosis of bone metastasis in prostate cancer. J Urol 155:1348-1351, 1996.

227. Yu H, Giai M, Diamandis EP, Katsaros D, Sutherland DJA, Levesque MA, Roagna R, Ponzone R, Sismondi P. Prostate-specific antigen is a new favorable prognostic indicator for women with breast cancer. Cancer Res 55:2104-2110, 1995.

228. Monne M, Croce CM, Yu H, Diamandis EP. Molecular characterization of prostate-specific antigen messenger RNA expressed in breast tumors. Cancer Res 54:6344-6347, 1994.

229. Yu H, Diamandis EP, Levesque M, Sismondi P, Zola P, Katsaros D. Ectopic production of prostate specific antigen by a breast tumor metastatic to the ovary. J Clin Lab Anal 8:251-253, 1994.

230. Yu H, Diamandis EP, Sutherland DJ. Immunoreactive prostate-specific antigen levels in female and male breast tumors and its association with steroid hormone receptors and patient age. Clin Biochem 27:75-79, 1994.

231. Fielder PJ, Rosenfeld RG, Graves HC, Grandbois K, Maack CA, Sawamura S, Ogawa Y, Sommer A, Cohen P. Biochemical analysis of prostate specific antigen-proteolyzed insulin-like growth factor binding protein-3. Growth Regul 4:164-172, 1994.

232. Killian CS, Corral DA, Kawinski E, Constantine RI. Mitogenic response of osteoblast cells to prostate-specific antigen suggests an activation of latent TGF-beta and a proteolytic modulation of cell adhesion receptors. Biochem Biophys Res Commun 192:940-947, 1993.

233. Cramer SD, Chen Z, Peehl DM. Prostate specific antigen cleaves parathyroid hormone–related protein in the PTH-like domain: Inactivation of PTHrP-stimulated cAMP accumulation in mouse osteoblasts. J Urol 156:526-531, 1996.

234. Rabbani SA, Desjardins J, Bell AW, Banville D, Mazar A, Henkin J, Goltzman D. An amino-terminal fragment of urokinase isolated from a prostate cancer cell line (PC-3) is mitogenic for osteoblast-like cells. Biochem Biophys Res Commun 173:1058-1064, 1990.

235. Liu DF, Rabbani SA. Induction of urinary plasminogen activator by retinoic acid results in increased invasiveness of human prostate cancer cells PC-3. Prostate 27:269-276, 1995.

236. Dunstan CR, Boyce R, Boyce BF, Garrett IR, Izbicka E, Burgess WH, Mundy GR. Systemic administration of acidic fibroblast growth factor (FGF-1) prevents bone loss and increases new bone formation in ovariectomized rats. J Bone Miner Res 14(6):953-959, 1999.

237. Matuo Y, Nishi N, Matsui S, Sandberg AA, Isaacs JT, Wada F. Heparin binding affinity of rat prostate growth factor in normal and cancerous prostate: Partial purification and characterization of rat prostatic growth factor in the Dunning tumor. Cancer Res 47:188-192, 1987.

238. Mansson PE, Adams P, Kan M, McKeehan WL. HBGF-1 gene expression in normal rat prostate and two transplantable rat prostate tumors. Cancer Res 49:2485-2494, 1989.

239. Nishikawa K, Yoshitake Y, Minemura M, Yamada K, Matuo Y. Localization of basic fibroblast growth factor (bFGF) in a metastatic cell line (AT-3) established from the Dunning prostatic carcinoma of rat: Application of a specific monoclonal antibody. Adv Exp Med Biol 324:131-139, 1992.

240. Nakamoto T, Chang CS, Li AK, Chodak GW. Basic fibroblast growth factor in human prostate cancer cells. Cancer Res 52:571-577, 1992.

241. Shain SA, Ke LD, Wong G, Karaganis AG. Rat prostate cancer cell line–specific production and apparent secretion of heparin-binding growth factors. Cell Growth Differ 3:249-258, 1992.

242. Izbicka E, Dunstan C, Esparza J, Jacobs C, Sabatini M, Mundy GR. Human amniotic tumor that induces new bone formation in vivo produces growth-regulatory activity in vitro for osteoblasts identified as an extended form of fibroblast growth factor. Cancer Res 56:633-636, 1996.

243. Jimi E, Shuto T, Ikebe T, Jingushi S, Hirata M, Koga T. Basic fibroblast growth factor inhibits osteoclast-like cell formation. J Cell Physiol 168:395-402, 1996.

244. Urist MR. Bone: Formation by autoinduction. Science 151:893-899, 1965.

245. Harris SE, Bonewald LF, Harris MA, Sabatini M, Dallas S, Feng JQ, Ghosh-Choudhury N, Wozney J, Mundy GR. Effects of transforming growth factor beta on bone nodule formation and expression of bone morphogenetic protein 2, osteocalcin, osteopontin, alkaline phosphatase, and type I collagen mRNA in long-term cultures of fetal rat calvarial osteoblasts. J Bone Miner Res 9:855-863, 1994.

246. Harris SE, Feng JQ, Harris MA, Ghosh-Choudhury N, Dallas MR, Wozney J, Mundy GR. Recombinant bone morphogenetic protein 2 accelerates bone cell differentiation and stimulates BMP-2 mRNA expression and BMP-2 promoter activity in primary fetal rat calvarial osteoblast cultures. Mol Cell Differ 3:137-155, 1995.

247. Maliakal JC, Asahina I, Hauschka PV, Sampath TK. Osteogenic protein-1 (BMP-7) inhibits cell proliferation and stimulates the expression of markers characteristic of osteoblast phenotype in rat osteosarcoma (17/2.8) cells. Growth Factors 11:227-234, 1994.

248. Sampath TK, Maliakal JC, Hauschka PV, Jones WK, Sasak H, Tucker RF, White KH, Coughlin JE, Tucker MM, Pang RH. Recombinant human osteogenic protein-1 (hOP-1) induces new bone formation in vivo with a specific activity comparable with natural bovine osteogenic protein and stimulates osteoblast proliferation and differentiation in vitro. J Biol Chem 267:20352-20362, 1992.

249. Shafritz AB, Shore EM, Gannon FH, Zasloff MA, Taub R, Muenke M, Kaplan FS. Overexpression of an osteogenic morphogen in fibrodysplasia ossificans progressiva. N Engl J Med 335:555-561, 1996.

250. Harris SE, Harris MA, Mahy P, Wozney J, Feng JQ, Mundy GR. Expression of bone morphogenetic protein messenger RNAs by normal rat and human prostate and prostate cancer cells. Prostate 24:204-211, 1994.

251. Pollard M, Luckert MS, Scheu J. Effects of diphosphonate and x-rays on bone lesions induced in rats by prostate cancer cells. Cancer 61:2027-2032, 1988.

252. Chen D, Feng JQ, Feng M, Harris MA, Mahy P, Mundy GR, Harris SE. Sequence and expression of bone morphogenetic protein 3 mRNA in prolonged cultures of fetal rat calvarial osteoblasts and in rat prostate adenocarcinoma PA III cells. DNA Cell Biol 14:235-239, 1995.

253. Harris SE, Boyce B, Feng JQ, Mahy P, Harris MA, Mundy GR. Antisense bone morphogenetic protein 3 (BMP 3) constructions decrease new bone formation in a prostate cancer model. J Bone Miner Res 7(Suppl 1):S115, 92A, 1992.

254. Yanagisawa M, Kurihara H, Kimura S, Tomobe Y, Kobayashi M, Mitsui Y, Yazaki Y, Goto K, Masaki T. A novel potent vasoconstrictor peptide produced by vascular endothelial cells. Nature 332:411-415, 1988.

255. Langenstroer P, Tang R, Shapiro E, Divish B, Opgenorth T, Lepor H. Endothelin-1 in the human prostate: Tissue levels, source of production and isometric tension studies. J Urol 151:495-499, 1993.

256. Takuwa Y, Ohue Y, Takuwa N, Yamashita K. Endothelin-1 activates phospholipase C and mobilizes Ca^{2+} from extra- and intracellular pools in osteoblastic cells. Am J Physiol 257:E797-E803, 1989.

257. Takuwa Y, Masaki T, Yamashita K. The effects of the endothelin family peptides on cultured osteoblastic cells from rat calvariae. Biochem Biophys Res Commun 170:998-1005, 1990.

258. Alam AS, Gallagher A, Shankar V, Ghatei MA, Datta HK, Huang CL, Moonga BS, Chambers TJ, Bloom SR, Zaidi M. Endothelin inhibits osteoclastic bone resorption by a direct effect on cell motility: Implications for the vascular control of bone resorption. Endocrinology 130:3617-3624, 1992.

259. Nelson JB, Hedican SP, George DJ, Reddi AH, Piantadosi S, Eisenberger MA, Simons JW. Identification of endothelin-1 in the pathophysiology of metastatic adenocarcinoma of the prostate. Nature Med 1:944-949, 1995.

260. Yamashita J, Ogawa M, Nomura K, Matsuo S, Inada K, Yamashita S, Nakashima Y, Saishoji T, Takano S, Fujita S. Interleukin 6 stimulates the production of immunoreactive endothelin 1 in human breast cancer cells. Cancer Res 53:464-467, 1993.

261. Yin JJ, Grubbs BG, Cui Y, Harris S, Harris MA, Garrett IR, Guise TA. Role of endothelin-1 (ET-1) in osteoblastic metastases to bone. Bone 23(Suppl):S377, 1998.

262. Chackal-Roy M, Niemeyer C, Moore M, Zetter BR. Stimulation of human prostatic carcinoma cell growth by factors present in human bone marrow. J Clin Invest 84:43-50, 1989.

263. Lang SH, Miller WR, Habib FK. Stimulation of human prostate cancer cell lines by factors present in human osteoblast-like cells but not in bone marrow. Prostate 27:287-293, 1995.

264. Kostenuik PJ, Sanchez-Sweatman O, Orr FW, Singh G. Bone cell matrix promotes the adhesion of human prostatic carcinoma cells via the alpha 2 beta 1 integrin. Clin Exp Metastasis 14:19-26, 1996.

265. Morton DM, Barrack ER. Modulation of transforming growth factor beta 1 effects on prostate cancer cell proliferation by growth factors and extracellular matrix. Cancer Res 55:2596-2602, 1995.

266. Stewart AF, Horst R, Deftos LJ, Cadman EC, Lang R, Broadus AE. Biochemical evaluation of patients with cancer-associated hypercalcemia: Evidence for humoral and nonhumoral groups. N Engl J Med 303:1377-1383, 1980.

267. Burtis WJ, Brady TG, Orloff JJ, Ersbak JB, Warrell RP Jr, Olson BR, Wu TL, Mitnick ME, Broadus AE, Stewart AF. Immunochemical characterization of circulating parathyroid hormone–related protein in patients with humoral hypercalcemia of cancer. [Abstract.] N Engl J Med 322:1106-1112, 1990.

268. Ackery D, Yardley J. Radionuclide-targeted therapy for the management of metastatic bone pain. Semin Oncol 20(2):27-31, 1993 (published erratum appears in Semin Oncol 20:551, 1993).

269. Robinson RG, Preston DF, Schiefelbein M, Baxter KG. Strontium 89 therapy for the palliation of pain due to osseous metastases. JAMA 274:420-424, 1995.

270. vanderPluijm G, Vloedgraven H, vanBeek E, vanderWee-Pals L, Löwik C, Papapoulos S. Bisphosphonates inhibit the adhesion of breast cancer cells to bone matrices in vitro. J Clin Invest 98:698-705, 1996.

271. Shipman CM, Rogers MJ, Apperley JF, Graham R, Russell G, Croucher PI. Anti-tumour activity of bisphosphonates in human myeloma cells. Leuk Lymphoma 32(1-2):129-138, 1998.

272. Shipman CM, Croucher PI, Russell RG, Helfrich MH, Rogers MJ. The bisphosphonate incadronate (YM175) causes apoptosis of human myeloma cells in vitro by inhibiting the mevalonate pathway. Cancer Res 58(23):5294-5297, 1998.

273. Hortobagyi GN, Theriault RL, Lipton A, Porter L, Blayney D, Sinoff C, Wheeler H, Simeone JF, Seaman JJ, Knight RD, Heffernan M, Mellars K, Reitsma DJ. Long-term prevention of skeletal complications of metastatic breast cancer with pamidronate. Protocol 19 Aredia Breast Cancer Study Group. J Clin Oncol 16(6):2038-2044, 1998.

274. Theriault RL, Lipton A, Hortobagyi GN, Leff R, Gluck S, Stewart JF, Costello S, Kennedy I, Simeone J, Seaman JJ, Knight RD, Mellars K, Heffernan M, Reitsma DJ. Pamidronate reduces skeletal morbidity in women with advanced breast cancer and lytic bone lesions: A randomized, placebo-controlled trial. Protocol 18 Aredia Breast Cancer Study Group. J Clin Oncol 17(3):846-854, 1999.

275. Diel IJ, Solomayer EF, Costa SD, Gollan C, Goerner R, Wallwiener D, Kaufmann M, Bastert G. Reduction in new metastases in breast cancer with adjuvant clodronate treatment. N Engl J Med 339:357-363, 1998.

276. Berenson JR, Lichtenstein A, Porter L, Dimopoulos MA, Bordoni R, George S, Lipton A, Keller A, Ballester O, Kovacs MJ, Blacklock HA, Bell R, Simeone J, Reitsma DJ, Heffernan M, Seaman J, Knight RD. Efficacy of pamidronate in reducing skeletal events in patients with advanced multiple myeloma. N Engl J Med 334:488-493, 1996.

277. Rodan GA, Fleisch HA. Bisphosphonates: Mechanisms of action. J Clin Invest 97:2692-2696, 1996.

278. Fleisch H. Bisphosphonates: Mechanisms of action. Endocr Rev 19:80-100, 1998.

279. Schmidt A, Rutledge SJ, Endo N, Opas EE, Tanaka H, Wesolowski G, Leu CT, Huang Z, Ramachandaran C, Rodan SB, Rodan GA. Protein-tyrosine phosphatase activity regulates osteoclast formation and function: Inhibition by alendronate. Proc Natl Acad Sci USA 93:3068-3073, 1996.

280. Rogers MJ, Watts DJ, Russell RGG, Ji X, Xiong X, Blackburn GM, Bayless AV, Ebetino FH. Inhibitory effects of bisphosphonates on growth of amoebae of the cellular slime mold *Dictyostelium discoideum.* J Bone Miner Res 9:1029-1039, 1994.

281. Russell RG, Rogers MJ. Bisphosphonates: From the laboratory to the clinic and back again. Bone 25(1):97-106, 1999.

282. Rogers MJ, Frith JC, Luckman SP, Coxon FP, Benford HL, Monkkonen J, Auriola S, Chilton KM, Russell RG. Molecular mechanisms of action of bisphosphonates. Bone 24(5 Suppl):73S-79S, 1999.

283. Berenson JR, Lichtenstein A, Porter L, Dimopoulos MA, Bordoni R, George S, Lipton A, Keller A, Ballester O, Kovacs M, Blacklock H, Bell R, Simeone JF, Reitsma DJ, Heffernan M, Seaman J, Knight RD. Long-term pamidronate treatment of advanced multiple myeloma patients reduces skeletal events. Myeloma Aredia Study Group. J Clin Oncol 16(2):593-602, 1998.

284. Coleman RE, Purohit OP, Vinholes JJ, Zekri J. High dose pamidronate. Clinical and biochemical effects in metastatic bone disease. Cancer 80:1686-1690, 1997.

285. Kanis JA, McCloskey EV, Powles T, Paterson AH, Ashley S, Spector T. A high incidence of vertebral fracture in women with breast cancer. Br J Cancer 79(7-8):1179-1181, 1999.

286. Sasaki A, Boyce BF, Story B, Wright KR, Chapman M, Boyce R, Mundy GR, Yoneda T. The bisphosphonate risedronate reduces metastatic human breast cancer burden in bone in nude mice. Cancer Res 55:3551-3557, 1995.

287. Warrell RP. Gallium nitrate for the treatment of bone metastases. Cancer 80:1680-1685, 1997.

288. Taube T, Kylmala T, Lamberg-Allardt C, Tammela TL, Elomaa I. The effect of clodronate on bone in metastatic prostate cancer. Histomorphometric report of a double-blind randomised placebo-controlled study. Eur J Cancer 30A:751-758, 1994.

289. Vinholes J, Guo C-Y, Purohit OP, Eastell R, Coleman RE. Metabolic effects of pamidronate in patients with metastatic bone disease. Br J Cancer 73:1089-1095, 1996.

290. Adami S. Bisphosphonates in prostate carcinoma. Cancer 80:1674-1679, 1997.

291. Krum H, Viskoper RJ, Lacourciere Y, Budde M, Charlon V. The effect of an endothelin-receptor antagonist, bosentan, on blood pressure in patients with essential hypertension. Bosentan Hypertension Investigators. N Engl J Med 338:784-790, 1998.

10 Pharmacologic Management of Bone Cancer Pain

Wen-hsien Wu, M.D., and Christina W. Chin, M.D.

Any tumor can metastasize to bone. As many as 70% of the patients with breast, prostate, lung, kidney, and thyroid primary tumors that metastasize are associated with bone metastases. In fact, bone metastasis is the most common cause of cancer-related pain, and bone pain is a common cause of disability. With aggressive treatment in a group of terminal patients, those least likely to be pain free were those with bone metastasis (10%) and prostate cancer (6%).[1] Cancer pain can be divided into acute, subacute, and chronic types. Acute pain is related to surgery, tumor invasion, obstruction of hollow organs, and pathologic fracture. Subacute pain involves gradual local tumor invasion before it reaches the bone. Chronic pain is associated with advanced, widespread bone metastasis. It is also possible to have mixed types of pain. One must remember that cancer-related pain can exist concurrently with preexisting, noncancer chronic pain. Therefore to construct an effective therapy for controlling bone pain, one must understand all aspects of the pain and the possible mechanisms involved in the nociception generation in the nervous system. It is also important to recognize the common pain syndromes involved in bone metastasis.

PHYSIOLOGIC MECHANISMS OF BONE PAIN

Several related areas warrant a brief review. Bone contains both myelinated A-δ and unmyelinated C fibers. These fibers are most dense in the compact bone. Other richly innervated tissues include periosteum and all periarticular structures except the articular cartilage. Therefore both cortex and bone marrow are pain sensitive. The vascular structure that feeds bone is innervated with its own neural network, but its role in the generation of pain remains unclear. Peripheral irritation may activate the nociceptors. The signals then travel through mainly unmyelinated C and myelinated A-δ fibers to the spinal cord. When the nociceptive input arrives in the spinal cord, it undergoes considerable modulation. If the nociception is strong enough (in signal amplitude, firing frequency, and duration of signal barrages), it irreversibly changes the spinal cord sensory processing apparatus. These changes include loss of interneuronal inhibition, activation of the wide dynamic range neurons (causing spontaneous firing), and loss of the descending inhibitory modulation. The input signals are transmitted unchecked to the central nervous system (CNS). The signals are then processed through the sensory/discriminatory, emotional/affective, and cognitive/behavioral domains, resulting in the interpretation and expression of pain.

Despite advances in knowledge the fact that not every patient with bone metastases has pain indicates that the basis for bone pain is still not fully understood. The mechanosensory system in the bone is still under intensive investigation.[2] New knowledge in bone biology will influence future approaches to bone metastases and bone pain.

Metastasis is a major problem in management. Carcinomas such as breast, prostate, lung, kidney, and thyroid tend to metastasize to the bone. Metastasis is a multifactorial phenomenon. Current research suggests that the complex process involves both biologic properties of the malignant cell and host tissue factors.[3] The cellular properties include the following:

1. Cell motility
2. Expression of matrix metalloproteinases (MMPs) that influence the cell's ability to degrade extracellular matrix components
3. Ability to cross basement membranes, gain access to vascular or lymphatic circulation, and egress in a remote organ site related to the motility and MMP expression
4. Endothelial adhesion mechanisms that facilitate distant vascular or lymphatic seeding
5. Chemotaxis conferring target organ selectivity
6. Selective cell adhesion to specific extracellular matrices or cellular components through cell surface receptors such as integrins
7. Ability to induce angiogenesis to support metastatic tumor growth
8. Local invasiveness related to MMPs and other proteases and possibly cytotoxic effects on the host tissue
9. Continued uncontrolled growth driven by a variety of molecular mechanisms, including locally secreted host and tumor cytokines

The host tissue factors are important because they influence the environment for seeding of tumor cells. These tissue factors may be a stronger determinant than the traditionally believed attributes of anatomy (e.g., vascular lymphatic distribution).[4] The secretion of MMPs is essential for local tissue invasion and penetration of basement membranes. MMP research is rapidly expanding and thus opening doors for manipulating metastasis. There are 14 best characterized MMPs that process varying substrate specificity and tissue expression. All MMPs have two highly conserved zinc-binding domains (a catalytic and a structural site) and two conserved calcium-binding domains. Thus they could be manipulated by chelating agents. The enzymes are all secreted in an inactive proenzyme form. Cleavage of the propeptide activates the MMP, which can then degrade substrate molecules. Furthermore, MMPs can cleave the proenzyme forms of one another and thus become activated in a cascade-type fashion. MMP expression is also regulated at the transcriptional level by growth factors, cytokines, and intracellular signaling molecules, including transforming growth factor beta (TGF-β), tumor necrosis factor alpha (TNF-α), and cyclic adenosine monophosphate (c-AMP).[5-8]

All MMP-secreting cells also secrete endogenous inhibitor proteins of these enzymes, namely tissue inhibitors of metalloproteinases (TIMPs). These TIMPs bind stoichiometrically to MMPs to maintain them in an inactive state. Thus the balance between TIMP and MMP expression ultimately controls the amount of matrix degradative activity. Overexpression of TIMP inhibits metastasis in animals, and underexpression enhances metastasis.[9,10] It has been suggested that MMP expression correlates with metastasis and prognosis in patients with several different cancers, as does underexpression of TIMP.[11-13]

Bone consists of bone matrix, osteoclasts, osteoblasts, resting surface cells, and osteocytes. A brief review will improve the design of treatment.

The osteoclast activity causes bone resorption.[14] Lytic bone metastases weaken bone, which leads to bone pain. Thus understanding the mechanisms in osteoclast-induced bone resorption becomes important in attempts to control bone metastases.[15]

The osteoclast is derived from hematopoietic progenitor cells. Osteoclast activation is thought to depend on its secreted products. Osteoclasts resorb bone by forming a "ruffled border" between folds of plasma membrane and mineralized bone. Adjacent to the ruffled border is a "clear zone" that contains actinlike filaments. At the ruffled border, acid and lysosomal hydrolases are secreted. The lysosomal hydrolases function optimally at an acid pH.

Osteoclast acid phosphatase is distinct from prostatic and lysosomal acid phosphatases and may catalyze pyrophosphate (P—O—P) removal before hydroxyapatite solubilization. The bisphosphonate (P—C—P) bond may inhibit this phosphatase-catalyzed reaction.

Osteoclastic bone resorption and motility are regulated by several factors. The best known is calcitonin. A calcitonin receptor has been sequenced and is homologous to the parathyroid hormone–related protein (PTHrP) receptor.[16] Elevated calcium levels inhibit osteoclast function. Zaidi et al.[17] explored the role of endothelial cell products. They reported that prostacyclin and endothelial cells may inhibit osteoclast function and that peroxides may increase motility. Gallwitz et al.[18] showed that 5-lipoxygenase metabolites of arachidonic acid stimulate isolated osteoclasts to resorb calcified matrices. This provides another hypothetical link between prostaglandins and osteoclast activity.

At a molecular level, osteoclastic bone resorption depends on the expression of the c-*src* protooncogene, which is related to the *src* oncogene found in the Rous sarcoma virus. Knockout mice deficient in the *src* gene develop osteopetrosis.[19] Osteoclasts from these mice are unable to form ruffled borders and resorption pits in response to parathyroid hormone and to interleukin-1. The c-*src* protooncogene encodes for the pp60[c-*src*] tyrosine kinase. In marrow cell cultures, calcitonin inhibits pp60[c-*src*] tyrosine kinase activity. Herbimycin A, a specific enzyme inhibitor, inhibits osteoclastic bone resorption in vitro and hypercalcemia in vivo.[20]

Osteoblasts are mesenchymal cells containing alkaline phosphates. They form bone and modulate osteoclastic activity. Osteoblasts produce osteopontin, osteocalcitonin, osteonectin, and type I alpha I procollagen, which are important for bone mineralization and have been used as markers of osteoblast activity. Osteoblast activity is regulated by hormones, such as growth hormone, and by local cytokine production.[21] Some local factors can stimulate osteoblastic osteogenesis. These factors include PTHrP, bone morphogenetic proteins, the TGF-β family, and insulinlike growth factors (IGF). The mechanism by which osteoblasts activate osteoclasts is still unclear.

Bone turnover can be studied with the use of certain markers, such as serum alkaline phosphatase, osteocalcin, urine calcium, urinary hydroxyproline, and cross-linked urinary pyridinium, on the basis of knowledge of bone formation and resorption.[22] These studies are informative in evaluating therapies directed at osteoclastic activity (e.g., bisphosphonates).

Bone biology is changed by bone metastases, which increase bone resorption. Weakened bone causes pain. Several possible mechanisms involved in osteoclastic bone resorption were discussed earlier; however, these mechanisms and the role of cytokines may differ for different tumors. Garrett[23] implanted VX2 carcinoma cells intraperitoneally in rabbits, which were sacrificed from 24 hours to 8 weeks later. Vigorous microscopic osteoclastic reactions were evident near the tumor cells with new periosteal bone formation. Galasko[24] further showed histologic osteoclastic proliferation and bone destruction in the bone specimens from 68 patients with different tumors.

Another hypothesis of bone pain involves sensitization of peripheral nerve endings by inflammation mediators (e.g., kinins). Prostaglandins (PGs) sensitize nerve endings, and increased PG production has been observed in bone metastases. PGs, particularly PGE_1 and PGE_2, are important because they are associated with the shaping of the bone and producing hyperalgesia.[25] Inhibitors of PG synthesis reduce pain and in some cases tumor growth in the bone as well.[25-30] In an early observation of rabbits with VX2 carcinoma cells implanted in the tibia the levels of PGE_2, bone destruction, and osteoclasts in tumorous bone were greater than in animals treated with indomethacin.[31] The effects of PGE_2 on osteoclasts and bone resorption are complex, however, and do not extrapolate to human breast cancer.[32] Despite this difficulty, certain data support the role of PGs in bone metastasis. For example, bone pain from osteoid osteoma is sensitive to aspirin and other nonsteroidal anti-inflammatory drugs (NSAIDs). This tumor has been shown to produce PGE_2 and PGI_2 levels 30 times normal.[33] Anti-PGE_2 antibodies were used to compare immunohistochemically osteomas from five patients with NSAID-sensitive pain with specimens from other bone tumors as controls. PGE_2 was detected in osteoblasts of all but two of the patients. Rich innervation of the arterioles in the osteoma patients was noted, suggesting innervation may be commensurate with PG production.

Prostaglandins also mediate hormonal response to certain tumors, such as the effect of prolactin on breast cancer cells.[34] It is not clear, however, whether the PG release associated with new bone formation or bone destruction actually causes bone pain. Other factors also may influence the pain in metastatic bone disease. Osteoclast activation factor (OAF), a nonprostaglandin substance, found in other metastatic tumors and multiple myeloma, is thought to be an algogenic agent. Mediators such as acetylcholine, histamine, serotonin, bradykinin, and substance P can activate nociceptors. Substance P can sensitize nociceptors and cause plasma extravasation through increased capillary permeability.

Bone macrophages, circulating factors (e.g., calcitonin), and changes in host cells, calcium metabolism, and hormone receptor status of the metastatic tumor cells contribute to pain production in bone metastasis.[35] Endocrine manipulation using diethylstilbestrol, steroids, calcitonin, hypophysectomy, and levodopa has been reported to relieve pain in patients with both endocrine- and nonendocrine-responsive bone disease. These findings support the concept that hormone interactions are also important in bone pain.[36-40] Bone marrow edema from bone metastasis and increased blood flow can cause rising intraosseous pressure and pain, particularly in the presence of sensitized nerve endings. Unfortunately, despite new understanding, clinical experience shows that some patients with bone metastasis have significant pain and that others rarely do.

PATIENT EVALUATION

Bone pain is a somatic nociceptive pain. As such, one can expect it to be localized to the tumor site(s) and to be worsened by weightbearing or movement (incidental pain). On examination, pain can be reproduced by local pressure or movement of the affected site.

In the evaluation of a patient, one must consider the site of the pain and other syndromes that can mimic bone pain. For example, midline back pain may come from cord compression, vertebral body collapse, vertebral body invasion, marked retroperitoneal adenopathy, degenerative joint disease, and osteoporosis. Hip pain may be caused by lumbosacral plexopathy, impending femoral fracture, referred pain from the lumbar spine, avascular necrosis of the hips, and myofascial pain from poor posture. Recent therapy is also pertinent. Patients with prostate or breast cancer may have increased bone pain following hormone manipulation, and patients receiving recombinant granulocyte colony stimulating factor (r-GCSF) may report low-back and hip pain. Radiation therapy increases pain in the radiated area in a small number of patients.

Patients with bone pain from metastases can present with additional symptoms. Patients with metastasis to the base of the skull may complain of headaches and cranial nerve abnormalities. Patients with metastasis to the clivus may complain of diplopia and a vertex headache. Patients with atlantoaxial destruction will present with a rigid neck, cervical muscle spasms, and severe neck and arm pain. Patients with massive tumor invasion to the chest wall may complain of an inability to stand up because of associated severe pain. Patients with extensive sacral involvement may complain of pelvic pain that occurs when they are standing.

A careful history and physical examination coupled with relevant radiologic imaging studies are often adequate to establish a diagnosis. In some patients it may be necessary to provide pain control first before any study or even examination can be performed. In these patients, fracture or impending fracture must be considered, and surgical evaluation may be warranted. Guidelines for evaluating the risk for impending fracture of the long bones have been proposed.[41] If a hip fracture is highly likely, then general anesthesia may be necessary to expedite evaluation and treatment. Whether surgery or radiation should be the primary means of treating impending fractures is unresolved.

TREATMENT MODALITIES

Many treatment modalities have been reported for controlling pain from bone metastases. Several problems among the older reports, however, make them difficult to interpret: the use of nonvalidated patient pain rating scales, no assessment of mobility, and no recording of concurrent analgesics. Many of these studies are single-arm studies in patients with either similar histology or with different histologic diagnoses. Some studies are involved in the measurement of bone turnover. These patients are difficult to study because they are ill, are often confounded with other acute medical problems, and may not have long enough survival for proper outcome evaluation. When these patients are being observed, it is important to assess for both constant and incidental pain.

Chemotherapy or Hormone Therapy

Treating the underlying disease is essential when it is sensitive to hormone manipulations (prostate cancer, breast cancer) or chemotherapy. Approximately 70% of patients with prostate cancer and bone pain and 33% of those with breast cancer and bone pain will experience pain relief with hormone manipulations. Doses of medroxyprogesterone acetate (MPA) at 1200 mg/d PO in seven patients with refractory prostate carcinoma and bone pain led to pain relief in six patients.[42]

Radiation

Radiation has been the traditional therapy for bone metastasis. It can be given as external beam radiation targeting a localized bone lesion or as hemibody irradiation (HBI) for multifocal disease. How radiation therapy relieves pain from bone lesions is still unknown. Pain relief may occur within several days, although a small number of patients may experience transient exaggeration of pain. Approximately 80% of patients have been reported to experience pain relief with radiation therapy. Lytic lesions, however, can still progress to pathologic fracture during radiation therapy.

External Beam Radiation Therapy

The optimal dose and schedule for external beam radiation therapy (EBRT) remains controversial.[43] The standard practice is 10 fractions with 3 Gy per fraction. However, there has been a trend toward shorter courses with larger fractions. A 1992 consensus statement pointed to the lack of definitive studies and allowed for treating patients with a short life expectancy with one fraction of 8 Gy.[44]

Hemibody Irradiation

HBI is indicated for widespread or multifocal disease. Salazar et al.[45] found HBI provided some pain relief in 73% of patients and complete pain relief in 20% of patients. Fifty percent of these patients responded within 48 hours, and 80% within 1 week. Doses greater than 6 Gy for the upper torso and 8

Gy for the lower torso only increased toxicity. The principal side effects are radiation sickness and radiation pneumonitis.

Radionuclide Therapy

Radionuclide therapy is an active area that has been the subject of reviews by Lewington[46] and Clarke.[47]

Strontium 89

[89]Sr is a pure beta emitter with a half-life of 50.5 days. It is selectively concentrated in osteoblastic lesions. Its use is indicated for patients with multifocal refractory bone pain. Contraindications include leukopenia (WBC <2400/µl) and thrombocytopenia (platelets <60,000/µl). A relative contraindication is urinary insufficiency, as the drug is excreted renally. Previous wide-field radiation is not a contraindication. Dosage is 40 to 80 µCi/kg IV. Side effects include thrombocytopenia and a 10% to 20% exaggeration of pain (in up to 1 month). Treatment for the side effects is dexamethasone, 2 mg PO qid.

Response rates to ^{89}Sr are reported to be approximately 50% for moderate to marked relief. There is no known predictor for favorable outcome. Lewington et al.[48] studied 32 patients with painful bone metastases from prostate cancer and observed complete clinical success in patients (11 of 32 with 21 of 32 dropout) given [89]Sr. Porter et al.[49] studied the effect of adjuvant ^{89}Sr in patients with localized painful bone metastases. There was no pain relief at the target site but a decreased rate of occurrence of new metastases in the ^{89}Sr arm. This aspect may represent a reduction in total health care cost.

[89]Sr has been compared to other radiation therapy modalities. Dearnaley et al.[50] found equivalent analgesia with ^{89}Sr and HBI in a retrospective case-controlled study. In a randomized three-arm study (n = 284; HBI, local EBRT and ^{89}Sr), Quilty et al.[51] showed that pain relief was equal at 65% in all three arms at 3 months. The only difference was a decrease in the number of new metastases in the ^{89}Sr arm (64% in HBI and EBRT patients and 42% in ^{89}Sr patients). [89]Sr has also been used to treat breast cancer and other primary tumors.[52]

Other Radionuclides

Other radionuclides include rhenium 186, samarium 153, and phosphorus 32.[53] Iodine 131 has been used for bone metastases from thyroid cancer. [32]P

has been available for four decades but is not widely used because of bone marrow toxicity.

Osteoclast Agents
Bisphosphonates

The bisphosphonates are a group of stable pyrophosphate (P—O—P) analogs characterized by a central carbon atom linking two phosphate groups (P—C—P) and two side chains of variable structure. The mechanism whereby bisphosphonates decrease bone resorption is unknown. These agents bind to hydroxyapatite in bone and decrease bone turnover. In bone marrow cultures a study of five different bisphosphonates showed that they inhibit the formation or proliferation of osteoclast-like mononuclear cells.[54,55] Bisphosphonates are indicated for Paget's disease and hypercalcemia of malignancy. Their use was reviewed by Averbuch.[56]

Renal failure may be caused by rapid injection of large doses of the bisphosphonates etidronate and clodronate. This could be prevented by IV fluid priming (500 ml over 2 hours). In 50% of patients a transient pyrexia of 1° to 2° C may last up to 3 days. Laboratory changes include reduced peripheral lymphocytes, elevated serum C reactive protein, and reduced serum zinc. Serum should be monitored for changes in calcium, phosphate, and magnesium levels. The infusion rate of pamidronate, however, does not affect body retention of pamidronate, and a dose of 60 mg can be given over 1 hour.[57]

Etidronate (1-hydroxyethylidene-1,1-diphosphonate). There have not been many reports on the use of etidronate for bone pain. Schnur[58] gave 13 patients 5 to 15 mg/kg/d for up to 4 weeks; all but one patient experienced pain relief. Smith[59] randomized 57 patients to four different treatment groups; patients were allowed to go on an open-label protocol if no relief was obtained. A low response rate of 14% was noted. Etidronate also significantly inhibited mineralization.

Clodronate (dichloromethylene-1,1-diphosphonate). Neri et al.[60] studied 20 postmenopausal women with skeletal metastases from breast cancer given clodronate 450 mg IV daily for 5 days and then with 100 mg IM for 10 days. Pain was reduced significantly in 15 patients. In a double-blind crossover study, Ernst et al.[61,62] studied 24 patients with metastatic bone disease. Patients received either 600 mg in 500 ml normal saline over 4 hours or placebo. On a visual analog scale, significant pain relief was seen with clodronate, but the percentage of responding patients was not given. Doses of 600 mg and 1500 mg may be equianalgesic.

Pamidronate (3 amino-1-hydroxypropylidene-1,1-diphosphonate). Reportedly, intravenous dosage of pamidronate has been increasing over the last few years. Thurlimann et al.[63] compared initial doses and continuing infusions of 60 and 90 mg of pamidronate. He found that an initial dose of 60 mg was equivalent to an initial dose of 90 mg but that subsequent infusions of 90 mg were needed for analgesia. In a study of patients with breast cancer metastatic to bone, doses of 60 or 90 mg of pamidronate reduced bone pain, but doses of 30 mg did not. A single dose of 120 mg as palliative therapy was associated with a 59% response rate in 34 patients with bone metastases.

Recently single-arm studies[64-67] have been performed, primarily in Europe, in patients with prostate cancer, breast cancer, and myeloma. An overall response rate of 50% in pain relief has been reported. Markers of bone turnover decrease in patients treated with pamidronate, but the relationship of this to pain relief is unclear from the papers. There is a need for randomized placebo-controlled trials.

Calcitonin

Calcitonin is a peptide hormone with 32 amino acids[68]; salmon calcitonin is the most potent form. Calcitonin inhibits osteoclast function.[69,70] This is accompanied by the production of c-AMP and by increased cytosolic calcium in the osteoclast.[69-72] Its mechanism of analgesia, however, may be independent of its effect on osteoclasts; calcitonin may alter binding of beta endorphins in the central nervous system.[70,73]

Calcitonin is indicated for malignant hypercalcemia,[71,72,74,75] Paget's disease, reflex sympathetic dystrophy, and osteoporotic vertebral collapse. Special concerns include anaphylactic reactions; a trial of 1 unit SC is recommended before treatment is started. Calcitonin is given subcutaneously; the ratio of intranasal to subcutaneous doses is 3 to 1.

Spaventi and Vrbanec[76] studied 25 patients with bone metastases from different primary tumors and gave 100 IU of salmon calcitonin daily for 1 to 2 months. By the sixth day, average pain intensity decreased on a scale of 3 from 2.5 to 1. Hindley et al.[77] randomized 32 patients to 200 IU SC × 6 to 8 doses vs. placebo. At 1 week, 5 of the 13 calcitonin patients but none of the 12 placebo patients experienced relief. Blomqvist et al.[78] randomized 49 patients with stable breast cancer metastasized to bone receiving antineoplastic therapy to salmon calcitonin 100 MRCU SC × 3 months or saline. No difference was seen in skeletal pain. In a randomized placebo-control study (33 patients), Gennari et al.[79] showed salmon calcitonin to be effective.

Most metastatic bone pain responds successfully to chemotherapy or radiation therapy in combination with nonsteroidal anti-inflammatory drugs (NSAIDs) and steroids. The pain will subside with successful treatment outcome. Pain control becomes imperative, however, prior to initiation of antitumor therapy or when treatment fails. A multidimensional approach for this type of pain management is the ideal. Treatment of primary tumor initially is with radiation therapy, chemotherapy or hormone manipulation, and orthopedic stabilization, which are followed by analgesia management. Psychological services may also be needed for associated depression, fear, anger, and death and dying issues.

ANALGESIC THERAPY

One must integrate all the information regarding the effectiveness of the traditional therapy aimed at the tumor, the possible mechanisms involved in nociceptive activation, factors causing sensitization signal transmission, the changes in the spinal cord, and the central nervous system (CNS) status (emotional/affective, cognitive/behavioral domains) to use analgesics and their adjunctive drugs effectively.

Nonsteroidal Anti-Inflammatory Drugs

NSAIDs are widely used for management of mild to moderate pain because they inhibit prostaglandin production and the inflammatory reaction induced by tumors. Actual clinical data on NSAIDs in bone pain are limited. Trials of published meta-analysis on NSAIDs have recommended that further clinical research is needed to establish efficacy of NSAIDs in bone pain. Commonly used NSAIDs are listed in Table 10-1.

Aspirin is the most commonly used NSAID. Pa-

Table 10-1   Dosing data for acetaminophen (APAP) and nonsteroidal anti-inflammatory drugs

Drug	Usual dose for adults and children ≥50 kg body weight	Usual dose for children[1] and adults[2] ≤50 kg body weight
Acetaminophen and over-the-counter NSAIDs		
Acetaminophen	650 mg q5h	10-15 mg/kg q4h
	975 mg q6h	15-20 mg/kg q4h (PR)
Aspirin	650 mg q4h	10-15 mg/kg q4h
	975 mg q6h	15-20 mg/kg q4h (PR)
Ibuprofen (Motrin, others)	400-600 mg q6h	10-15 mg/kg q6-8h
Prescription NSAIDs		
Carprofen (Rimadyl)	100 mg tid	
Choline magnesium trisalicy-late (Trilisate)	1,000-1,500 mg tid	25 mg/kg tid
Choline salicylate (Arthropan)	870 mg q3-4h	
Diflunisal (Dolobid)	500 mg q12h	
Etodolac (Lodine)	200-400 mg q6-8h	
Fenoprofen calcium (Nalfon)	300-600 mg q6h	
Ketoprofen (Orudis)	25-60 mg q6-8h	
Ketorolac tromethamine (Toradol)	10 mg q4-6h to a maximum of 40 mg/d	
Magnesium salicylate (Doan's, Magan, Mobidin, others)	650 mg q4h	
Meclofenamate sodium (Meclomen)	50-100 mg q6h	
Mefenamic acid (Ponstel)	250 mg q6h	
Naproxen (Naprosyn)	250-275 mg q6-8h	5 mg/kg q8h
Naproxen sodium (Anaprox)	275 mg q6-8h	
Sodium salicylate (Generic)	325-650 mg q3-4h	
Parenteral NSAIDs		
Ketorolac tromethamine (Toradol)	60 mg initially; then 30 mg q6h IM; not to be given longer than 5 d	

tients with cancer, however, are frequently at increased risk of bleeding from the disease process and from treatment-related thrombocytopenia.

Acetaminophen is a weaker anti-inflammatory drug than aspirin; however, it carries less gastric irritation, erosion, and bleeding. It rarely causes thrombocytopenia.

Mefenamic acid has less of an analgesic effect than commonly used fenoprofen, diflunisal, naproxen, and naproxen sodium.

Indomethacin is both analgesic and anti-inflammatory and is more potent than aspirin. It reduces the elevated serum calcium levels in patients with metastatic cancer. Gastrointestinal side effects are fairly common, occurring in approximately half the patients, and in 20% of patients are severe enough to require its discontinuation. The side effects of gastric ulceration, frontal headache, and hematopoietic reaction may complicate its use.

Ketorolac is a fairly recent addition to the list of NSAIDs. It is available in intravenous or oral formulation. Because it causes gastrointestinal irritation, therapy should be limited to 5 days in either formulation.

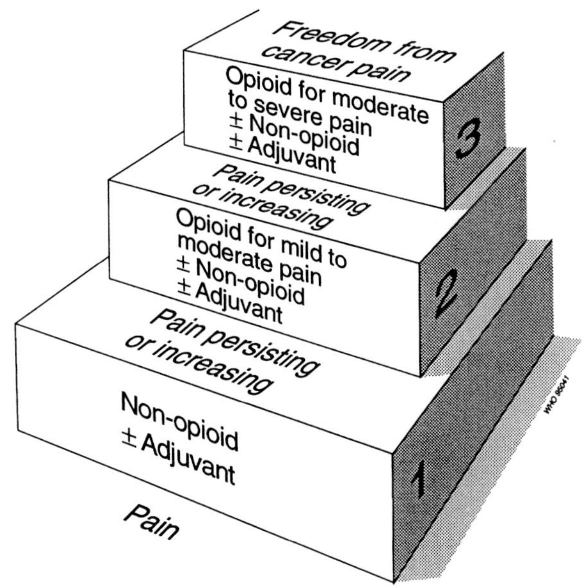

Fig. 10-1   The WHO three-step analgesic ladder. (Reproduced by permission of WHO from Cancer Pain Relief, 2nd ed. Geneva: World Health Organization, 1996.)

Celecoxib, a new NSAID, is a selective cyclo-oxygenase-2 inhibitor. Its lack of cyclo-oxygenase-1 inhibition prevents the gastric irritation caused by other NSAIDs.

When an NSAID becomes less effective, a narcotic should be added to it, not replace it, because the combined therapy usually yields a better treatment outcome. A combination of NSAIDs is not recommended, since they compete for the protein-binding site. Combination preparations of opioid (CNS and peripheral nervous system [PNS] mechanisms) and NSAID (PNS mechanism) to treat metastatic bone pain are a logical approach. The daily toxic dose limits of the NSAID, however, should be strictly observed. For example, Percocet consists of oxycodone 5 mg and acetaminophen 650 mg. When a daily dose requirement exceeds 3000 mg of acetaminophen, there is risk of liver damage. Therefore at a higher dose range it is recommended that the opioid component be separated from that of the NSAID.

Opioid Analgesics

Opioid analgesics are essential in managing cancer-related bone pain. They are described in the discussions that follow.

The three-step ladder World Health Organization (WHO) approach (Fig. 10-1) should not be followed in sequence in cases of severe pain. Instead, an opioid should be used as the initial analgesic. A strong opioid should be used initially to control severe pain. The commonly used opioids

are shown in Table 10-2. Morphine sulfate is the gold standard. On the basis of its long clinical experience and according to the available research data, it has been the most frequently prescribed opioid. Oral administration is preferred whenever possible. If parenteral dosing is necessary, intravenous or subcutaneous administration is preferable. Intramuscular opioid administration is suboptimal because of erratic drug absorption. An aggressive approach in preventing expected side effects and in treating actual opioid-induced toxicities is mandatory.

Opioid should be administered around the clock to prevent breakthrough pain. A knowledge of the pharmacokinetics of each compound is necessary to properly administer the various preparations. In general, short-acting opioids are effective for approximately 4 hours and therefore should be prescribed initially at 4-hour intervals. One third to one half of the 4-hour dose should be prescribed as needed every 1 to 2 hours for breakthrough pain. If the pain is not effectively controlled, the doses given can be increased 33% to 50%, regardless of the dose given. This will quickly establish the effective daily dosage. Intravenous titration can also be used to rapidly establish the effective dose. Once the daily dose is established, a long-acting preparation can be used instead with a short-acting opioid of the same class for breakthrough pain.

It is emphasized that there is no ceiling dose of opioids. The right dose is the effective dose with no or controllable side effects. The primary reason to change to a different opioid formulation is because the side effects cannot be controlled, not because "too high a dose" is reached. Individual variations among patients in side effect profiles are common and unpredictable.

Meperidine should not be used regularly on a long-term basis (more than several days). Accumulation of the toxic metabolite normeperidine can result in CNS excitation, with agitation, confusion, and seizures. This occurs particularly in the elderly and in those with compromised renal functions. Similarly, levorphanol and morphine must be used cautiously in patients with nephropathies. Both compounds have toxic metabolites normally ex-

Table 10-2 Oral and parenteral narcotic analgesics for severe pain

Narcotic agonists	Route	Equianalgesic dose (mg)*	Duration (h)	Plasma half-life (h)	Comments
Morphine	IM	10	4-6	2-3.5	Standard for comparison; available in slow-release tablets
	PO	60	4-7		
Codeine	IM	130	4-6	3	Biotransformed to morphine; useful as initial narcotic analgesic
	PO	200+	4-6		
Oxycodone	IM	15		—	Short acting; available as 5 mg dose in combination with aspirin and acetaminophen
	PO	30	3-5		
Heroin	IM	5	4-5	0.5	Illegal in United States; high solubility for parenteral administration
	PO	60	4-5		
Levorphanol (Levodromoran)	IM	2	4-6	12-16	Good oral potency; requires careful titration in initial dosing because of drug accumulation; more soluble than morphine
	PO	4	4-7		
Hydromorphone (Dilaudid)	IM	1.5	4-5	2-3	Available in high-potency in injectable form (10 mg/ml) for cachectic patients and as rectal suppositories
	PO	7.5	4-6		
Oxymorphone (Numorphan)	IM	1	4-6	2-3	Available in parenteral and rectal suppository form only
	PR	10	4-6		
Meperidine (Demerol)	IM	75	4-5	3-4 (normeperidine 12-16)	Contraindicated in patients with renal disease; accumulation of active toxic metabolite, normeperidine, produces CNS excitation
	PO	300+	4-6		
Methadone (Dolophine)	IM	10		15-30	Good oral potency; requires careful titration in initial dosing to avoid drug accumulation
	PO	20			

*Based on single-dose studies in which an intramuscular dose of each drug listed was compared to morphine for the establishment of its relative potency. Oral doses are those recommended when change from parenteral to oral routes is made. For patients without prior narcotic exposure the recommended oral starting dose is 30 mg for morphine, 5 mg for methadone, 2 mg for levorphanol, and 4 mg for hydromorphone.

creted by the kidney, and build-up can result in CNS toxicity.

Equianalgesia from either oral or parenteral opioid is associated with similar side effects. Mixed agonist-antagonist is not recommended for long-term use. Table 10-2 lists the morphinelike agonists, the equianalgesic doses with oral and parenteral use, the half-life, time to peak effect, and the duration of activity.

Several issues involved in long-term use of narcotics warrant discussion. These are tolerance, physical dependence, and addiction. Long-term use of narcotics in cancer pain can be associated with development of tolerance and physical dependence. Psychological dependence (addiction) is rare.

Tolerance may be defined as the need for increased amounts of opioids to maintain the same analgesic effectiveness when the pain stimulus remains constant. Most chronic, stable, cancer-related pain can be controlled with stable doses of opioids for prolonged periods. Tolerance may slowly develop in some patients and may require a gradual increase in opioid dose.[38] Sudden development of frequent breakthrough pain is commonly associated with disease progression, not tolerance.

One should not deprive the patient of adequate analgesia because of the suspicion of tolerance. Tolerance does not hamper the therapy. Simply increasing the dose will satisfy the need as a result of tolerance. In incurable cancer, pain relief and improvement of quality of life are the main therapeutic goals. Physical dependency is characterized by withdrawal symptoms upon rapid dose reduction; symptoms include sympathetic hyperactivation, such as sweating, agitation, nausea, vomiting, and diarrhea. Opioid withdrawal usually can be prevented by giving 10% to 20% of the maintenance daily dosage, which is usually not a problem in patient management.

Addiction or psychological dependence is a state in which the patient is seeking or abusing a drug, not for pain relief but to satisfy a craving, while fully recognizing the detrimental effect of the drug. It was the experience of a large series of cancer patients with moderate to severe pain that long-term administration of narcotics did not cause significant problems in clinical management, even in the presence of tolerance and withdrawal symptoms.

Addictive behavior was identified only in 3% to 5% of the population. This population had a history of drug abuse or of recreational medication use.[80] We also demonstrated in a prospective study in noncancer chronic pain that long-term use of narcotics did not produce significant management problems. Most people will receive a fixed dosage of narcotic, with a small percentage requiring an increase because tolerance develops. The addictive population is easily identified. The most commonly displayed addictive behaviors are request for early prescription refill on two or more occasions, report of lost or stolen medication on two or more occasions, theft of prescription pad, alteration of prescription, use of multiple pharmacies, seeking medication from other physicians, and failure to return unused medication. Inadequate dosing of opioid produces "spiraling down" effects (depression, inactivity, and awakening due to pain) in noncancer pain patients. When an adequate narcotic dose was achieved, all "spiraling down" effects vanished.[81,82]

Addiction is a commonly feared side effect of opioids. This pathologic drug-seeking behavior is rare in patients taking opioids for cancer pain analgesia. An estimated occurrence is less than 1 in 3000 patients. This is quite different than the physical dependence that occurs in most patients who take opioids in an around-the-clock fashion for more than 2 to 3 weeks. If a patient's pain is relieved by some other means, however, the opioids can be discontinued quickly and safely without significant withdrawal response. This is accomplished by decreasing the dose of opioids by about one half to one third every 1 to 2 days until the oral equivalent of 30 mg of morphine per day is achieved. Opioids can then be stopped without difficulty.

Patients who are suboptimally treated (i.e., for pain control rather than pain prevention) and require regular dosing to relieve pain may present with a "pseudoaddiction" syndrome. The patient may become disruptive or manipulative and may appear to have drug-seeking behavior. Appropriate opioid administration to completely relieve the pain would be the proper approach to curtail this "pseudoaddiction."

Choice, Potency, and Conversion of Opioids

The choice of opioid for cancer pain follows no exact pattern or logic. Drug potency is not necessarily relevant to drug selection; rather it is a convenient expression of the relative affinity of receptor binding. If the patient requires 60 mg of codeine, it can simply be replaced by 10 mg of morphine. It must be remembered that the individual variation of sensitivity to an opioid can be as much as sixfold, and furthermore the side effect profile of an opioid can vary among individuals. Therefore in each patient one must weigh the therapeutic and side effects to have a successful treatment outcome. There are pragmatic aspects in selection of an opioid, such as how many pills the patient can take at a given time. Certain medications are not recommended for long-term use; for example, meperidine (Demerol) because of its active toxic metabolite, normeperidine. The half-life of this metabolite is 12 to 16 hours, and it can induce neurologic symptoms of hyperactivity, such as mood elevation, tremors, multifocal myoclonus, and seizures. Methadone is long acting, with the analgesic effect lasting for 6 to 8 hours while the metabolite lingers on for 16 to 24 hours. Therefore after the initial titration for several days, the dosage may have to be reduced to avoid accumulation of the metabolite. One should use methadone with caution in patients with renal insufficiency.

Once the adequate daily opioid dose has been established, conversion from short-acting to continuous release preparations is often desirable to reduce the frequency of drug administration. The conversion factor from oral to parenteral dose is approximately 3 to 1. For breakthrough pain a short-acting opioid can be given at one sixth to one quarter of the 12-hour continuous release dose every 2 to 3 hours. The conversion factors from morphine to other opioids are given in Table 10-2. Approximately two thirds of this oral equivalent dose is then used initially to allow for the possibility of a lack in cross-tolerance between different opioid preparations. Subsequent upward dose titration can then follow.

Alternative Routes of Opioid Administration

Fentanyl is a lipophilic compound. Transdermal administration is most useful for the patient with fairly constant pain who is comatose, cannot take oral medications, or does not comply with drug regimens. The cutaneous patch usually is changed every 72 hours, but for some patients it appears to be effective for only 48 hours because of tolerance or changes in skin conditions. The onset of action is 14 to 18 hours. Steady state kinetics occur at 36 to 48 hours. Because it is stored in the adipose tissues, it takes about 24 hours to dissipate after removal of the patch. All patients using transdermal fentanyl must also be given some short-acting opioid for breakthrough pain. Sustained-release compounds (oral or transdermal) should not be used to titrate analgesia or for the patient with unpredictable pain.

The rectal route of administration (suppositories) is useful in patients with dysphagia or lack of subcutaneous tissue or venous access. Suppositories are available for hydromorphone, oxymorphone, and morphine. Equianalgesic dosing to oral preparations is used. Although the oral sustained-release preparations are not approved for rectal use, there is some substantiating clinical evidence that rectally administered MS Contin (morphine) is as effective at equianalgesic doses as those given orally.

Although oral administration is the easiest and most widely accepted route, subcutaneous administration and intravenous infusion also are acceptable. Patient-controlled analgesia (PCA), usually by continuous infusion with bolus dosing as necessary, can be given intravenously or subcutaneously. It is predominately used when oral or transdermal pain management is not possible because of uncontrollable side effects or an inability to take oral medications. In special conditions, PCA can be used to rapidly titrate analgesia. PCA is only indicated for a relatively small percentage of patients because of its cost and the relative difficulty in maintenance as compared to oral or transdermal administration.

Intraspinal (epidural and intrathecal) administration of opioids may be effective when other routes of administration have failed or when side effects are uncontrollable. Preservative-free morphine hydromorphone and fentanyl are most commonly administered by this route. They can be given by bolus or continuous infusion. Externalized catheters can be used for several days for radiation therapy or clinical trial for efficacy. The catheter can be tunneled subcutaneously and then externalized and used for months with adequate care.[83,84] The catheter also can be implanted and connected to a subcutaneous access port to receive the drug.[85] Permanently implanted catheters can be connected to an implantable infusion pump system, which can be used for protracted therapy.[86-90] The primary indication for epidural or intrathecal administration of opioids is for patients with cancer pain below the midthoracic area and for those who have failed previous oral or transdermal opioid drug trials because of unmanageable side effects. Plasma levels are significantly lower when opioid is given intraspinally rather than orally or intravenously, resulting in fewer side effects. Concomitant administration of clonidine epidurally (FDA approved) or intrathecally (under investigation) can reduce the requirement of opioid.

Intraventricular or cisternal administration via Ommaya reservoir has been reported to be of some benefit for intractable pain. It is most often used for cervicofacial pain, cervicobrachial pain, and other pains unresponsive to conservative measures.

Management of Opioid Side Effects

Opioid-related side effects are usually preventable or controllable. All opioids possess similar side effect profiles; however, there is considerable individual variability in occurrence and severity. To reduce side effects, sometimes a sequential trial of different opioids is required. All the opioid side effects except constipation abate with time.

There is no correlation between the opioid plasma level and its therapeutic and side effects. *The right dose is the dose that works.*

The Myths of Frequent Respiratory Depression and Addiction or Psychological Dependency

Opioids act on the brain stem respiratory center to decrease responsiveness to CO_2 tension. Pain is a natural antagonist to respiratory depression. Significant respiratory depression is uncommon unless the pain is totally controlled and the patient becomes overly sedated. Opioids may be used safely after a careful titration to achieve analgesia in patients with pulmonary diseases. Naloxone can be used, if necessary, to reverse *significant* opioid-induced respiratory depression. If used, an ampule of 0.4 mg naloxone should be diluted with 10 ml of normal saline and given at 1 ml IV every 1 to 2 minutes. It can be repeated or given by IV infusion (0.004 mg/kg/min). It may be given more rapidly for severe respiratory depression. Too-rapid administration of large doses of this drug could precipitate a withdrawal response in an opioid-dependent patient. Since the half-life of naloxone is about 30 minutes and is usually significantly less than that of the opioids, repeat doses or even a naloxone drip may be necessary.

Adjuvant Drugs to Narcotic Therapy

Adjuvant drugs have been developed for clinical indications other than analgesia. Except for methotrimeprazine (phenothiazine analgesic), they are not as effective as narcotics in relieving pain. In many instances there are no efficacy studies for the coanalgesic properties, particularly in cancer pain patients. The selection of an adjuvant must be individualized using the simplest and most potent combination of drugs.

Steroids

Steroids are the most commonly used adjuvant in managing pain from metastatic bone disease. The exact mechanism of the analgesic effect is not clearly understood. It was thought that its anti-inflammatory and antitumor effects were at least partially responsible in most (85%) of the patients with spinal cord compression from epidural mass. Dexamethasone 100 mg IV as part of the regular therapy protocol provided significant pain relief and a marked reduction in analgesic requirement.[91] The steroid's ability to produce euphoria and increase appetite and weight gain contribute greatly to the cancer patient's sense of well-being. Two studies showed prolonged survival time and reduction in the narcotic dosage.[92,93] In the patient with epidural compression and pain the initial dose usually is 100 mg of IV dexamethasone, followed by a tapering schedule with maintenance at approximately 16 mg during radiation therapy. This would achieve significant pain relief. Dexamethasone possesses approximately 8 times the anti-inflammatory activity of prednisone without its mineralocorticoid property. In a prospective study,[94] dexamethasone seemed to be more effective than prednisone against nerve compression pain, but the side effects profiles are similar. The most common side effects of NSAIDs are gastric ulceration and gastrointestinal bleeding. Therefore their concomitant use should be avoided.

Tricyclic Antidepressants

A tricyclic antidepressant (TCA) is commonly used for neuropathic pain. It suppresses the influx calcium channel current.[95] There is no ceiling analgesic effect of TCA in neuropathic pain. The nortriptyline effect is mediated by its inhibitory effect on serotonin metabolism in the central nervous system. Antidepressants have been used as coanalgesics in combination with morphine. An evening dose usually helps sleep because of its potent analgesic and sedative effect. In the presence of depression, as much as 300 mg orally per day may be required.

Antihistamines

The antihistamine hydroxyzine specifically possesses analgesic properties. A dose of 100 mg of parenteral hydroxyzine possesses analgesic activity approaching that of 8 mg of parenteral morphine.[96] Hydroxyzine has an additive analgesic effect when used in combination with opioids.[97] Hydroxyzine also possesses antiemetic and antianxiety properties. A dose of 25 to 30 mg of hydroxyzine can be used as a coanalgesic with a narcotic. Ondansetron, a 5-hydroxytryptamine ($5HT_3$) inhibitor (an antiemetic), has recently been found to possess sodium channel current inhibition properties.[98] Therefore this drug potentially can be used as a local anesthetic to treat neuropathic pain, which is frequently a component of cancer pain. Clinical trials, however, have not been performed.

Phenothiazines

Methotrimeprazine (Levoprome) possesses the strongest analgesic property in this class of drugs. An analgesic dose of intramuscular methotrimeprazine equal to that of morphine is 1 to 1. It is particularly valuable in managing cancer bone pain in special circumstances, such as patients tolerant of the narcotic but with bowel obstruction and respiratory depression. In patients with pain and uncontrolled narcotic-induced nausea, vomiting, or anxiety, it is effective as an analgesic, antiemetic, and sedative. An initial test dose of 5 mg IM should be used to evaluate the sedative and hypotensive effect. The dose of 10 to 20 mg IM is relatively commonly used. Variations in individual responses may be marked. Side effects include postural hypotension and excessive sedation. Tolerance to this side effect does develop with repeated administration. Extrapyramidal effect can also occur, but the incidence is unknown.

Chlorpromazine is used in terminal illness and cancer pain and does not produce an additive analgesia. It is used as a tranquilizer and antiemetic.

Anticonvulsants

Phenytoin and carbamazepine inhibit sodium and some channel current. They are used to treat neuropathic pain, such as postherpetic neuralgia, diabetic neuropathy, and deafferentation pain.[99] They have not been effective in treating bone pain, except when it is associated with radiculopathy. Carbamazepine is particularly useful in treating acute shocklike neuralgia as seen in patients with cranial or high cervical neck pain caused by tumor infiltration or traumatic neuroma. It is also used in patients with phantom limb pain secondary to traumatic neuroma. The dosage of carbamazepine begins at 100 mg PO per day and slowly increases to 800 mg per day over a 7- to 10-day period. The blood count should be taken 2 weeks after the initiation of therapy and at regular intervals during therapy to monitor potential side effects.

Gabapentin (Neurontin) is structurally related to the neurotransmitter gamma-aminobutyric acid (GABA) but does not interact with the GABA receptor. It is not converted metabolically into GABA or GABA agonist, and it is not an inhibitor of GABA uptake or degradation. In radioligand binding assays (up to 100 μmol/L), gabapentin did not exhibit affinity to many common receptors, including benzodiazepine, glutamate, N-methyl-D-aspartate (NMDA), alpha 1-, alpha 2-, or beta-adrenergics, histamine H_1, 5-HTS_1, 5-HTS_2, opiate μ, δ or κ, voltage-sensitive Ca^{2+} channel and voltage-sensitive Na^+ channel. The mechanism of its anticonvulsant action is unknown.

Daily doses of up to 2700 mg have been used without significant side effects. Gabapentin is not substantially metabolized in humans and is eliminated by renal excretion as an unchanged drug. Thus renal insufficiency prolongs its plasma half-life. Gabapentin does not alter the pharmacokinetics and pharmacodynamics of other anticonvulsants, such as phenytoin, carbamazepine, valproic acid, and phenobarbital. Cimetidine reduces creatinine clearance (by 10%), which reduces gabapentin clearance. The small reduction in gabapentin clearance is not likely to be important clinically.

Butyrophenone

Haloperidol (Haldol), a butyrophenone, may be used as a coanalgesic or for treatment of side effects from methadone.[100] Haloperidol may also be used to manage confusion, hallucinations, overwhelming pain, nausea, and vomiting.[101] It is the drug of choice for cancer patients with acute psychosis or agitated delirium.

Central Nervous System Stimulants

Dextroamphetamine (Dexedrine) (10 mg IM)[102] produced an additive analgesic effect when used with morphine in a single-dose study of postoperative pain. It is also used (2.5 to 5 mg twice daily) to reduce the sedative effect of long-term opioid therapy. There are no controlled studies of long-term use of a CNS stimulant in cancer pain management.

Snow used cocaine to treat bone pain.[103] Twycross[104] reported that adding cocaine in 10 mg increments per dose of the Bromptom cocktail resulted in a small but statistically significant increase in alertness, but discontinuing cocaine had no detectable effect. In a controlled study of morphine and cocaine, however, Kaiko et al.[105] showed that cocaine (10 mg oral) alone or as an additive to morphine exhibits no analgesic effect. The perceived CNS excitatory effect was thought to be from blockade of dopamine reuptake, resulting in elevation of excitatory agonists. Recently cocaine was found to depress the $GABA_A$ current of hippocampal neurons.[106] The clinical significance of this depression is debatable.

Nerve Blocks and Neurolysis

Diagnostic nerve blocks are useful in defining specific neural involvement or in assessing the outcome of planned neurolytic blocks. Nerve blocks are most effective in controlling acute radicular pain associated with a rib fracture or nerve root compression.

Epidural and intrathecal blocks are effective for pain from bilateral innervation, such as vertebral or sacral metastases, or from "midline" pain.[38,107]

CONCLUSION

Management of pain is one of the most important treatments the clinician performs for the cancer patient. In skeletal metastases the wide variety of treatment modalities discussed in this chapter are available to the clinician. Psychological drug dependence is not a major problem; therefore relief of pain to allow a functional level of independence for the patient should be the goal of the oncology team.

ACKNOWLEDGMENT

We are grateful to Ms. Rhonda Smith for her excellent assistance in typing this manuscript.

REFERENCES

1. Morris JN, Mor V, Goldberg RJ, Sherwood S, Greer DS, Hiris J. The effect of treatment setting and patient characteristics on pain in terminal cancer patients: A report from the National Hospice Study. J Chronic Dis 39:27-35, 1986.
2. Cowin SC, Moss-Salentjin L, Moss ML. Candidates for the mechanosensory system in bone. J Biomech Eng 113:191-197, 1991.
3. Rosier RN, Hicks DG, Teot LA, Puzas JE, O'Keefe RJ. Mechanisms of bone metastasis. In Progress in Pain Res Mgmt, Assessment and Treatment of Cancer Pain. Seattle: IASP Press, 1998, pp 257-268.
4. Kuratsu S, Uchida A, Araki N. Mechanism of organ selectivity in the determination of metastatic patterns of Dunn osteosarcoma. Trans Ortho Res Soc 17:196, 1992.
5. Overall CM. Regulation of tissue inhibitor of matrix metalloproteinase expression. Ann NY Acad Sci 732:51-64, 1994.
6. Mann EA, Hibbs MS, Spiro JD, Bowik C, Wang XZ, Clawson M, Chen LL. Cytokine regulation of gelatinase production by head and neck squamous cell carcinoma: The role of tumor necrosis factor-alpha. Ann Otol Rhinol Laryngol 104:203-209, 1995.
7. Tanaka K, Iwamoto Y, Ito Y, Ishibashi T, Nakabeppu Y, Sekiguchi M, Sugioka Y. Cyclic AMP-regulated synthesis of the tissue inhibitors of metalloproteinases suppresses the invasive potential of the human fibrosarcoma cell line HT1080. Cancer Res 55:2927-2935, 1995.
8. Callaghan MM, Lovis RM, Rammohan C, Lu Y, Pope RM. Autocrine regulation of collagenase gene expression by TNF-alpha in U937. J Leukoc Biol 59:125-132, 1996.
9. Montgomery AM, Mueller BM, Reisfeld RA, Taylor SM, DeClerck YA. Effect of tissue inhibitor of the matrix metalloproteinases-2 expression on the growth and spontaneous metastasis of a human melanoma cell line. Cancer Res 54:5467-5473, 1994.

10. Watanabe M, Takahashi Y, Ohta T, Mai M, Sasaki T, Seiki M. Inhibition of metastasis in human gastric cancer cells transfected with tissue inhibitor of metalloproteinase 1 gene in nude mice. Cancer 77(8 Suppl):1676-1680, 1996.

11. Baker T, Tickle S, Wasan H, Docherty A, Isenberg D, Waxman J. Serum metalloproteinases and their inhibitors: Markers for malignant potential. Br J Cancer 70:506-512, 1994.

12. Naylor MS, Stamp GW, Davies BD, Balkwill FR. Expression and activity of MMPS and their regulators in ovarian cancer. Int J Cancer 58:50-56, 1994.

13. Onisto M, Riccio MP, Scannapieco P, Caenazzo C, Griggio L, Spina M, Stetler-Stevenson WG, Garbisa S. Gelatinase A/TIMP-2 imbalance in lymph-node-positive breast carcinomas, as measured by RT-PCR. Int J Cancer 63:621-626, 1995.

14. Zaidi M, Pazianas M, Shankar VS, Bax BE, Bax CM, Bevis PJ, Stevens C, Huang CL, Blake DR, Moonga BS, et al. Osteoclast function and its control. Exp Physiol 78:721-739, 1993.

15. Coleman RE, Purohit OP. Osteoclast inhibition for the treatment of bone metastases. Cancer Treat Rev 19:79-103, 1993.

16. Lin HY, Harris TL, Flannery MS, Aruffo A, Kaji EH, Gorn A, Kolakowski LF Jr, Lodish HF, Goldring SR. Expression cloning of an adenylate cyclase–coupled calcitonin receptor. Science 254:1022-1024, 1991.

17. Zaidi M, Alam AS, Bax BE, et al. Role of the endothelial cell in osteoclast control: New perspectives. Bone 14:97-102, 1992.

18. Gallwitz WE, Mundy GR, Lee CH, Qiao M, Roodman GD, Raftery M, Gaskell SJ, Bonewald LF. 5-lipoxygenase metabolites of arachidonic acid stimulate isolated osteoclasts to resorb calcified matrices. J Biol Chem 268:10087-10094, 1993.

19. Soriano P, Montgomery C, Geske R, Bradley A. Targeted disruption of the c-*src* proto-oncogene leads to osteopetrosis in mice. Cell 64:693-702, 1991.

20. Yoneda T, Lowe C, Lee CH, Gutierrez G, Niewolna M, Williams PJ, Izbicka E, Uehara Y, Mundy GR. Herbimycin A, a pp60[c-src] tyrosine kinase inhibitor, inhibits osteoclastic bone resorption in vitro and hypercalcemia in vivo. J Clin Invest 91:2791-2795, 1993.

21. Zheng MH, Wood DJ, Papadimitriou JM. What's new in the role of cytokines on osteoblast proliferation and differentiation? Pathol Res Pract 188:1104-1121, 1992.

22. Delmas PD. Biochemical markers of bone turnover. I. Theoretical considerations and clinical use in osteoporosis. Am J Med 20(Suppl 2):11S-16S, 1993.

23. Garrett IR. Bone destruction in cancer. Semin Oncol 20(Suppl 2):4-9, 1993.

24. Galasko CS. Mechanisms of bone destruction in the development of skeletal metastases. Nature 263:507-508, 1976.

25. Powles TJ, Clark SA, Easty GC, Neville AM. The inhibition by aspirin and indomethacin of osteolytic tumour deposits and hypercalcaemia in rats with Walker tumour and its possible application to human breast cancer. Br J Cancer 28:316-321, 1973.

26. Day SB, Laird Myers WB, Stansly P, et al. Factors influencing development of bone metastases. In Day SB, ed. Cancer Invasion and Metastases: Biologic Mechanisms and Therapy. New York: Raven Press, 1977.

27. Ferreira SH, Nakamura M, de Abreu Castro MS. The hyperalgesic effects of prostacycline and prostaglandin E2. Prostaglandins 16:31-37, 1978.

28. Brodie GN. Indomethacin and bone pain. [Letter.] Lancet 1:1160, 1974.

29. Gasic GJ, Gasic TB, Murphy S. Anti-metastatic effect of aspirin. Lancet 2:932-933, 1972.

30. Stoll BA. Indomethacin in breast cancer. Lancet 2:384, 1973.

31. Galasko CS, Bennett A. Relationship of bone destruction in skeletal metastases to osteoclast activation and prostaglandins. Nature 263:508-510, 1976.

32. Bennett A. The role of biochemical mediators in peripheral nociception and bone pain. Cancer Surveys 7:55-67, 1988.

33. Greco F, Tamburrelli F, Ciabattoni G. Prostaglandins in osteoid osteoma. Int Orthop 15:35-37, 1991.

34. Sacks PV. Prolactin, prostaglandin, and bone pain of metastatic breast cancer. [Letter.] Lancet 2:1385, 1974.

35. Bockman RS, Laird Myers WB. Osteotropism in human breast cancer. In Day SB, ed. Cancer Invasion and Metastases: Biologic Mechanisms and Therapy. New York: Raven Press, 1977.

36. Miles J, Lipton S. Mode of action by which pituitary alcohol injection relieves pain. In Bonica JJ, Albe-Fessard D, eds. Advances in Pain Research and Therapy. New York: Raven Press, 1976.

37. Minton JP. Proceedings: The response of breast cancer patients with bone pain to L-dopa. Cancer 33:358-363, 1974.

38. Foley KM. The treatment of cancer pain. N Engl J Med 313:84-95, 1985.

39. Moricca G. Chemical hypophysectomy for cancer pain. In Bonica JJ, ed. Advances in Neurology. New York: Raven Press, 1974.

40. Tolis GJ. L-dopa for pain from bone metastasis. [Letter.] N Engl J Med 292:1352-1353, 1975.

41. Mirels H. Metastatic disease in long bones: A proposed scoring system for diagnosing impending pathologic fractures. Clin Orthop 249:256-264, 1989.

42. Sasagawa I, Satomi S. Effect of high dose medroxyprogesterone acetate on plasma hormone levels and pain relief in patients with advanced prostate cancer. Br J Urol 65:278-281, 1990.

43. Bates T. A review of local radiotherapy in the treatment of metastases and cord compression. Int J Radiat Oncol Biol Phys 23:217-221, 1992.

44. Bates T, Yarnold JR, Blitzer P, Nelson OS, Rubin P, Maher J. Bone metastasis consensus statement. Int J Radiat Oncol Biol Phys 23:215-216, 1992.

45. Salazar OM, Rubin P, Hendrickson FR, Komaki R, Poulter C, Newall J, Asbell SO, Mohiuddin M, Van Ess J. Single-dose half-body irradiation for palliation of multiple bone metastases from solid tumors. Cancer 58:29-36, 1986.

46. Lewington VL. Targeted radionuclide therapy for bone metastases. Eur J Nucl Med 20:66-74, 1993.

47. Clarke SEM. Radionuclide therapy in oncology. Cancer Treat Rev 20:51-71, 1994.

48. Lewington VJ, McEwan AJ, Ackery DM, Bayly RJ, Keeling DH, Macleod PM, Porter AT, Zivanovic MA. A prospective, randomized double-blind crossover study to examine the efficacy of strontium-89 in pain palliation in patients with ad-

vanced prostate cancer metastatic to bone. Eur J Cancer 27: 954-958, 1991.

49. Porter AT, McEwan AJ, Powe JE, Reid R, McGowan DG, Lukka H, Sathyanarayana JR, Yakemchuk VN, Thomas GM, Erlich LE, et al. Results of a randomized phase-III trial to evaluate the efficacy of strontium-89 adjuvant to local field external beam irradiation in the management of endocrine resistant metastatic prostate cancer. Int J Radiat Oncol Biol Phys 25:805-813, 1993.

50. Dearnaley DP, Bayly RJ, A'Hern RP, Gadd J, Zivanovic MM, Lewington VJ. Palliation of bone metastases in prostate cancer. Hemibody irradiation or strontium-89? Clin Oncol (R Coll Radiol) 4:101-107, 1992.

51. Quilty PM, Kirk D, Bolger JJ, Dearnaley DP, Lewington VJ, Mason MD, Reed NS, Russell JM, Yardley J. A comparison of the palliative effects of strontium-89 and external beam radiotherapy in metastatic prostate cancer. Radiother Oncol 31:33-40, 1994.

52. Kovner F, Ron IG, Levita M, Chaitchik S. Strontium-89 therapy in patients with carcinoma of unknown origin and incurable pain from bone metastases. J Pain Symptom Manage 8:47-51, 1993.

53. Freeman LM, Blaufox MD, eds. Radionuclide therapy of intractable bone pain. Semin Nucl Med 22:1-58, 1992.

54. Hughes DE, Mian M, Guilland-Cumming DF, Russell RGG. The cellular mechanism of action of bisphosphonates. Drugs Exp Clin Res 17:109-114, 1991.

55. Hughes DE, MacDonald BR, Russell RG, Gowen M. Inhibition of osteoclast-like cell formation by bisphosphonates in long-term cultures of human bone marrow. J Clin Invest 83(6):1930-1935, 1989.

56. Averbuch SD. New bisphosphonates in the treatment of bone metastases. Cancer 72:3443-3452, 1993.

57. Leyvraz S, Hess U, Flesch G, Bauer J, Hauffe S, Ford JM, Burckhardt P. Pharmacokinetics of pamidronate in patients with bone metastases. J Natl Cancer Inst 84:788-792, 1992.

58. Schnur W. Relief of metastatic bone pain with etidronate disodium. Ohio State Med J 83:62-65, 1987.

59. Smith JA. Palliation of painful bone metastases from prostate cancer using sodium etidronate: Results from a randomized prospective, double-blind, placebo-controlled study. J Urol 141:85-87, 1989.

60. Neri B, Gemelli MT, Sambataro S, Colombi L, Benvenuti F, Ludovici M, Pacini P. Subjective and metabolic effects of clodronate in patients with advanced breast cancer and symptomatic bone metastases. Anticancer Drugs 3:87-90, 1992.

61. Ernst DS, MacDonald RN, Paterson AH, Jensen J, Brashear P, Bruera E. A double-blind, crossover trial of intravenous clodronate in metastatic bone disease. J Pain Symptom Manage 7:4-11, 1992.

62. Ernst DS, Brashear P, Paterson A, et al. Controlled trial of intravenous clodronate in patients with metastatic bone disease and pain. Proc Am Soc Clin Oncol 13:431, A1478, 1994.

63. Thurlimann B, Wessler F, Radziwill A, et al. Pamidronate in patients with malignant osteolytic bone disease and pain: A dose finding study. Proc Am Soc Clin Oncol 12:432, 1993.

64. Glover D, Lipton A, Keller A, Miller AA, Browning S, Fram RJ, George S, Zelenakas K, Macerata RS, Seaman JJ. Intravenous pamidronate disodium treatment of bone metas-

tases in patients with breast cancer. Cancer 74:2949-2455, 1994.

65. Purohit OP, Dickson I, Anthony C, Coleman R. The effect of a single pamidronate (APD) infusion on metastatic bone pain, quality of life (QOL), and markers of bone resorption. Proc Am Soc Clin Oncol 13:430, A1475, 1994.

66. Conte PF, Giannessi PG, Latreille J, et al. Delayed progression of bone metastases with pamidronate therapy in breast cancer patients: A randomized, multicenter phase III trial. Ann Oncol 5(Suppl 7):S41-S44, 1994.

67. Houston SJ, Rubens RD. The systemic treatment of bone metastases. Clin Orthop 312:95-104, 1995.

68. Deftos LJ. Calcitonin secretion in humans. In Cooper CW, ed. Current Research on Calcium Regulating Hormones. Austin: University of Texas Press, 1987, pp 79-100.

69. Deftos LJ, Glowacki J. Mechanisms of bone metabolism. In Kem DC, Frohlick E, eds. Pathophysiology. Philadelphia: JB Lippincott, 1984, pp 445-468.

70. Moonga BS, Alam AS, Bevis PJ, Avaldi F, Soncini R, Huang CL, Zaidi M. Regulation of cytosolic-free calcium in isolated rat osteoclasts by calcitonin. J Endocrinol 132:241-249, 1992.

71. Deftos LJ. Medullary thyroid carcinoma. New York: S Karger, 1983, pp 1-114.

72. Deftos LJ. Calcitonin and medullary thyroid carcinoma. In Bennett JC, Plum F, eds. Cecil Textbook of Medicine, 20th ed. Philadelphia: WB Saunders, 1996, pp 1372-1375.

73. Deftos LJ. Pituitary cells secrete calcitonin in the reverse hemolytic plaque assay. Biochem Biophys Res Commun 146: 1350-1356, 1987.

74. Deftos LJ, Roos B. Medullary thyroid carcinoma and calcitonin gene expression. In Peck WA, ed. Bone and Mineral Research. Amsterdam: Excerpta Medica, 1989, pp 267-316.

75. Fischer JA, Born W. Calcitonin gene products: Evolution, expression and biological targets. Bone Miner 2:347-353, 1987.

76. Spaventi S, Vrbanec D. Effect of calcitonin on the skeleton and bone pain in patients with osteolytic metastases. Acta Med Iugosl 41:33-42, 1987.

77. Hindley AC, Hill EB, Leyland MJ, Willes AE. A double-blind controlled trial of salmon calcitonin in pain due to malignancy. Cancer Chemother Pharmacol 9:71-74, 1982.

78. Blomqvist C, Elomaa I, Porkka L, Karonen SL, Lamberg-Allardt C. Evaluation of salmon calcitonin treatment in bone metastases from breast cancer—a controlled trial. Bone 9:45-51, 1988.

79. Gennari C, Chierichetti MS, Piolini M, Vibelli C, et al. Analgesic activity of salmon and human calcitonin against cancer pain: A double-blind, placebo-controlled clinical study. Curr Ther Res 38:298-308, 1985.

80. Portenoy RK, Foley KM. Chronic use of opioid analgesics in non-malignant pain: Report of 38 cases. Pain 25:171-186, 1986.

81. Ciccone DS, Bandilla EB, Just N, Secoy J, Wu W. Prospective assessment of opioid therapy for chronic nonmalignant pain. Paper presented at Conference on Pain Management and Chemical Dependency: Evolving Perspectives, New York, New York, November, 1996.

82. Ciccone DS, Bandilla EB, Just N, Secoy J, Wu W. Patterns of opioid use among patients with chronic noncancer pain:

Preliminary results of a prospective study. Paper presented at 14th Annual Scientific Meeting of the American Pain Society, Los Angeles, California, November, 1995.

83. Du Pen SL, Du Pen AR, Polissar N, Hansberry J, Kraybill BM, Stillman M, Panke J, Everly R. Implementing guidelines for pain management: Results of a randomized controlled clinical trial. J Clin Oncol 17:361-370, 1999.

84. Du Pen SL. Epidural techniques for cancer pain management: When, why, and how? Curr Rev Pain 3(3):183-189, 1999.

85. Mennan D, Lagares-Garcia JA, Kurek S, Craig D, Green J, Fritz W. Managing intractable pain with an intrathecal catheter and injection port: Technique and guidelines. Am Surg 65:1054-1060, 1999.

86. Krames ES. Practical issues when using neuraxial infusion. [Review.] Oncology (Huntingt) 13(5 Suppl 2):37-44, 1999.

87. Plummer JL, Cherry DA, Cousins MJ, Gourlay GK, Onley MM, Evans KH. Long-term spinal administration of morphine in cancer and non-cancer pain: A retrospective study. Pain 44(3):215-220, 1991.

88. Schultheiss R, Schramm J, Neidhardt J. Dose changes in long- and medium-term intrathecal morphine therapy of cancer pain. Neurosurgery 31:664-670, 1992.

89. Winkelmuller M, Winkelmuller W. Long-term effects of continuous intrathecal opioid treatment in chronic pain of nonmalignant etiology. J Neurosurg 85:458-467, 1996.

90. Anderson VC, Burchiel KJ. A prospective study of long-term intrathecal morphine in the management of chronic nonmalignant pain. Neurosurgery 44:289-301, 1999.

91. Greenberg HS, Kim JH, Posner JB. Epidural spinal cord compression from metastatic tumor: Results from a new treatment protocol. Ann Neurol 8:361-366, 1980.

92. Schell HW. The risk of adrenal corticosteroid therapy in far-advanced cancer. Am J Med Sci 252:641-649, 1966.

93. Schell HW. Adrenal corticosteroid therapy in far advanced cancer. Geriatrics 27:131-141, 1972.

94. Twycross RG, Lack SA. Symptom control in far-advanced cancer: Pain relief. London: Pittman Books, 1983.

95. Choi J, Huang G, Shafik E, Wu W, McArdle J. Imipramine's selective suppression of an L-type calcium channel in neurons of murine dorsal root ganglia involves G proteins. J Pharmacol Exp Ther 263:49-53, 1992.

96. Beaver WT, Feise G. Comparison of analgesic effects of morphine sulfate, hydroxyzine, and their combination in patients with postoperative pain. In Bonica JJ, Albe-Fessard D, eds. Advances in Pain Research and Therapy. New York: Raven Press, 1976.

97. Halpern LW. Psychotropics, ataractics, and related drugs. In Bonica JJ, Albe-Fessard D, eds. Advances in Pain Research and Therapy. New York: Raven Press, 1979.

98. Ye JH, Mui WC, Ren J, Hunt TE, Wu W, Zbuzek VK. Ondansetron exhibits the properties of a local anesthetic. Anesth Analg 85:1116-1121, 1997.

99. Swerdlow M, Stjernsward J. Cancer pain relief—an urgent problem. World Health Forum 3:325, 1982.

100. Hanks GW, Thomas PJ, Trueman T, Weeks E. The myth of haloperidol potentiation. Lancet 2:523-524, 1983.

101. Breivik H, Rennemo F. Clinical evaluation of combined treatment with methadone and psychotropic drugs in cancer patients. Acta Anaesthesiol Scand 74(Suppl):135-140, 1982.

102. Forrest WH Jr, Brown BW Jr, Brown CR, Defalque R, Gold M, Gordon HE, James KE, Katz J, Mahler DL, Schroff P, Teutsch G. Dextroamphetamine with morphine for the treatment of postoperative pain. N Engl J Med 296:712-715, 1977.

103. Snow H. The opium-cocaine treatment of malignant disease. Br Med J 1:1019, 1987.

104. Twycross RG. Value of cocaine in opiate containing elixirs. Br Med J 2:1348, 1977.

105. Kaiko RF, Kanner R, Foley KM, Wallenstein SL, Canel AM, Rogers AG, Houde RW. Cocaine and morphine interaction in acute and chronic cancer pain. Pain 3(1):35-45, 1987.

106. Ye JH, Liu PL, Wu W, McArdle JJ. Cocaine depresses $GABA_A$ current of hippocampal neurons. Brain Res 770:169-175, 1997.

107. Pilon RN, Baker AR. Chronic pain control by means of an epidural catheter: Report of a case with description of the method. Cancer 37:903-905, 1976.

Radiation Therapy

Rodney J. Ellis, M.D., and Timothy J. Kinsella, M.D.

Radiation therapy for the treatment of metastatic cancer frequently involves irradiation of bone lesions. The incidence of bone metastases varies with tumor histology but has been reported to occur in 23% to 84% of cancer patients studied.[1-4] Autopsy series have shown that bone is the third most frequent site of metastatic disease, after lung and liver. Although authorities agree that the cancers that metastasize most frequently to bone are breast, prostate, and lung cancers, other less common cancers that metastasize to bone include myeloma and lymphomas.[5]

Although approximately half of the patients who undergo radiation therapy are treated with palliative intent, the majority of these patients are treated for lesions that cause pain related to the destruction of bone.[3,6,7] Metastatic bone lesions represent a systemic disease for which a cure is rarely obtained. However, as in curative treatment, proper management often requires a multidisciplinary approach, combining the efforts of the orthopedic surgeon, the medical oncologist, and the radiation oncologist.

Although the majority of bone metastases are not intrinsically painful, they can cause pain by any of several mechanisms, including local bone pain, pain radiating to a local region, referred pain to nearby sites, nerve compression, and muscle spasms. Pain produced by bone metastases may be only partially responsive to narcotics or nonsteroidal anti-inflammatory drugs.[8] Therefore radiotherapy is most commonly used to relieve pain and to prevent further disease progression at the involved site or sites.

Various techniques have been developed to deliver radiation for bone metastases; however, the standards for this therapy are still not clearly defined and accepted. Part of the difficulty in defining the most effective radiation treatment for bone metastases is defining objective and easily reproducible criteria for assessment of response.[9] Because osseous lesions are either osteolytic or osteoblastic, both bone scans and plain films may be required for accurate analysis of disease extent. Although bone scans can be useful to detect bone metastases, plain films or magnetic resonance imaging (MRI) may be more accurate for following the response to irradiation.[10-13] Patient response to therapy also may be difficult to define, depending on the timing of the posttreatment assessment and on whether the response is scored by the patient or by the health care providers.[14] The focus of this chapter will be to provide a general overview of radiation therapy for metastatic cancers involving bone.

HISTORICAL REVIEW

After Roentgen's discovery of the x-ray in 1895, Becquerel discovered radioactivity in Paris in 1896. The isolation of radium by Marie Curie in 1898 then quickly led to the use of radiation to treat malignant disease. Early attempts to use x-rays were limited to superficial tumors, such as skin cancer and laryngeal carcinomas. The treatment of deep-tissue tumors was limited by the low energy of existent cathode tubes and often resulted in excessive skin doses and treatment-related toxicity. Although brachytherapy became useful for the treatment of deeper tumors, such as cervical cancer or prostate carcinoma, the treatment of bone metastasis in the early part of the century consisted mainly of the use of opium derivatives or other pain medicines to sedate the patient and help reduce pain.[15,16]

The development of higher-energy radiation therapy units saw the beginning of the widespread use of radiation to treat painful bone metastases. Orthovoltage units came first, and they were followed by megavoltage radiation, such as the cobalt 60 units that became popular in the 1950s. These units were capable of the deep tissue penetration needed to provide relief from the pain of bone metastases and to prevent further disease progression. With the advent of linear accelerators, the energies available for photon therapy have increased, thereby allowing increased skin sparing while increasing the dose to the tumor and decreasing both side effects and the risk of complications in normal tissues.

TREATMENT REGIMENS

Palliative radiation for bone metastases is usually delivered to a local field limited to the involved site of a lesion, with appropriate margins identified to prevent a geographic miss. Although most lesions can be adequately visualized with the use of conventional simulation, lesions involving adjacent soft tissue may require complex computerized treatment planning to assure proper coverage of both the bone and soft tissue components. There has been no standardization of total dose or optimal number of radiation treatments, although a final report of an expert panel sponsored by the American College of Radiology (ACR) was published recently.[17] The recommendations of the expert panel will be highlighted in this chapter.

Frequency

Various regimens of radiotherapy are currently used, depending on the clinical scenario. The term *standard fractionation* usually refers to daily treatments delivered 5 days per week, Monday through Friday, at a daily dose of 180 to 200 cGy. The most commonly used treatment schedules for palliative therapy are "hypofractionated therapy," in which daily doses greater than 200 cGy are delivered. Because of the increased daily fraction size delivered in hypofractionated treatments, the total number of fractions are reduced, thus shortening the total number of treatments. Decreasing the number of treatments is often advantageous for debilitated patients for whom ambulation is difficult. Although not routinely recommended by the expert panel from the ACR, some European treatment centers often recommend a single fraction of radiation of up to 800 cGy for patients receiving palliative radiation.[17-20] The use of multiple daily fractions, termed either *accelerated* or *hyperfractionated radiation,* also has been explored.

"Accelerated fractionation" describes the delivery of multiple daily fractions, commonly of 150 cGy to 200 cGy each, so that the total prescribed dose may be delivered in a reduced amount of time compared with standard fractionation. However, as the dose delivered per fraction is increased, so are the late effects of treatment, such as fibrosis and tissue necrosis. Therefore the acute toxicity of accelerated regimens has limited their widespread clinical application.

Hyperfractionation also commonly delivers two or even three daily fractions; however, each treatment is reduced in size from standard fractionation. Ideally, hyperfractionation with smaller doses allows delivery of a higher total dose of radiation to a tumor while decreasing the late effects of treatment.

Although hyperfractionation or accelerated regimens appear to be gaining acceptance as curative therapy, they do not seem to have any advantage in the palliative setting because many patients treated with a palliative intent are not expected to live long enough to suffer the late effects of radiotherapy.[14,21,22] Again, a hyperfractionated approach was not recommended by the expert panel report on bone metastases.[17]

Dosage

The prescribed total radiation dose varies, depending on the clinical situation and the fractionation schedule chosen by the radiation oncologist. It is generally accepted that a dose of at least 5000 cGy should be prescribed to eradicate microscopic disease, as in the postoperative curative setting for head and neck carcinomas.[23] As the volume of tumor increases from microscopic to gross disease, the required amount of radiation must also increase to ensure that the disease will be eradicated. However, as the total dose is increased, the acute and late complications of treatment also increase. Therefore, in a palliative setting where the goal of treatment is either pain relief or prevention of disease progression, lower total doses are usually prescribed to obtain the treatment goal without causing a significant risk of treatment-related morbidity. The dose required to accomplish this goal is often controversial but typically ranges between 2000 cGy and 5000 cGy, depending on the involved site as well as the responsiveness of the particular tumor type to radiation.[18] According to the ACR expert panel report, doses in the range of 2000 cGy in 5 fractions, 3000 cGy in 10 fractions, or 3500 cGy in 14 fractions are acceptable in most circumstances. Daily doses of greater than 400 cGy were not recommended as a standard.[17]

Patient Variables

Patient factors may also affect decisions regarding the prescribed radiation dose. The duration of response to a course of radiation tends to be longer for both increased total dose and increased total number of fractions.[24] For example, a patient with breast carcinoma that recurs several years after initial treatment in the form of a solitary bone metastasis may continue to live for many years and may therefore benefit from a more protracted standard course of therapy to a higher total dose (e.g., 3500 to 3750 cGy in 14 to 15 fractions). Conversely, an elderly patient with multifocal disease involving both soft tissue and painful bone metastasis may obtain relief after 2000 cGy in five fractions to the involved site. Although the second patient may be more likely to have late treatment-related morbidity or to have pain recur at the tumor site as a result of disease progression, he or she will most likely succumb to progressive disease before either event occurs.[21] An attempt to deliver standard daily fractions in such a clinical scenario may cause unnecessary discomfort because of the daily trips to the radiation treatment facility, as well as treatment-related discomfort, such as positioning on a hard, uncomfortable radiation treatment table.

Retreatment

For patients who have recurrent pain at a previously irradiated site, reirradiation may be possible. Patients may be expected to have a high response rate to retreatment (50% to 80%); however, they also may be at a higher risk of complications if the first course of treatment delivered higher total doses.[25] If the patient is expected to live longer than 3 to 4 months, a total dose of 3000 cGy to the retreatment site might be used with 200 cGy fractions to limit acute and late (>6 months) toxicities to adjacent soft tissues.

Clinical Studies

The Radiation Therapy Oncology Group conducted a randomized trial (RTOG 74-02), published by Tong et al.,[1] that evaluated various fractionation schedules for patients with osseous metastases. A total of 1016 patients were entered into the trial. The patients were divided into two groups. Group 1 consisted of 266 patients, each with a solitary painful osseous metastasis, while group 2 included 750 patients with multiple osseous metastases but with only one painful site to receive treatment. The patients in group 1 were randomly assigned to receive either 4050 cGy in 3 weeks (270 cGy per fraction) or 2000 cGy in 1 week (400 cGy per fraction). The patients in group 2 were randomly assigned to one of four arms, receiving 3000 cGy (300 cGy per fraction) in 2 weeks, 1500 cGy (300 cGy per fraction) in 1 week, 2000 cGy (200 cGy per fraction given twice a day) in 1 week, or 2500 cGy (250 cGy per fraction given twice a day) in 1 week. Nearly 90% of the patients evaluated reported some pain relief, and 54% obtained complete relief. The initial analysis for evaluable group 1 patients (146/266) with solitary lesions failed to show any advantage for either treatment arm, in either duration of relief or relapse of pain in the treatment site. However, a significantly higher incidence of pathologic fractures was noted in patients participating in the protracted treatment arm of 4050 cGy (18% vs. 4%, P = 0.02). A trend toward faster relief was noted for the 2000 cGy regimen (P = 0.06); however, this trend was believed possibly to be attributable to a bias in the method of data collection. Analysis of the treatment results for group 2 likewise failed to show a benefit with any of the four treatment arms in terms of duration of pain relief, recurrence of pain in the treatment field, or risk of pathologic fracture. Analysis of the rate of relief for patients in group 2 showed that complete pain relief occurred most quickly in the 1500 cGy arm and most slowly in the 2500 cGy arm.[1]

A reanalysis of the RTOG 74-02 study was published by Blitzer[24] in 1985, 3 years after the first report. In Blitzer's report the two groups of patients were combined, and a logistic regression technique was applied for a multivariant statistical analysis. End points for the analysis included narcotic score, combined pain and narcotic score, and incidence of retreatment. A statistically significant correlation was found between the number of fractions delivered in relation to complete pain relief. Blitzer concluded that protracted dose-fractionation schedules are more effective for relief of bone pain than short-course schedules. Blitzer does admit that, although combining both groups improves the statistical power of the study, it may also bias the treatment results, especially if there were inherent differences between the two groups of patients.[24]

The results of a series of three trials evaluating single-fraction treatments has been published by the Royal Marsden Hospital in London. The first trial was a randomized study comparing a single 800 cGy radiation dose with a "conventional" course of 3000 cGy in 10 fractions (300 cGy per fraction).[19] No difference in results was reported; both groups achieved an overall response rate of 85%, with a complete response rate of 27%. Neither skeletal site nor tumor histology influenced the results.[19] A second study by the same group evaluated treatment results using a smaller fraction size of 400 cGy in a single fraction in a phase II trial. The complete response rate for this lower dose was 5%, with an overall response rate of 43%.[20] The third study was a prospective randomized trial that evaluated 400 cGy vs. 800 cGy single doses for metastatic bone pain.[18] One hundred thirty-three patients received an 800 cGy dose, and 137 patients were given a single dose of 400 cGy. Although a statistically significant higher response rate was noted for the higher single fraction of 800 cGy assessed 4 weeks after treatment (69% vs. 44%), the complete response rates of the two groups were nearly identical (39% vs. 36%). Patients given the lower dose of 400 cGy did, however, require more frequent retreatment than the group treated with 800 cGy (20% vs. 9%), and at 12 weeks after treatment the complete response rate continued to favor the 800 cGy treatment regimen, even with retreated patients included from the 400 cGy arm.[18]

Most recently, Niewald et al.[26] reported the results of a randomized trial comparing rapid-course radiation and standard radiation therapy. One hundred patients were randomized, with 51 patients receiving 2000 cGy in 5 fractions (400 cGy per fraction) and 46 patients treated with 3000 cGy in 15 daily fractions (200 cGy per fraction). Once again, no significant differences were found in the frequency of pain relief, duration of pain relief, improvement of mobility, recalcification, frequency of pathologic fractures, or survival rates. A slight trend favored the standard treatment in terms of lack of recalcification and frequency of pain relief (partial pain relief 83% vs. 68%, complete relief 22% vs. 14%). The conclusion was that 2000 cGy in five fractions should be accepted as the standard treatment because of the limited life expectancy of these patients and to reduce their hospital stays.[26] This study adds to the list of studies that fail to demonstrate a significant advantage of any identified treatment schedule.[27-29]

American College of Radiologists' Guidelines

The ACR radiotherapy recommendations were recently published to help provide treatment guidelines.[17] The guidelines were based on recommendations of an expert panel after evaluation of the currently available literature. With the use of a series of 25 clinical "variants" believed to represent most situations that radiation oncologists in the United States commonly encounter, the treatment recommendations of the panel experts were obtained by a survey. Dose prescriptions ranging from 20 Gy in five fractions, 30 Gy in 10 fractions, to 35 Gy in 14 fractions were recommended as acceptable in most circumstances. Singe doses of >4 Gy were discouraged except possibly in the setting of rib metastases, and total doses >35 Gy in 14 fractions were thought to be appropriate only in the setting of metastatic renal cell carcinoma or for women with solitary metastases and a long disease-free interval after an initial diagnosis of breast cancer. Although the expert panel believed that rapid schedules are acceptable for patients with a life expectancy of less than 3 months, guidelines for choosing patients with short life expectancy are lacking.[17]

HEMIBODY RADIATION

An alternative form of external beam radiation involving the treatment of larger volumes to encompass multiple bone metastases is termed hemibody irradiation (HBI) or wide-field radiotherapy. HBI may be used to treat the upper, middle, or lower body, either alone or sequentially, depending on the extent of disease. The treatment usually delivers between 600 and 1000 cGy as a single fraction.[30,31] Many patients experience rapid relief of pain, often within 48 hours; however, the adverse side effects of this form of therapy can limit its clinical application.

Indications

HBI is generally offered to patients who have multiple symptomatic bone metastasis or to debilitated patients with multiple metastasis for whom daily travel for treatments would be difficult. Not only has it been shown to be effective in achieving rapid pain relief for most patients, but it also has been shown to prevent progression in asymptomatic sites identified by bone scans. The use of HBI does not limit the ability to deliver further localized radiation therapy to sites that fail to respond completely or that recur after treatment.

Drawbacks

Acute side effects may occur within 1 to 2 hours of treatment and can last up to 2 weeks. An acute radi-

It has been estimated that $900 million dollars is spent annually on palliative radiotherapy, the majority of which is for bone metastases.[47] It can be assumed that more than 1,200,000 new cases of cancer will be diagnosed each year, and approximately half of these patients will eventually require palliative therapy for disease progression.[7] With the treatment of metastatic breast cancer as an example of overall treatment cost, in 1990 it was estimated that the average monthly cost of hospital treatment was $2000 and that treatment of skeletal disease was responsible for 63% of that monthly cost. Because more than 350,000 patients worldwide die each year of either breast or prostate cancer, it is evident that early intervention to treat pain and to prevent disease progression should decrease overall health care costs by preventing additional hospitalizations.[21]

The quality of life for patients with metastatic disease also must be addressed in an evaluation of the overall cost of treatment. Although narcotics may be effective for pain relief, they do not prevent disease progression and cannot be effective in maintaining ambulation if painful lesions result in pathologic fractures. Recently, bisphosphonates have proved to be useful in treating bone metastases by delaying disease progression and decreasing pain; however, approximately half of the patients so treated did not experience pain relief and still required additional chemotherapy or radiation to achieve relief.[14,48-51]

Additional studies will be needed to resolve the issues concerning the appropriate uses of radiotherapy for osseous metastases. Recently, a patterns-of-care study has been published; this used the results of a national survey of radiation oncologists in the United States to determine the most frequent approaches to treatment of bone metastases. Local-field therapy continues to be the most frequent form of radiotherapy prescribed, being used either alone or in combination with other therapies in 54% and 74% of patients, respectively. Furthermore, protracted regimens continue to be prescribed by 90% of the physicians polled in 97% of their cases, with the most common schedule being 30 Gy in 10 fractions used by 77% of physicians in 64% of cases. Although HBI is still used infrequently (1% to 2% of all cases), systemic radionuclides, such as strontium 89 (4 to 10.8 mCi), appear to be

prescribed more frequently, either alone or in addition to local therapy (21% and 40%, respectively).[52] Currently the RTOG is conducting a trial (RTOG 97-14) designed to assess the quality of life as well as the relief of symptoms for patients with osseous metastatic lesions from either breast or prostate cancer. It is hoped that as we continue to expand and develop the multidisciplinary approach of cancer management to include palliative treatment for metastatic lesions, we will be able to provide maximum relief of symptoms while also reducing the overall cost for the large group of cancer patients with metastatic osseous lesions.

REFERENCES

1. Tong D, Gillick L, Hendrickson FR. The palliation of symptomatic osseous metastases: Final results of the Radiation Therapy Oncology Group. Cancer 50:893-899, 1982.
2. Harvey HA. Issues concerning the role of chemotherapy and hormonal therapy of bone metastases from breast carcinoma. Cancer 80(8 Suppl):1646-1651, 1997.
3. Nightengale B, Brune M, Blizzard SP, Ashley-Johnson M, Slan S. Strontium chloride Sr 89 for treating pain from metastatic bone disease. Am J Health Syst Pharm 52:2189-2195, 1995.
4. Patterson AHG. Bone metastases in breast cancer, prostate cancer and myeloma. Bone 8(Suppl 1):17-22, 1987.
5. Mundy G. Mechanisms of bone metastasis. Cancer 80(8 Suppl):1546-1556, 1997.
6. Lewington VJ. Cancer therapy using bone-seeking isotopes. Phys Med Biol 41:2027-2042, 1996.
7. Ciezki J, Macklis RM. The palliative role of radiotherapy in the management of the cancer patient. Semin Oncol 22(Suppl 3):82-90, 1995.
8. Twycross RG. Management of pain in skeletal metastases. Clin Orthop 312:187-196, 1996.
9. Nielson OS, Munro AJ, Tannock IF. Bone metastasis: Pathophysiology and management policy. J Clin Oncol 9:509-524, 1991.
10. Hortobagyi GN, Libshitz HI, Seabold JE. Osseous metastases of breast cancer: Clinical, biological, radiographic, and scintigraphic evaluation of response to therapy. Cancer 53:577-582, 1984.
11. Yankelevitz DF, Henschke CI, Nisce L, Yi Y, Cahill P. Effect of radiation therapy on thoracic and lumbar bone. AJR Am J Roentgenol 157:87-92, 1991.
12. Fossa SD, Winderen M. Does decreased skeletal uptake of ^{99m}Tc-methylene bisphosphonate in irradiated bone indicate the absence of bone metastases? Radiother Oncol 27:63-65, 1993.
13. Steiner RM, Mitchell DG, Rao VM, Schweitzer ME. Magnetic resonance imaging of diffuse bone marrow disease. Radiother Oncol 27:63-65, 1993.
14. Hoegler D. Radiotherapy for palliation of symptoms in incurable cancer. Curr Probl Cancer 21:129-183, 1997.
15. Perez CA, Brady LW, Roti Roti JL. Overview. In Perez CA,

Brady LW, eds. Principles and Practice of Radiation Oncology. Philadelphia: Lippincott-Raven, 1997, pp 1-78.

16. Hilaris BS, Mastoras DA, Shih LL, Bodner WR. History of brachytherapy: The years after the discovery of radium and radioactivity. In Nag S, ed. Principles and Practice of Brachytherapy. Armonk, NY: Futura Publishing, 1997, pp 13-26.

17. Rose CM, Kagan AR. The final report of the expert panel for the Radiation Oncology Bone Metastasis Work Group of the American College of Radiology. Int J Radiat Oncol Biol Phys 40:1117-1124, 1998.

18. Hoskins PJ, Price P, Easton D, Regan J, Austin D, Palmer S, Yarnold JR. A prospective randomized trial of 4Gy or 8Gy single doses in the treatment of metastatic bone pain. Radiother Oncol 23:74-79, 1992.

19. Price P, Hoskins PJ, Easton D, Austin D, Palmer SG, Yarnold JR. Prospective randomized trial of single and multifraction radiotherapy schedules in the treatment of painful bony metastases. Radiother Oncol 6:247-255, 1986.

20. Price P, Hoskins PJ, Easton D, Austin D, Palmer SG, Yarnold JR. Low dose single fraction radiotherapy in the treatment of metastatic bone pain: A pilot study. Radiother Oncol 12:297-300, 1988.

21. Coleman RE. Skeletal complications of malignancy. Cancer 80(8 Suppl):1588-1594, 1997.

22. Rosenthal DI. Radiologic diagnosis of bone metastases. Cancer 80(8 Suppl):1595-1606, 1997.

23. Ang KK, Kaanders J, Peters LJ. Modes of therapy. In Cooke DB, Zinner SR, Klass FM, Martin JH, eds. Radiotherapy for Head and Neck Cancers. Philadelphia: Lea & Febiger, 1994, pp 3-4.

24. Blitzer PH. Reanalysis of the RTOG study of the palliation of symptomatic osseous metastasis. Cancer 55:1468-1472, 1985.

25. Mithal NP, Needham PR, Hoskin PJ. Retreatment with radiotherapy for painful bone metastases. Int J Radiat Oncol Biol Phys 29:1011-1014, 1994.

26. Niewald M, Tkocz HJ, Abel U, Scheib T, Walter K, Nieder C, Schnabel K, Berberich W, Kubale R, Fuchs M. Rapid course radiation vs. more standard treatment: A randomized trial for bone metastases. Int J Radiat Oncol Biol Phys 36:1085-1089, 1996.

27. Madsen EL. Painful bone metastasis: Efficacy of radiotherapy assessed by the patient: A randomized trial comparing 4 Gy × 6 versus 10 Gy × 2. Int J Radiat Oncol Biol Phys 9:1775-1779, 1983.

28. Cole DJ. A randomized trial of a single treatment versus conventional fractionation in the palliative radiotherapy of bone metastases. Clin Oncol 1:59-62, 1989.

29. Rasmusson B, Vejborg I, Jensen AB, Andersson M, Banning AM, Hoffman T, Pfieffer P, Nielson HK, Sjogren P. Irradiation of bone metastases in breast cancer patients: A randomized trial with one year follow-up. Radiother Oncol 34:179-184, 1995.

30. Salazar OM, Rubin P, Hendrickson FR, Komaki R, Poulter C, Newall J, Asbell SO, Mohiuddin M, Ess JV. Single-dose halfbody irradiation for palliation of multiple bone metastases from solid tumors: Final Radiation Therapy Oncology Group report. Cancer 58:29-36, 1986.

31. Douglas P, Rossier P, Mirimanoff RO, Coucke PA. Third-body irradiation as an effective palliative treatment for painful multiple bone metastases resistant to chemo- or hormonal treatment. Radiother Oncol 28:76-78, 1993.

32. Kuban DA, Schellhammer PF, El-Mahdi AM. Hemibody irradiation in advanced prostatic carcinoma. Urol Clin North Am 18:131-137, 1991.

33. Jones PW, Bogardus CR, Anderson DW. Significance of initial "performance status" in patients receiving halfbody radiation. Int J Radiat Oncol Biol Phys 10:1947-1950, 1984.

34. Zelefsky MJ, Scher HI, Forman JD, Linares LA, Curley T, Fuks Z. Metastatic prostate cancer: A comparison of single dose and fractionated regimens. Int J Radiat Oncol Biol Phys 17:1281-1285, 1989.

35. Salazar OM, Scarantino CW, Rubin P, Feldstein ML, Keller BE. Total (half-body) systemic irradiation for occult metastases in non-small cell lung cancer: An Eastern Cooperative Oncology Group Pilot report. Cancer 46:1932-1944, 1980.

36. Reed RC, Lowery GS, Nordstrom DG. Single high dose-large field irradiation for palliation of advanced malignancies. Int J Radiat Oncol Biol Phys 9:1243-1246, 1988.

37. Nag S, Shah V. Once-a-week lower hemibody irradiation (HBI) for metastatic cancers. Int J Radiat Oncol Biol Phys 12:1003-1005, 1986.

38. Andriole GL, Catalona WJ. Hemibody irradiation in advanced prostatic carcinoma. Urol Clin North Am 18:131-137, 1991.

39. Poulter CA, Cosmatos D, Rubin P, Urtasun R, Cooper JS, Kuske RR, Hornback N, Coughlin C, Weigensberg I, Rotman M. A report of RTOG 8206: A phase III study of whether the addition of single dose hemibody irradiation to standard fractionated local field irradiation is more effective than local field irradiation alone in the treatment of symptomatic osseous metastases. Int J Radiat Oncol Biol Phys 23:207-214, 1992.

40. Serafini AN. Current status of systemic intravenous radiopharmaceuticals for the treatment of painful metastatic bone disease. Int J Radiat Oncol Biol Phys 30:1187-1194, 1994.

41. Janjan NA. Radiation for bone metastases, conventional techniques and the role of systemic radiopharmaceuticals. Cancer 80(8 Suppl):1628-1645, 1997.

42. Ben-Josef E, Filizack L, Davis L, Porter AT. Repeated administration of strontium-89 for palliation of painful osseous metastases. Proc Am Soc Clin Oncol 16(A204):59, 1997.

43. Tu S, Delpassand ES, Jones D, Amato RJ, Ellerhorst J, Logothetis CJ. Strontium-89 combined with doxorubicin in the treatment of patients with androgen-independent prostate cancer. Urol Oncol 2:191-197, 1996.

44. Preston D, Clark-Snow R, Crispen RG, Fabian CJ, Hapgood M, Schiefelbein M, Simonich WL. Safety of strontium-89 in metastatic breast cancer: Incidence of and risk factors for grade III-IV myelotoxicity. Proc Am Soc Clin Oncol 16(A657):187, 1997.

45. Wehbe T, Akerley W, Safran H, Cummings F, Rege V, Sambandam S, Maynard J, Leone L. Strontiun-89, estramustine and vinblastine (SEV) in hormone refractory prostate carcinoma (HRPC): Concurrent chemoradiotherapy. Proc Am Soc Clin Oncol 16(A1110):312, 1997.

46. Dahut W, Arcenas A, Feldman S, Hoffmeister K, Chen A, Powers A, Simonich WL. Strontium-89 (Sr-89 Metastron) and estramustine (EM) in hormone refractory prostate cancer (HRPC): A phase II study. Proc Am Soc Clin Oncol 16(A1182):331, 1997.

47. Hanks G. The crisis in health care cost in the United States: Some implications for radiation oncology. Int J Radiat Oncol Biol Phys 23:203-206, 1992.

48. Kanis JA, McCloskey EV. Clodronate. Cancer 80(8 Suppl):1691-1694, 1997.

49. Adami S. Bisphosphonates in prostate carcinoma. Cancer 80(8 Suppl):1674-1679, 1997.

50. Coleman RE, Purohit OP, Vinholes JJ, Zekri J. High dose pamidronate: Clinical and biochemical effects in metastatic bone disease. Cancer 80(8 Suppl):1686-1690, 1997.

51. Body JJ. Clinical research update: Zoledronate. Cancer 80(8 Suppl):1699-1701, 1997.

52. Ben-Josef E, Shamsa F, Williams AO, Porter AT. Radiotherapeutic management of osseous metastases: A survey of current patterns of care. Int J Radiat Oncol Biol Phys 40:915-921, 1998.

Nonoperative vs. Operative Treatment of Bone Metastases

William M. Parrish, M.D., and Joseph Benevenia, M.D.

Bone metastasis may be the first sign of disseminated disease in many cancer patients. This is especially true in patients with so-called "bone-seeking" tumors: breast, prostate, lung, and renal cell carcinomas. Once metastatic bone disease has developed, the prognosis for cure is generally poor. The adverse effects of bone metastasis can be many and can significantly alter a patient's quality of life. These effects include pain, bone loss and fracture, hypercalcemia, spinal cord compression, and psychological depression.

Treatment of a patient with metastatic bone disease should give consideration to each of these effects.

PATIENT EVALUATION AND FOLLOW-UP

Effective care of patients with bone metastasis should begin at the time the primary neoplasm is diagnosed. Early recognition of metastatic bone disease will provide the best opportunity for treatment. Thorough evaluation and treatment of patients with metastatic bone disease should be a multidisciplinary effort. The team should include specialists in medical oncology, radiation therapy, diagnostic radiology, nuclear medicine, orthopedic surgery, pain management, and physical medicine and rehabilitation. Close collaboration between team members will result in optimal care for the patient. Coordination of these multidisciplinary specialties into an organized clinic has been done with positive results.[1] Evaluation and staging of patients with cancer should include a thorough history and physical examination with attention given to any reference to a symptom or physical sign of early bone metastasis. Imaging studies should include a total-body bone scan as part of the workup to look for metastatic lesions. A skeletal survey may be needed for patients with renal cell carcinoma or multiple myeloma because a bone scan may be falsely negative.

Prospective screening for recurrence or metastasis with the use of serum tests such as prostate-specific antigen (PSA) or thyroid hormone testing is possible for patients with prostate and thyroid cancers. The use of urinary N-telepeptide analysis has shown some predictive value in detecting bone metastasis. N-telepeptides are breakdown products of collagen, which are excreted in urine and increase with osteolysis of bone.[2,3,4]

The goals of treatment for patients with metastatic bone disease should be to relieve pain, prevent development of pathologic fractures, improve quality of life by maintaining mobility, and perhaps prolong survival.[5] These goals should be obtained in as noninvasive a manner as possible.

OPERATIVE VS. NONOPERATIVE CARE

The treatment provided for a patient with metastatic bone disease depends on many factors, including extent of disease, type of cancer, physical condition of the patient, social issues, and the patient's desires.

The prime consideration in treating a bone lesion nonoperatively is the risk of fracture from the lesion. The "Harrington criteria" have been used to try to predict impending fractures in femoral lesions. These criteria suggest that bone with a lytic lesion 2.5 cm in diameter, involving 50% or more

Table 12-1   ECOG performance status

Grade	ECOG
0	Fully active, able to carry out all predisease performance without restriction
1	Restricted in physically strenuous activity but ambulatory and able to carry out work of a light or sedentary nature (e.g., light housework, office work)
2	Ambulatory and capable of all self-care but unable to carry out any work activities; up and about more than 50% of waking hours
3	Capable of only limited self-care; confined to bed or chair more than 50% of waking hours
4	Completely disabled; cannot carry on any self-care; totally confined to bed or chair
5	Dead

of the cortex or involving the calcar of the femur, is at significant risk of fracture.[6] Although this may be true, these criteria alone should not dictate operative treatment.

Criteria also have been established by the Eastern Cooperative Oncology Group in an attempt to grade patients' performance on the basis of their functional status (Table 12-1).[7] Although this grading system may not provide a definitive basis for determining how to best treat a patient with metastatic bone disease, it does provide a means of organizing the approach to these patients on the basis of their functional expectations. This is not to say that patients in grades 3 or 4 are not candidates for aggressive treatment. Although these patients are functionally limited, they may have a relatively long life expectancy, and consideration of pain control and prevention of impending fractures is important.

If the lesion is radiosensitive, as in the breast or prostate, and the patient's overall health is good enough to allow him or her to limit weightbearing with crutches or a walker while receiving radiation therapy, then nonoperative treatment may be used for a femoral lesion. Conversely, a patient with the same defect arising from a renal cell metastasis would not be expected to have a predictable response to radiation, and surgery might be indicated. In this case, even wide resection may be considered.

The patient with disseminated disease who is unable to ambulate safely with assistance is not likely to be a candidate for nonoperative management. Every effort should be made to avoid fracture if possible, and this patient may present too great a risk for nonoperative care. The anatomic site of the lytic lesion is also important. A large lytic lesion of the proximal humerus in the nondominant arm is much more safely treated nonoperatively than a corresponding lesion in the femoral neck. Likewise, diaphyseal lesions and some spinal column lesions may be amenable to orthotic support while adjuvant therapy is administered (Fig. 12-1).

Each patient with metastatic bone disease is an individual, and his or her treatment should reflect that fact. Careful consideration must be given to

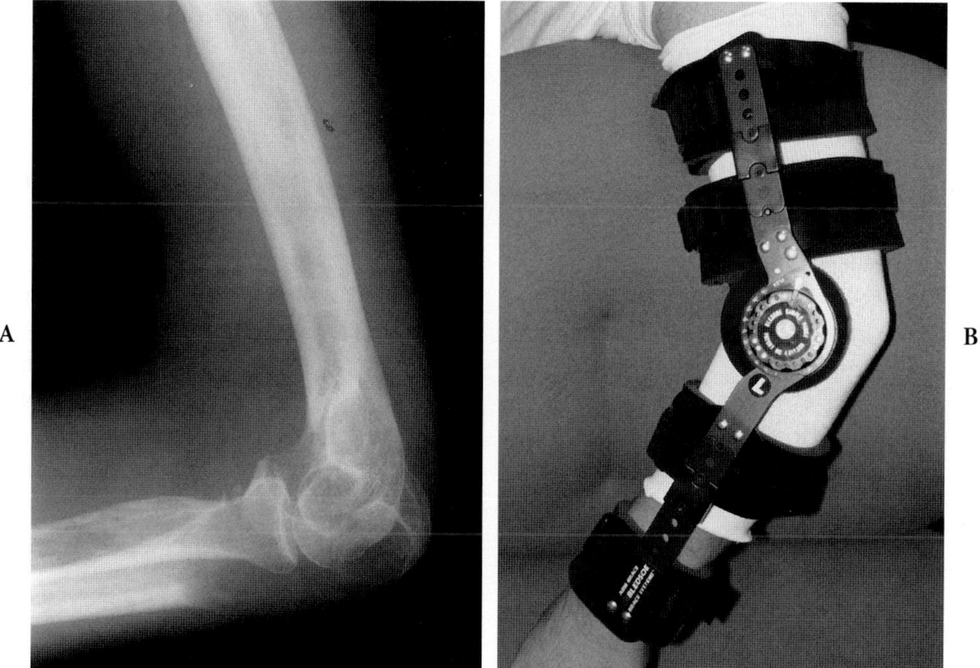

Fig. 12-1   **A,** Fifty-year-old white man with end-stage metastatic renal cell carcinoma. **B,** Stabilization with a locked elbow brace provided pain control.

the patient's health, type of tumor, and the risks and consequences of fracture. This will enable the treating physician to choose treatment that is best for that individual patient, whether operative or nonoperative.

OPTIONS FOR NONOPERATIVE CARE
Radiation

External beam radiation has been an important treatment measure for patients with metastatic bone disease. This treatment provides pain relief in the majority of patients, generally within 2 to 4 weeks of treatment.[5,8] Breast cancer and prostate cancer can be expected to respond reliably to external beam radiation. This is *not* true of renal cell cancer and lung cancers. Patients with these types of metastatic lesions can be treated with external beam therapy but must be watched closely for progression of their disease. The dose of radiation needed to achieve arrest of tumor growth and pain relief may be as little as 8 Gy delivered in one dose. Dropping that dose to 4 Gy was not as effective in relieving pain in one study.[9]

Systemic radiotherapy with radioisotopes has been used in the treatment of breast, prostate, and follicular cell thyroid carcinomas.[10,11] Response rates for treatment of breast and prostate carcinomas with strontium 99 have been reported to be as high as 70% to 80%.[12,13] Radioactive iodine is routinely used for treatment of patients with follicular cell carcinomas of the thyroid. Other radionucleotides have also been evaluated as possible systemic agents. These include samarium 153 and rhenium 186. Radiotherapy options are covered more extensively in Chapter 11, "Radiation Therapy."

Minimally Invasive Radiologic Procedures

In patients with metastatic spine disease, vertebrae at high risk for pathologic fractures have been stabilized with fluoroscopically guided percutaneous injection of methyl methacrylate into the vertebral body. This procedure is called vertebroplasty and often significantly reduces pain associated with pathologic fracture of the vertebral body. Vertebroplasty is performed utilizing fluoroscopy for placement of a large-bore 12-gauge needle through which the cement is injected. The procedure is carried out with sedative and local anesthetic and is generally well tolerated by the patient. Significant relief of pain and improvement of stability have been reported in patient groups.[14,15] Reported complications have been few but may include pulmonary embolus, infection, sciatica, and difficulty in swallowing because of extravasation of cement.

The concept of vertebroplasty is now being extended to treatment of extremity lesions. Injection of methyl methacrylate into contained painful supraacetabular lesions has resulted in significant pain relief and avoidance of surgical intervention for patients in the Cancer Center at Penn State University (Fig. 12-2).

This concept has been taken a step further with the addition of radiofrequency ablation of metastatic lesions followed by percutaneous cementation for structural support. Dupuy et al.[16] reported their experience of combining radiofrequency ablation and methyl methacrylate cementation at the 1998 meeting of the Radiologic Society of North America. They report marked pain relief in 90% of the patients treated in this fashion. Lesions up to 8 cm in diameter were treated with success.

Percutaneous stabilization techniques with methyl methacrylate show early promise of offering a reliable, effective treatment alternative for patients with metastatic disease of an extremity. This should be followed closely as further treatments using these techniques emerge.

Medical Management: Bisphosphonate Therapy

The use of bisphosphonate therapy to treat osteolytic metastatic disease has aroused much recent interest and shown some early promise. Bisphosphonate therapy is now used routinely in cancer centers as a standard part of treatment for osteolytic metastatic disease. Bisphosphonates decrease bone resorption by inhibiting osteoclast activity. The exact mechanism by which this occurs is not fully understood.[17]

Bisphosphonate therapy may decrease the number of fractures in osteolytic disease by one half.[18,19] Although morbidity associated with skeletal metastasis has been shown to be reduced in patients with breast cancer, there is no clear evidence that length of survival is increased. Bisphosphonate treatment is discussed extensively in Chapter 9.

A

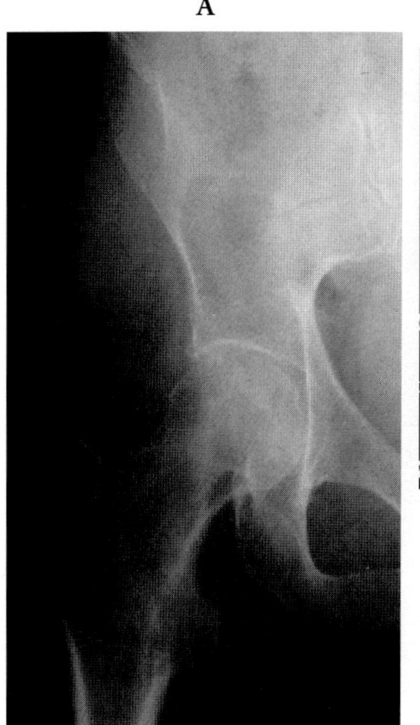

B

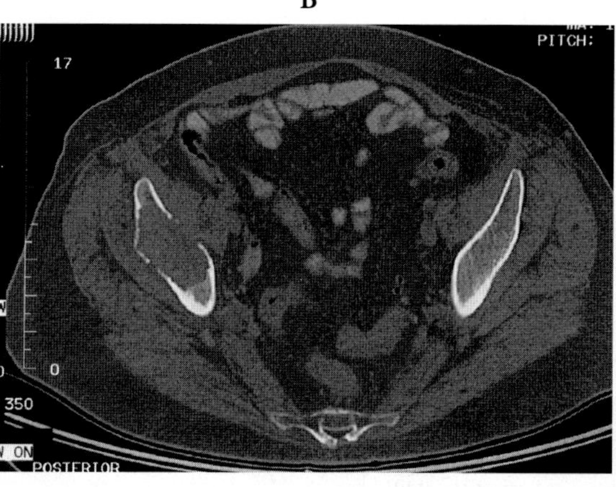

C

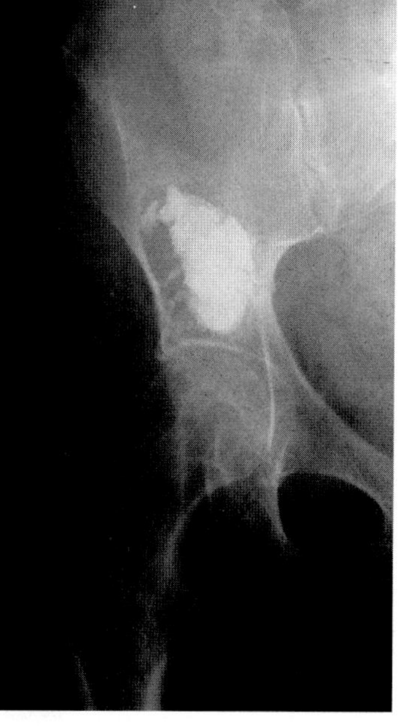

Fig. 12-2   **A,** Sixty-six-year-old woman with metastatic renal cell cancer and right hip pain in spite of radiation. **B,** CT scan demonstrating large supraacetabular lesion. **C,** Plain film demonstrating methyl methacrylate acetabuloplasty. Patient had complete relief of her hip pain.

Orthotics and Bracing

The many assistive devices available to aid the patient with metastatic disease in activities of daily living may decrease the need for operative intervention. These include ambulatory aids, such as wheelchairs, walkers, crutches, canes, and quadripod canes. Patients must be evaluated individually as to the type of ambulatory aid that is appropriate for them. Likewise, assistive devices such as hospital beds, overhead trapezes, toilet seat extensions, and shower seats may make safe, nonoperative care possible by simplifying activities of daily living.

The use of orthotic devices and bracing may be useful in providing external support for pathologic fractures while the patient is undergoing adjuvant therapy. This is especially helpful for metastatic lesions of the mid-diaphysis of the humerus. The goal of the orthotic or bracing device should be to stabilize the fracture site and provide pain relief during treatment. Some metastatic lesions may be so destructive that surgical reconstruction is not possible. In this case, a brace may be required permanently (Fig. 12-3).

Many types of orthotic devices for stabilization of impending fracture are available. The spine can be braced with cervical collars or a variety of braces for the thoracolumbar spine (Fig. 12-4). Classic fracture braces for long bones are also available (Fig. 12-5, *A*). Bracing does not have to be complex. A simple knee immobilizer, with or without hinges, may be all that is needed to provide support for patients with grade 3 or 4 disease (Fig. 12-5, *B* and *C*). Although metastatic disease rarely occurs distal to the elbow or knee, simple bracing with a forearm splint or an ankle-foot orthosis is available for patients with disease in these locations (Fig. 12-6).

Use of an orthotic device requires education of the patient and his or her family. The patient must understand how to apply the brace effectively and tension it appropriately. If the brace is applied too loosely, not enough support will be obtained. Conversely, overtightening of the brace may cause venous occlusion, resulting in painful swelling or, if prolonged, the development of a neuropraxia. Skin care is also important. The skin beneath the orthosis must be checked regularly for signs of breakdown or irritation. Adjustment of the brace by the fitting orthotists may be needed periodically if the circumference of the extremity changes.

Consultation with a physical therapist or an occupational therapist can be helpful. These professionals work with patients to help them reach their

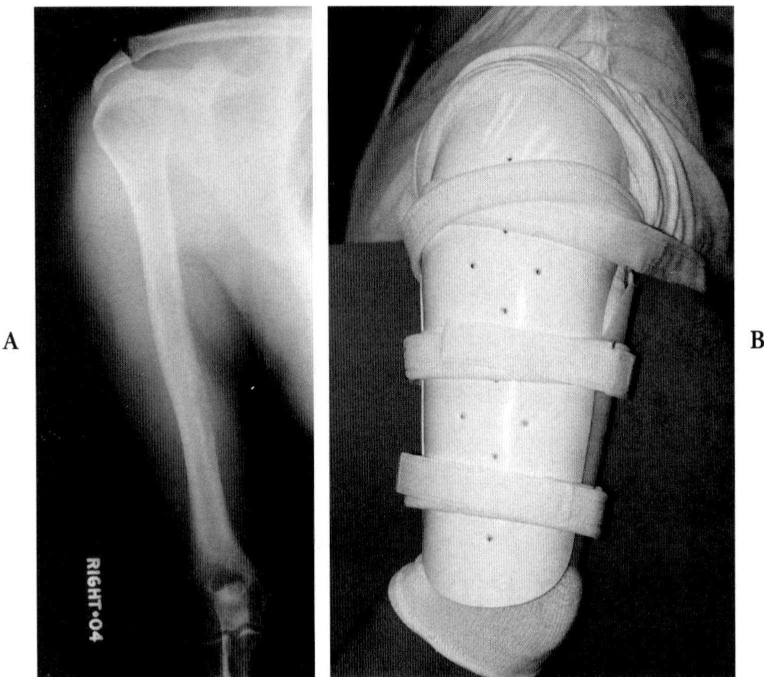

Fig. 12-3   A, Sixty-year-old woman with mid-diaphyseal humeral metastasis. **B,** Humeral fracture brace used successfully while patient received adjuvant radiation therapy.

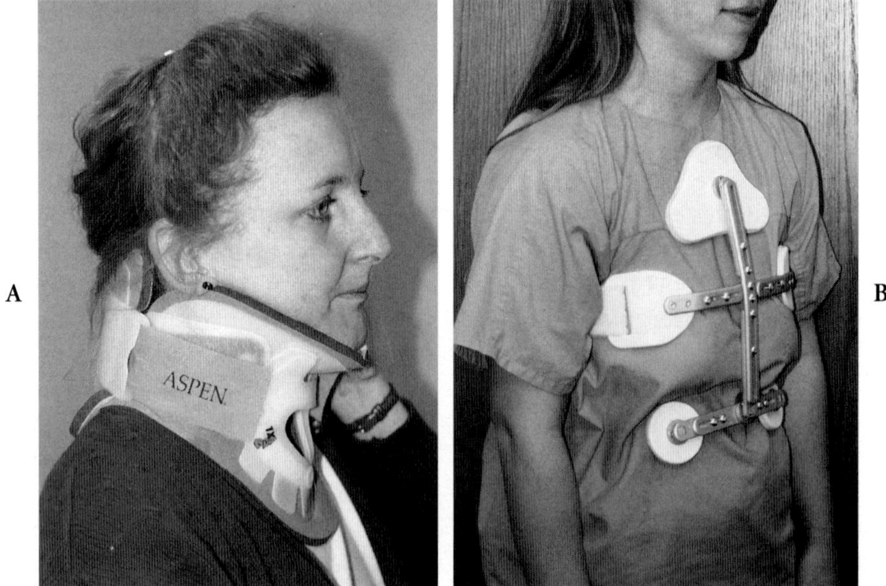

Fig. 12-4   A, Cervical collar for external bracing of the cervical spine. **B,** Cash type of brace used to provide support for compression fractures.

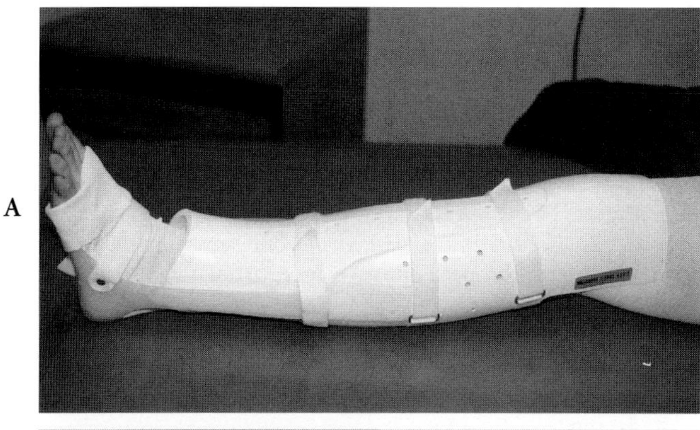

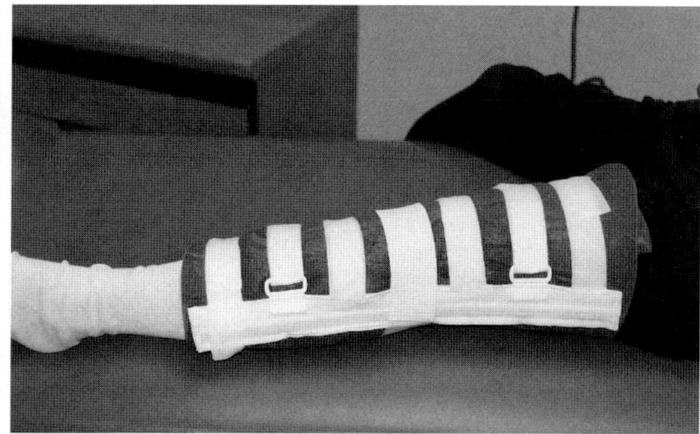

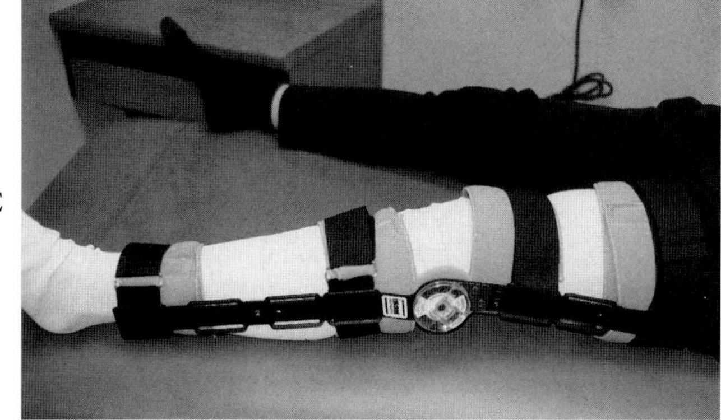

Fig. 12-5 **A,** Example of a tibial fracture brace that can be used for support while a patient is receiving adjuvant therapy. Similar braces are available for the femur and humerus. **B,** Simple knee immobilizer. **C,** Hinged-knee immobilizer, which allows motion of the knee joint or can be locked in a position of comfort.

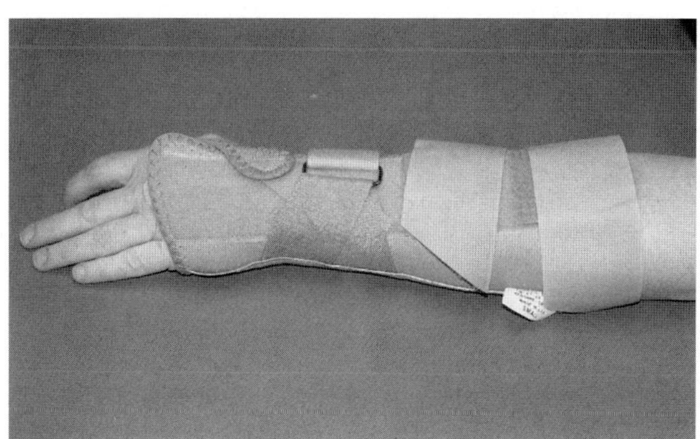

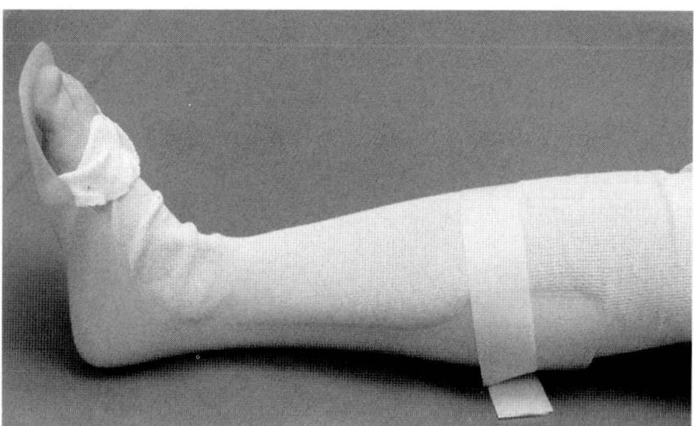

Fig. 12-6 **A,** Forearm splint for stabilization of the wrist. **B,** Ankle-foot orthosis used for support of the ankle joint.

maximum potential within their physical and psychological limitations. Often the therapist's input is much more effective than that of a family member for keeping a patient active and mobile while he or she has the ability. Physical and occupational therapists can also be very valuable to the family for teaching assisted methods to accomplish activities of daily living.

HOSPICE CARE

Treatment of the terminally ill patient with metastatic disease should be directed at providing pain relief in the least invasive way possible. Hospice care may make it possible for the patient to be at home rather than in an institution during their final days. Hospice care can include nursing assistance, housekeeping assistance, and emotional support for the patient and the family.

If outpatient hospice care is not available, some hospitals provide palliative care units in which terminal care is delivered in a more relaxed, less institutional setting than the traditional hospital room. These rooms are designed to give patients and their families privacy while providing professional care as needed to assist them.[20,21]

Care of the terminally ill pediatric patient is not the same as that of a terminally ill adult. The pediatric patient will have different emotional needs than a dying adult and is more likely to have parents present with an interest in sharing in the personal care. This can be difficult for hospital staff to recognize and accept. Hospice and hospital staff workers should be comfortable dealing with pediatric patients and should be familiar with pediatric treatment in general when caring for terminally ill pediatric patients.[22]

CONCLUSION

The decision to treat a metastatic lesion of bone in an operative or nonoperative fashion is multifaceted. The individual needs of each patient must be considered and specific realistic goals developed. The primary goal of treatment should be the relief of pain with stabilization of impending fractures in as noninvasive a manner as possible. A knowledge of nonoperative treatment alternatives and close collaboration with other members of the multidisciplinary team will provide the best opportunity to meet these goals and provide the patient with the best possible care.

REFERENCES

1. Janjan NA, Payne R, Gillis T, Podoloff D, Libshitz HI, Lenzi R, Theriault R, Martin C, Yasko A. Presenting symptoms in patients referred to a multidisciplinary clinic for bone metastases. J Pain Symptom Manage 16(3):171-178, 1998.
2. Demers LM, Costa L, Chinchilli VM, Gaydos L, Curley E, Lipton A. Biomechanical markers of bone turnover in patients with metastatic bone disease. Clin Chem 41(10):1489-1494, 1995.
3. Schlosser K, Scigalla P. Biochemical markers as surrogates in clinical trials in patients with metastatic bone disease and osteoporosis. Scand J Clin Lab Invest Suppl (Norway) 227:21-28, 1997.
4. Vinholes JJ, Purohit OP, Abbey ME, Eastell R, Coleman RE. Relationships between biomechanical and symptomatic response in a double-blind randomized trial of pamidronate for metastatic bone disease. Ann Oncol (Netherlands) 8(12):1243-1250, 1997.
5. Nielsen OS. Palliative treatment of bone metastases. Acta Oncologica 5(Suppl 35):58-60, 1996.
6. Harrington KD. New trends in the management of lower extremity metastases. Clin Orthop (169):53-61, 1982.
7. Oken M, Creech R, Tormey D, Horton J, Davis T, McFadden E, Carbone P. Toxicity and response criteria of the Eastern Cooperative Oncology Group. Am J Clin Oncol 5:649-655, 1982.
8. Nielsen OS, Munro AJ, Tannock IF. Bone metastases: Pathophysiology and management policy. J Clin Oncol 9(3):509-524, 1991.
9. Hoskin PJ, Price P, Easton D, Regan J, Austin D, Palmer S, Yarnold JR. A prospective randomised trial of 4 Gy or 8 Gy single doses in the treatment of metastatic bone pain. Radiother Oncol 23(2):74-78, 1992.
10. Houston SJ, Rubens RD. The systemic treatment of bone metastases. Clin Orthop (312):95-104, 1995.
11. Taub M, Begas A, Love N. Advanced prostate cancer: Endocrine therapies and palliative measures. Postgrad Med 100(3):139-140, 143-6, 152 passim, 1996.
12. Laing AH, Ackery DM, Bayly RJ, Buchanan RB, Lewington VJ, McEwan AJ, Macleod PM, Zivanovic MA. Strontium-89 therapy for pain palliation in prostatic skeletal malignancy. Br J Radiol 64:816-822, 1991.
13. Robinson RG, Spicer JA, Preston DF, Wegst AV, Martin NL. Treatment of metastatic bone pain with strontium-89. Nucl Med Biol 14:219-222, 1987.
14. Cotton A, Dewatre F, Cortet B, Assaker R, Leblond D, Duquesnoy B, Chastanet P, Clarisse J. Percutaneous vertebroplasty for osteolytic metastases and myeloma: Effects of the percentage of lesion filling and the leakage of methyl methacrylate at clinical follow-up. Radiology 200(2):525-530, 1996.

15. Weill A, Chiras J, Simon JM, Rose M, Sola-Martinez T, Enkaoua E. Spinal metastases: Indications for and results of percutaneous injection of acrylic surgical cement. Radiology 199(1):241-247, 1996.

16. Dupuy DE, Safran H, Mayo-Smith WW, Goldberg SN. Radiofrequency ablation of painful osseous metastatic disease. Presented at the 1998 Scientific Program, Radiological Society of North America, McCormick Place, Chicago, Ill., Dec. 2, 1998.

17. Mundy GR. Pathophysiology of bone metastasis. Presented at Biologic Concepts in Cancer With Clinical Implications for the Year 2000 and Beyond. Penn State Geisinger's Milton S. Hershey Medical Center, Hershey, Pa., Oct. 15, 1998.

18. Hortobagyi GN, Theriault RL, Porter L, Blayney D, Lipton A, Sinoff C, Wheeler H, Simeone JF, Seaman J, Knight RD. Efficacy of pamidronate in reducing skeletal complications in patients with breast cancer and lytic bone metastases. N Engl J Med 335:1785-1791, 1996.

19. Berenson JR, Lichtenstein A, Porter L, Dimopoulos MA, Bordoni R, George S, Lipton A, Keller A, Ballester O, Kovacs MJ, Blacklock HA, Bell R, Simeone J, Reitsma DJ, Heffeman M, Seaman J, Knight RD. Efficacy of pamidronate in reducing skeletal events in patients with advanced multiple myeloma. N Engl J Med 334:488-493, 1996.

20. Fulton JP. Palliative care for cancer patients—Current issues. Med Health 81(8):276-277, 1998.

21. Martin EW. Inpatient hospice care: A new option for the terminally ill. Rhode Island Med 78(4):118-119, 1995.

22. Finlay I, McQuillan R, Webb D. Paediatric palliative care: The role of an adult palliative care service. [Letter.] Palliat Med 9(2):166-167, 1995.

Palliative Care of the Terminal Patient

Doreen M. Oneschuk, M.D., and Eduardo Bruera, M.D.

the absence of radiculopathy, the pain from vertebral metastases can be referred to the limbs and aggravated by straight leg raising.[20] The main complications of vertebral metastases are vertebral collapse, radiculopathy, and epidural spinal cord compression. Collapse of vertebral bodies is particularly frequent in the thoracic spine and may acutely aggravate the pain syndrome by impinging on the nerve roots and causing skeletal deformities, elevating the risk of epidural spinal cord compression. Radiculopathies can develop at any level; the pain is felt on the spine, deep in the muscles innervated by the affected root, and in the corresponding dermatome. Pain from the presence of a radiculopathy is usually exacerbated by increased intraspinal pressure from coughing, sneezing, and straining.[17,20] For radicular pain a "burning" or "tingling" nature to the pain may be described, as well as occasional paroxysms of lancinating pain. Sensory or motor deficits are further indicators of nerve involvement and level of involvement.[13]

TREATMENT OPTIONS FOR BONE PAIN

To optimize quality of life for patients with cancer, well-tolerated, repeatable, and effective treatments for bone pain are necessary.[12] Treatment modalities may be limited to the exclusive use of analgesics, such as opioids, but may commonly involve combination treatment regimens, including the use of corticosteroids, bisphosphonates, hormonal therapy or chemotherapy, radiotherapy, orthopedic interventions, and anesthetic or neurosurgical procedures.

Opioid Analgesics

Opioid analgesics remain the mainstay for control of both diffuse bone pain and pain in isolated areas of bone.[13] Bone pain typically responds well to opioids.[21,22] A majority of patients will likely require a strong opioid agonist such as morphine, hydromorphone, oxycodone, fentanyl, or methadone. Because most patients experience continuous pain, an around-the-clock dosing of an opioid is advised, in addition to a breakthrough or rescue dose on an as-needed basis. The dose can then be titrated to achieve adequate pain control. At the same time, measures to prevent common side effects such as

constipation and nausea should be applied. In addition, knowledge of common neuropsychiatric side effects, such as opioid-induced delirium, hallucinations, myoclonus, and excessive sedation, and their management strategies, is essential.[23] Oral administration is preferred, although on occasion an alternative route is required. The subcutaneous route has been shown to be as effective as the intravenous route and more convenient. Other options include rectal and transdermal formulations.

With regard to incident pain, titration of opioids may prove difficult. Patients may require short-acting breakthrough or rescue doses of analgesics to provide pain relief that breaks through the chronic daily pain.[6,11] It is frequently recommended that these breakthrough doses be given before an activity that may elicit pain. Unfortunately most patients with incidental pain receive limited benefit from currently available breakthrough analgesics because the duration of pain is shorter than the latency for analgesia.[24] Newer, highly liposoluble opioids, such as transmucosal fentanyl, could prove particularly useful in the management of incidental bone pain.[25,26] In cases in which severe sedation arises as a symptom of dose-limiting opioid toxicity during the intervals between incident pain the addition of a psychostimulant could be considered. By reducing sedation and thereby improving analgesia, psychostimulants may allow patients to tolerate a higher dose of opioids.[24]

Nonsteroidal Anti-inflammatory Drugs

Although the World Health Organization[1] advises these medications as the first-line approach for the management of mild to moderate cancer pain, strong, methodologically sound studies have yet to establish evidence-based support in favor of nonsteroidal anti-inflammatory drugs in cancer pain.[27] Moreover, the use of nonsteroidal anti-inflammatory drugs carries the risk of development of adverse reactions, those of the most concern in cancer patients being gastrointestinal, renal, and hematologic reactions. Nonsteroidal anti-inflammatory drugs may cause renal insufficiency by impairing intrarenal blood flow by inhibition of prostacyclin, a renovasodilator. Thus renal impairment can result in opioid metabolite accumulation, giving rise to various neuropsychiatric toxicities.[28,29] A new generation of nonsteroidal anti-inflammatory drugs capable of selectively inhibiting cyclo-oxygenase 2 (COX 2) is available. These agents will probably not have the traditional side effects related to COX 1 inhibition, and it is hoped that they will be combined successfully with opioids.[30]

Corticosteroids

Corticosteroids appear to be effective in reducing bone pain from a variety of solid tumors. Apart from their adjuvant analgesic properties, corticosteroids have various other potential benefits for patients with advanced disease, including improvement in appetite, decrease in nausea, and an improvement in the sensation of well-being.[31] The ideal type and optimal dose of corticosteroid has not been well established, and dose recommendations are mainly based on uncontrolled anecdotal reports and clinical experience. Recommended corticosteroids and doses are 4 to 8 mg of dexamethasone orally or subcutaneously two to three times per day, 20 to 40 mg of prednisone orally two to three times per day, or 16 to 32 mg of methylprednisolone orally two to three times per day.[32] Dexamethasone appears to be preferred because of its ease of administration on a twice-daily basis, in addition to its minimal to absent mineralocorticoid effects. If effectiveness is demonstrated, the corticosteroid dose should gradually be tapered to the lowest possible effective dose or, if possible, be discontinued to avoid long-term adverse effects.[13] Corticosteroids also have been found to be beneficial in the treatment of spinal cord compression and should be initiated early when spinal cord compression is suspected.[33] In patients with a relatively long expected survival, maintenance therapy with corticosteroids should be carefully weighed against the potential side effects, including immunosuppression, avascular necrosis, edema, hyperglycemia, proximal myopathy, and neuropsychiatric side effects.[34] With regard to the latter, delirium has been found to be more common than mood disorders in cancer patients taking dexamethasone.[35] Because steroid myopathy can contribute further to decreased ambulation and immobility, one should observe closely for this side effect in particular. If it arises, consideration can be given to discontinuing the corticosteroid, which of-

ten results in complete reversibility of the problem.[36] Another option for those who are benefitting from the use of a corticosteroid is to change to a nonfluorinated steroid, such as methylprednisolone or prednisone.[37]

Bisphosphonates

Bisphosphonates are pyrophosphate analogs that are thought to inhibit osteoclast-mediated bone resorption.[38] Clodronate and pamidronate are the bisphosphonates that have been studied and used most extensively in malignant disease to date; however, newer bisphosphonates with greater potency, including alendronate, risedronate, ibandronate, and zolendronate, are now available.[39] Numerous methodologically sound research studies have better defined the potential positive effects on bone metastases, including increased pain relief,[40-42] increased time to progression of disease,[40] decreased median time to first skeletal event,[43] and decreased skeletal events.[41]

This subject is discussed in more detail in Chapter 9 of this book.

Hormonal Therapy and Chemotherapy

Adequate assessments of pain relief and effect on quality of life in patients treated with different chemotherapy and hormonal therapy regimens for bone metastases from breast, lung, and prostate cancer, lymphoma, and multiple myeloma are lacking. There is no clear evidence that hormonal therapy or quick chemotherapy has an analgesic effect per se. When tumors respond to these treatments, however, pain can be significantly decreased.[44] Hormonal therapy can sustain symptom relief in patients with widespread painful bone metastases from prostate cancer.[45-47] Hormonal therapy has few side effects, making it the preferable palliative treatment modality in hormone-responsive tumors such as those of the breast and prostate.[44]

Chemotherapy has been used with limited success in the palliative treatment of pain associated with bone metastases.[48,49] Because the toxicity of chemotherapy is severe, particularly in patients with advanced cancer who are already debilitated, there is little justification for using it to relieve pain unless there is a significant chance of obtaining an objective response.[44]

Radiotherapy and Radioisotopes

External beam irradiation is a well-established treatment of choice for localized bone pain due to metastatic disease.[50] Traditionally, radiation has been administered in multiple fractions over several days to weeks, although current evidence indicates that single fractions are as effective as multiple fractions when pain relief is the goal.[51-54] Moreover, single fractions are less demanding on both the patient and the resources. It appears that the relapse rate of bone pain after single doses is similar to that after multiple doses, and reirradiation of an area with a single fraction is feasible, particularly if there was a good response after the first treatment. A small portion of initial nonresponders may respond to a second dose of radiation. In addition, most studies suggest that there is no difference in frequency of acute toxicity between single and multiple fractions. The role of prophylactic radiotherapy has not been well defined, although there may be a place for it in the treatment of sites that appear to be at high risk of developing a pathologic fracture. Several retrospective studies have emphasized the importance of postoperative radiotherapy. Postoperative radiation has been thought to promote bone healing and prevent tumor progression within the area of metastatic invasion and possibly to prevent metastases in the immediate region surrounding the tumor. Furthermore, it is believed that postoperative radiotherapy aids in regaining use of the extremity and leads to a decrease in further reoperations at the site.[55,56]

Another treatment option used to control pain due to metastatic disease is the systemic administration of bone-seeking radioisotopes, such as strontium chloride (^{89}Sr) and phosphorus (^{32}P).[57-59] A placebo-controlled trial and a large randomized trial involving patients with metastatic prostate cancer suggest beneficial analgesic effects from the use of strontium.[60,61] Disadvantages of strontium therapy include the potential for severe hematologic toxicity, delay in pain relief, and high cost.[58] Other isotopes, such as sumarium (^{153}Sm) and rhenium (^{186}Re), which appear to have a better side effect profile, a shorter half-life, and a higher percentage of bone uptake, are being investigated.[58,62] Randomized control trials of radioisotopes vs. bisphosphonates in the treatment of metastatic bone pain are required.

COMMON COMPLICATIONS ASSOCIATED WITH BONE METASTASES
Hypercalcemia

Hypercalcemia occurs in approximately 10% to 40% of cancer patients during their illness trajectory,[63] and it is probably the most common metabolic complication of malignant disease. It is of clinical importance because of the morbidity associated with it.[12] Hypercalcemia is frequently a cause of symptoms in patients with terminal cancer. Hypercalcemia encompasses a wide range of clinical presentations that may be quite nonspecific and can be confused with manifestations of the underlying cancer or its treatment. As hypercalcemia most commonly disturbs neurologic, gastrointestinal, cardiovascular, and renal function, common clinical features of hypercalcemia include fatigue, anorexia, bone pain, constipation, nausea, vomiting, altered mental status, lethargy, polydipsia, polyuria, and intravascular volume depletion. Neurologic symptoms can progress to seizures, coma, and death, and cardiac manifestations can include arrhythmia or a classic shortening of the QT interval on electrocardiograms.[64,65] Symptoms tend to be most prominent in patients who have a rapid increase in serum calcium levels, as well as those with the highest calcium levels, and are often more apparent in elderly patients than in younger patients. In cancer patients, hypercalcemia is commonly steadily progressive, and the patients may experience symptoms with a relatively low serum calcium concentration.[66] If the patient has symptoms of hypercalcemia, treatment is warranted with follow-up observation of improvement or alleviation of symptoms. If the symptoms of hypercalcemia are not responsive to treatment, future treatment of episodes of hypercalcemia may not be warranted. When hypercalcemia occurs in a patient who is unresponsive or ill because of other medical problems, treatment of the hypercalcemia is not required.

Pathologic Fractures

Pathologic fractures have been reported in 8% to 30% of patients with bone metastases,[67,68] although the true incidence of pathologic fractures in patients with bone metastases is somewhat uncertain and depends on whether rib and vertebral fractures are also considered. Vertebral collapse is probably underreported in most series.[12] Pain on activity should always be regarded as a sign of possible abnormal osseous structures with a potential for fracture.[69] A pathologic fracture typically results in a sudden exacerbation of pain, although it is important to recall that not all bone metastases are painful and that pathologic fractures can occur without preceding pain.[13] Proximal parts of long bones are generally more commonly involved, and the bones with a high propensity to fracture more often are the femur (50%) and the humerus (15%).[68] Rib fractures and vertebral collapse can result in loss of height, kyphoscoliosis, and a degree of restrictive lung disease. Epidural extension of tumor in the spine or pathologic fractures of a long bone, however, appear to cause the most disability. The probability of a pathologic fracture increases with the duration of metastatic involvement and therefore, somewhat paradoxically, is more common in patients with disease confined to bone who have a relatively good prognosis. Because the development of a fracture is so devastating to a cancer patient, increased emphasis is now being placed on attempts to predict which metastatic sites are at risk of fracture, the use of prophylactic surgery, and the long-term administration of bisphosphonates.[70]

Neurologic Complications and Spinal Cord Compression

Neuropathic and bone pain frequently coexist when spinal disease extends to compress or invade nerve roots of the spinal cord, as may occur with epidural spinal cord compression complicating vertebral bone metastases or osteophytic compression of spinal nerve roots.[6] Motor, sensory, and autonomic signs may arise with invasion of the epidural space and compression of the spinal cord. Cord compression occurs in approximately 5% of cancer patients, and a local or radicular pain may be the only sign of compression before the development of sudden paralysis.[71] Close monitoring is necessary in patients with vertebral bone metastases, regardless of whether they have back pain; however, when the development of back pain in a cancer patient coincides with a plain spinal radiograph abnormality, it should serve as a warning of the possible development of spinal cord compression.[12] Although pain is the first and most common presenting feature of spinal cord compression, one

also needs to look for motor weakness, paresthesia, sensory deficits, and bladder and bowel impairment.[71] Neurologic recovery is inversely related to the degree of pretreatment neurologic impairment, and the proportion of patients who are ambulatory after treatment declines from more than 80% for patients who are ambulatory at the initiation of therapy to less than 50% if they are paraparetic, and less than 10% if they are paraplegic.[33] The keys to successful rehabilitation are early diagnosis, high-dose corticosteroids, and rapid assessment and urgent referral for either spinal stabilization and decompression or radiotherapy.[72]

ORTHOPEDIC MANAGEMENT

Current techniques for surgical management of pathologic fractures are extremely effective in alleviating pain and allowing patients to resume an ambulatory status, often without the need for external support. This in turn has significantly improved the quality of the remaining months or years for these persons. The long-term survival of patients after their first pathologic fracture associated with cancer has more than tripled for the most common cancers during the past 25 years. Surgical techniques for stabilizing pathologic or impending fractures must be individualized for the area of involvement, the particular qualities of the bone involved, and the potential for involvement of adjacent soft tissue structures.[73] Various factors are weighed in determining whether a patient should have surgery; these include the overall prognosis, fitness for surgery, and the degree of pain or functional loss. As with any treatment modality, the potential benefits to be gained with surgery need to be weighed against the potential risks.[67] An expected survival of only weeks to months is not necessarily a contraindication to surgery. Even in bedridden terminal patients, orthopedic procedures may improve some degree of function and ease the nursing care of the patient. In many cases, particularly those involving pathologic fractures of the hips and lower extremities, surgery offers the only definitive therapy to control pain and provide mobility.[67] Fixation for lower-extremity long bones, such as the femur, must be able to withstand weightbearing stresses. Upper-extremity pathologic fractures are often subjected to distractive forces inherent in lifting and pulling, in addition to heavy compressive forces, particularly in patients who require crutches or other devices to assist them in walking. Most malignant pathologic fractures of the pelvis, long bones, or spine are amenable to effective stabilization, leading to resumption of weightbearing ambulation in all but a few patients, good or excellent pain relief in the vast majority, and thus improved quality of life.[73] Prophylactic stabilization has been advocated in patients at high risk of pathologic fracture.[74]

ANESTHETIC AND NEUROSURGICAL PROCEDURES

Various anesthetic procedures are available to alleviate malignant bone pain, including local anesthetic nerve and plexus blocks, in addition to the use of epidural or intrathecal routes of opioid administration.[75] Drawbacks to the use of spinal/epidural opioids include high costs, invasiveness of the procedure, potential for catheter dislodgment or blockage, and risk of spinal infections.[21,76] With regard to neurosurgical procedures, percutaneous cordotomy can be considered when other treatment modalities have failed for management of unilateral incidental pain below the waist.[77,78] Neurologic complications of this procedure include hemiparesis, urinary retention, and the risk of unmasking pain on the contralateral side of the body.[79] Rhizotomy can be considered for refractory chest or limb pain. Similar to a cordotomy, this procedure is not without potential side effects, including paresis, sphincter dysfunction, and impairment of touch, proprioception, and dysesthesias.[77]

REHABILITATION

Rehabilitation in patients with advanced cancer differs from traditional rehabilitation in that it does not necessarily achieve the return of the patient to work or even to his or her home. It may, however, help to relieve discomfort and improve quality of life by reducing the negative effects of physical dependence.[80]

The functional status of a patient should demand the same disciplined approach to assessment and communication as that for other symptoms such as pain and nausea. In addition, the patient, the family, and the respective health care providers should be attentive to the continuous shift in both symptom and functional status of the patient as a result of the changing and progressive course of the illness.[81]

Although a recent report suggested poor success with rehabilitation in patients with an Eastern Cooperative Oncology Group performance score of 3 or more,[82] the need and motivation for rehabilitation in the terminally ill are high. Other studies indicate that most patients are excellent candidates for active rehabilitation programs after surgical treatment for pathologic fractures or spinal cord compression.[80,83] In one study, 54 patients with metastatic bone disease were followed prospectively to assess the risk of pathologic fracture during rehabilitation. Sixteen fractures were observed in 12 patients. Only one fracture occurred while the patient was undergoing rehabilitation, and this was a fourth lumbar vertebral compression fracture that did not affect the clinical course of the patient. Patients in the fracture group were generally younger, female, and in a more advanced stage of disease with lytic metastases in a previous site of pathologic fracture.[83] Patients with pathologic fractures from malignant disease with residual functional deficits are an obvious group for whom multidisciplinary rehabilitation programs might be appropriate. Another study looked at 58 patients with 62 pathologic fractures secondary to metastatic disease who were admitted to a rehabilitation hospital during a 5-year period. In addition to the significant number of patients[34] who were discharged home, there was a significant improvement in transfers, ambulation, and the ability to perform activities of daily living. Patients with a poor rehabilitation outcome included those with hypercalcemia and those requiring parenteral opioids.[84] Another study assessed 301 terminal cancer patients who received physical therapy in a hospice facility during a period of 6½ years. The objectives were to determine whether physical therapy in the terminal stage can be significantly effective for the dying patient. The investigation was made by assessing the activities of daily living of the patients and by evaluating a questionnaire sent to the families. Almost all patients experienced at least some relief from various types of discomfort, including pain, dyspnea, leg edema, constipation, and other impairments of their activities of daily living. Two hundred thirty-nine patients showed improvement in activities of daily living, in addition to the average transfer and locomotion score on the Barthel mobility index. It seemed that patients who had more fully discussed the physical therapy program with the therapist believed that the rehabilitation was effective and satisfactory. Families who actively participated in the rehabilitation process assessed it as more effective, more satisfactory to the patient, and more useful in overall patient care than did families who did not participate at all. Patients with paralysis, especially with paraplegia caused by spinal metastases, showed less improvement. Because such patients are likely to have severe disability, bedsores, restricted range of motion, and phlebitis, physical therapy is even more important to enable them, as much as possible, to gain control and independence. Because the result indicated greater improvement in patients who experienced rehabilitative care more frequently or at an earlier stage, it is strongly recommended that active rehabilitation services be started soon after admission to an inpatient facility or hospice.[85] Besides the risk of progressive muscle weakness, muscle atrophy, and osteoporosis, prolonged bed rest does not appear to benefit the patient with already established fractures, particularly when it seems that fractures clearly related to mobilization are unlikely to occur. It appears that fractures may occur even if the patient is on bed rest.[83,86]

With regard to rehabilitation in those with spinal cord injury, a 12-year retrospective review of 27 patients admitted to a rehabilitation facility for care of spinal cord injuries secondary to cancer revealed an overall 1-year survival rate of 58%. In the complete spinal cord injury group with a 38% 1-year survival after discharge, only one of three patients was independent at 1 year. Therefore functional independence appears to be an unrealistic goal in most of these patients. It was thought that proper attention to the prevention of skin, bowel, and bladder problems would probably avoid readmissions to the hospital and minimize discomfort in these patients and thus should be the rehabilitation goal. On the other hand, patients in this study with incomplete injuries had a much better prognosis. Skills, self-care, and ambulation were well maintained throughout the 1-year follow-up. The

nine patients with incomplete injuries but no useful motor function below the level of the injury were the group that benefitted the most from rehabilitation because of their greater deficits.[87] Another retrospective review of 70 patients with spinal cord compression due to tumor who were referred to a rehabilitation hospital in the United States revealed 26 home discharges, 15 transfers to other facilities, and 29 deaths. Of the 26 patients who went home, 24 participated in transfers, all were mobile at least at the wheelchair level, and 13 of 14 improved in Kenny scores. Of the 34 patients who were not discharged home, only 5 showed improvement in mobility and transfers. In addition, patients discharged to home used fewer or no parenteral opioids and had a lower incidence of incontinence.[88]

REHABILITATION THERAPY AND REHABILITATIVE AIDS

Rehabilitation in palliative care may satisfy different purposes in the same patient, such as restoring independence, limiting the damage of a hypokinetic syndrome, and providing psychological support. It also provides a rhythm to the patient's stay and strengthens desired goals.[89] The focus of the rehabilitation team is that of attempting to obtain a maximum level of functioning for their patients within the limits imposed by their patient's disease process.[90] The rehabilitative role also serves to reduce the degree to which disabilities become permanent and interfere with everyday life.[91] Physiotherapy is most likely to be helpful when an improvement in function can be anticipated after recent surgery or medical treatment.[92] Exercise can prevent pain and loss of movement from stiff joints, increase muscle strength, and improve vitality by stimulating lung and circulatory function. Without mobility, there may be dependence on others for personal care, with consequent loss of privacy, dignity, and self-esteem. Many factors may have an adverse effect on mobility, including pain, weakness, loss of balance, loss of confidence, dyspnea, stiffness, contractures, constipation, and diarrhea. Consequently a proactive approach to identifying and monitoring these symptoms is imperative. Many patients lose their mobility unnecessarily, either because they give up and take to their beds prematurely or because they are overprotected by caring relatives. It is for this reason that caregivers should be involved as much as possible in the rehabilitation program,[93] including identifying needs, setting goals, and determining the treatment and techniques.[94] If a pathologic fracture does occur and is treated with or without operative repair, appropriate exercise will be needed with attempts at gradual improvement in mobility. Initial therapy can include simple active leg exercises. While the quadriceps will contract against gravity, standing with assistance (if necessary) can be attempted, followed by walking. When the patient has regained mobility, attention can be paid to other weak areas that then can be exercised accordingly. Rollator walking frames, other walking aids, reclining armchairs, and wheelchairs may be required and are useful in aiding mobility and relieving pain during weightbearing.[95] Soft or lightweight rigid collars, lively or rigid splints, lightweight orthoses, or slings provide support and alleviate pain in regions of the spine or fractured or edematous arms and reduce neural stretch in the lower extremities. Along with ambulation, correct positioning in bed, wheelchair, or other chair can do much to alleviate pain, aid in breathing, improve sleep, and prevent deformities and pressure ulcers.[95-97] Deformities may lead to unnecessary discomfort and distress, making simple nursing procedures difficult.[95] Patients with advanced cancer and bone metastases are prone to the development of pressure ulcers. Contributing factors include lack of exercise and anorexia, where weight loss reduces the amount of protective subcutaneous fat. Atrophy of the muscles also can lead to the emergence of bone prominences and risk damage to the overlying skin.[92,95] Thus proper lifting, handling, and movement that avoid direct friction on the skin (which can easily occur during sliding transfers) is required. Special mattresses and cushions can aid comfort, allay pain, and help prevent pressure ulcers by minimizing pressure on the body.[95] In a study of 68 patients in a hospital-based palliative care setting, 24 (35%) developed pressure ulcers during their hospital stay. The 24 patients with pressure ulcers identified in the study had a total of 42 pressure ulcers. The most frequent skin breakdown occurred on the coccyx[17] and the buttocks.[15] Risk factors identified for development of

pressure ulcers in this setting included cognitive status, continence, nutrition, and sensory awareness.[98]

Incidental pain can compromise independence in essential activities of daily living, such as transferring, toileting, sitting, walking, and lying down.[99] Many of these activities, such as walking and toileting, can become even more difficult or impossible when steroid myopathy develops with the use of corticosteroids. Pathologic fracture of the proximal third of the humerus or aseptic necrosis of the head of the humerus from prolonged steroid therapy use can result in shoulder and arm pain that complicates such functions as dressing and personal care. With movement-induced pain, transcutaneous electrical nerve stimulation (TENS) can complement bracing and other strategies.[97] In patients with spinal cord compression or paraplegia the treatment program can be focused on building power in the arms, hands, and shoulder girdle so that transfers from bed to wheelchair or toilet can be achieved. Use of such aids as sliding boards is also helpful. Passive movements to paralyzed legs can help prevent joint stiffening and contractures.[93] A systematic and frequent reevaluation of functional performances of advanced cancer patients receiving rehabilitation is important to detect even minimal benefit from rehabilitation interventions.[89] The Edmonton Functional Assessment Tool (EFAT) was developed to evaluate the extent to which patients actually perform functional activities in a palliative care setting. It was deemed a suit-

---

EFAT Considers Ten Functions

Communication
Pain
Mental status
Dyspnea
Sitting or standing balance
Mobility
Walking or wheelchair locomotion
Activities of daily living
Fatigue
Motivation

able measure of functional status in palliative care because a change in functional status was demonstrated over time and because repeated assessments were possible without additional burden to the patient, the family, or the team.[100] Therefore the EFAT has been suggested as a reliable outcome measure to evaluate the efficiency of rehabilitation in a palliative care context. The EFAT considers the 10 functions listed in the box on p. 186.[100]

DELIRIUM

Some 80% to 90% of palliative patients experience some symptoms of delirium shortly before death.[101,102] Delirium is defined as a transient organic brain syndrome characterized by the acute onset of disordered attention (arousal) and cognition, accompanied by disturbances of psychomotor behavior and perception.[103] Three clinical variances of delirium have been described on the basis of the type of arousal disturbance: hypoalert-hypoactive, hyperalert-hyperactive, and mixed type.[104,105] In hypoactive delirium the patient may be classically described as "pleasantly confused," may be minimally verbally responsive, or may be unresponsive. With hyperactive delirium the patient may be physically and psychologically restless, with thrashing, moaning, groaning, or other behaviors that could be and usually have been interpreted as signs of pain.[106] Another concern for a patient in an agitated delirium is that thrashing around can increase bone pain and possibly cause pathologic fractures.[107] Assessing the intensity of pain when patients are in an agitated delirium becomes a problem as well as a source of disagreement among staff members, contributing to family stress because of varying interpretations of the patient's condition. The data of Bruera et al.[108] suggest that most of the patients, if they recover, will not remember having had any pain during their confusional episode, and that staff members from palliative care units are probably overestimating the level of pain and overtreating the patients with extra doses of opioids. This situation can serve as a source of potential conflict between the family, who may interpret agitated delirium as a manifestation of pain, and the staff.[108] Therefore, in the presence of delirium, the family may require counseling provided by the health care staff.[107]

PSYCHOLOGICAL CONSEQUENCES FOR THE PATIENT AND FAMILY

Suffering may arise from the perceived loss of a physical, psychological, or a social resource. The patient sometimes perceives physical incapability for a desired activity as a threat to the self and experiences diminished integrity of his or her person. This awareness is part of suffering. Those patients who successfully control their emotions and mentation, even as physical capabilities and energy precipitously decline, gain a sense of mastery over their dying that may contribute positively to the family's ability to cope.[109] Patients with advanced cancer may require management of many different symptoms to ameliorate their discomfort and improve their quality of life.[110] Patients with overwhelming physical symptoms and functional limitations are much more likely to report severe levels of psychological distress. For example, clinically significant pain nearly doubles the likelihood of a major psychiatric complication of cancer, especially depressive disorders and confusional states.[111] Thus, from the outset, the treatment plan for cancer patients should include proactive pain and symptom control options. It should also include attempts to minimize helplessness or perceived helplessness by engaging psychosocial resources. Because active coping helps preserve self-worth,[109] learning coping skills such as relaxation and meditation also can help patients continue to function effectively.

The dimensions of family functioning include integrating the past, solving problems, dealing with feelings, making use of resources, considering others, portraying family identity, and fulfilling and tolerating differences. In palliative care, these dimensions enable the palliative care practitioner to individualize interventions to meet the needs of each family at its level of functioning.[112] Families experience a number of demands, such as completing practical tasks of daily living and at the same time providing physical care of the patient.[113] For family caregivers, it may be impossible to anticipate the emotional and psychological changes that precede death.[110] For many, the most distressing symptom is pain. Caregivers do not want their loved ones to suffer; however, they may fear oversedation, wanting to keep their loved one alert for interactions, or they may fear enhancing death by giving too much medication. On the other hand, they may be fearful of giving too little medication.[114] Families are frequently even more distressed than the patient and require a great deal of time and attention if they are to accept the reality of the illness and become supportive of each other and of the patient.[115] In one study, as the patients' activity levels decreased, the caregivers' psychological needs increased.[116] In another study, the quality of life experienced by the patient was found to be related to the health status of the family members. These findings are consistent with the family systems theory that postulates that a change in one family member impinges on the well-being of other family members. The strong correlation between the patient's symptom distress and his or her quality of life suggests that alleviation of symptom distress may indirectly affect the health status of family members.[117] Thus, addressing caregivers' informational and psychological needs during the care of their loved ones is vital.

HOME VS. HOSPICE VS. IN-HOSPITAL CARE

One cannot simply say that home care is better than hospice care or that hospice care is better than in-hospital palliative care. It all depends on the patient, the course of the disease, the changing circumstances of each patient, availability of extended family support in the community, and possibly on the particular geographic community itself.[118] Patients should be able to move freely between home, the hospice, and a tertiary palliative care unit, depending on the needs at that moment, and with minimal disruptions (Fig. 13-1). This requires availability of resources in another setting when needed, easy flow of communication, documentation, and avoidance of duplication.[115] Communication between the four settings described in Fig. 13-1 requires frequent assessment of symptoms, such as those described in the box on p. 179, and then criteria for each of the arrows shown in Fig. 13-1 that connect each of the settings.

Coordinated care, including that of supportive family members, is often required to enable loved ones to stay and die at home. This usually includes the availability of more than one caregiver at home.[119] For home management, certain skills required by families to manage their loved one's care have been identified. These include pain management (i.e., oral or parenteral medications), nutritional needs (i.e., tube feedings), respiratory comfort (i.e., use of oxygen), wound care (i.e., pressure ulcers), and bowel and bladder management.[114] Family members may require instruction in the use of equipment and supplies to control symptoms, such as hospital beds, bedside commodes, Hoyer lifts, wheelchairs, and intravenous poles, all of which can be intimidating and overwhelming.[110] For a palliative home care program to succeed, there must be regular visits by trained nurses, physicians, and preferably social workers who are competent in managing common palliative care symptoms and who must be able to respond to emergencies at any time. It is imperative that the

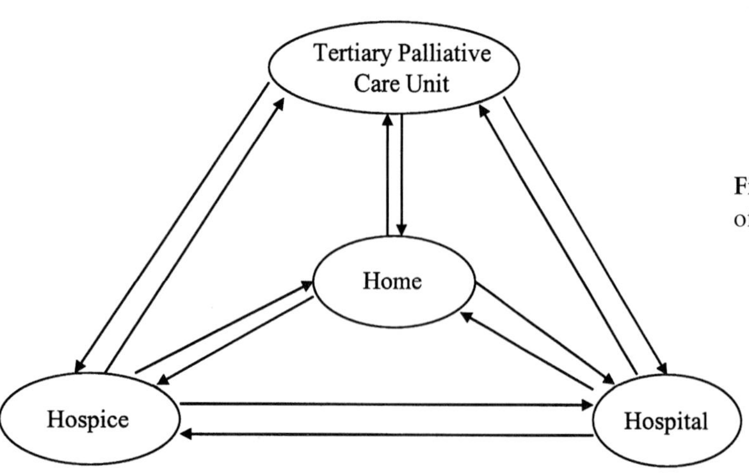

Fig. 13-1   Four different settings for the delivery of palliative care services.

family be involved, their questions answered, and their fears dealt with. Cultural differences must also be recognized and respected. These measures will help to avoid caregiver distress and "burnout."[118] Twenty-four-hour accessibility via telephone calls and home visits can reduce a family's fears and uncertainty while caring for their loved ones.[120]

Other factors that can have an impact on the decision for home involvement may include the effect on children and financial considerations.[110] Although it is often reassuring for a relative to have home care staff in the home to lessen responsibility, the loss of privacy and the sense of intrusion may become an issue.[121] Advantages to home care include reduced health costs and minimized demands on acute care beds. Further advantages to the patient include familiar and comfortable surroundings and probably greater time spent with family members.[118] Although patients may hope to end their lives in their own homes, they are often conscious of putting excessive strain on relatives. For this reason, patients and relatives may be reassured by knowing that inpatient care is available if required.[122] Families may not be able to endure the physical and psychological strain encountered when caring for an increasingly dependent and debilitated relative. At this point, the needs and wishes of the family may need to take priority over those of the patient. If the burden of care becomes too great, the patient may need to be institutionalized for the remainder of the terminal phase. These situations require careful thought and discussion by all parties involved in the care: patients, family members, and health care professionals.[123] Very often this will involve admission to a long-term palliative care or hospice site; however, when severe physical symptoms of the patient or significant psychosocial distress of the patient or the family arises, a tertiary palliative care unit with access to an interdisciplinary team may be required. Staff members, such as social workers, pastoral counselors, and care aids, play a pivotal role in this setting, especially in their capacity to provide psychosocial support. More than ever, these families have a great need for support, to be kept informed, and to feel and be treated as if they were active and equal participants in the care planning process. To fulfill families' needs, special communication skills and extra time on the part of the entire team are re-

quired.[124] Patient and family conferences with the unit health team in attendance should be scheduled at various times throughout the patient's stay. These conferences can strengthen health care provider and family ties, reduce the risk of miscommunication, and provide a therapeutic milieu for family counseling.[125]

CONCLUSION

Appropriate palliative care of patients with bone metastases includes assessment and management of both complicating physical and psychological symptoms. Bone pain, the development of pathologic fractures, and possible spinal cord compression compromise mobility, activities of daily living, and ultimately quality of life. Although a successful outcome may not always be achieved, rehabilitation should be offered to the majority of these patients. Their place of care, whether home-, hospice-, or hospital-based, will depend on availability of home care services, the patient's disabilities, and the wishes of the patient and his or her family.

REFERENCES

1. Foley K. The treatment of cancer pain. N Engl J Med 313:84-95, 1985.
2. Galasko CSB. Skeletal metastases. Clin Orthop 210:18-30, 1986.
3. Bruera E, Lawlor P. Cancer pain management. Acta Anaesthesiol Scand 41:146-153, 1997.
4. McGuire DB. Comprehensive and multidimensional assessment and measurement of pain. J Pain Symptom Manage 7:312-319, 1992.
5. Fallon MT, Hanks GW. Control of common symptoms in advanced cancer. Ann Acad Med Singapore 23:171-177, 1994.
6. Payne R. Mechanisms and management of bone pain. Cancer 80(Suppl 8):1608-1613, 1997.
7. Folstein MF, Folstein S, McHugh PR. Mini-mental state: A practical method for grading the cognitive state of patients for the clinician. J Psychiatr Res 12:189-198, 1975.
8. Ewing JA. Detecting alcoholism: The CAGE questionnaire. JAMA 252:1905-1907, 1984.
9. Foley KM. Pain syndromes in patients with cancer. In Portenoy RK, Kanner R, eds. Pain Management: Theory and Practice. Philadelphia: FA Davis, 1996, pp 191-215.
10. Front D, Schneck SO, Frankel A, Robinson E. Bone metastases and bone pain in breast cancer: Are they closely associated? JAMA 242(16):1747-1748, 1979.
11. Portenoy RK, Hagen NA. Breakthrough pain: Definition, prevalence and characteristics. Pain 41:273-281, 1990.
12. Coleman RE. Skeletal complications of malignancy. Cancer 80(Suppl 8):1588-1594, 1997.

Malignancies such as breast cancer develop in a two-step process: initiation and promotion. During initiation, irreversible genetic changes take place as a result of exposure to any of multiple substances such as chemicals or viruses. Initiation, however, does not by itself lead to cancer. Cancer evolves following the process of promotion. Although not all the steps in cancer promotion are understood, an essential feature is cellular proliferation. Agents that stimulate cellular proliferation include growth factors, hormones, and oncogenes. Estrogen and progesterone are the primary hormones that stimulate breast epithelial proliferation. Both stimulatory and inhibitory growth factors are elaborated by breast cancer cells in response to these hormones. Such factors include epidermal growth factor (EGF), fibroblast growth factor (FGF), and insulin-like growth factors. These growth factors act by binding to specific cell membrane receptors. The ability to measure estrogen and progesterone receptors in breast cancer tissues has provided the first scientific basis for systemic therapy of breast cancer. Analysis of these hormone receptors as well as analysis of growth factor receptors such as *HER2/neu,* an epithelial growth factor family member, provides important prognostic and therapeutic information.[1]

GENETICS AND EPIDEMIOLOGY

The breast cancer proto-oncogenes *BRCA1* and *BRCA2* are associated with breast and ovarian cancer.[2,3] These genes were discovered in studies of familial clustering. *BRCA1,* a susceptibility gene for early-onset breast cancer, is strongly associated with the breast-ovarian cancer syndrome, with strong data showing that mutations of *BRCA1* are accountable. Mutations of *BRCA1* convey an 85% lifetime risk of breast cancer as well as a 50% to 60% lifetime risk of ovarian cancer. *BRCA2* also increases susceptibility to early-onset breast cancer and has an associated 85% lifetime risk of breast cancer. Interestingly, *BRCA2* does convey an increased risk of male breast cancer that ordinarily occurs at an incidence one hundredth that of female breast cancer. *BRCA2* also is seemingly associated with an increased risk of prostate cancer.

Despite the intensive search and investigation into genes regulating the occurrence and behavior of breast cancer, thus far it appears that the involvement of such genes as *BRCA1* and *BRCA2* accounts for only 5% of breast cancer in the American public. Other factors that may contribute to breast cancer are undergoing careful scrutiny, including exposure to pesticides and other chemicals in the environment, dietary habits,[4] and other environmental factors. Researchers have been intrigued by the incidence of breast cancer among women who have lived their entire lives in Japan compared to the incidence among Japanese women who have migrated to Hawaii or who were born and raised in California.[5] The incidence of breast cancer in Japanese women who never left their country is small. The incidence of breast cancer in Japanese women who migrated to Hawaii or California is modest, but women of Japanese extraction born and raised in California have the same breast cancer incidence as any other American, with an expected lifetime incidence of 1 in 9, rapidly approaching 1 in 8. The presumed cause for this phenomenon is the dietary habits of these women: the traditional Japanese diet is high in soy and rice and low in beef, and the traditional American diet is high in fat and meat.

Similarly the incidence of breast cancer among women living on Long Island is much higher than in nearly any other region in the United States.[6,7] One theory explaining this extraordinary incidence is the widespread use of pesticides and herbicides on the farms of this region.[8] The large population of Ashkenazi Jewish women, in whom a genetic predisposition to breast cancer has been identified, likely contributes to the incidence.[9]

RISK FACTORS

Major risk factors for breast cancer include female gender, age, family history, and prior history of either breast cancer or cellular atypia. As in the case with most epithelial cancers, the risk of breast cancer increases with age. Two thirds of women diagnosed with breast cancer are above the age of 60.

Minor risk factors include early age at menarche, late menopause, conception of first child at greater than 30 years of age or nulliparity, obesity, history of benign breast disease, and prolonged exposure to hormones, such as in use of oral contraceptives.[10] The risk that a particular woman will develop breast cancer can be assessed using the Gail model.[11]

A woman living in the United States has a lifetime risk of about 1 in 9 of developing breast cancer. In 1998 an estimated 180,300 new cases of invasive breast cancer will be diagnosed.[12]

Breast cancer can be classified as noninvasive or invasive on the basis of whether it is histologically confined to the lumen of the breast duct. Noninvasive breast cancers are increasingly being diagnosed because of the routine use of mammography. The most common of these noninvasive cancers include ductal carcinoma in situ (DCIS), lobular carcinoma in situ (LCIS), and comedocarcinoma. All noninvasive forms of breast cancer have an excellent prognosis, as they rarely, if ever, metastasize. The most common form of breast cancer is infiltrating ductal carcinoma, which comprises slightly more than half of all breast cancer diagnoses. Less common forms of invasive breast cancer include medullary carcinoma, lobular carcinoma, and mucinous carcinoma. Tubular carcinomas, while invasive histologically, almost never metastasize.

CHEMOPREVENTION

The NSABP (National Surgical Adjuvant Breast and Bowel Project) recently reported that tamoxifen used as chemoprevention in women at high risk of developing breast cancer, compared to an untreated control population, demonstrated a one-third reduction in cancer incidence.[13] Even with early analysis the tamoxifen also reduced the incidence of bone events such as pathologic fracture. Adverse effects associated with this chemopreventive use of tamoxifen included thromboembolic disease and uterine cancer. Similarly, a trial of raloxifene, an antiosteoporotic agent, also demonstrated a remarkable reduction in the incidence of breast cancer in those women receiving it vs. untreated controls.[14] Interest in raloxifene specifically is spurred by its lack of association with uterine cancer as well as by its positive effects on bone mineral density.[15] A randomized prospective trial comparing tamoxifen and raloxifene is in the final stages of completion. Unfortunately the role of tamoxifen or raloxifene as effective chemoprevention is somewhat clouded by two negative trials, one from England[16] and the other from Italy,[17] which failed to show a chemopreventive effect of tamoxifen vs. an untreated control.

BREAST CANCER STAGING

Staging is the most important element in treatment planning for women with breast cancer. The TNM system is used internationally. Early localized breast cancer (stages 1 and 2) is characterized by tumors less than 5 cm without fixed, palpable nodes or evidence of distant metastasis. The more advanced cancers, stages 3 and 4, include larger tumors or tumors with skin invasion, fixed palpable lymph nodes, or evidence of distant metastasis. Reevaluation of the disease stage and tumor characteristics following surgery permits a more precise prediction of outcome. Primary prognostic factors include actual tumor size and the presence and extent of lymph node involvement. Regardless of the type of surgery (lumpectomy or mastectomy), prognosis is best for women with small primary tumors (less than 2 cm) and negative lymph nodes, with more than three fourths of these patients being alive and free of disease 10 years later. By contrast, when lymph nodes contain tumor cells, nearly 50% of women will relapse. The more lymph node involvement, the more likely relapse will follow. A less favorable outcome occurs when four or more lymph nodes are involved. Recently surgeons began investigating the use of sentinel node biopsy, similar to the approach taken in melanoma. Sentinel node biopsy is quickly moving toward becoming a standard of care because of the surgeon's desire to avoid the lymphedema that often follows lymph node dissection. The effect of sentinel node biopsy on prognosis in breast cancer and its treatment, however, is currently unclear.[18,19]

The evaluation of a patient with newly diagnosed breast cancer is rapidly evolving as a result of the adoption of evidence-based medicine. While it was once routine to obtain a bone scan on all women newly diagnosed with breast cancer, the false positive rates are such that this practice has now been abandoned. Indeed, in the evaluation of a newly diagnosed breast cancer patient the minimalist approach predominates so that only those tests necessary for preoperative evaluation and the other treatment modalities involved, including radiation and chemotherapy, are recommended.

Mammography is essential now not only for diagnosis but also for treatment planning of radiation therapy.

Increased attention to pathologic analyses of the cancer is necessary as testing for hormone receptors such as estrogen and progesterone and the *HER2/neu* receptor help plan appropriate systemic therapy. Although there are several tumor markers described in breast cancer, including CEA, CA15.3, and CA27/29, their positive and negative predictive values are such that they have not been incorporated into routine practice.[20]

EVALUATION

Patients with newly diagnosed metastatic breast cancer are evaluated to determine the extent of the disease. Useful studies to determine the extent of the disease include chest radiograph, bone scan, liver function studies, and computed tomography (CT) of head, chest, abdomen, and pelvis.

Breast cancer metastases in bone may be lytic, blastic (Fig. 14-1, *A*), or, most commonly, mixed (Fig. 14-1, *B* and *C*). Areas of bones normally occupied by red marrow in adults are most commonly affected, such as the skull (Fig. 14-1, *D*), axial skele-

A   B   C

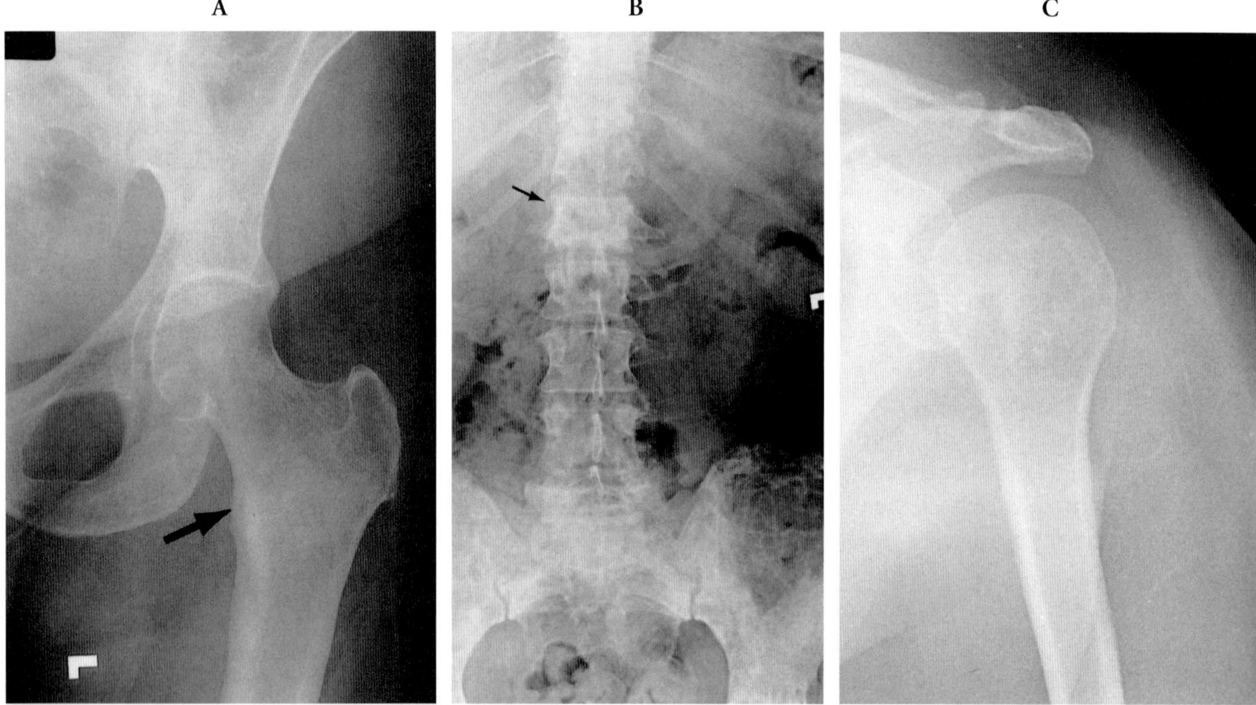

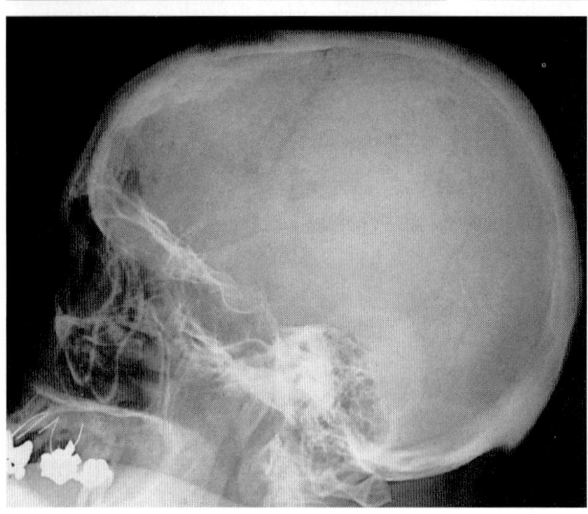

D

Fig. 14-1   **A,** Anteroposterior radiograph of the proximal femur demonstrates a poorly marginated sclerotic lesion in a 58-year-old woman with a 2-year history of breast carcinoma metastatic to the skeleton. **B,** Anteroposterior radiograph of the lumbar spine demonstrates an expansile lytic lesion in the left iliac wing and the characteristic ivory vertebrae at L1. Metastatic breast cancer presents radiographically as lytic, sclerotic, or mixed lesions, and multiple radiographic appearances can be seen in the same patient. **C,** The proximal humerus demonstrates a mixed lytic and sclerotic appearance. In patients with metastatic breast cancer the proximal long bones frequently are involved. The humerus is usually involved later in the disease process. **D,** Lateral radiograph of the skull demonstrates lytic bone destruction in the frontal skull. Bone metastases in breast carcinoma occur roughly in proportion to sites of red marrow in adults.

ton, and proximal long bones. Disease may occur in multiple bones concurrently or as a single focus.

Distinguishing between osteoporosis and metastatic breast cancer as the cause of skeletal abnormalities presents special challenges, particularly in the postmenopausal woman presenting with vertebral compression fractures and a history of breast cancer. An understanding of the type of breast cancer (invasive vs. noninvasive) and consequently the degree of suspicion that metastatic breast cancer is the cause is helpful. Magnetic resonance imaging (MRI) may be helpful in difficult cases; although the fractured vertebral body will show marrow changes regardless of the cause, marrow changes in adjacent vertebral bodies or other red marrow sites suggest metastatic breast cancer.

Radiographic evidence of bone response to systemic therapy or even to bisphosphonates may not be seen for weeks or even months. Lack of improvement on plain radiographs of lytic bone disease due to breast cancer should not be taken as a treatment failure. Rather the entire picture, including response of visceral disease and reduction of overall bone pain, should be considered.

TREATMENT

Patients with limited extent, no evidence of impending organ failure, and disease that is likely to be hormone responsive, especially those with soft tissue or bone metastasis, often are treated initially with hormone therapy.[21] As their disease progresses, hormone responders are treated with second- and third-line hormone treatments and often gain months or years of high-quality life. Eventually most women develop hormone-refractory metastases that are best treated with chemotherapy.

Endocrine Therapy

Initial endocrine therapy for premenopausal patients includes an antiestrogen such as tamoxifen (Nolvadex) or toremifene (Fareston).[22] Alternatives with equivalent benefit include surgical oophorectomy and medical oophorectomy with a luteinizing hormone–releasing hormone agonist (LHRH) such as goserlin (Zoladex). Initial endocrine therapies for postmenopausal patients also include tamoxifen or toremifene. Second-line therapies include the aromatase inhibitor anastrozole (Arimidex).[23] Third-line hormonal therapy employs a progestin such as megestrol (Megace) or medroxy-

progesterone (Provera).[21] The toxicities of tamoxifen and toremifene include deep venous thrombosis, hot flashes, and endometrial abnormalities including uterine cancer. Side effects of anastrozole are minimal, whereas side effects for progestins include weight gain and fluid retention.

Chemotherapy

Patients with intermediate- or high-risk categories of metastasis usually are offered chemotherapy as the first systemic treatment. If patients have estrogen-receptor-positive tumors, they may be offered hormone therapy in addition to chemotherapy or after chemotherapy as maintenance therapy. Several standard regimens are used for treatment of stage 4 breast cancer. They include CAF (cyclophosphamide, methotrexate, 5-fluorouracil [5-FU]), CMF (cyclophosphamide, methotrexate, 5-FU), AP (doxorubicin [Adriamycin], paclitaxel [Taxol]), and AT (doxorubicin, docetaxel [Taxotere]). These regimens are associated with myelosuppression and some degree of nausea and vomiting. Doxorubicin-containing regimens always produce alopecia and can produce cardiotoxicity. Clinical trials suggest that regimens containing a taxane such as paclitaxel or docetaxel along with the anthracycline doxorubicin are rapidly becoming first-line chemotherapy.

Growth Factors

Growth factors and their receptors are known to play critical roles in cell growth and differentiation. Abnormal expression of human epithelial growth factor receptor 2 (HER2) contributes to transformation and tumorigenesis. A newly developed humanized monoclonal antibody to this receptor, trastuzumab (Herceptin), has been introduced into clinical use.[24] Trastuzumab is active by itself as palliative therapy for women with metastatic breast cancer and significantly more active when combined with chemotherapies such as doxorubicin, the taxanes, or cyclophosphamide.[25] Remarkably, trastuzumab is relatively free of acute side effects. Unfortunately there is a significant incidence of cardiotoxicity associated with this drug, especially when the patient has had or is concurrently receiving doxorubicin.

Breast cancer is the first solid tumor that has had drugs developed to specific cancer targets. Tamoxifen, which blocks the estrogen receptor, an essential physiologic factor in breast cancer development, and trastuzumab, which binds the *HER2/neu* receptor necessary for tumorigenesis, are highly effective treatments without the noxious toxicities commonly associated with cancer treatment, such as alopecia, myelosuppression, and nausea and vomiting.

Autologous Stem Cell Support

Over the past decade there has been a great deal of interest in the role of high-dose chemotherapy with autologous stem cell support.[26] This form of therapy is not standard clinical practice at this time. Following a highly enthusiastic initial introduction, recent studies suggest little advantage to this approach over modern chemotherapy. Several randomized clinical trials testing the value of this approach are coming to completion.

Bisphosphonates

The bisphosphonates, a new class of pyrophosphate analog, bind to bone to alter the classic bone resorption-remodeling cycle. Working through mechanisms that have yet to be fully elucidated, the bisphosphonates appear to interfere with the efficacy of osteoclastic resorption and also to have an effect on osteoblasts. First-generation bisphosphonates (etidronate) were plagued by multiple side effects on normal and diseased bone. Newer bisphosphonates, however, have greater potency with a lower side effect profile. The most widely studied bisphosphonate for breast cancer is pamidronate. A randomized, double-blind study of pamidronate[27] showed that skeletal events (fracture, need for radiation or surgery) could be significantly reduced in patients with lytic bone metastases from breast cancer who were undergoing concurrent treatment with hormone therapy. There was less bone pain and less need for analgesics in the pamidronate-treated group.

Poor bioavailability and gastrointestinal side effects limit the use of oral bisphosphonates. It has been suggested, however, that use of oral clodronate in patients with breast cancer not only decreases the number of skeletal events but also potentially decreases the incidence of new lytic disease.[28] Further studies are needed to clarify the role of bisphosphonates as antitumor drugs and to define the appropriate dosage and duration of treatment. Bisphosphonate therapy, however, should be

strongly considered for patients with symptomatic lytic bone metastases due to breast cancer.

Radiation

The role of radiation in the management of symptomatic metastasis to bone in breast cancer is well established.[29,30] Most symptomatic bone metastases in breast cancer can be palliated by external beam radiation. Radiation delivers the expectation of symptomatic relief. Typical courses of external beam radiation include 25 to 30 Gy fractionated over a period of 2 weeks. Current investigation includes other radiation schedules, including single-fraction radiation, which increases the ease of administration.

Surgery
Preoperative Evaluation

The orthopedic surgeon involved in evaluating and treating the patient with symptomatic bone metastasis from breast cancer should recognize his or her part as a member of a multidisciplinary team. Consideration must be given to use of less invasive methods of control of symptomatic disease, such as improved analgesics, radiation therapy, or bisphosphonates.

Some bone metastasis, however, will not be amenable to other modalities, and surgical stabilization of impending or actual fractures can markedly relieve symptoms and improve quality of life in selected patients. Patients with weightbearing pain refractory to other treatments, large symptomatic lytic defects with significant threat of fracture, or with frank long bone fractures are good candidates for consideration of surgical interventions. Specific regional considerations and implant selection for management are covered in other chapters.

Preoperative assessment of the potential surgical patient with metastatic breast cancer should always include consultation with the treating medical oncologist, who can (1) provide an estimate of longevity, (2) discuss systemic treatment and associated perioperative risks, and (3) orchestrate the patient's associated care and help make the appropriate decisions regarding which modality may be appropriate. Estimated longevity must be such that patients can reap the benefits of stabilization, particularly when weighed against the rigors of the planned perioperative course. In general estimated survival should be at least 6 weeks. Patients with metastatic breast cancer often live years or even decades following diagnosis of metastatic bone disease. Concurrent chemotherapy, whether intravenous or oral, may affect perioperative planning. Treatment with tamoxifen increases a woman's chances of thromboembolic events, and appropriate perioperative prophylaxis should be considered. On the other hand, systemic therapy with taxanes or many combination chemotherapy regimens can cause neutropenia and thrombocytopenia. Careful timing of surgical procedures when possible can lessen the risk of infection and bleeding associated with acute marrow toxicity from these drugs. Finally, local disease may not be most appropriately controlled with an operation. In the patient with rapidly progressive disease, systemic treatment considerations may override the immediate skeletal considerations when the patient as a whole is evaluated.

Because breast cancer metastasis to bone may involve multiple sites, preoperative orthopedic evaluation should also include some evaluation of long bones other than the presenting symptomatic site. Surgical intervention in the extremities will usually involve altered weightbearing patterns, and if increased loading of other long bones is anticipated postoperatively, preoperative assessment to ensure their structural integrity can avert a postoperative fracture at another site. If the patient has had a recent bone scan, adequate information may be available, otherwise a long-bone survey in appropriate patients should be considered.

Biopsy and Pathology Evaluation

Patients with a history of breast cancer with no histologic documentation of metastasis who present with a bone lesion and who are approached surgically should have the goal of tissue diagnosis added to the goal of surgical stabilization. Particularly for the older patient with a history of noninvasive breast cancer, the possibility of a second cancer should be carefully entertained.

At the time of operation, coordination with both the medical oncologist and the pathologist can ensure optimal and cost-effective care. Surgical intervention for stabilization sometimes offers an important opportunity for the oncologist to attain information helpful to directing the patient's systemic treatment regimens. With the increasing numbers of tests available on breast cancer tissue, those that may be helpful to the medical oncologist in prescribing future care should be ordered first. Tests such as estrogen and progesterone receptors can help assess the likelihood of hormonal treatment responsiveness, and the presence of the *HER2/neu* antigen may be helpful in assessing the possible efficacy of Herceptin.

CONCLUSION

Breast cancer is one of the most common causes of musculoskeletal metastatic disease. Many of the patients survive for years with known skeletal metastases. Chemotherapy, hormonal therapy, and osteoclast inhibitors all play a role in the treatment of these patients. The lesions also usually respond well to radiation. Surgery usually is reserved for pathologic fractures and large lytic bone lesions. The length of survival continues to increase for patients with metastatic breast cancer. With continued advances in the management of the skeletal metastatic disease, many patients are able to lead active and rewarding lives.

REFERENCES

1. Slamon DJ, Godolphin W, Jones LA, Holt JA, Wong SG, Keith DE, Levin WJ, Stuart SG, Udove J, Ullrich A, et al. Studies of the HER-2/neu proto-oncogene in human breast and ovarian cancer. Science 244(4905):707-712, 1989.
2. Miki Y, Swensen J, Shattuck-Eidens D, Futreal A, Harshman K, Tavtigian S, Liu Q, Cochran C, Bennett M, Ding W, Bell R, Rosenthal J, Hussey C, Tran T, McClure M, Frye C, Hattier T, Phelps R, Haugen-Strano A, Katcher H, Yakumo K, Gholami Z, Shaffer D, Stone S, Bayer S, Wray C, Bogden R, Dayananth P, Ward J, Tonin P, Narod S, Bristow P, Norris F, Helvering L, Morrison P, Rosteck P, Lai M, Barrett J, Lewis C, Neuhausen S, Cannon-Albright L, Goldgar D, Wiseman R, Kamb A, Skolnick M. A strong candidate for the breast and ovarian cancer susceptibility gene *BRCA-1*. Science 266:66-71, 1994.
3. Marcus JN, Watson P, Page DL, Narod SA, Lenoir GM, Tonin P, Linder-Stephenson L, Salerno G, Conway TA, Lynch HT. Hereditary breast cancer: Pathobiology, prognosis, and *BRCA1* and *BRCA2* gene linkage. Cancer 77:697-709, 1996.
4. Holmes MD, Hunter DJ, Colditz GA, Stampfer MJ, Hankinson SE, Speizer FE, Rosner B, Willett WC. Association of dietary intake of fat and fatty acids with risk of breast cancer. JAMA 281:914-920, 1999.
5. Buell P. Changing incidence of breast cancer in Japanese-American women. J Natl Cancer Inst 51:1479-1483, 1973.
6. Kulldorff M, Feuer EJ, Miller BA, Freedman LS. Breast cancer clusters in the northeast United States: A geographic analysis. Am J Epidemiol 146(2):161-170, 1997.
7. Lewis-Michl EL, Melius JM, Kallenbach LR, Ju CL, Talbot TO, Orr MF, Lauridsen PE. Breast cancer risk and residence near

industry or traffic in Nassau and Suffolk Counties, Long Island, New York. Arch Environ Health 51(4):255-265, 1996.

8. Stellman SD, Djordjevic MV, Muscat JE, Gong L, Bernstein D, Citron ML, White A, Kemeny M, Busch E, Nafziger AN. Relative abundance of organochlorine pesticides and polychlorinated biphenyls in adipose tissue and serum of women in Long Island, New York. Cancer Epidemiol Biomarkers Prev 7:489-496, 1998.

9. Gilbert F, Dabney MK, Diemer K, Ludwig S, Rosenthal G, Osborne MP. *BRCA1/BRCA2* mutations and breast cancer in Ashkenazi Jewish women. Ann NY Acad Sci 833:198-203, 1997.

10. Dickson RB, Lippman ME, Harris JR, Morrow M, Norton L. Cancer of the breast. In Devita VT, Hellman S, Rosenberg SA, eds. Cancer, Principles and Practice of Oncology, 5th ed. Philadelphia: Lippincott-Raven, 1997, pp 1541-1616.

11. Gail MH, Brinton LA, Byar DP, Corle DK, Green SB, Schairer C, Mulvihill JJ. Projecting individualized probabilities of developing breast cancer for white females who are being examined annually. J Natl Cancer Inst 81:1879-1886, 1989.

12. Singletary SE, Bevers T, Dempsey P, Farrar B, Garber J, Harris R, Helvie M, Jacobs M, Pass H, Smith MLP, Tarantolo S, Venta L. NCCN practice guidelines: Screening for and evaluation of suspicious breast lesions. Oncology 12(11A):89-141, 1998.

13. Fisher B, Costantino JP, Wickerham DL, Redmond CK, Kavanah M, Cronin WM, Vogel V, Robidoux A, Dimitrov N, Atkins J, Daly M, Wieand S, Tan-Chiu E, Ford L, Wolmark N, and other National Surgical Adjuvant Breast and Bowel Project investigators. Tamoxifen for the prevention of breast cancer: Report of the National Surgical Adjuvant Breast and Bowel Project P-1 study. J Natl Cancer Inst 90:1371-1388, 1998.

14. Jordan C, Glusman JE, Eckert S, Lippman M, Powles T, Costa A, Morrow M, Norton L. Incident primary breast cancers are reduced by raloxifene: Integrated data from multicenter, double-blind, randomized trials in ~12,000 postmenopausal women. Proc Am Soc Clin Oncol 17:122A, 1998.

15. Delmas PD, Bjarnason NH, Mitlak BH, Ravoux AC, Shah AS, Huster WJ, Draper M, Christiansen C. The effects of raloxifene on bone mineral density, serum cholesterol, and uterine endometrium. N Engl J Med 337:1641-1647, 1997.

16. Powles T, Eeles R, Ashley S, Easton D, Change J, Dowsett M, Tidy A, Viggers J, Davey J. Interim analysis of the incidence of breast cancer in the Royal Marsden Hospital Tamoxifen Randomised Chemoprevention Trial. Lancet 352:98-101, 1998.

17. Veronesi U, Maisonneuve P, Costa A, Sacchini V, Maltoni C, Robertson C, Rotmensz N, Boyle P, on behalf of the Italian Tamoxifen Prevention Study. Prevention of breast cancer with tamoxifen: Preliminary findings from the Italian randomised trial among hysterectomized women. Lancet 352: 93-97, 1998.

18. Krag D, Weaver D, Ashikaga T, Moffat F, Klimberg VS, Shriver C, Feldman S, Kusminsky R, Gadd M, Kuhn J, Harlow S, Beitsch P. The sentinel node in breast cancer—a multicenter validation study. N Engl J Med 339:941-946, 1998.

19. McMasters KM, Giuliano AE, Ross MI, Reintgen DS, Hunt KK, Byrd DR, Klimberg VS, Whitworth PW, Tafra LC, Edwards MJ. Sentinel-lymph-node biopsy for breast cancer—not yet the standard of care. N Engl J Med 339:990-995, 1998.

20. Recommended breast cancer surveillance guidelines. American Society of Clinical Oncology. J Clin Oncol 15:2149-2156, 1997.

21. Parazzini F, Colli E, Scatigna M, Tozzi L. Treatment with tamoxifen and progestins for metastatic breast cancer in postmenopausal women: A quantitative review of published randomized clinical trials. Oncology 50:483-489, 1993.

22. Update: NCCN practice guidelines for the treatment of breast cancer. Oncology 13(5A):41-66, 1999.

23. Goss PE, Gwyn KM. Current perspectives on aromatase inhibitors in breast cancer. J Clin Oncol 12:2460-2470, 1994.

24. Cobleigh M, Vogel CL, Tripathy D, Robert NJ, Scholl S, Fehrenbacher L, Paton V, Shak S, Lieberman G, Slamon D. Efficacy and safety of Herceptin (humanized anti-HER2 antibody) as a single agent in 222 women with HER2 overexpression who relapsed following chemotherapy for metastatic breast cancer. Proc Am Soc Clin Oncol 17:97A, 1998.

25. Slamon D, Leyland-Jones B, Shak S, Paton V, Bajamonde A, Fleming T, Eiermann W, Wolter J, Baselga J, Norton L. Addition of Herceptin (humanized anti-HER2 antibody) to first line chemotherapy for HER2 overexpressing metastatic breast cancer (HER2+/MBC) markedly increases anticancer activity: A randomized, multinational controlled phase III trial. Proc Am Soc Clin Oncol 17:98A, 1998.

26. Eddy DM. High-dose chemotherapy with autologous bone marrow transplantation for the treatment of metastatic breast cancer. J Clin Oncol 10:657-670, 1992.

27. Theriault RL, Lipton A, Hortobagyi GN, Leff R, Gluck S, Stewart JF, Costello S, Kennedy I, Simeone J, Seaman JJ, Knight RD, Mellars K, Heffernan M, Reitsma DJ. From the Protocol 18 Aredia Breast Cancer Study Group. Pamidronate reduces skeletal morbidity in women with advanced breast cancer and lytic bone lesions: A randomized, placebo-controlled trial. J Clin Oncol 17(3):846-854, 1999.

28. Diel IJ, Solomayer EF, Costa SD, Gollan C, Goerner R, Wallwiener D, Kaufmann M, Bastert G. Reduction in new metastases in breast cancer with adjuvant clodronate treatment. N Engl J Med 339:357-363, 1998.

29. Tong D, Gillick L, Hendrickson FR. The palliation of symptomatic osseous metastases: Final results of the radiation therapy oncology group. Cancer 50:893-899, 1982.

30. Blitzer PH. Reanalysis of the RTOG study of the palliation of symptomatic osseous metastasis. Cancer 55:1468-1472, 1985.

Endocrine Cancer

Michael A. Samuels, M.D., *and Timothy J. Kinsella,* M.D.

Endocrine cancers comprise a diverse group of tumors. Endocrine tumors originate in tissues that secrete hormones, the chemical substances that travel via the bloodstream to alter the function of target tissues elsewhere in the body. These tumors include those that originate in the thyroid, parathyroid, and pituitary glands as well as in the islet cells of the pancreas (gastrinoma), the adrenal medulla (pheochromocytoma), the adrenal cortex, and the gastrointestinal tract or other locations (carcinoid tumors).

The tumors in these groups are not uniform in their ability to cause paraneoplastic syndromes. Such activity is the hallmark of the pancreatic islet cell tumors, pheochromocytomas, parathyroid carcinomas, and carcinoid tumors. The others generally are hormonally silent.

The focus of this chapter concerns the potential for and treatment of endocrine tumors metastatic to bone. With the exception of thyroid carcinomas, these malignant tumors are not widely recognized for their propensity to metastasize to bone. The world literature regarding the management of thyroid bone metastases with surgery and radioactive iodine is plentiful; otherwise, the literature on endocrine bone metastases is relatively sparse, consisting mainly of case reports and small retrospective patient series from single institutions. We have used this chapter to consolidate this literature so the clinician can draw appropriate conclusions concerning the evaluation and treatment of the patient with endocrine bone metastases. Where possible, the chapter delineates the relative roles of therapeutic modalities, including surgery, radiation therapy, chemotherapy, radioactive isotope therapy, and noncytotoxic pharmacologic therapy.

Thyroid Carcinoma

DIFFERENTIATED THYROID CARCINOMA

Cancer of the thyroid gland accounts for 90% of all endocrine malignant tumors,[1] with an estimated incidence of 17,200 cases in the United States in 1998. There is a female-to-male predominance of almost 3 to 1.[2] Pathologic subtypes include papillary, mixed papillary-follicular, follicular, Hürthle cell, medullary, and anaplastic tumors. As a group,

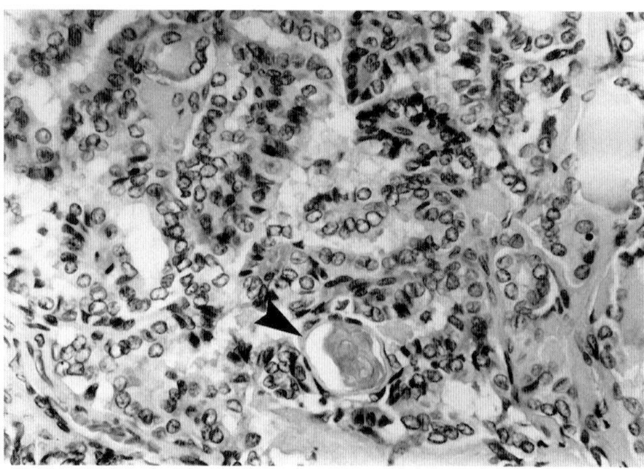

Fig. 15-1   Papillary thyroid carcinoma. Note the papillary configuration of tumor cells, optically clear-appearing nuclei, nuclear grooving, and psammoma body *(arrow)*.

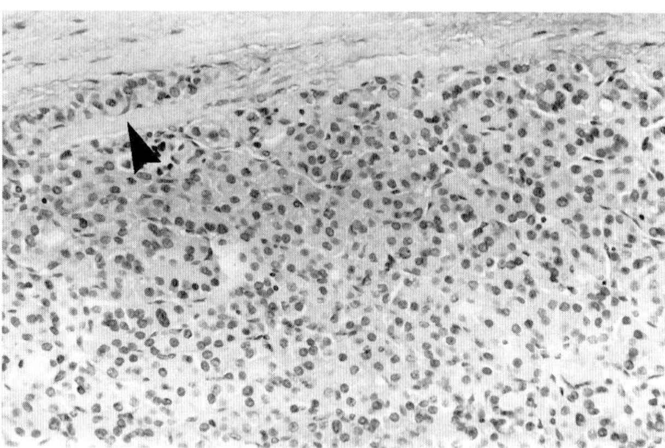

Fig. 15-2   Follicular thyroid carcinoma. Note the crowding of follicles, hypercellularity, and capsular invasion *(arrow)*.

thyroid cancers are especially relevant to this text because they comprise one of the five most common tumors to metastasize to bone.[3]

Although their clinical behavior differs, papillary (Fig. 15-1), follicular (Fig. 15-2) and Hürthle cell types are often grouped as differentiated thyroid cancer (DTC).

Incidence and Patterns of Spread

DTCs comprise the majority of cases overall, and bone metastases are rarely seen. In a series of 600 patients operated on for DTC in France, Proye et al.[4] found bone disease in 28 (4.7%). Bone metastases were detected in 1.3% of patients with papillary carcinoma and 7% of patients with follicular carcinoma. Of the overall group, 19 of 28 were diagnosed at the outset, and 9 of 28 relapsed in bony sites with an average lag time of 4.5 years after surgery. Fifteen of the nineteen patients who had bone involvement at diagnosis presented with bone pain as their chief complaint. Seventy-five percent of the patients with bone metastases had multiple lesions. The lesions tended to affect the axial skeleton, with sites as follows: vertebra 29%, pelvis 22%, ribs 21%, femur 15%, and skull 13%. Almost half had other synchronous or metachronous metastatic disease, especially lung involvement.

Ruegemer et al.[5] described a cohort of 988 patients with DTC who underwent primary surgical management at the Mayo Clinic from 1946 to 1970. The distribution of pathologic subtypes included 859 (87%) with papillary histologic features, 100 (10%) with follicular tumors, and 29 (3%) with Hürthle cell (a variant of follicular) tumors. Of this overall group, 85 (9%) had diagnoses of distant metastases during life. By subtype, metastases were seen in 7% of those with papillary disease, 19% of those with follicular disease, and 34% of those with Hürthle cell tumors. At the time of diagnosis of the first metastasis, the lungs only were involved in 53%, the bones only in 20%, and multiple organs in 16%. Overall mortality rates 5 and 10 years after the diagnosis of metastases were 65% and 75%, respectively. Age at the time of first diagnosis of metastatic disease and multiple organ involvement were the only significant factors associated with cancer death.

An Israeli series by Zohar and Strauss,[6] in contrast to the Proye study, focused on occult distant metastases in DTC. After total thyroidectomy in 187 patients with DTC, total-body ^{131}I scanning revealed 11 patients (5.9%) with occult metastases. As expected, organs involved were bone, lung, or both. Seven patients had papillary disease, and four had follicular disease. Pathologic factors associated with these cases included multicentric disease within the thyroid, total involvement of the gland, and extracapsular extension of tumor. Seven of the eleven patients (64%) died during the first 3 years after resection.

Using the same Mayo Clinic data set as Ruege-mer, Hay and colleagues[3] noted that the median time from diagnosis of thyroid cancer to skeletal spread was 2 years, although in two patients with papillary disease, bone metastases were diagnosed 21 and 26 years after their initial diagnoses. Despite these statistical outliers, 95% of the patients with skeletal spread died of their thyroid cancer.

Yamashita et al.[7] compared 50 patients with metastatic papillary carcinoma and 50 patients with localized disease. Multivariate analysis showed only extranodal extension of tumor to be a significant prognostic indicator of distant metastases ($P = 0.0045$). The odds ratio of extranodal invasion in distant metastasis was 9. The risk of death in the group with extranodal involvement was higher than for those patients without this feature ($P < 0.01$).

Two available series have examined the risk of distant metastases, including bone involvement, in small carcinomas of the thyroid. Rosen et al. from Toronto examined a group of 99 patients with tumors <15 mm in diameter, and found two with bone metastases.[8] Noguchi et al. from Japan assembled a series of 867 patients with carcinomas <10 mm who were treated surgically. With a mean follow-up of 2 years, two patients experienced relapse in bone.[9] The risk of metastases in small carcinomas, therefore, appears to be lower than in larger tumors.

Evaluation
Imaging

Many authors have described whole-body imaging for metastases in DTC, using ^{131}I as part of a combined diagnostic and therapeutic strategy. As suggested by Leger,[10] patients first undergo total thyroidectomy. An ablative dose of 3.7 GBq (100 mCi) is then administered to eradicate postoperative thyroid remnants. An imaging dose of 0.2 to 0.4 GBq (5.4 to 10.8 mCi) is then used to localize distant metastases, including bone disease. If metastases are found, a second treatment dose of 3.7 to 7.4 GBq (100 to 200 mCi) is administered in an attempt to eradicate the metastases.

Tenenbaum and colleagues[11] noted the difficulty of using the technique described to provide precise localization of DTC bone metastases, especially in the thorax. To improve upon it, they performed a study that added technetium 99m hydroxymethylene diphosphonate (^{99m}Tc-HMDP) scanning to ^{131}I scanning. They divided patients into two groups. Group 1 consisted of 15 patients with known DTC bone metastases. They were treated with 3.7 GBq (100 mCi) ^{131}I. They were dosed 4 to 5 days later with 740 MBq (20 mCi) ^{99m}Tc-HMDP. Whole-body scans with simultaneous acquisition of iodine and technetium images were obtained with a large-field-of-view camera fitted with a high-energy collimator. Technetium uptake was abnormal in 47 of 63 localizations. The superimposition of the techniques permitted an accurate localization in 80% of the spinal metastases and 46% of osseous thoracic localizations, even in the presence of lung metastases, which can be a confounding factor. In group 2, nine patients with bone pain, neurologic signs, or elevated serum thyroglobulin were known to have DTC bone metastases without iodine uptake. Technetium uptake was positive in 37 of 38 localizations, with 1 false negative area. The authors concluded that ^{99m}Tc-HMDP scanning was useful in both groups.

In a study from Japan, Kobayashi et al.[12] undertook an even more highly controlled examination of the role of technetium scanning in DTC after total thyroidectomy. In their study, the Tc compound used was ^{99m}Tc-methoxyisobutylisonitrile (MIBI). Twenty-seven patients with thyroid carcinoma were evaluated (23 patients with papillary adenocarcinoma, 3 with follicular disease, and 1 unknown). All cases were confirmed by surgery. Twenty-four patients then underwent ^{131}I therapy with 4.5 to 5.5 GBq (122 to 149 mCi) administered. Whole-body scintigrams were obtained 7 to 10 days later. Thirty minutes after an injection of ^{99m}Tc-MIBI (740 MBq or 20 mCi), single-photon emission computed tomography (SPECT) imaging was performed with a three-head gamma camera. Abnormal accumulation of ^{99m}Tc-MIBI was noted in 14 patients, with all lesions confirmed on computed tomography (CT) or magnetic resonance imaging (MRI). In 11 of the 13 patients with negative Tc scans, anatomic imaging was also negative. In patients with follicular disease, strong accumulation of both technetium and iodine was seen. In papillary metastases showing substantial uptake of technetium, iodine uptake was also present. The authors concluded that ^{99m}Tc-MIBI SPECT imaging is more sensitive than anatomic imaging for soft tissue metastases of DTC.

Finally, Miyamoto and colleagues[13] compared nuclear imaging techniques of metastatic DTC lesions in 27 patients. Twelve patients had known bone metastases. Agents used included ^{99m}Tc-MIBI, ^{201}Tl, and ^{131}I. Technetium detected 93.5% of the bone metastases, whereas thallium detected 90.3% and iodine detected 85.1%. Although the results were relatively comparable with each agent, the authors preferred the image quality with technetium and suggested it for the postoperative follow-up of patients with thyroid cancer.[13]

Proye et al.[4] note in their article that all the bone metastases in their series that were visible on plain film (25 of 28 patients) appeared as osteolytic lesions. Hay et al.[3] echoed this finding, adding that varying degrees of internal septation are seen in the lesions, which are usually round or ovoid. Often there is bone expansion with cortical thinning, destruction, or breakthrough with adjacent soft-tissue extension. With therapy and healing, however, these lesions often show evidence of remineralization and become sclerotic in appearance.

Serum Markers in Metastatic Disease to Bone

The normal serum thyroglobulin level ranges from 1 to 43 ng/ml. Transient elevations of thyroglobulin levels may occur after procedures that include fine-needle aspiration of the thyroid, surgery or irradiation of the gland, and administration of thyrotropin-releasing hormone (TRH) or thyroid-stimulating hormone (TSH). The thyroglobulin level decreases on administration of thyroid hormone. The presence of antithyroglobulin antibodies may cause a false elevation or decrease of serum thyroglobulin levels. High levels of thyroglobulin may be seen in benign thyroid diseases, such as Graves' disease, thyroiditis, and multinodular goiter. These confounding factors prevent measurement of serum thyroglobulin from being a useful tool in the initial diagnosis of thyroid carcinoma.[14]

The serum thyroglobulin level may be used as an indicator of the risk of occult metastatic disease in DTC or as a clue to the organ of origin of known metastases. Edmonds and Willis[15] from Middlesex, England, measured serum thyroglobulin levels in 40 patients with metastatic thyroid carcinoma. Eighteen of this group had levels greater than 400 µg/L. The authors used the marker as a screening tool in 128 patients with newly diagnosed DTC. In five patients with metastases, elevated thyroglobulin levels pointed to a thyroid origin for the metastases rather than a concurrent primary tumor.[15]

In a case report, Girelli et al.[16] discussed a patient in whom follicular carcinoma was treated with surgery and radioactive iodine, followed by hormone suppression. Serial serum thyroglobulin measurements showed a stable level of less than 1 ng/ml. Twelve years after surgery, thyroglobulin levels increased over an 18-month period to 149 ng/ml. CT detected an isolated adrenal metastasis. Adrenalectomy was performed, and pathologic study showed follicular disease with Hürthle cells. Follow-up serum measurements demonstrated a decrease in thyroglobulin levels to 0.9 ng/ml. This report points to the potential role of this serum marker in the monitoring of DTC patients.

In general, the most important role for measurement of serum thyroglobulin levels is to complement nuclear scanning as a method of detecting recurrent and metastatic disease in patients after thyroidectomy and radioiodine ablation of residual thyroid tissue, even in the presence of thyroid hormone suppression.

Fine-Needle Aspiration Biopsy of Potential Thyroid Bone Metastases

Some patients will present with bone metastases from an unknown primary tumor. Fine-needle aspiration biopsy (FNAB) of the bone may be used to make a definitive diagnosis and to select treatment. Dhimes and colleagues[17] described the typical cytologic findings in bone metastatic follicular carcinoma of tumor cell clusters in a follicular pattern with peripherally situated, pink-stained vacuoles on May-Grünwald-Giemsa stain. They pointed to the peripheral vacuoles as the significant morphologic finding indicating a thyroid origin for the metastatic tissue.

Flow Cytometric DNA Analysis of Thyroid Metastases

Several investigators have examined both primary and metastatic thyroid carcinoma tissues by flow cytometric DNA analysis and have correlated these findings with survival data.

Joensuu et al.[18] examined cellular DNA content from paraffin-embedded tissue blocks from thyroidectomy specimens in 125 patients. Aneuploidy

was seen in only 24% of the papillary carcinoma cases but in 56% of the follicular and 57% of the medullary cases. Aneuploidy was more common in elderly patients, in cases with moderately or poorly differentiated tumors, and in cases with tumor penetration through the thyroid capsule. All factors reached statistical significance. Patients with aneuploid tumors had a significantly inferior rate of survival than those with diploid tumors (P <0.0001). The authors conclude that the increasing incidence of aneuploidy in elderly patients may explain their generally poorer prognosis as compared with younger patients.

Using flow cytometric techniques, Hrafnkelsson and colleagues[19] from Iceland examined paraffin-embedded thyroidectomy specimens from 150 patients with papillary carcinomas. Their results were consistent with those of Joensuu et al. in that aneuploidy was seen more frequently in elderly patients and in non-well-differentiated tumors. They also found aneuploidy to be associated with male sex and tumors with high S-phase fractions.

A study of follicular neoplasms in men older than 50 years was undertaken by Hruban et al.[20] from Memorial Sloan-Kettering Cancer Center. DNA analysis of paraffin-embedded primary thyroidectomy and resected metastatic tissues showed a higher rate of aneuploidy or tetraploidy in metastases (50%) compared with a rate of 27% in the thyroidectomy specimens of patients without metastases.

A Japanese case report by Komatsu and colleagues[21] takes this analysis to a higher level of complexity. The investigators obtained specimens from the primary tumor and each metastatic site in a 56-year-old woman with papillary thyroid carcinoma involving lymph nodes, lungs, and sternal bone. The primary tumor contained populations of diploid cells and aneuploid cells with a DNA index of 1.3. The lymph node foci contained only the diploid populations, but the lung and bone metastases contained both the diploid and aneuploid populations.

An interesting study of patients with radiation-associated DTC was performed by Komorowski et al.[22] from Wisconsin. DNA analysis of thyroidectomy specimens from 16 patients with DTC and a prior history of low-dose head or neck irradiation was obtained and compared with results from 37 DTC patients with no history of prior irradiation.

The proportions of papillary, follicular and medullary cancers in each group were similar. None of the 16 radiation-associated tumors was aneuploid, whereas 10 of the 37 specimens without a history of irradiation were aneuploid. Since the authors' original hypothesis was that irradiation caused thyroid cancer by inducing chromosomal aberrations, the results were unexpected. Of course, more subtle DNA changes undetectable by flow cytometry may have been present in the radiation-associated specimens. It is also important to note that the incidence of radiation-associated DTC is decreasing in the United States because radiation has not been used to treat benign childhood diseases for about 40 years.[23]

Overall, it seems reasonable to conclude from the flow cytometry literature that aneuploidy is associated with aggressive malignant behavior in DTC and is an independent risk factor for decreased survival. Primary thyroid tumors that metastasize to bone are more likely to contain aneuploid populations than tumors that do not metastasize to organs other than lymph nodes. In a single patient with bone metastases, the bone lesions are likely to contain aneuploid cells if they were present in the primary tumor.

Treatment
Radioiodine

Schlumberger and colleagues from the Institut Gustave-Roussy[24] describe the techniques involved in ^{131}I therapy for metastatic DTC. They recommend a dose of 100 to 150 mCi in adults and of 1 mCi per kilogram of body weight in children. To provide TSH stimulation, levothyroxine therapy is discontinued for 3 weeks and patients are given T_3 for that time. The latter is then withdrawn for 14 days. TSH levels are measured, and if they are high enough, the treatment dose of radioiodine is administered. A posttreatment scan follows 5 days later. Treatments may be repeated every 3 to 6 months until all areas of uptake resolve. Ninety percent of patients who achieve complete remission do so with a cumulative dose of 600 mCi or less. Patients with nonfunctioning metastases invariably have a poor prognosis.

The efficacy of radioiodine treatment of bone metastases from DTC is controversial. First, there is not a strict correlation between uptake of ^{131}I in a metastatic focus and elimination of pain or radiographic improvement (control of the metastasis). In a study by Mizukami and colleagues[25] from Japan, 32 patients with DTC bone metastases were evaluated with ^{131}I scanning. Bone lesions in 22 patients (69%) showed uptake.

In a series from M.D. Anderson Cancer Center, Wood and colleagues[26] noted a median survival of 49 months in patients who received ^{131}I treatment and of 52 months in those who did not. It is difficult to draw any conclusion from these results, however, because almost all patients received multimodality therapy.

In the series by Proye et al.,[4] bone lesions in only 12 of 28 patients showed radioiodine uptake. Three patients whose metastases showed uptake were treated with radioiodine only. One cure and one partial remission were observed. Nineteen additional patients received combined modality treatment that included [131]I. There were five partial remissions and one cure. In the 16 patients without uptake, no cures were seen unless radioiodine was used. The mean isotope dose was 7000 MBq (189 mCi). When survivals were examined, the authors concluded that ^{131}I, either combined or alone, improves the survival rate of patients, even if they are not cured of bone metastases, until the eleventh year. This conclusion is supported by Lee and Lore,[14] who suggest that ^{131}I should be the initial treatment of all functioning bone metastases, with the initial dose no less than 200 mCi.[14]

Hay et al.[3] point to less positive results in the treatment of thyroid carcinoma bone metastases with radioiodine. They note series showing effective palliation in only one third to one fourth of patients. They also comment that Hürthle cell tumors, although a variant of follicular cancers, rarely take up radioiodine. This limits the usefulness of ^{131}I in the treatment of recurrent or metastatic Hürthle cell disease.

Occasional serious complications have been observed after radioiodine therapy. Sartorelli et al.[27] followed up 94 patients with metastatic DTC after thyroidectomy, ^{131}I ablation of thyroid remnants, and ^{131}I treatment for the metastases. They noted only 6% of the patients with complete and permanent control of their bone disease. Three patients (3%) had severe complications due to radioiodine, including one patient with acute leukemia, one patient with macroscopic hematuria with radiation cystitis, and one patient with bladder cancer. Three additional patients had grade III or IV thrombocytopenia.

External Irradiation

Lee and Lore[14] suggest that radioiodine treatment should be the initial therapy for all functioning metastatic bone lesions, with an initial dose of no less than 200 mCi. External irradiation is used for DTC bone metastases in patients with multiple lesions (which renders surgical resection inappropriate) in whom radioiodine treatment has been ineffective. Total external beam doses of 50 to 60 Gy using conventional fractions are recommended, presumably because DTC is relatively clinically radioresistant, and protracted fractionation schedules should provide prolonged control of pain in these patients with relatively long life expectancies, compared with abbreviated radiotherapy courses. Schlumberger et al.[24] also recommend the use of external irradiation to complement radioiodine and suggest doses of 40 to 45 Gy. Such treatment does not preclude repeat ^{131}I treatment in the future.

Wood et al.[26] and Simpson[28] confirm the efficacy of external beam radiotherapy, usually combined with ^{131}I, in providing long-term palliation of symptoms but do not suggest total doses or fractionation schemes. Hay et al.[3] recommend external radiotherapy in patients with symptomatic lesions or in those with an inadequate response to ^{131}I or a lack of radioiodine uptake. Since the natural history of DTC lesions is long, they suggest high-dose, protracted fractionation courses in those cases. They note that several patients from their institution who were treated in this way remained free of disease for 10 to 15 years before they died of unrelated causes. With anaplastic disease the expected survival is short, and Hay et al. recommend administering lower total doses in 5 to 10 fractions in 1 to 2 weeks. Significant relief of pain is seen in about 80% of patients, and plain film evidence of bone healing is seen in more than 90% of patients.

Surgical Resection

Roher and colleagues[29] from Düsseldorf discuss the rationale for surgical resection of DTC bone metastases. In their center, 78% of primary bone metastases were treated operatively, a very high proportion. They note high survival rates of 33% to 60% at 5 years in these patients, making it important to control symptoms and prevent pathologic fractures over long periods of time. They claim that surgical treatment of DTC bone metastases improves quality of life in these patients, regardless of any influence on survival. Iwamoto et al.[30] from Kyushu University support this concept, comparing the long-term survival seen in these patients with that seen in women with bone metastases from breast carcinoma and describing aggressive surgical resection in both patient groups, especially for lesions involving the spine and long bones.

Hay and colleagues[3] from the Mayo Clinic describe specific indications for surgical resection. First, in any case of unifocal dissemination (solitary bone metastasis), aggressive surgical management is indicated. Surgical resection of bone metastases is an especially relevant concept in thyroid cancer, since of the five most common types of metastatic bone tumor, a unifocal metastatic bone lesion is most common with thyroid cancer. In patients with multifocal bone involvement, surgical considerations encompass both prophylactic and definitive management. Candidates include those with lytic lesions larger than 2.5 cm, destruction of the cortical diameter by 50% or more, or lesions that continue to cause pain after radioiodine therapy. In patients with an established pathologic fracture, open reduction with internal fixation provides pain control and improves mobility.

Embolization of bone metastases is recommended by Schlumberger et al.,[24] particularly for painful vertebral lesions. It may be used in cases of persistent bone pain after external irradiation has proved unhelpful, and it may be repeated.

An interesting case report involving an alternative local therapy is presented by Nakada et al.[31] from Sapporo. They describe a 62-year-old woman with metastatic papillary disease involving the sternum, for whom palliative radioiodine and external radiation treatment had proved ineffective in reducing pain. The lesion was treated with percutaneous ethanol injection therapy (PEIT) four times, twice with ultrasound guidance and twice with CT guidance. The pain completely disappeared. A posttreatment CT scan and radioisotope imaging showed a significant decrease in the tumor volume.

The serum thyroglobulin level fell to one twentieth of the pretreatment level. The authors suggest that PEIT is a valuable technique for the treatment of thyroid carcinoma bone metastases that are refractory to radioiodine.

Chemotherapy

The use of chemotherapy to treat DTC bone metastases is rarely discussed in the literature. Wood et al.[26] note that this modality was reserved until all other forms of therapy had failed to halt progression of metastatic growth. No complete response was seen with any single agent or combination regimen. This finding is in contrast to the clear efficacy of certain chemotherapy regimens in anaplastic disease, which will be discussed later.

Lee and Lore[14] recommend consideration of a number of chemotherapeutic agents, including doxorubicin, bleomycin, and cisplatin in "selected patients" with advanced disease. Schlumberger et al.[24] note a less than 20% response rate for doxorubicin, which they consider the most active agent available.

MEDULLARY THYROID CARCINOMA

Medullary thyroid cancer (MTC) arises from the parafollicular or "C cell" and has features unlike those of DTC (Fig. 15-3). It represents 4% to 10% of all thyroid carcinoma cases[14] and is characterized by the production of calcitonin, which is present at elevated levels in patients with active disease and may be used as a tumor marker.

Medullary disease may be sporadic (80% to 90% of cases)[14] or associated with multiple endocrine neoplasia (MEN) syndrome type IIA or IIB. Patients with sporadic or type IIB–associated disease appear to have a poorer prognosis than patients with type IIA–associated disease.[32]

A retrospective study of 202 patients treated for MTC at M.D. Anderson Cancer Center from 1943 to 1987 was undertaken by Samaan and colleagues.[33] They compared prognosis in MEN II cases as compared with sporadic cases. Although patients with familial disease survived longer than those with sporadic disease, this difference disappeared once adjustments were made for the older age and more advanced tumors seen in the sporadic group. They also conclude that radiotherapy is ineffective in MTC on the basis of the inability of

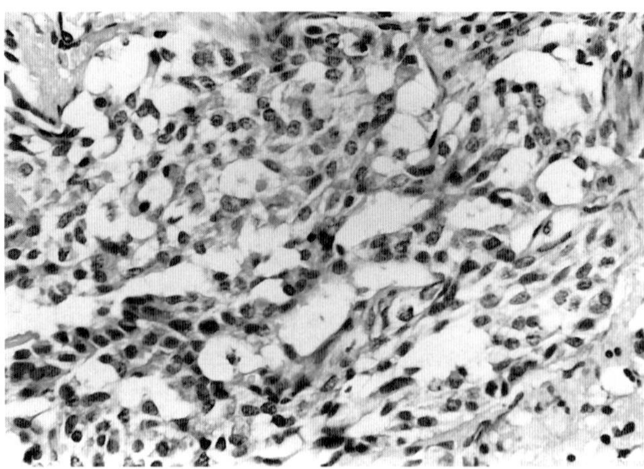

Fig. 15-3   Medullary thyroid carcinoma. This high-power view demonstrates finely dispersed nuclear chromatin. A nesting growth pattern and amyloid deposition (not shown) are characteristic of MTC.

postoperative external radiation treatment to the primary tumor bed to improve survival. The authors note that patients with bone metastases often have elevated carcinoembryonic antigen (CEA) levels.

Bone metastases in MTC may be either osteolytic or osteoblastic on plain radiographs. Ahuja and Ernst[34] reported a case of a 32-year-old man who had extensive metastases at the time of diagnosis. The bone metastases had an osteoblastic appearance, which the authors assume was due to biologically active tumor calcitonin. The patient died 15 years after the diagnosis of the advanced tumor. The authors speculate that the long survival time may indicate that the prognosis is better for osteoblastic than for osteolytic metastases.

Hay et al.[3] note that bone metastases from MTC are often slow growing and that sometimes surgical resection is indicated for these lesions.

The only available study that specifically examines the role of radiotherapy in bone metastases from MTC was presented by Sarrazin and colleagues[35] from Paris. The investigators used external irradiation to treat 10 patients with bone metastases. A dose of 30 Gy in 10 fractions was delivered with a cobalt 60 treatment unit. All 10 patients experienced relief of bone pain. Median survival in this group was 18 months.

Despite doubts concerning the radiosensitivity of MTC, external radiotherapy remains the palliative treatment of choice for bone metastases in this disease.

ANAPLASTIC THYROID CARCINOMA

Anaplastic (or undifferentiated) thyroid cancer (Fig. 15-4) is a highly malignant neoplasm that affects mainly elderly patients, with a female-to-male ratio of 2:1. It is one of the most aggressive neoplasms affecting human beings.[36] It spreads rapidly to regional lymph nodes and causes distant metastases, especially to lung and bone.[37] Local recurrence in a matter of weeks after resection of neck disease is often seen. The only treatment to demonstrate significant effectiveness has been a multimodality approach consisting of multiagent chemotherapy with aggressive radiotherapy. The most influential study in this area was reported by Kim and Leeper[38] from Memorial Sloan-Kettering Cancer Center. The authors treated 19 patients with anaplastic disease with twice daily external radiotherapy to a total dose of 57.6 Gy and weekly doxorubicin chemotherapy at a dose of 10 mg/m^2. Complete responses were seen in 84% of the patients. Long-term local control was achieved in 68% of the patients. Median survival was 1 year. Progression of distant disease was seen in all three patients with distant metastases, however. The authors conclude that chemotherapy alone has little effect in anaplastic disease.

In the series reported by Hay et al.[3] from the Mayo Clinic, 93 of 1142 patients with thyroid cancer had anaplastic histologic features. Despite the aggressive behavior of these tumors and the fact that pulmonary metastases developed in 30%, only 5% of the patients had bone metastases. The authors suggest that this was due to the extremely short survival of these patients, who did not live long enough to experience tumor spread to bone.

There is little evidence in the literature concerning the efficacy of palliative radiotherapy in metastatic anaplastic bone disease. This may be due to the extremely short survivals seen in most series and the predominance of death due to locally progressive disease in the neck. In a series of 37 patients with anaplastic tumors, Kobayashi and colleagues[39] from Osaka noted no neck recurrences in patients who received twice daily radiotherapy but a 50% rate of local recurrence in patients who underwent daily radiotherapy, despite complete surgi-

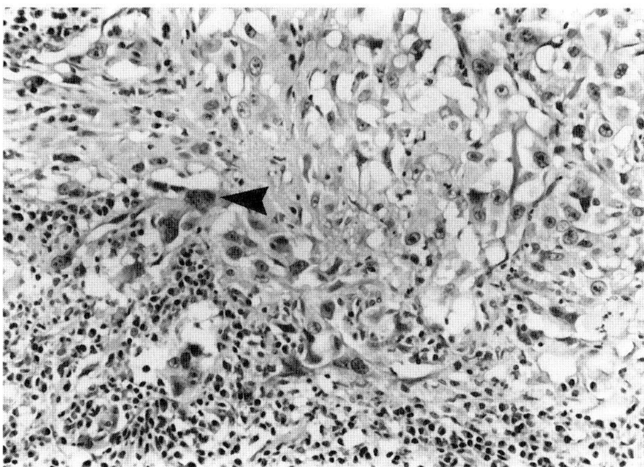

Fig. 15-4   Anaplastic thyroid carcinoma. Note the predominance of epithelioid cells showing bizarre, pleomorphic nuclei *(arrow)* and prominent nucleoli.

cal resections in the latter group. On the basis of this data and data from other series, the authors contend that hyperfractionated radiotherapy is a prerequisite for adequate control of anaplastic disease. Although there is no published experience to support this, it might be appropriate to treat anaplastic bone metastases with twice daily techniques as well.

Parathyroid Carcinoma

Parathyroid carcinoma is rare, affecting approximately 2.3% of all patients with hyperparathyroidism.[40] The median age at diagnosis is 45 years,[41] with a female-to-male ratio of nearly 1:1. Clinical features of the disease include a palpable neck mass and findings of severe hyperparathyroidism, including hypercalcemia, nephrolithiasis, renal failure, bone abnormalities, peptic ulcer symptoms, and pancreatitis. Recurrent laryngeal nerve palsy is sometimes seen, and this finding in combination with hyperparathyroidism should raise the suspicion of parathyroid carcinoma.[42] The serum calcium level averages about 15.[40,43,44] Parathormone levels average five times normal.[44]

Primary treatment of parathyroid carcinoma involves en bloc surgical resection of the primary tumor mass and adjacent thyroid lobe. In a review of 70 cases, Schantz and Castleman[43] noted 18 cases (30%) with regional or distant metastases. Of the 70 cases, 5 (7%) showed spread to bone. Other sites of distant spread included lung and liver. Five- and ten-year survival rates in a series of 62 cases reviewed by Shane and Bilezikian[44] were less than 50% and 35%, respectively.

The radiographic findings of bone changes due to severe hyperparathyroidism are well established and include osteitis fibrosa cystica, subperiosteal bone resorption, diffuse osteoporosis, "salt and pepper" skull, and absence of the lamina dura.[44] However, these findings are unrelated to invasion of bone by parathyroid carcinoma itself. Lytic lesions appearing to be "brown tumors" of parathyroidism may actually harbor metastatic cells, and FNAB as well as surgical resection may be used to make this diagnosis.[45] A case report[46] notes that ^{99m}Tc-MIBI scanning revealed bone metastases when [201]thallium chloride scanning failed. Technetium 99m-sestamibi has been reported to detect bone metastases.[42] Nuclear bone scans may provide false negative results if patients are receiving treatment with bisphosphonates (etidronate or pamidronate) for treatment of hypercalcemia. These compounds must be discontinued, because they compete for bone uptake with the scanning compounds.[47]

DNA analysis by flow cytometry has demonstrated an increased incidence of aneuploidy in metastatic deposits as compared with primary parathyroid tumors.[48] When primary tumors are analyzed, those from patients in whom metastatic disease later developed showed higher rates of aneuploidy than did those from patients whose disease remained localized.[49] S-phase status may also be a useful marker for prognosis in parathyroid carcinoma, with high S-phase measurements indicating rapid tumor proliferation and aggressive behavior.[50]

Virtually all investigators point to surgery as the only consistently effective treatment of distant metastases, including those to bone, in parathyroid carcinoma. Shane and Bilezikian[44] explain that metastatic parathyroid carcinoma has a long natural history. Surgical resection of metastases, although not curative, may lead to clinical improvement for long time periods, and vigorous attempts at resection are therefore indicated. A case report from Japan[51] describing resection of an iliac metastasis recommended CT-guided transcutaneous tumor marking to facilitate localization of bone me-

tastases at surgery. Sandelin and colleagues[47] from Ann Arbor, Michigan, recommend selective venous sampling as the single most informative technique in localizing occult, functioning areas of metastatic disease in order to plan surgical resection.

The literature fails to demonstrate endorsement of the use of external radiotherapy in treating either local or distant disease recurrence, with most investigators calling it "ineffective."[40,41,44,52-54] The only statement pointing to the successful use of radiotherapy comes from Wynne et al.[55] from the Mayo Clinic, who describe a patient who appeared cured of local disease invading the trachea after radiation treatment.

Chemotherapy for parathyroid carcinomas has been investigated most prominently by Bukowski and colleagues[56] at the Cleveland Clinic. They reported a case in which a patient with pulmonary metastases achieved a complete response to treatment with fluorouracil, cyclophosphamide, and dacarbazine. The response lasted 15 months. Calandra et al.[53] present another interesting case report in which a patient had a significant biochemical response to treatment with dacarbazine alone. Overall, though, it is fair to summarize the chemotherapy literature on metastatic parathyroid carcinoma as sparse and preliminary at best.

Malignant Gastrinoma

Gastrinomas (Fig. 15-5) are non-β-islet cell tumors, generally located in the pancreas or duodenum, that secrete gastrin. The clinical syndrome of overproduction of gastric acid leading to peptic ulcer disease, often accompanied by diarrhea, was initially described by Zollinger and Ellison in 1955.[57] Gastrinomas may be sporadic, or they may be associated with MEN I syndrome.

Differentiation between benign and malignant disease rests on demonstration of metastases, most often to the liver. Approximately two thirds of gastrinomas are malignant and have metastasized at diagnosis.[58,59] Although in past decades most patients died of the sequelae of gastric hypersecretion, improved medical control of this problem in the current era has resulted in most patients dying of their metastases. Cure rates of metastatic disease at 5 years do not exceed 30% to 50%.[60]

Metastatic disease most often involves the liver,

abdominal or extra-abdominal lymph nodes, or bone.[60] In approximately 12% of patients with liver metastases, the disease spreads to bone.[61]

Imaging of metastatic gastrinoma includes the use of CT and MRI.[58] Somatostatin receptor scintigraphy has proved useful in the localization of primary tumors for surgical resection as well as in the localization of metastases for surgical, radiation, or chemoembolization therapy.[62] Intraoperative ultrasonography, selective abdominal angiography, selective venous sampling for gastrin from portal venous tributaries, and venous sampling for gastrin after intra-arterial secretin injection are more invasive techniques available to localize gastrinoma metastases in the abdomen.[63]

Although solitary bone metastases may be resected, most patients with bone involvement have multiple lesions. The palliative treatment of choice in these cases is external irradiation. Barton et al.[61] described a series of six such patients. The metastases appeared as both osteolytic and osteoblastic on plain film radiographs. All lesions involved the central skeleton. Most were painful. In two cases, patients had hypercalcemia without elevated parathormone levels. The authors note poor responses to cytotoxic chemotherapy, including streptozocin, 5-fluorouracil, doxorubicin, and dacarbazine. In the four patients who received external radiotherapy, generally 30 Gy, effective relief of pain was seen. Five of six patients died of their disease, with an average survival of 3.3 years from date of diagnosis, compared with a similar cohort of patients with

metastatic gastrinoma without bone metastases, who had an average survival of 7 years. The authors conclude that bone metastases are associated with a poor prognosis in metastatic gastrinoma. Other series and case reports confirm the palliative effectiveness of external irradiation in this situation.[64-66]

The mainstay of therapy for metastatic gastrinoma has been surgical resection of metastases (principally intra-abdominal) and medical treatment with H_2-blocking drugs or omeprezole to reduce acid production. Cytotoxic chemotherapy has been used to slow tumor progression. The principal drugs have been streptozocin and fluorouracil.[67] A prospective study of 21 patients from France,[68] however, failed to confirm the efficacy of this approach. Kim and colleagues[66] from Loyola University examined a retrospective series of 20 patients and noted the best results with dacarbazine, which produced a 50% response. However, these series concentrated on evaluation of tumor mass and gastrin levels, not on reduction of symptoms of bone metastases. Valette and colleagues[69] from Lyon presented a case report of a patient with a large, painful iliac metastasis from gastrinoma, in which treatment with 5-fluorouracil and streptozocin followed by 45 Gy external irradiation and doxorubicin and cisplatin failed. The lesion was treated with arterial infusion of doxorubicin followed by arterial embolization. Two sessions were required. Pain resolved in 2 months, and CT showed a dramatic response. The patient died of widespread metastases 17 months after the last embolization without iliac progression of disease.

Malignant Carcinoid Tumors

Carcinoid tumors (Fig. 15-6) are histologically related to islet cell tumors and most frequently originate in the gastrointestinal tract or bronchus. Carcinoid tumors may originate less frequently in a variety of other sites, as well. Malignant carcinoids are differentiated from benign lesions only by the presence of metastases. Tumors derived from the embryologic foregut (bronchus, stomach, and pancreas) and the hindgut (descending colon and rectum) have a higher propensity to metastasize than those from the midgut (mainly the appendix).[70]

Carcinoid tumors are associated with the "carcinoid syndrome," which includes cutaneous flush-

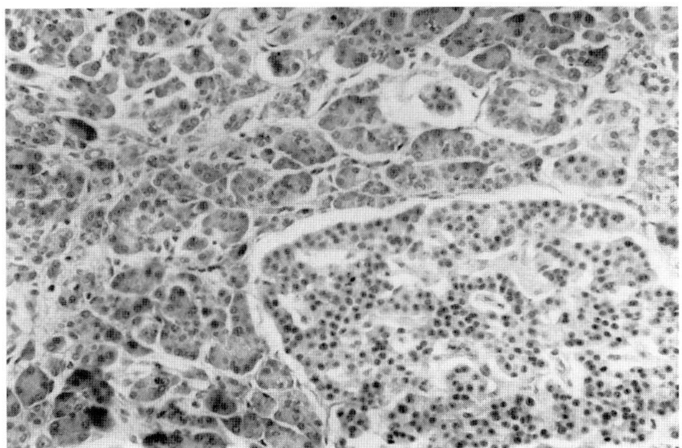

Fig. 15-5 Malignant gastrinoma. The tumor shows an acinar-like growth pattern and prominent nucleoli. Note entrapped, normal-appearing islet cells *(lower right).*

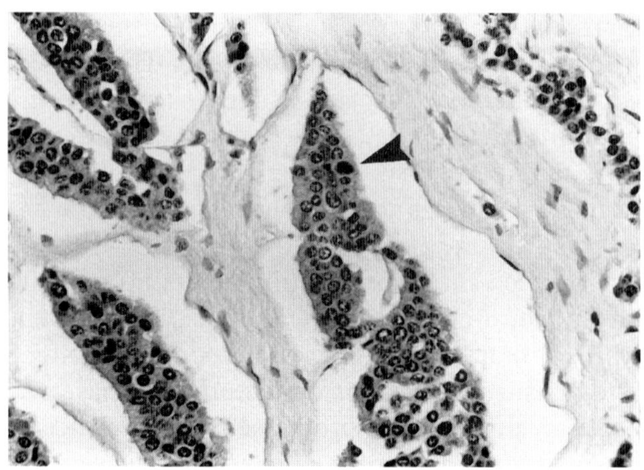

Fig. 15-6   Malignant carcinoid tumor. Note the trabecular growth pattern, pleomorphic, hyperchromatic nuclei, and frequent mitoses *(arrow)*.

ing, diarrhea, valvular heart disease, asthma or wheezing, and facial telangiectasia.[71] The syndrome is a sign of advanced, and often metastatic, disease.

Although metastases to liver and lymph nodes are most common, spread to bone is seen in carcinoid tumors originating in many sites. Origins include bronchus,[72-74] thymus,[75-77] stomach,[78] gallbladder,[79] distal small bowel and cecum,[80] and testis.[81] Bone metastases generally appear as osteoblastic lesions on plain radiographs[70,74] and involve the axial skeleton. A case report, however, discusses a patient with bronchial carcinoid with both an osteolytic metastasis in the clavicle and an osteoblastic metastasis in the humerus from the same primary tumor.[82] Ashraf,[72] in another case report, makes the point that the radiologic constellation of a bone lesion in association with a lesion in the lung usually points to lung carcinoma with spread to bone. However, if the bone metastasis is osteoblastic, the primary tumor may actually be a bronchial carcinoid tumor rather than a carcinoma.

The primary treatment of metastatic carcinoid tumors is surgery, which has been applied to bone metastases as well as to intra-abdominal disease,[81,83] often in the setting of a solitary metastasis or when tissue is needed to make a diagnosis. In cases in which metastasis to bone is occult, the bone involvement may be responsible for persistent symptom of carcinoid syndrome after resection of the primary tumor, lymph node, or liver involvement.[80] Nakagawa and colleagues[75] from Osaka published a

discussion of three cases of thymic carcinoid with metastases, in which two patients achieved disease control with surgery and postoperative radiotherapy. In their report, which included a review of 160 published cases, the investigators conclude that the combination of surgery plus postoperative radiotherapy is more effective than surgery alone in the locally advanced or metastatic setting. They also recommend radiotherapy alone for unresectable metastases. Other investigators have confirmed the efficacy of external irradiation in this setting.[77,84] Cytotoxic chemotherapy may also be used in patients with multiple bone lesions. A Japanese report by Sakai et al.[78] documented a patient who achieved a complete response after receiving six cycles of cisplatin, etoposide, cyclophosphamide, epirubicin, and vincristine. This was followed by high-dose chemotherapy and an autologous peripheral blood stem cell transplant. The authors recommend this combination for patients with carcinoid tumors for whom the prognosis is poor.

Malignant Pheochromocytoma

Pheochromocytomas (Fig. 15-7) are neoplasms that originate in the enterochromaffin cells of the adrenal medulla. The tumors generally produce catecholamines and may cause severe hypertension. Although studies vary, as many as half of all pheochromocytomas may be malignant on the basis of development of metastases.[71] Histologic evaluation of resected pheochromocytomas is inadequate to differentiate benign from malignant tumors. In a series of 98 patients from the Mayo Clinic[85] who underwent complete resection of localized, noninvasive, histologically benign pheochromocytomas and paragangliomas, 88 (90%) had nonfamilial, sporadic disease. Nine patients (9%) had MEN II disease. In six patients (6.5%) recurrent pheochromocytoma developed after they had achieved normal postoperative urinary catecholamine levels. Distant metastases developed in four of these six patients. The authors emphasize that lifelong follow-up is necessary for all patients after resection of pheochromocytoma.

In a series of 20 patients in France with malignant pheochromocytomas[86] the timing of development of metastases was highly variable. Metastases were seen at presentation in 11 patients, within

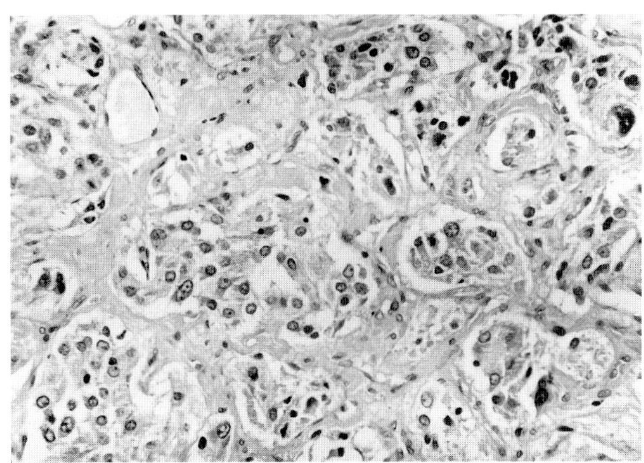

Fig. 15-7 Malignant pheochromocytoma. Note the classic "Zellballen" pattern with rounded nests of large tumor cells separated by stroma.

3 years in 7 patients, and at 9 and 28 years in 2 patients. Again, histologic study was not helpful. Catecholamine overproduction was seen in all patients, predominantly affecting norepinephrine. Serum levels of neuron-specific enolase (NSE), neuropeptide Y, and procalcitonin were frequently elevated.

The finding of elevated NSE levels in malignant disease was echoed by Japanese investigators.[87] In a case report of a patient who underwent resection of an apparently localized pheochromocytoma, norepinephrine levels fell postoperatively but NSE levels remained high. The patient had widespread metastases to lung, liver, and bone. The authors suggested that serum NSE may be a useful marker for differentiating malignant from benign pheochromocytoma.

Unlike routine histologic examination, DNA analysis demonstrates differences between malignant and benign pheochromocytomas. Nativ and colleagues[88] from the Mayo Clinic performed DNA analysis on paraffin-embedded tissue samples from 184 patients with pheochromocytomas and paragangliomas. Diploid, tetraploid, and aneuploid findings each represented one third of the samples. All patients with metastases, however, had tetraploid or aneuploid findings.

Bone is the most common site of distant metastasis from pheochromocytoma. As a result of improvements in medical control of hypercatecholaminemia, bone lesions have become a more prominent cause of morbidity in the disease. Most bone lesions involve the axial skeleton. On plain radiographs the lesions usually appear expansile and mixed lytic-sclerotic. Standard bone scanning has been used to detect bone lesions, but ^{131}I-meta-iodobenzylguanidine (MIBG) scanning generally has been considered the most suitable technique for imaging of primary and metastatic pheochromocytomas.[89]

An alternative nuclear scanning agent to ^{131}I-MIBG is ^{123}I-MIBG. Advantages include a lower false negative rate, superior image quality, and the fact that ^{123}I permits SPECT imaging, which can reveal additional anatomic information.[90] The timing of imaging after injection may be significant, as noted in a report from Australia.[91] Although many centers delay imaging until 24 hours after injection, the authors detected a bone metastasis on a scan at 5 hours, which was not visualized at 24 hours. Yet another nuclear imaging approach in the quest for greater sensitivity is intraoperative ^{125}I-MIBG scanning. In a case-control study from France,[92] this technique demonstrated the ability to detect pheochromocytoma deposits, including those in bone, undetected by preoperative ^{131}I-MIBG scans. This allowed the surgeon to attempt a more complete resection of the disease.

Radiopharmaceuticals may be used for treatment as well as for imaging of metastatic pheochromocytomas.[86,93,94] However, results include mainly partial responses without long-term duration, and bone lesions appear to respond less frequently than metastases to other organs.[93]

Surgical resection of pheochromocytomas involving bone is unusual but may be appropriate in some patients for whom bone stabilization is required. Extended symptom-free survival after surgical resection has been reported.[95] Preoperative embolization may be performed as an adjunct to surgery in selected cases.[96]

External irradiation can effectively palliate symptoms from pheochromocytoma bone metastases. A case report from Tokyo,[97] however, discusses a patient who had acutely exacerbated hypertension, tachycardia, and a low-grade fever after beginning radiotherapy (20 Gy). The authors suggest that this syndrome, which was correlated with increased levels of serum catecholamines, was due to radiation-induced tissue destruction with release of these agents into the bloodstream. They recommend pretreatment with adrenergic blocking agents or α-methyl tyrosine, as well as careful monitoring of the patient's general condition during radiation therapy.

The role of chemotherapy in metastatic pheochromocytoma is poorly defined. Chemotherapy has been used alone or combined with surgery[86] or with external radiotherapy.[98] Agents include streptozocin, cyclophosphamide, vincristine, and dacarbazine. No drug has demonstrated a promising response rate.

Adrenocortical Carcinoma

Adrenocortical carcinoma (ACC) is an uncommon and aggressive cancer that originates in the adrenal cortex. Incidence of this tumor is approximately 2 per million in the world population, or 0.05% to 0.2% of all cancers.[99] One of the largest series in the literature was described by Luton et al.[100] from Paris. They studied 105 patients who were referred to the Hospital Cochin from 1963 to 1987. The patients' mean age was 46 years and the female-to-male ratio was 2.5:1. Thirty percent of the patients had distant metastases at diagnosis. Eighty patients underwent surgery, and 59 also received mitotane (o,p'-DDD) chemotherapy. Overall, tumor dissemination occurred in 82% of the patients, and the median survival for the entire group was 14.5 months.

A study of 42 patients from Roswell Park[101] noted that 52% of the patients had distant metastases at diagnosis. Sites of metastatic involvement were retroperitoneal lymph nodes in 68%, lung in 71%, liver in 42%, and bone in 26%. A comparable series of 77 cases from M.D. Anderson Cancer Center[102] showed that metastases developed in 78% of the patients with a similar distribution of metastatic sites (lung, liver, peritoneal and pleural surfaces, lymph nodes, and bone). Five-year survival was 30%.

Imaging of ACC uses standard anatomic techniques, including plain film radiographs, CT, and MRI. Nuclear agents used for detection of bone lesions include routine bone scanning with technetium 99m.[103] An agent specific for imaging of ACC is 6-β-^{131}I-iodomethyl-19-norcholesterol, which can detect primary lesions, as well as metas-

tases to lymph nodes, parenchymal organs, and bone. This agent makes it possible to perform a whole-body scan to evaluate a patient for metastatic disease.[104,105]

DNA analysis of ACC has not proved helpful. A study of 14 patients from M. D. Anderson Cancer Center in which surgical specimens underwent flow cytometry showed all 14 to be aneuploid, eliminating this feature as a prognostic factor.[106]

Treatment of locally recurrent and metastatic ACC includes surgical resection, external irradiation, and chemotherapy. Surgery is generally used for nonbone recurrences, including metastases to lymph nodes, lung, and liver, and appears more effective than the other modalities.[107-109] For bone metastases, especially in cases of multiple lesions, external radiotherapy can effectively palliate symptoms.[108,109] Mitotane is the most widely used systemic agent in patients with distant disease. Several reports note that mitotane does not improve survival,[100,107] whereas other investigators report small numbers of patients with objective responses and prolonged survivals with this medication.[110-112] Mitotane may have a beneficial effect on bone lesions.[112] Traditional cytotoxic chemotherapeutic agents have not proved useful in the treatment of ACC metastases.[109-111]

Pituitary Carcinomas

Most pituitary neoplasms are intrasellar adenomas. Adenomas may infiltrate bone or dura and are then classified as invasive adenomas. Pituitary carcinomas are defined as tumors with subarachnoid, brain, or systemic metastasis. Pituitary tumors include those that produce growth hormone, prolactin, adrenocorticotropic hormone (ACTH), follicle-stimulating hormone (FSH), luteinizing hormone (LH), thyroid-stimulating hormone (TSH), tumors with mixed hormone production, and tumors without hormone production.[113]

Pituitary adenomas far outnumber pituitary carcinomas. A review of the world literature reveals only a handful of cases of pituitary carcinoma, and even fewer with bone metastases. The available cases with bone involvement will be described here.

Mixson and colleagues[114] from the National Institutes of Health described a 42-year-old woman who underwent surgery for a TSH-secreting pituitary adenoma. The tumor progressed locally 1 year later and was treated with external irradiation and octreotide with a partial response. Four years later, a large sacral metastasis as well as pulmonary nodules developed. Biopsy of the sacral mass demonstrated the pituitary origin of the tumor. Treatment with 5-fluorouracil, cyclophosphamide, and doxorubicin again resulted in a partial response. A pleural effusion containing the same malignant cells developed. The authors note that the response to octreotide and chemotherapy is encouraging and that this case (reported in 1993) represents the first report of a TSH-secreting pituitary carcinoma.

Casson et al.[115] reported a case of a patient with an ACTH-producing pituitary tumor. He underwent surgical resection but had local recurrence, which was treated with repeat resection and external irradiation. ACTH levels remained elevated. Liver, bone, and lymph node metastases developed, and the patient died soon after suffering a spinal cord compression. Immunoperoxidase staining demonstrated ACTH in the pituitary recurrence and metastases.

Walker and colleagues[116] from London described three patients with malignant prolactinomas with extracranial metastases. One of the patients had biopsy-proven bone recurrence 15 years after therapy to the primary tumor with external irradiation, bromocriptine, resection, and chemotherapy. The other two patients had recurrence in liver, lungs, and lymph nodes. In all three patients, palliative measures were unsuccessful.

Dayan et al.[117] presented the case of a patient with a growth-hormone–producing tumor that metastasized to the cervical spine. The patient was cured by surgical resection of the lesion. Geroulanos[118] presented a case report of a patient with a chromophobe carcinoma with metastases to liver and bone.

Given the rarity of bone metastases from pituitary carcinomas, it is not possible to draw reliable conclusions from the literature regarding management of this clinical situation.

ACKNOWLEDGMENTS

The authors acknowledge the efforts of Drs. Joseph Tomashefski and Mahmood Aijazi in providing the photomicrographs included in the text. They also acknowledge the research assistance of Ms. Bonnie Hami.

REFERENCES

1. Brage ME, Simon MA. Evaluation, prognosis, and medical treatment considerations of metastatic bone tumors. Orthopedics 15(5):589-596, 1992.

2. Landis SH, Murray T, Bolden S, Wingo PA. Cancer statistics, 1998. CA Cancer J Clin 48(1):6-29, 1998.

3. Hay ID, Rock MG, Sim FH, Swee RG, Unni KK, Gunderson LL. Thyroid cancer. In Sim FH, ed. Diagnosis and Management of Metastatic Bone Disease: A Multidisciplinary Approach. New York: Raven Press, 1988, pp 305-317.

4. Proye CA, Dromer DH, Carnaille BM, Gontier AJ, Goropoulos A, Carpentier P, Lefebvre J, Decoulx M, Wemeaux JL, Fossati P. Is it still worthwhile to treat bone metastases from differentiated thyroid carcinoma with radioactive iodine? World J Surg 16(4):640-645, 1992.

5. Ruegemer JJ, Hay ID, Bergstralh EJ, Ryan JJ, Offord KP, Gorman CA. Distant metastases in differentiated thyroid carcinoma: A multivariate analysis of prognostic variables. J Clin Endocrinol Metab (67)3:501-508, 1988.

6. Zohar Y, Strauss M. Occult distant metastases of well-differentiated thyroid carcinoma. Head Neck 16(5):438-442, 1994.

7. Yamashita H, Noguchi S, Murakami N, Kawamoto H, Watanabe S. Extracapsular invasion of lymph node metastasis is an indicator of distant metastasis and poor prognosis in patients with thyroid papillary carcinoma. Cancer 80(12): 2268-2272, 1997.

8. Rosen IB, Azadian A, Walfish PG. Adverse aspects of small thyroid cancer and need for retreatment. Head Neck 17(5): 373-376, 1995.

9. Noguchi S, Yamashita H, Murakami N, Nakayama I, Toda M, Kawamoto H. Small carcinomas of the thyroid: A long-term follow-up of 867 patients. Arch Surg 131(2):187-191, 1996.

10. Leger AF. Distant metastasis of differentiated thyroid cancers: Diagnosis by 131 iodine (I 131) and treatment. Ann Endocrinol (Paris) 56(3):205-208, 1995.

11. Tenenbaum F, Schlumberger M, Bonnin F, Lumbroso J, Aubert B, Benali H, Parmentier C. Usefulness of technetium-99m hydroxymethylene diphosphonate scans in localizing bone metastases of differentiated thyroid carcinoma. Eur J Nucl Med 20(12):1168-1174, 1993.

12. Kobayashi M, Mogami T, Uchiyama M, Moriya E, Mori Y, Ohtani Y, Kawakami K, Asahara R. Usefulness of 99mTc-MIBI SPECT in the metastatic lesions of thyroid cancer. Nippon Igaku Hoshasen Gakkai Zasshi 57(3):127-132, 1997.

13. Miyamoto S, Kasagi K, Misaki T, Alam MS, Konishi J. Evaluation of technetium-99m-MIBI scintigraphy in metastatic differentiated thyroid carcinoma. J Nucl Med 38(3):352-356, 1997.

14. Lee KY, Lore JM. The treatment of metastatic thyroid disease. Otolaryngol Clin North Am 23(3):475-493, 1990.

15. Edmonds CJ, Willis CL. Serum thyroglobulin in the investigation of patients presenting with metastases. Br J Radiol 61(724):317-319, 1988.

16. Girelli ME, Casara D, Rubello D, Piccolo M, Piotto A, Pelizzo MR, Busnardo B. Metastatic thyroid carcinoma of the adrenal gland. J Endocrinol Invest 16(2):139-141, 1993.

17. Dhimes P, Carabias E, Lozano F, DeAgustin P. Microinvasive follicular thyroid carcinoma detected by fine-needle aspiration skeletal metastases: A case report. Acta Cytol 41(2):565-568, 1997.

18. Joensuu H, Klemi P, Eerola E, Tuominen J. Influence of cellular DNA content on survival in differentiated thyroid cancer. Cancer 58(11):2462-2467, 1986.

19. Hrafnkelsson J, Stal O, Enestrom S, Jonasson JG, Bjornsson J, Olafsdottir K, Nordenskjold B. Cellular DNA pattern, S-phase frequency and survival in papillary thyroid cancer. Acta Oncol 27(4):329-333, 1988.

20. Hruban RH, Huvos AG, Traganos F, Reuter V, Lieberman PH, Melamed MR. Follicular neoplasms of the thyroid in men older than 50 years of age: A DNA flow cytometric study. Am J Clin Pathol 94(5):527-532, 1990.

21. Komatsu M, Kobayashi S, Sugenoya A, Masuda H, Takahashi S, Iida F, Ito N. An autopsied case of papillary thyroid carcinoma showing DNA heterogeneity: Comparison of DNA content between primary focus and metastatic focus. Nippon Geka Gakkai Zasshi 93(2):208-211, 1992.

22. Komorowski RA, Deaconson TF, Vetsch R, Cerletty JM, Wilson SD. DNA content in radiation-associated thyroid cancer. Surgery 104(6):992-996, 1988.

23. Mehta MP, Goetowski PG, Kinsella TJ. Radiation-induced thyroid neoplasms 1920-1987: A vanishing problem? Int J Rad Oncol Biol Phys 16(6):1471-1475, 1989.

24. Schlumberger M, Challeton C, DeVathaire F, Parmentier C. Treatment of distant metastases in differentiated thyroid carcinoma. J Endocrinol Invest 18:170-172, 1995.

25. Mizukami Y, Michigishi T, Nonomura A, Hashimoto T, Terahata S, Noguchi M, Hisada K, Matsubara F. Distant metastases in differentiated thyroid carcinomas: A clinical and pathologic study. Hum Pathol 21(3):283-290, 1990.

26. Wood WJ, Singletary SE, Hickey RC. Current results of treatment for distant metastatic well-differentiated thyroid carcinoma. Arch Surg 124(12):1374-1377, 1989.

27. Sartorelli B, Glanzmann C, Lutolf UM. Long-term results following radioiodine treatment of patients with metastasizing follicular and papillary thyroid carcinoma. Schweiz Rundsch Med Prax 79(49):1523-1530, 1990.

28. Simpson WJ. Radioiodine and radiotherapy in the management of thyroid cancers. Otolaryngol Clin North Am 23(3):509-521, 1990.

29. Roher HD, Goretzki PE, Wahl RA. Surgery of metastases of differentiated thyroid cancers. Langenbecks Arch Chir 371(2):103-113, 1987.

30. Iwamoto Y, Sugioka Y, Chuman H, Shiba K, Yuge I. Surgical treatment of metastatic tumors of long bones and the spine. Adv Exp Med Biol 324:295-303, 1992.

31. Nakada K, Kasai K, Watanabe Y, Katoh C, Kanegae K, Tsukamoto E, Itoh K, Tamaki N. Treatment of radioiodine-negative bone metastasis from papillary thyroid carcinoma with percutaneous ethanol injection therapy. Ann Nucl Med 10(4):441-444, 1996.

32. Carney JA, Seizmore GW, Hayles AB. C-cell disease in thyroid gland in MEN type IIB. Cancer 44:2173-2183, 1979.

33. Samaan NA, Schultz PN, Hickey RC. Medullary thyroid carcinoma: Prognosis of familial versus nonfamilial disease and the role of radiotherapy. Horm Metab Res Suppl 21:21-25, 1989.

34. Ahuja S, Ernst H. Osteoblastic bone metastases in medullary thyroid carcinoma. Strahlenther Onkol 167(9):549-552, 1991.

35. Sarrazin D, Fontaine F, Rougier P, Gardet P, Schlumberger M, Travagli JP, Bounik H, Parmentier C, Tubiana M. The role of external radiotherapy in the treatment of medullary thyroid carcinoma. Bull Cancer (Paris) 71(3):200-208, 1984.

36. Nel CJC, Heerden JA, Goellner JR, Gharib H, McConahey WM, Taylor WF, Grant CS. Anaplastic carcinoma of the thyroid: A clinicopathologic study of 82 cases. Mayo Clin Proc 60:51-58, 1985.

37. Busnardo B, Girelli ME, Nacamulli D, Pelizzo MR, Danielle O, Rigon A. Undifferentiated carcinoma of the thyroid gland. Chir Ital 46(4):37-41, 1994.

38. Kim JH, Leeper RD. Treatment of locally advanced thyroid carcinoma with combination doxorubicin and radiation therapy. Cancer 60:2372-2375, 1987.

39. Kobayashi T, Asakawa H, Umeshita K, Takeda T, Maruyama H, Matsuzuka F, Monden M. Treatment of 37 patients with anaplastic carcinoma of the thyroid. Head Neck 18(1):36-41, 1996.

40. Wang C, Gaz R. Natural history of parathyroid carcinoma. Am J Surg 149(4):522-527, 1985.

41. Hakaim AG, Esselstyn CB. Parathyroid carcinoma: 50-year experience at The Cleveland Clinic Foundation. Cleve Clin J Med 60:331-335, 1993.

42. Shane E. Parathyroid carcinoma. Curr Ther Endocrinol Metab 6:565-568, 1997.

43. Schantz A, Castleman B. Parathyroid carcinoma: A study of 70 cases. Cancer 31(3):600-605, 1973.

44. Shane E, Bilezikian JP. Parathyroid carcinoma: A review of 62 patients. Endocr Rev 3(2):218-226, 1982.

45. Sulak LE, Brown RW, Butler DB. Parathyroid carcinoma with occult bone metastases diagnosed by fine-needle aspiration cytology. Acta Cytol 33(5):645-648, 1989.

46. Koyano H, Shishiba Y, Shimizu T, Suzuki N, Nazakawa H, Tachibana S, Murata H, Furui S. Successful treatment by surgical removal of bone metastasis producing PTH: New approach to the management of metastatic parathyroid carcinoma. Intern Med 33(11):697-702, 1994.

47. Sandelin K, Thompson NW, Bondeson L. Metastatic parathyroid carcinoma: Dilemmas in management. Surgery 110(6):978-986, 1991.

48. Obara T, Fujimoto Y, Kanaji Y, Okamoto T, Hirayama A, Ito Y, Kodama T. Flow cytometric analysis of parathyroid tumors: Implication of aneuploidy for pathologic and biologic classification. Cancer 66(7):1555-1562, 1990.

49. Obara T, Fujimoto Y, Hirayama A, Kanaji Y, Ito Y, Kodama T, Ogata T. Flow cytometric DNA analysis of parathyroid tumors with special reference to its diagnostic and prognostic value in parathyroid carcinoma. Cancer 65(8):1789-1793, 1990.

50. Sandelin K. Parathyroid carcinoma. Cancer Treat Res 89:183-192, 1997.

51. Van Heerden JA, Roland CF, Carney JA, Sheps SG, Grant CS. Long-term evaluation following resection of apparently benign pheochromocytomas/paragangliomas. World J Surg 14(3):325-329, 1990.

52. Fujimoto Y, Obara T. How to recognize and treat parathyroid carcinoma. Surg Clin North Am 67(2):343-357, 1987.

53. Calandra DB, Chejfec G, Foy BK, Lawrence AM, Paloyan E. Parathyroid carcinoma: Biochemical and pathologic response to DTIC. Surgery 96(6):1132-1137, 1984.

54. Flye MW, Brennan MF. Surgical resection of metastatic parathyroid carcinoma. Ann Surg 193(4):425-435, 1981.

55. Wynne AG, van Heerden J, Carney JA, Fitzpatrick LA. Parathyroid carcinoma: Clinical and pathologic features in 43 patients. Medicine (Baltimore) 71(4):197-205, 1992.

56. Bukowski RM, Sheeler L, Cunningham J, Esselstyn C. Successful combination chemotherapy for metastatic parathyroid carcinoma. Arch Intern Med 144(2):399-400, 1984.

57. Zollinger RM, Ellison EH. Primary peptic ulcerations of the jejunum associated with islet cell tumors of the pancreas. Ann Surg 142:709, 1955.

58. Tjon A, Tham RT, Falke TH, Jansen JB, Lamers CB. CT and MR imaging of advanced Zollinger-Ellison syndrome. J Comput Assist Tomogr 13(5):821-828, 1989.

59. Park HM, Gudkese DB, Clark SA, Nelson R. Skeletal metastasis from gastrinoma: An uncommon manifestation of pancreatic endocrine tumor. Clin Nucl Med 11(11):799-800, 1986.

60. Mignon M, Cadiot G, Marmuse JP, Lewin MJ. Is gastrinoma a medical disease? Yale J Biol Med 69(3):289-300, 1996.

61. Barton JC, Hirschowitz BI, Maton PN, Jensen RT. Bone metastases in malignant gastrinoma. Gastroenterology 91(5):1179-1185, 1986.

62. Horing E, Rath U, Rucker S, von Gaisberg U, Meincke J, Walendzik J, Dorr U, Bihl H. Somatostatin receptor scintigraphy in the primary diagnosis and follow-up care of gastrinoma. Dtsch Med Wochenschr 119(11):367-374, 1994.

63. Vinayek R, Frucht H, Chiang HC, Maton PN, Gardner JD, Jensen RT. Zollinger-Ellison syndrome: Recent advances in the management of gastrinoma. Gastroenterol Clin North Am 19(1):197-217, 1990.

64. Gery B, Roussel A, Valla A. Usefulness of radiotherapy in treatment of advanced gastrinomas. Radiother Oncol 27(3):259-260, 1993.

65. Pederson RT, Haidak DJ, Ferris RA, Macdonald JS, Schein PS. Osteoblastic bone metastasis in Zollinger-Ellison syndrome. Radiology 118(1):63-64, 1976.

66. Kim DG, Chejfec G, Prinz RA. Islet cell carcinoma of the pancreas. Am Surg 55(6):325-332, 1989.

67. Ruffner BW. Chemotherapy for malignant Zollinger-Ellison tumors: Successful treatment with streptozotocin and fluorouracil. Arch Intern Med 136(9):1032-1034, 1976.

68. Ruszniewski P, Hochlaf S, Rougier P, Mignon M. Intravenous chemotherapy with streptozotocin and 5 fluorouracil for hepatic metastases of Zollinger-Ellison syndrome: A prospective multicenter study in 21 patients. Gastroenterol Clin Biol 15(5):393-398, 1991.

69. Valette PJ, Souquet JC, Chayvialle JA. Arterial chemoinfusion and embolization of iliac metastasis from pancreatic islet cell carcinoma. AJR Am J Roentgenol 153(6):1318, 1989.

70. Peavy PW, Rogers JV, Clement JL, Burns JB. Unusual osteoblastic metastases from carcinoid tumors. Radiology 107(2):327-330, 1973.

71. Norton JA, Doppman JL, Jensen RT. Cancer of the endocrine system. In DeVita VT, Hellman S, Rosenberg SA, eds. Cancer: Principles and Practice of Oncology. Philadelphia: JB Lippincott, 1989, pp 1269-1344.

72. Ashraf MH. Bronchial carcinoid with osteoblastic metastases. Thorax 32(4):509-511, 1977.

73. Katakami N, Matsumoto H, Ishihara K, Umeda B. Successful treatment of carcinoid syndrome in two cases of bronchial carcinoid. Nippon Kyobu Shikkan Gakkai Zasshi 33(11):1313-1318, 1995.

74. Taillandier J, Alemanni M. Osteonecrosis, metastases and bronchial carcinoid. Rev Rhum Mal Osteoartic 59(2):140-143, 1992.

75. Nakagawa K, Yasumitsu T, Kotake Y, Iwasaki T, In K. Thymic carcinoid tumor: Report of 3 operative cases. Nippon Kyobu Geka Gakkai Zasshi 40(10):1955-1961, 1992.

76. Valli M, Fabris GA, Dewar A, Chikte S, Fisher C, Corrin B, Sheppard MN. Atypical carcinoid tumor of the thymus: A study of eight cases. Histopathology 24(4):371-375, 1994.

77. Georgy BA, Casola G, Hesselink JR. Thymic carcinoid tumors with bone metastases: A report of two cases. Clin Imaging 19(1):25-29, 1995.

78. Sakai K, Nomura H, Nogami T, Saeki T, Etoh Y, Imamura H, Kamio T, Suko S, Tokunaga H, Suko H. A case of complete remission of gastric endocrine cell carcinoma with multiple bony metastasis by combination chemotherapy and high-dose chemotherapy with autologous peripheral blood stem cell transplantation. Gan To Kagaku Ryoho 24(15):2277-2280, 1997.

79. Kumar S, Agarwal S, Bhargava SK, Minocha VR. Malignant carcinoid tumor of the gallbladder: A case report and review of the literature. Trop Gastroenterol 13(2):78-84, 1992.

80. Dilawari RA, Douglass HO. Gastrointestinal carcinoids: Extrahepatic metastases and symptomatology following resection. J Surg Oncol 11(3):243-248, 1979.

81. Shimura S, Uchida T, Shitara T, Nishimura K, Murayama M, Honda N, Koshiba K. Primary carcinoid tumor of the testis with metastasis to the upper vertebrae: Report of a case. Nippon Hinyokika Gakkai Zasshi 82(7):1157-1160, 1991.

82. Norman A, Greenspan A, Steiner G. Case report 173: Verified osteolytic metastasis in the clavicle from a bronchial carcinoid tumor and probable osteoblastic metastasis in the humerus from the same lesion. Skeletal Radiol 7(2):155-157, 1981.

83. Kirkpatrick DB, Dawson E, Haskell CM, Batzdorf U. Metastatic carcinoid presenting as a spinal tumor. Surg Neurol 4(3):283-287, 1975.

84. Tochner ZA, Kinsella TJ, Glatstein E. Hepatic irradiation in the management of metastatic hormone-secreting tumors. Cancer 56(1):20-24, 1985.

85. Van Heerden JA, Roland CF, Carney JA, Sheps SG, Carney CS. Long-term evaluation following resection of apparently benign pheochromocytomas/paragangliomas. World J Surg 14(3):325-329, 1990.

86. Schlumberger M, Gicquel C, Lumbroso J, Tenenbaum F, Comoy E, Bosq J, Fonseca E, Ghillani PP, Aubert B, Travagli JP. Malignant pheochromocytoma: Clinical, biological, histologic and therapeutic data in a series of 20 patients with distant metastases. J Endocrinol Invest 15(9):631-642, 1992.

87. Ikeda I, Okuno T, Terao T, Masuda M, Hirokawa M. A case of malignant pheochromocytoma with high levels of serum

neuron-specific enolase (NSE) and calcitonin. Hinyokika Kiyo 40(9):813-816, 1994.

88. Nativ O, Grant CS, Sheps SG, O'Fallon JR, Farrow GM, van Heerden JA, Lieber MM. The clinical significance of nuclear DNA ploidy pattern in 184 patients with pheochromocytoma. Cancer 69(11):2683-2687, 1992.

89. Lynn MD, Braunstein EM, Wahl RL, Shapiro B, Gross MD, Rabbani R. Bone metastases in pheochromocytoma: Comparative studies of efficacy of imaging. Radiology 160(3): 701-706, 1986.

90. Lynn MD, Shapiro B, Sisson JC, Beierwaltes WH, Meyers LJ, Ackerman R, Mangner TJ. Pheochromocytoma and the normal adrenal medulla: Improved visualization with I-123 MIBG scintigraphy. Radiology 155(3):789-792, 1985.

91. Lau AK, Roach PJ. Bone metastases in pheochromocytoma: Optimal timing of I-123 MIBG scintigraphy. Clin Nucl Med 21(4):316-318, 1996.

92. Proye CA, Carnaille BM, Flament JB, Hossein-Foucher CA, Lecouffe PP, Marchandise XM, Lennquist S. Intraoperative radionuclear 125I-labeled metaiodobenzylguanidine scanning of pheochromocytomas and metastases. Surgery 111(6):634-639, 1992.

93. Sisson JC, Shapiro B, Beierwaltes WH, Glowniak JV, Nakajo M, Mangner TJ, Carey JE, Swanson DP, Copp JE, Satterley WG. Radiopharmaceutical treatment of malignant pheochromocytoma. J Nucl Med 25(2):197-206, 1984.

94. Fischer M. Nuclear medicine diagnosis and treatment in pheochromocytoma and neuroblastoma. Bildgebung 56(4): 141-145, 1987.

95. Krodel A, Lohscheidt K, Muller-Hocker J. Surgical therapy of polytopic vertebral metastasis in malignant pheochromocytoma. Z Orthop Ihre Grenzgeb 133(2):176-179, 1995.

96. Chiras J, Cognard C, Rose M, Dessauge C, Martin N, Pierot L, Plouin PF. Percutaneous injection of an alcoholic embolizing emulsion as an alternative preoperative embolization for spine tumor. Am J Neuroradiol 14(5):1113-1117, 1993.

97. Teno S, Tanabe A, Nomura K, Demura H. Acutely exacerbated hypertension and increased inflammatory signs due to radiation treatment for metastatic pheochromocytoma. Endocr J 43(5):511-516, 1996.

98. Araki T, Chigusa I, Saitoh K. A case of malignant ectopic pheochromocytoma with bone metastasis. Hinyokika Kiyo 35(6):1005-1007, 1989.

99. Jensen JC, Pass HI, Sindelar WF, Norton JA. Recurrent or metastatic disease in select patients with adrenocortical carcinoma. Arch Surg 126(4):457-461, 1991.

100. Luton JP, Cerdas S, Billaud L, Thomas G, Guilhaume B, Bertagna X, Laudat MH, Louvel A, Chapuis Y, Blondeau P. Clinical features of adrenocortical carcinoma, prognostic factors, and the effect of mitotane therapy. N Engl J Med 322(17):1195-1201, 1990.

101. Didolkar MS, Bescher RA, Elias EG, Moore RH. Natural history of adrenal cortical carcinoma: A clinicopathologic study of 42 patients. Cancer 47(9):2153-2161, 1981.

102. Nader S, Hickey RC, Sellin RV, Samaan NA. Adrenal cortical carcinoma: A study of 77 cases. Cancer 52(4):707-711, 1983.

103. Pacheco EJ, Moreno AJ, Jimenez C, Carpenter A, Steinbaum S, Brady K. Fortuitous imaging of a primary adrenocortical carcinoma with Tc-99m HDP. Clin Nucl Med 20(10):906-908, 1995.

104. Seabold JE, Haynie TP, DeAsis DN, Samaan NA, Glenn HJ, Jahns MF. Detection of metastatic adrenal carcinoma using ^{131}I-6-beta-iodomethyl-19-norcholesterol total body scans. J Clin Endocrinol Metab 45(4):788-797, 1977.

105. Drane WE, Graham MM, Nelp WB. Imaging of an adrenal cortical carcinoma and its skeletal metastasis. J Nucl Med 24(8):710-712, 1983.

106. Lee JE, Berger DH, el-Naggar AK, Hickey RC, Vassilopoulou-Sellin R, Gagel RF, Burgess MA, Evans DB. Surgical management, DNA content, and patient survival in adrenal cortical carcinoma. Surgery 118(6):1090-1098, 1995.

107. Hajjar RA, Hickey RC, Samaan NA. Adrenal cortical carcinoma: A study of 32 patients. Cancer 35(2):549-554, 1975.

108. Cohn K, Gottesman L, Brennan M. Adrenocortical carcinoma. Surgery 100(6):1170-1177, 1986.

109. Pommier RF, Brennan MF. An eleven-year experience with adrenocortical carcinoma. Surgery 112(6):963-970, 1992.

110. Decker RA, Kuehner ME. Adrenocortical carcinoma. Am Surg 57(8):502-513, 1991.

111. Linos DA, Vassilopoulos PP, Papadimitriou J, Tountas K. The surgical management of adrenal cortical carcinoma. Int Surg 71(2):104-106, 1986.

112. Katsumi T, Murayama K. A case of non-functioning adrenal cortical carcinoma with pulmonary and bone metastases. Hinyokika Kiyo 35(11):1893-1895, 1989.

113. Scheithauer BW, Kovacs KT, Laws ER, Randall RV. Pathology of invasive pituitary tumors with special reference to functional classification. J Neurosurg 65(6):733-744, 1986.

114. Mixson AJ, Friedman TC, Katz DA, Feuerstein IM, Taubenberger JK, Colandrea JM, Doppman JL, Oldfield EH, Weintraub BD. Thyrotropin-secreting pituitary carcinoma. J Clin Endocrinol Metab 76(2):529-533, 1993.

115. Casson IF, Walker BA, Hipkin LJ, Davis JC, Buxton PH, Jeffreys RV. An intrasellar pituitary tumor producing metastases in liver, bone and lymph glands and demonstration of ACTH in the metastatic deposits. Acta Endocrinol (Copenh) 111(3):300-304, 1986.

116. Walker JD, Grossman A, Anderson JV, Ur E, Trainer PJ, Benn J, Lowy C, Sonksen PH, Plowman PN, Lowe DG. Malignant prolactinoma with extracranial metastases: A report of 3 cases. Clin Endocrinol (Oxf) 38(4):411-419, 1993.

117. Dayan C, Guilding T, Hearing S, Thomas P, Nelson R, Moss T, Bradshaw J, Levy A, Lightman S. Biochemical cure of recurrent acromegaly by resection of cervical spinal canal metastases. Clin Endocrinol (Oxf) 44(5):597-602, 1996.

118. Geroulanos S. Chromophobe carcinoma of the pituitary gland with metastases in liver and bones. Schweiz Med Wochenschr 99(50):1817-1824, 1969.

CHAPTER

16

Cancer of the Gastrointestinal Tract

Leonard L. Gunderson, M.D., Michael J. O'Connell, M.D., Douglas J. Pritchard, M.D., Michael G. Haddock, M.D., and Franklin H. Sim, M.D.

In the United States, malignant tumors arising in the gastrointestinal tract (esophagus, stomach, pancreas, biliary tract, liver, small bowel, colon, rectum, and anus) have the second highest incidence of invasive cancers involving any organ system. In 1998 the following numbers of new cases of cancer of the gastrointestinal (GI) tract were anticipated in the United States, according to specific primary site[1]: colon, 95,600; rectum, 36,000; pancreas, 29,000; stomach, 22,600; liver and biliary tract, 20,600; esophagus, 12,300; small intestine, 4500; and anus and anal canal, 3300. Most of these malignancies are adenocarcinomas that arise from the epithelium, glands, or ducts of the affected organ. Although neuroendocrine tumors (carcinoid and islet-cell carcinomas), lymphomas, squamous cell carcinomas, and sarcomas can also arise from the GI tract, they account for fewer than 10% of the malignant GI tract cancers.

The mainstay of therapy for resectable GI tract carcinomas is surgical resection. For locally unresectable, nonmetastatic GI tract cancers, therapy is combined-modality chemoirradiation, which can be given either as primary treatment or as preoperative treatment before an attempt at resection, intraoperative irradiation, or both.[2-6] For resected, high-risk GI tract carcinomas, adjuvant postoperative chemoirradiation (concurrent and maintenance chemotherapy) has reduced local relapse and improved survival in randomized trials for rectal, pancreatic, and gastric cancers.[3,6-14] Adjuvant postoperative multidrug chemotherapy has improved survival (disease-free and overall) in randomized trials for node-positive colon cancers.[15-18] Concurrent chemoirradiation has become the standard of care for the initial treatment of cancers of the anal canal (surgery is reserved for salvage treatment), with local control in approximately 80% of patients and 5-year survival in approximately 70%.[19-21] Combination chemoirradiation (concurrent and maintenance chemotherapy) has also demonstrated the ability to cure 25% to 30% of patients with esophageal cancer who are not good candidates for or who reject surgical resection.[22,23] With GI tract lymphomas, chemotherapy, irradiation, or combinations thereof can achieve high local control and reasonable survival without surgical resection.

For patients with metastatic GI tract cancers, both irradiation and chemotherapy can provide palliative benefits. Irradiation alone or in conjunction with concomitant chemotherapy is most commonly employed as a palliative therapy for locally unresectable or locally recurrent lesions or for distant metastases that produce significant symptoms in a limited anatomic distribution (e.g., brain, bone, or occasionally liver). Chemotherapy alone is usually employed as a palliative modality for disseminated metastatic GI tract cancer to the liver, lung, or peritoneal cavity, or in combination with irradiation for metastases to brain or bone.

INCIDENCE

The frequency of clinically evident bone metastasis at the time of initial disease progression, after potentially curative surgical resection in patients with gastric or colorectal cancer, is seen in Table 16-1.[24] These data were derived from patients participating in surgical adjuvant research protocols sponsored by Mayo Clinic and the North Central Cancer Treatment Group (NCCTG). Although 4% to 18% of patients with disease relapse had evidence of bone metastasis at the time of initial tumor progression, they represented only 2% to 6% of all patients undergoing a curative resection.

The problem of musculoskeletal involvement by GI tract cancers is most evident among patients with local or regional relapse in a presacral tumor bed from a primary rectal or sigmoid cancer. The iliopsoas or posterior abdominal muscles can also be involved in local regional relapse of a colon cancer (cecum, ascending, descending, and transverse colon). With presacral relapse, direct invasion of the sacrum may occur. Severe pain and dysfunction are commonly a result of infiltration of sacral or lumbar nerve roots or bone destruction.

Among patients with advanced metastatic GI tract cancer, only a few will have clinically apparent bone metastasis. Table 16-2 summarizes the incidence of bone metastasis at the start of chemotherapy and at the time of progression of malignant disease for a group of patients with gastric, pancreatic, and colorectal cancers treated on research protocols sponsored by the Mayo Clinic and the NCCTG. Only 5% to 10% of patients had clinically apparent metastatic osseous lesions during the course of their disease.

Table 16-1   Clinically evident bone metastasis in patients with gastrointestinal cancer at time of initial tumor progression after potentially curative surgical resection*

Site of primary carcinoma	No. of patients (%)		
	Curative resection	Postsurgical tumor progression (all sites)	Bone metastasis
Stomach	54	25 (46.3)	2 (3.7)
Colon	306	119 (38.9)	5 (1.6)
Rectum	102	34 (33.3)	6 (5.9)

From O'Connell MJ, Gunderson LL, Beabout JW, Pritchard DJ, Wold LE. Gastrointestinal cancer. In Sim F, ed. Diagnosis and Management of Metastatic Bone Disease: A Multidisciplinary Approach. New York: Raven Press, 1988, pp 291-296. Used by permission.
*Surgical adjuvant research protocols sponsored by the Mayo Clinic and the North Central Cancer Treatment Group (NCCTG).

Table 16-2   Clinically evident bone metastasis in patients with advanced GI tract cancer treated with chemotherapy*

Site of primary tumor	Total treated	No. of patients with bone metastasis (%)		
		Start of chemotherapy	Time of progression	Total
Stomach	111	5 (4.5)	1 (0.9)	6 (5.4)
Pancreas	106	2 (1.9)	6 (5.7)	8 (7.6)
Colorectal	300	17 (5.7)	13 (4.3)	30 (10.0)

From O'Connell MJ, Gunderson LL, Beabout JW, Pritchard DJ, Wold LE. Gastrointestinal cancer. In Sim F, ed. Diagnosis and Management of Metastatic Bone Disease: A Multidisciplinary Approach. New York: Raven Press, 1988, pp 291-296. Used by permission.
*Research protocols sponsored by the Mayo Clinic and the North Central Cancer Treatment Group (NCCTG).

PATTERNS OF SPREAD

Carcinomas of the GI tract spread by four major routes: direct extension into contiguous structures and lymphatic, hematogenous, and peritoneal metastasis. The degree of both direct extension and lymphatic metastasis of a GI tract cancer influences whether the primary malignancy can be completely resected. The presence of both high-risk pathologic features also increases the risk of blood-borne or peritoneal metastasis at some point in the natural history of the disease.

The frequency of involvement of specific anatomic sites by metastatic disease varies according to the type and location of the primary carcinoma within the GI tract, as well as the initial TNM (tumor, node, metastasis) extent of the primary malignancy. For both colon and rectal cancer the risk of subsequent blood-borne spread is 40% to 50% in patients with T3-4 N1-2 lesions (MAC C_2 or C_3) vs. 20% to 25% in those with T3-4 N0 or T1-2 N1-2 lesions (MAC B_2, B_3, C_1).

The most common sites of metastatic disease from GI tract cancers include the liver, lung, peritoneal cavity, and retroperitoneal nodes. The liver is a site of blood-borne spread from all GI tract primary lesions and is the highest risk site for lesions with portal venous drainage (stomach, pancreas, biliary tract, colon, small bowel, rectum, and anus). The lung is a primary venous drainage site for only esophageal and rectal cancers. Lung may also become at risk with GI tract cancers at other sites that have local tumor extension to involve adjacent organs or structures with venous drainage to the lung (e.g., posterior extension of pancreatic cancer, involvement of the bladder by sigmoid cancer). The peritoneal cavity and retroperitoneal lymph nodes can become involved by metastatic disease from primary lesions in the abdomen or pelvic portion of the GI tract. The peritoneal cavity is at negligible risk, however, with esophageal primary malignancies that do not extend to involve the stomach. Celiac adenopathy can occur with esophageal lesions at any level, but this is a reasonably high risk only with distal esophageal lesions.

The skeletal system is among sites infrequently involved at the time of initial diagnosis of metastatic GI tract cancer. Other infrequent sites of metastasis include the brain and spinal cord.

DIAGNOSTIC AND SCREENING CONSIDERATIONS

In view of the low rate of bone metastasis from GI tract cancers, routine screening of the skeletal system is not employed as a component of follow-up examinations. For patients with musculoskeletal symptoms, initial screening is usually done with computed tomography (CT) and skeletal radiographs. Magnetic resonance imaging (MRI) may be useful in determining the extent of muscle and skeletal involvement. If radiographic findings are equivocal or if metastatic disease has never been histologically confirmed, biopsy is employed to establish the diagnosis of osseous metastasis.

TREATMENT

The prognosis and survival of patients with bloodborne or peritoneal metastasis from GI tract malignancies vary by site of malignancy and by histologic findings. Upper GI tract carcinomas (gastric, pancreas, liver) have a much shorter natural history than lower GI tract cancers (colorectal, anus). With metastatic lower GI tract cancer, survival at 1 or 2 years would not be unusual with chemotherapy treatment. If the metastasis is solitary (liver, lung, central nervous system), 5-year survival of 20% to 40% has been reported after surgical resection. In metastatic upper GI tract carcinomas, death commonly occurs within 3 to 6 months of diagnosis of the metastatic disease. Survival and prognosis in metastatic gastric cancer are slightly more favorable than in metastatic pancreatic ductal carcinomas because of better response rates to multidrug chemotherapy (3 months' extension of median survival). The longer natural history of islet-cell and carcinoid tumors and of lymphoma and the availability of systemic treatment tools result in better prognosis and survival of patients with these less-common GI tract malignancies.

The role of surgery, irradiation, and chemotherapy is dependent on the extent of musculoskeletal involvement by tumor and the absence or presence of disease elsewhere. The localized involvement of bone by GI tract cancers is usually most effectively managed by external beam irradiation, with or without concomitant and maintenance chemotherapy. Disseminated involvement of the skeleton is treated primarily with systemic chemotherapy. If weightbearing long bones are involved, however, orthopedic procedures and external irradiation may be indicated to prevent pathologic fractures. Distal sacrectomy may have a role in selected patients who have locally recurrent rectal cancer with direct invasion of the sacrum.

Systemic Therapy

Cytotoxic chemotherapy can produce objective tumor responses and symptomatic benefit in 10% to 75% of patients with malignant neoplasms of the gastrointestinal tract. The probability of response is dependent on the site of origin and the histologic type of tumor. GI tract lymphomas that metastasize are potentially curable with the use of intensive combination chemotherapy regimens, supplemental low-dose irradiation, or both.[25,26] Approximately 70% of patients with islet-cell carcinoma have objective tumor responses with streptozocin and doxorubicin. The median time to progression is more than 2 years, and this treatment is associated with improved survival.[27] With metastatic colorectal[28,29] and gastric cancers,[30,31] 15% to 40% of patients have temporary objective tumor responses (approximate median duration, 4 to 8 months) when various multidrug chemotherapy regimens are used. The rate of complete response, however, is usually less than 10%, and a sustained complete response is unusual. For pancreatic ductal carcinomas, results in the management of metastatic disease remain dismal.[32,33] Although a randomized trial comparing gemcitabine and 5-fluorouracil (5-FU) revealed an advantage to gemcitabine in response rates and quality of life, a meaningful survival benefit was not achieved.[33] Efforts are under way to combine gemcitabine, 5-FU, and cisplatin in an attempt to improve the systemic effect of chemotherapy. Therapy with gemcitabine plus 5-FU or cisplatin, or both, is also being evaluated in combination with irradiation for locally unresectable pancreatic cancers.

There are not enough patients with GI tract cancer who have measurable metastatic lesions within the osseous system to determine whether metastatic skeletal deposits are more or less sensitive to chemotherapy than are metastatic lesions in other anatomic locations. Clinicians should be aware, however, that a differential systemic response (i.e., response in one location but not another) can also occur.

Palliative Irradiation

Bone metastasis from GI tract cancer is uncommon, but when it occurs, it is usually in conjunction with other blood-borne metastasis. When irradiation is chosen to treat a metastatic bone problem, several goals are apparent and must be given priority in any clinical situation.[34-43] Pain, loss of structural integrity, and neurologic compromise are the most common problems, and reversal of these processes is the intent of treatment. The ability to reverse the process and relieve these symptoms, however, must be considered in relation to the cost, time, and inconvenience of treatment and the life expectancy and functional level of the patient. Acute morbidity should be minimized, and in patients in whom prolonged survival is a possibility, late effects should be considered.

With metastatic gastric or pancreatic cancers, life expectancy is usually a few months, and rapid irradiation treatment schedules are indicated. For such patients, reasonable schedules include 2000 cGy (20 Gy) in 5 fractions for 1 week or 3000 cGy (30 Gy) in 10 fractions for 2 weeks. In patients with end-stage disease in whom transportation is a problem, even single-fraction irradiation can provide palliative benefit.[34,40]

The natural history of metastasis from colorectal cancer differs in that patients more frequently survive for 1 to 2 years. More aggressive radiation

regimens may be appropriate in such patients in whom a maximal and prolonged effect of irradiation is warranted to minimize the morbidity related both to pain and to structural and neurologic function. In our experience and that of others,[43] such patients may benefit from a more protracted, higher-dose course of irradiation in the range of 4000 to 5000 cGy (40 to 50 Gy). In the randomized study done by the Radiation Therapy Oncology Group (RTOG), whereas the initial analysis showed no benefit to more protracted treatment,[42] in a reanalysis there was an advantage overall, most notably in patients with solitary metastasis, when a dose of 4050 cGy (40.5 Gy or 2.7 Gy $\times$ 15) was used.[43] Complete pain relief was achieved in 55% of patients with 40.5 Gy, compared with 37% in whom complete relief was achieved when 2000 cGy in 1 week (20 Gy or 4 Gy $\times$ 5) was used.[43] For patients in whom the only known disease is a solitary metastatic bone lesion and the interval from diagnosis of the primary tumor is prolonged, doses of radiation with the potential for permanent local control may be indicated (6000 cGy [60 Gy] in standard fractionation), depending on the tolerance of the surrounding organs or tissues.

When high-dose irradiation or reirradiation is used, multiple field techniques with careful beam-shaping devices are indicated to minimize the treatment of normal tissues. Other options to consider include bowel displacement with the patient in the prone position or with bladder distention or with both and the use of false tabletop techniques to allow anterior small bowel displacement.[44,45]

If maintenance chemotherapy is planned, radiation fields should be conservative, and an attempt should be made to treat less than 25% to 30% of bone marrow reserves. This more conservative approach will allow such patients to be eligible for phase I-II chemotherapy studies.

During protracted high-dose treatment of larger areas, peripheral blood cell counts should be monitored weekly or as necessary to avoid morbidity related to count suppression in an already compromised patient. This monitoring is especially important for patients who are receiving concomitant chemotherapy, have had recent systemic chemotherapy, or have multiple sites that have been previously irradiated. If the abdominal cavity is included in the external-beam irradiation (EBRT) field, GI tract toxic effects (nausea, vomiting, or diarrhea with resultant loss of weight) can occur. In addition to the use of tailored fields to minimize the effect on normal tissues, reduced fraction size and premedication with antiemetics can be helpful. Such symptoms will rapidly resolve after irradiation is completed.

Irradiation as a Component of Curative Treatment

There are two situations in which attempts at curative treatment may be justified despite bone involvement by GI tract malignancies. One is the rare circumstance of a solitary metastatic bone lesion in the absence of other metastatic lesions or local recurrence. The second is sacral or coccygeal involvement (or both) as the result of adherence to or invasion of bone by direct tumor extension from a tumor bed or by nodal recurrence from colon or rectal cancer.[5,7,46,47] In both instances a combination of operative resection and irradiation (preoperative or postoperative) would be used if surgical resection was technically feasible; it is difficult to deliver curative doses of radiation safely because of adjacent loops of dose-limiting small bowel.

With presacral recurrence from rectal or sigmoid colon cancer, a presurgical diagnostic study is done to rule out extrapelvic disease. The diagnostic study includes chest film, liver function studies, carcinoembryonic antigen (CEA) determination, and CT of the abdominal-pelvic region (which may need to include bone windows to determine the extent of sacral involvement). If the results are negative for metastasis, a course of preoperative irradiation with concomitant chemotherapy is usually given. In patients not previously irradiated, multiple field techniques are used to deliver 4500 cGy (45 Gy) in 25 fractions for 5 weeks to both the recurrent tumor region and nodal drainage sites and to deliver 540 to 900 cGy (5.4 to 9 Gy) in 3 to 5 fractions to a reduced field, for a total dose within the boost field of 5040 to 5400 cGy.[5,44,45] The higher dose is given only if small bowel can be excluded. The concomitant chemotherapy during irradiation would consist of either protracted venous infusion of 5-FU (225 mg/m^2/d, 5 to 7 days a week throughout the entire course of irradiation or until intolerance) or a bolus dose of 5-FU plus leucovorin for 4 consecutive days during weeks 1 and 5 of irradiation (5-FU, 400 mg/m^2/d and leucovorin, 20

mg/m^2/d). In previously irradiated patients the preoperative irradiation dose is restricted to 20 to 30 Gy in 10 to 15 fractions, and concomitant chemotherapy is usually a protracted venous infusion of 5-FU, 225 mg/m^2/d.[47]

A diagnostic study to rule out extrapelvic metastatic disease is repeated 3 to 4 weeks after completion of preoperative chemoirradiation. If the extrapelvic metastatic disease is not found, the patient is reevaluated for potential gross total tumor resection. For patients in whom sacral involvement is suspected, MRI may give additional information to the CT findings for determining the superior extent of disease and therefore the feasibility of distal sacrectomy.

If the lesion, as seen on CT, MRI, or both, can be removed totally and the sacrum preserved, the operation proceeds under the direction of the colorectal or urologic surgeon.[5] The radiation oncologist is consulted in the operating room regarding intraoperative radiotherapy (IORT) supplemented with intraoperative electron radiotherapy (IOERT),[2-7,46,47] high-dose rate (HDR) brachytherapy (HDR-IORT),[48] or brachytherapy with a permanent or temporary implant.[49,50]

If sacral resection is likely on the basis of preoperative CT or MRI, the patient is evaluated by a multidisciplinary team including a colorectal surgeon, orthopedic oncologist, radiation oncologist, and urologic surgeon or neurosurgeon, or both, depending on the superior extent of dissection.[46] If the superior extent of disease will allow distal sacrectomy with preservation of S2, abdominal exploration is done to rule out intra-abdominal disease. An aggressive pelvic operation ensues if there is no evidence of peritoneal seeding, liver metastasis, or para-aortic adenopathy. If surgical margins are positive or narrow (less than 2 cm), those margins are marked with small hemoclips and supplemental IORT is given with IOERT or HDR-IORT if either is technically feasible. An irradiation boost with afterloading brachytherapy or further external-beam radiotherapy (EBRT) is used if IORT is not technically feasible, and dose-limiting small bowel can be displaced with a vascularized omental pedicle or rectus abdominus flap. The EBRT component starts as early as 2 weeks postoperatively if healing is satisfactory. The radiation oncologist must be a participating member of the operating room team to help determine whether additional irradiation is indicated and which of the irradiation methods should be used.

Surgical Management
Bone Metastases

Although relatively few patients with cancers of the GI tract have bone metastasis, skeletal involvement can cause significant clinical problems and loss of quality of life. Management of these skeletal lesions poses a challenge to the orthopedic surgeon to provide pain relief and maintain a functional life. When metastasis threatens the structural integrity of a weightbearing bone and pathologic fracture is imminent, prophylactic surgical fixation should be considered because it provides an improved and faster functional recovery (Fig. 16-1). Obviously, if a pathologic fracture occurs in a long bone, open reduction and internal fixation may be indicated.

Significant advances have been made in the management of pathologic fractures with the development of improved fixation devices and prosthetic implants and, in extensive cases, with the use of methylmethacrylate.[50] The principle of surgical treatment is to provide stable and durable fixation. Because fixation failure is known to increase with

time and is usually a result of disease progression,[51] postoperative irradiation is used to achieve or improve local disease control.

The specific surgical treatment varies with the location of the lesion, the extent of bone destruction, and the general condition of the patient. In lesions involving long bones such as the femur, tibia, and humerus, internal fixation with third-generation intramedullary rods is preferred because of their load-sharing function. Modular prosthetic arthroplasty is a useful technique for patients with extensive lesions involving the hip, knee, or shoulder. Fortunately, these developments have resulted in significant advances in orthopedic management of these patients and allow achievement of the goal of stable, duration fixation to improve the quality of life.

Sacropelvic Resection for Locally Recurrent Anorectal Cancer

The outlook for patients with cancers of the sigmoid colon or rectum who have sacral involvement by direct extension of locally recurrent disease is generally poor if palliative irradiation is used as the only component of treatment. In addition, local

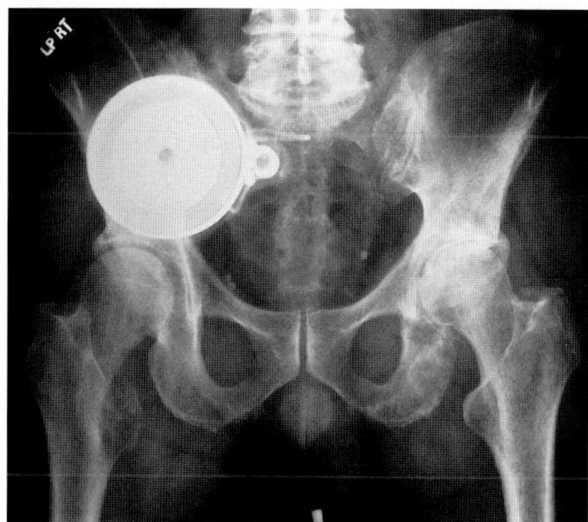
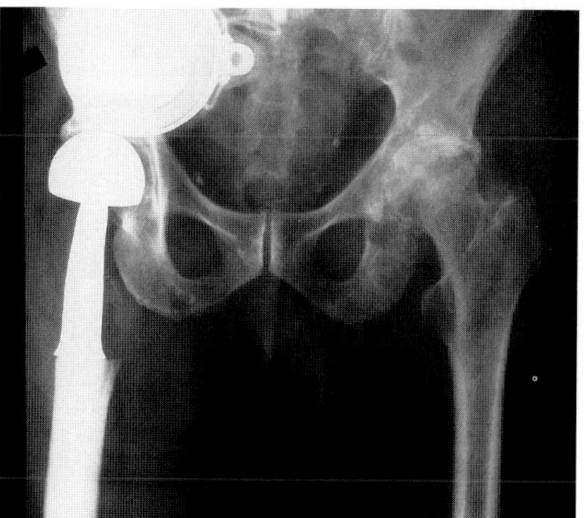

Fig. 16-1   A, Anteroposterior view of the pelvis and proximal femur, showing destructive lesion of the lesser trochanter and medial cortex of the proximal femur, with an impending pathologic fracture from metastatic adenocarcinoma of the colon. A large lesion in the pelvis had been treated with curettage of the tumor and cementation. **B,** Anteroposterior view of the pelvis and proximal femur, after resection of proximal femur and reconstruction arthroplasty with a custom type of bipolar endoprosthesis. (From O'Connell MJ, Gunderson LL, Beabout JW, Pritchard DJ, Wold LE. Gastrointestinal cancer. In Sim F, ed. Diagnosis and Management of Metastatic Bone Disease: A Multidisciplinary Approach. New York: Raven Press, 1988. Used by permission.)

disabling complications and neurogenic intractable pain are common.

Recent advances suggest that such lesions may be amenable to abdominosacral resection. Pelvic CT, with and without bone windows, and MRI are helpful in defining the precise extent of tumor involvement and the feasibility of sacrectomy as a treatment component (Fig. 16-2).

Careful patient selection is necessary to ensure a favorable outcome. Usually surgery is contraindicated when gross total resection is not considered possible on the basis of the preoperative imaging studies. Contraindications for sacrectomy usually include pelvic sidewall involvement, extension into the sciatic notch, proximal extension involving S1, or encasement of the iliac vessels.

The surgical approach is technically demanding. The sequential anterior and posterior approach is usually preferred at our institution (Figs. 16-3 and 16-4), but the simultaneous anterior and posterior approach can also be used effectively. In the sequential approach, anterior exploration is carried out by the colorectal or general surgeon to rule out an extrapelvic metastasis (liver metastasis, peritoneal bleeding, or retroperitoneal adenopathy), to mobilize visceral structures, to establish the anterior and lateral margins of the resection, and to devascularize the pelvis by ligation of the internal iliac vessels for lesions that extend above S3. In addition, a myocutaneous rectus abdominus flap is harvested for use in the closure of the posterior sacral incision. After the anterior wound is closed,

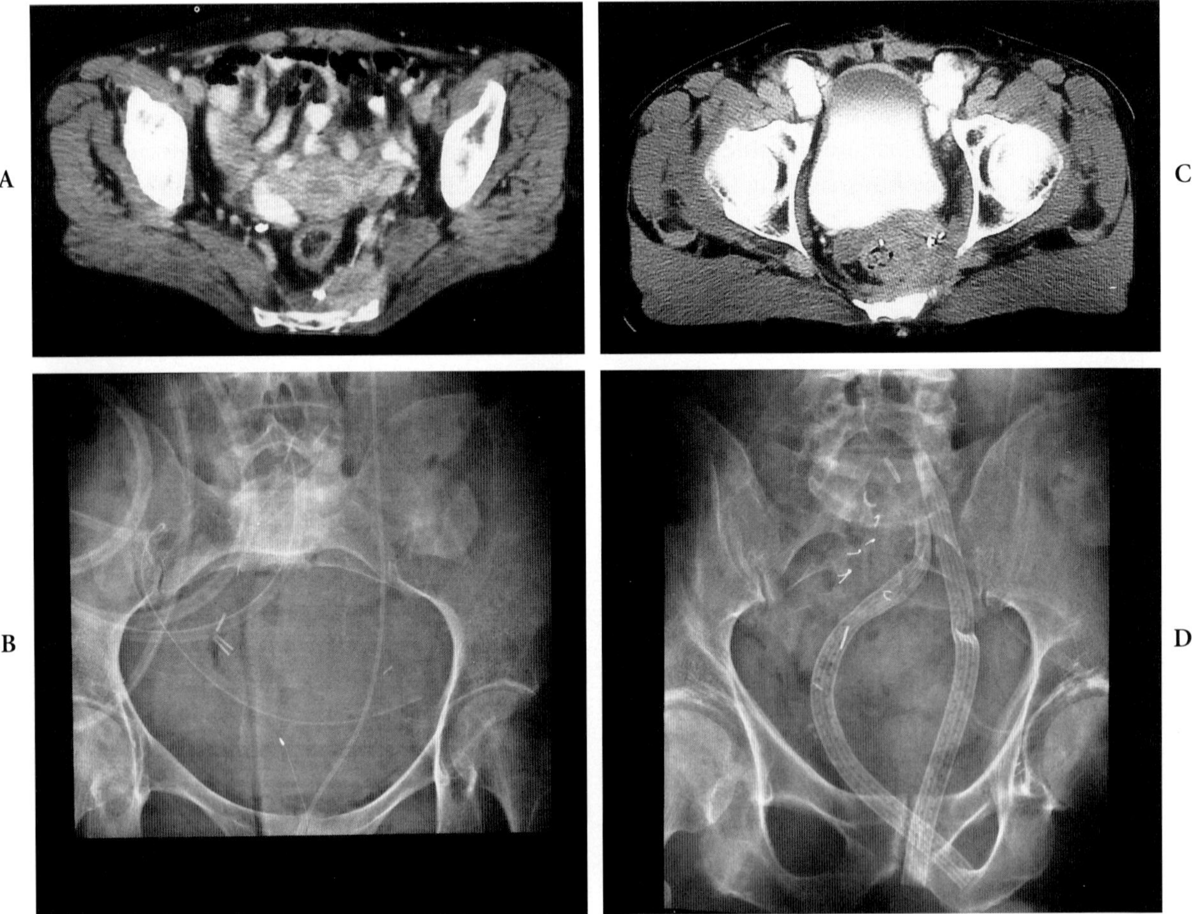

Fig. 16-2   A, CT of the pelvis and sacrum, showing locally recurrent anorectal cancer eroding into the left sacrum. **B,** Anteroposterior pelvis film obtained after sacral resection. **C,** CT of the pelvis, demonstrating locally recurrent sigmoid cancer involving the sacrum and left ischial spine. **D,** Anteroposterior pelvis film obtained after resection of the sacrum and left ischial spine.

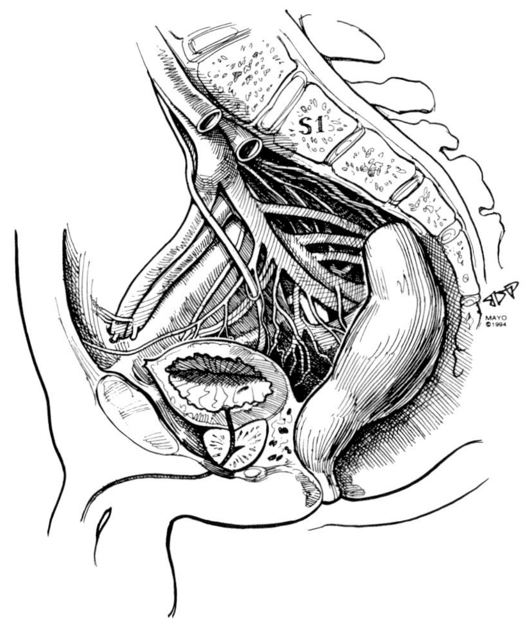

Fig. 16-3 Distal sacrectomy: operative technique, anterior approach (surgical anatomy). The anterior approach ensures that no extrapelvic disease exists and allows several preparatory steps for the sacral resection (anterior and lateral dissection, delineation of proximal sacral margin, parasacral vascular ligation, stoma formation, omental or rectus abdominus flap creation).

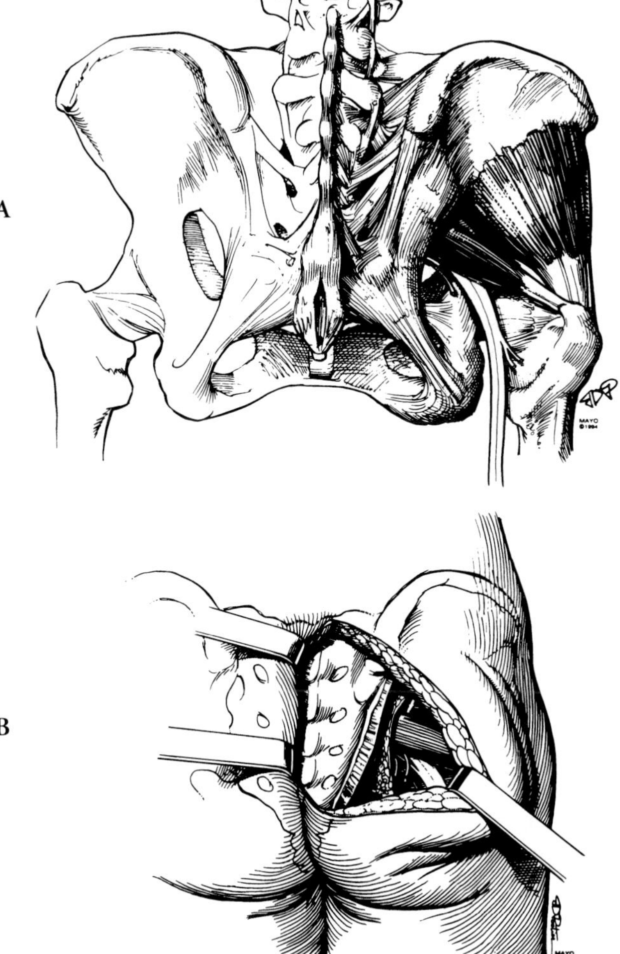

Fig. 16-4 Distal sacrectomy: operative techniques, posterior approach. **A,** Anatomic relationships; **B,** operative anatomy; **C,** distal sacral resection. For removal of the sacrum and presacral tumor posteriorly, the gluteal muscle must be dissected from the sacrum and the sciatic nerve identified. The sacrotuberous and sacrospinous ligaments, pyriform muscle, and endopelvic fascia are divided. The dural sac is then ligated and the sacrum transected after mobilization of nerve roots. (**A** and **B** from Magrini S, Nelson H, Gunderson LL, Sim H. Sacropelvic resection and intraoperative electron irradiation in the management of recurrent anorectal cancer. Dis Colon Rectum 39:1-8, 1996. **A** to **C** used by permission of the Mayo Foundation.)

38. Delclos L. New and old concepts in radiotherapeutic treatment. Int J Radiat Oncol Biol Phys 1:1217-1220, 1976.

39. Hendrickson FR, Shehata WM, Kirchner AB. Radiation therapy for osseous metastasis. Int J Radiat Oncol Biol Phys 1: 275-278, 1976.

40. Penn CRH. Single dose and fractionated palliative irradiation for osseous metastases. Clin Radiol 27:405-408, 1976.

41. Gilbert HA, Kagan AR, Nussbaum H, Rao AR, Satzman J, Chan P, Allen B, Forsythe A. Evaluation of radiation therapy for bone metastases: Pain relief and quality of life. AJR Am J Roentgenol 129:1095-1096, 1977.

42. Tong D, Gillick L, Hendrickson FR. The palliation of symptomatic osseous metastases. Cancer 50:893-899, 1982.

43. Blitzer PH. Reanalysis of the RTOG study of the palliation of symptomatic osseous metastasis. Cancer 55:1468-1472, 1985.

44. Gunderson LL, Russell AH, Llewellyn HJ, Doppke KP, Tepper JE. Treatment planning for colorectal cancer: Radiation and surgical techniques and value of small bowel films. Int J Radiat Oncol Biol Phys 11:1379-1393, 1985.

45. Gunderson LL, Martenson JA. Cancers of the colon and rectum. In Levitt S, ed. Technological Basis of Radiation Therapy: Practical Clinical Applications, 2nd ed. Philadelphia: Lea & Febiger, 1992, pp 342-350.

46. Magrini S, Nelson H, Gunderson LL, Sim H. Sacropelvic resection and intraoperative electron irradiation in the management of recurrent anorectal cancer. Dis Colon Rectum 39:1-8, 1996.

47. Haddock MG, Gunderson LL, Wolff BG, Sim FH, Wieand HS, Nelson H, Devine RM, Robinow SJ, Dozois RR. Salvage of locally recurrent rectal cancer with resection and IORT after prior adjuvant irradiation ± chemotherapy. Int J Radiat Oncol Biol Phys. In press.

48. Martinez A, Edmundson GK, Cox RS, Gunderson LL, Howes AE. Combination of external beam irradiation and multiple-site perineal applicator (MUPIT) for treatment of locally advanced or recurrent prostatic, anorectal, and gynecologic malignancies. Int J Radiat Oncol Biol Phys 11:391-398, 1985.

49. Martinez A, Goffinet DR, Fee W, Goode R, Cox RS. [125]Iodine implants as an adjuvant to surgery and external beam radiotherapy in the management of locally advanced head and neck cancer. Cancer 51:973-979, 1983.

50. Sim FH. Management of lesions of hip and acetabulum. American Academy of Orthopaedic Surgeons 65th Annual Meeting, Instructional Course Lecture, 1998.

51. Yazawa Y, Frassica FJ, Chao EY, Pritchard DJ, Sim FH, Shives TC. Metastatic bone disease: A study of the surgical treatment of 166 pathologic humeral and femoral fractures. Clin Orthop 251:213-219, 1990.

52. Wanebo HJ, Koness RJ, Vezeridis MP, Cohen SI, Wrobleski DE. Pelvic resection of recurrent rectal cancer. Ann Surg 220: 586-597, 1994.

53. Wanebo HJ, Gaker DL, Whitehill R, Morgan RF, Constable WC. Pelvic recurrent of rectal cancer: Options for curative resection. Ann Surg 205:482-495, 1987.

Gynecologic Cancer

Julian C. Schink, M.D., and Howard H. Bailey, M.D.

Each year more than 75,000 gynecologic cancers are diagnosed in the United States. This means that every 6 minutes a new gynecologic cancer is diagnosed, with 25,000 of these women dying each year. For the survivors and for those who die of this disease, orthopedic complications of these cancers are relatively rare. Generally speaking, the musculoskeletal problems associated with gynecologic malignancy can be broken down into three categories: the consequence of direct tumor invasion, the consequence of metastatic disease, and the sequelae of treatment of the primary or metastatic disease. In this chapter we will explore the common gynecologic malignancies and describe the recognized musculoskeletal manifestations of these malignancies.

ENDOMETRIAL CANCER

Endometrial cancer is the most common gynecologic malignancy, occurring in approximately 37,000 women in the United States each year. This cancer arises from the endometrial cavity lining the uterus in women with a median age of 61 years. The risk factors for endometrial cancer are unopposed estrogen and medical conditions that increase circulating estrogen levels, including hypertension, diabetes, obesity, and anovulation. Because most women with endometrial cancer have irregular vaginal bleeding, this cancer is usually diagnosed at a relatively early stage, with 80% of women having stage I disease. A small fraction of women have advanced disease at presentation or aggressive histologic features that ultimately result in metastatic disease. It is primarily these women with metastatic disease or at high risk of having metastatic disease who are likely to have musculoskeletal complications of endometrial cancer.

The initial treatment of endometrial carcinoma involves total abdominal hysterectomy with bilateral salpingo-oophorectomy and, in most cases, pelvic and periaortic lymph node dissection. Although the therapeutic benefit of the lymph node dissection has been debated, it is clearly helpful in defining the extent of treatment that women with endometrial cancer need.[1] The primary mode of spread for endometrial cancer is via the pelvic lymphatic vessels. The obturator, iliac, and presacral lymph nodes are the most likely sites of metastatic nodal disease. A small number of women with endometrial cancer will ultimately have hematogenous metastases. These usually arise in women with high-risk histologic findings such as carcinosarcoma, clear cell carcinoma, and glassy cell carcinoma.

Adjuvant radiotherapy is frequently prescribed for women with nodal metastasis and for women at high risk of having nodal metastasis. In women who have undergone thorough lymph node staging, the radiation field is generally directed at the regions with known nodal metastasis and one node group higher. In women who have not had lymph node staging done but are considered at high risk of having lymph node metastasis because of deep myometrial invasion or poorly differentiated tumors, the radiation field is generally confined to the pelvis.

Approximately 1% to 2% of women with endometrial cancer have stage IV disease at presentation. Stage IV disease may include bone metastasis either by direct extension into the pubic symphysis or by extension of nodal metastasis into the sacrum or other pelvic bones. Rarely, women have had isolated bone metastasis as their first sign of endometrial carcinoma.[2,3] Most of these women will have stenosis of the endocervical canal or some other condition that prevents vaginal bleeding, thus allowing the uterine tumor to grow and spread extensively before diagnosis. Furthermore, most of these women with metastatic disease at presentation will have fairly high-risk histologic findings, such as a grade III tumor or clear cell carcinoma. It is rare for a woman to have an isolated bone metastasis, either to the femur or to the vertebral column, and no other evidence of metastatic disease. Most practitioners would combine locally directed therapy to include total abdominal hysterectomy, bilateral salpingo-oophorectomy, and lymph node staging with directed radiation for patients with bone metastasis. Consideration of systemic chemotherapy would also be entertained by some practitioners for patients who have isolated bone metastasis when first seen. The benefit of adjuvant systemic chemotherapy in the management of high-risk endometrial cancer has not been established but is the subject of a Gynecologic Oncology Group phase III trial.

The most common sites of metastasis or recurrence of endometrial cancer include the pelvic and periaortic lymph nodes, the vagina, the lungs, and the liver. The musculoskeletal manifestations are most commonly seen in association with either bone metastasis in women with advanced disease or local complications of regionally advanced disease. The manifestations of regional metastasis are usually either from pelvic nodal metastasis or from periaortic metastasis.

Pelvic lymph node metastases most commonly occur in the obturator fossa. These metastatic tumors may cause an obturator neuropathy and an associated motor deficit. Furthermore, massively enlarged obturator lymph nodes may cause external iliac vein obstruction with resultant thrombosis or venous occlusion. External iliac nodal metastases may grow into the psoas muscle, causing pain from the direct invasion. In the most extreme cases these metastases may extend through the psoas muscle and directly invade or impinge on the femoral nerve. The management of these pelvic recurrences has generally involved resection, followed by either intraoperative or external beam radiotherapy. The prognosis for these patients is not good; a large percentage ultimately manifest widespread systemic disease.

Periaortic nodal metastases occur in the lymph nodes that lie between the aorta and the anterior surface of the vertebrae. As these lymph nodes grow, they cause either direct invasion of the vertebral body or, more commonly, involvement of the nerve roots, resulting in neurogenic pain and lumbosacral neuropathies. Surgical resection of these periaortic nodes, particularly if they include nerve root invasion, is much more difficult than removing pelvic lymph nodes. Periaortic disease is also associated with a high incidence of systemic metastasis. Periaortic recurrence is often an incurable condition treated with only palliative intent because of the high likelihood of systemic metastasis and the surgical challenge of resection in patients with this disease and significant comorbidities, such as obesity, hypertension, and diabetes. Optimal palliative treatment would generally involve a combination of locally targeted radiotherapy and systemic chemotherapy, either simultaneously or sequentially. The most active chemotherapy drugs are the platinum analogs and doxorubicin. The use of paclitaxel is rapidly emerging as an attractive and relatively well-tolerated chemotherapy option. Megestrol acetate has a 20% response rate for these patients, lower than chemotherapy, but it has an excellent therapeutic index and is often a first choice in patients with advanced disease.

Complications of Treatment

The musculoskeletal complications of our therapies for endometrial cancer can be separated into three categories. The first category is complications associated with the standard surgical procedure, which is total abdominal hysterectomy with bilateral salpingo-oophorectomy and pelvic and periaortic lymph node dissection. At the time of surgical resection, femoral nerve injury can occur from direct compression of the nerve by either the Balfour retractor or another fixed retractor such as the Buchwalter retractor. When these retractors are used in massively obese patients, direct compression of the femoral nerve may occur, although this complication is relatively rare, occurring in fewer than 1% of patients. At the time of pelvic lymph node dissection, the nodes in the obturator fossa anterior to the obturator nerve are removed. Injury to the obturator nerve is a recognized but rare complication of this procedure.

The second type of treatment-related complication with musculoskeletal manifestations in endometrial carcinoma has to do with estrogen deprivation. Many patients with endometrial cancer develop the disease because of high circulating levels of endogenous estrogen, so they are generally not at great risk of having complications of estrogen deficiency. However, because endometrial carcinoma is highly curable, many of these women do live for a long time afterward and may be subsequently denied estrogen replacement. They may then have late sequelae of estrogen deficiency, including osteoporosis and fracture (Fig. 17-1). Ninety percent of recurrences of endometrial cancer occur within 3 years of diagnosis, so many gynecologic oncologists are relatively comfortable in prescribing estrogen to women 3 to 5 years after their initial diagnosis. The safety of prescribing estrogen to women after treatment of endometrial cancer is the subject of an ongoing Gynecologic Oncology Group trial.

The third manifestation of treatment-related toxic effects results from complications of radiation therapy. The most common radiation fields in endometrial carcinoma include the pelvis and occasionally the periaortic lymph nodes. Standard radiation doses to the pelvis are between 45 and 50 Gy, and periaortic radiation is generally limited to 45

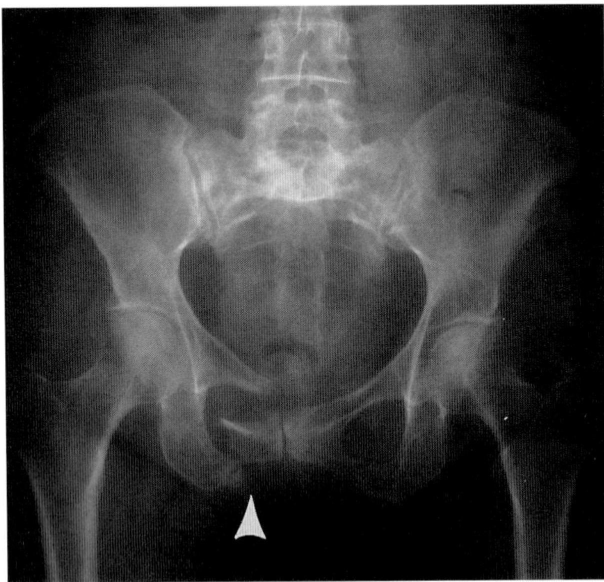

Fig. 17-1 Anteroposterior radiograph of the pelvis of a woman with a history of endometrial carcinoma and osteoporosis. A pelvic ring stress fracture is seen *(arrowhead).* The fracture became an asymptomatic fibrous nonunion.

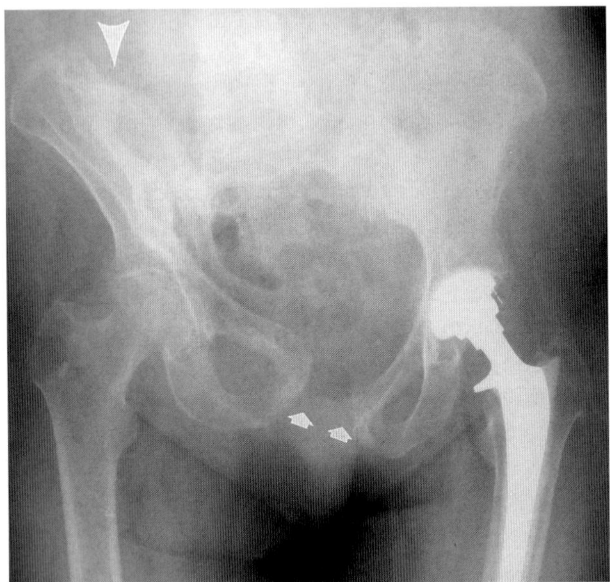

Fig. 17-2 Anteroposterior radiograph of the pelvis of a patient with a history of endometrial carcinoma and pelvic radiation. She previously had hip pain caused by avascular necrosis. A total hip replacement was performed. An unstable pelvic ring fracture with a symphysis diastasis *(small arrows)* and an iliac wing fracture *(arrowhead)* later developed.

Gy. Women with nodal metastases may receive a boost to approximately 60 Gy or even as high as 65 Gy to a small field. The consequences of this pelvic radiation can include radiation necrosis of the pubic symphysis or radiation exacerbation of lymphedema, pelvic ring fractures, and osteonecrosis of the femoral heads (Fig. 17-2). Because hypertension and diabetes are common comorbidities in these patients and are associated with radiation complications, it is not surprising that radiation necrosis may subsequently develop within the treatment field.

Uterine sarcoma is a rare uterine malignancy, making up 3% to 5% of all uterine cancers. Unfortunately, uterine sarcoma is generally much more aggressive than the more common endometrial carcinoma. Types of uterine sarcoma consist of uterine leiomyosarcoma, endometrial stromal sarcoma, and carcinosarcoma. Uterine leiomyosarcoma and endometrial stromal sarcomas are more commonly associated with hematogenous metastasis and thus isolated bone metastasis. There are several reports in the literature of isolated vertebral metastasis occurring in women who have been treated for uterine leiomyosarcoma. Metastases from uterine sarcoma are generally treated with focally directed radiotherapy with or without systemic chemotherapy. Although uterine sarcoma is often a systemic disease, the benefit of adjuvant systemic chemotherapy has not been demonstrated.

OVARIAN CANCER

Epithelial ovarian cancer is the leading cause of death from gynecologic cancer in the United States. Each year, approximately 25,000 new cases are diagnosed and 15,000 women die.[4] It is estimated that 1 in 70 American women will have ovarian cancer in her lifetime. The incidence of ovarian cancer increases with age. The incidence for women aged 40 to 44 years is 15 per 100,000; the incidence peaks in women aged 70 to 74 years, at 57 per 100,000. The median age of diagnosis is 63 years, and approximately half of patients are 65 years of age or older.[4] Risk factors for epithelial ovarian cancer somewhat mirror risk factors for breast cancer and include nulliparity, the use of ovulation-inducing drugs, and a history of breast cancer. Factors associated with a decreased risk include a history of multiple pregnancies and oral contraceptive use. Hereditary cancer syndromes, including ovarian cancer, have been established but will not be reviewed in this chapter.

Epithelial ovarian cancer can spread by one of three methods: exfoliation and implantation throughout the intraperitoneal surfaces, through the lymphatic system, and through the blood. Thus more than 75% of patients with ovarian cancer have disease metastatic throughout the peritoneal cavity at presentation. The most common presenting symptom is abdominal discomfort or pain. An elevated concentration of CA 125 (a monoclonal antibody raised against the cell surface glycoprotein found on the cell surface of various epithelial cells) is helpful but is not diagnostic for ovarian cancer because several benign and other malignant conditions can produce an elevation.[5] One of the most important factors in the successful treatment of epithelial ovarian cancer is adequate and aggressive surgical staging and tumor debulking if necessary. The primary reason is the chemoresponsiveness of epithelial ovarian cancer. Surgical staging helps identify those early-stage patients who might benefit from systemic chemotherapy and aggressive surgical debulking. This is important because the volume of residual disease after cytoreductive surgery is directly correlated with survival.[4] The cornerstone of treatment of metastatic ovarian cancer is combination chemotherapy. Response rates for current chemotherapy regimens are >75% in metastatic ovarian cancer, and significant survival advantages have been observed in some chemotherapy regimens.[6] The effectiveness of systemic chemotherapy in the recurrent setting depends on whether the patient has been exposed to platinum-based chemotherapy and whether it was effective. Thus it is important to remember that even in the recurrent setting there may be effective palliative options for epithelial ovarian cancer. Another option is radiation therapy, which has significant value in the palliative setting of ovarian cancer and may even have curative potential in the setting of microscopic disease only.[4]

Musculoskeletal Manifestations

The likelihood that orthopedic problems will develop as a direct result of ovarian cancer is rare. An autopsy study of the sites of metastases in epithelial ovarian cancer noted the following incidences: peritoneum, 80%; lymph nodes, abdominal, 60%;

pelvis, 50%; thorax, 30%; neck, 15%; small bowel, 45%; large bowel, 50%; liver, 50%; lung, 30%; pleura, 30%; and brain, bone, and pericardium, <5%.[7]

Abdul-Karim et al.[8] reviewed autopsies performed between 1948 and 1984 on 305 patients with primary carcinomas of the cervix, endometrium, ovary, fallopian tubes, vulva, and vagina. Skeletal metastases were detected before death and at autopsy in 49 total cases (16%) at the following sites: cervix, 20; endometrium, 17; ovary, 7; vulva, 4; and fallopian tube, 1. No patients had bone metastases as the only manifestation of metastatic disease. The authors also reviewed the incidence of osseous metastases from ovarian cancer. They quoted an incidence of 0% to 14%, with most studies noting an incidence of <5%. Their limited experience suggested that osseous metastases were a late manifestation of the disease, with poor survival time (<6 months) after diagnosis of osseous metastases. The most common site of metastases from ovarian carcinomas in their study was the vertebrae (Fig. 17-3). Other sites included the ribs, skull, pelvis, and femur. For the clinician, the incidence of certain metastatic sites during the course of the disease more accurately reflects the likelihood of encountering a problem than autopsy studies. Dauplat et al.[9] reviewed the clinical history of 255 patients with metastatic ovarian carcinoma who had stage IV disease. Of the 255 patients, 97 (38%) had the following stage IV diseases during the course of the carcinoma: malignant pleural effusions, 63; parenchymal liver metastases, 24; parenchymal lung metastases, 18; distant lymph node metastases, 18; subcutaneous nodules, 9; malignant pericardial effusion, 6; metastases to the central nervous system, 5; and bone metastases, 4. Risk factors for stage IV disease were bulky abdominal disease and positive retroperitoneal lymph nodes. Kumar et al.[10] reviewed 103 patients with ovarian cancer for a 3-year period and observed 4 cases (3 carcinomas, 1 germ cell cancer) of symptomatic bone metastases. All four patients had severe localized bone pain and bone swelling.

Because orthopedic specialists frequently are asked for their interpretation of bone scintigraphy results, we report on articles detailing soft tissue localization of radiotracer in patients with ovarian carcinoma. Bader[11] described a patient with known widespread ovarian carcinoma who, on bone scintigraphy, showed intense uptake in the area of the

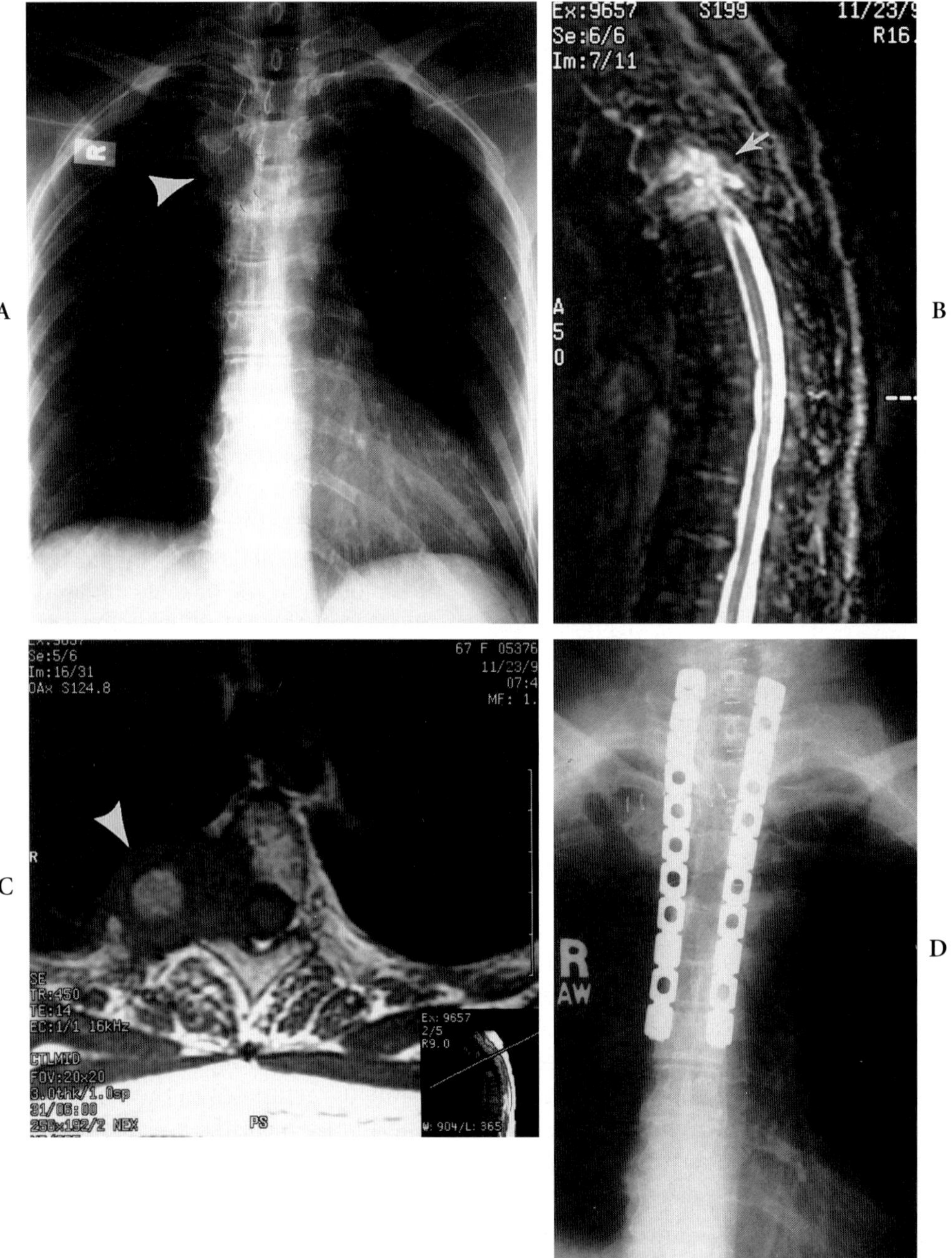

Fig. 17-3 **A,** Radiograph of the chest of a patient with a history of ovarian carcinoma. Destruction of the thoracic vertebrae with a soft tissue mass is seen *(arrowhead).* **B,** Sagittal magnetic resonance image, revealing tumor compressing spinal cord at the third thoracic vertebra with a soft tissue mass *(arrow).* **C,** Axial T1-weighted magnetic resonance image, showing soft tissue mass *(arrowhead)* with destruction of the vertebral body. **D,** The patient had an increasing neurologic deficit. An operative decompression with posterior stabilization was performed. The pathologic changes were consistent with the prior ovarian cancer.

transverse colon. Metastatic carcinoma surrounding the transverse colon was confirmed by computed tomography (CT) and single-photon emission computed tomography. Uysal et al.[12] and Ranner et al.[13] also described the detection of soft tissue metastases from ovarian carcinoma on bone scintigraphy. They noted similar cases of intense uptake of tracer in the soft tissues, corresponding to the liver, pelvis, and peritoneal surfaces, confirmed by CT or surgical biopsy. Ranner et al. hypothesized that the psammoma bodies throughout the tumor tissue were the substrate for the extraosseous tracer uptake. However, despite the observations noted here, bone scintigraphy is not considered part of the standard staging of ovarian cancers, including germ cell and stromal cell tumors. Mettler et al.[14] described their institutional experience with performing radiographic bone surveys or bone scintigraphy examinations on 104 patients with ovarian carcinoma. Of the 106 bone scans performed, 4 patients had positive scans for osseous metastases and 2 had equivocal scans. Of the 4 positive scans, 3 were obtained at initial diagnosis. In this series, fewer than 3% of the patients had osseous metastases at the initial staging. The three patients mentioned had stage III, grade 3 adenocarcinomas and also had corresponding bone pain. The authors did not observe soft tissue localization of disease, as mentioned earlier. Radiographic bone surveys or serum alkaline phosphatase levels were not any more helpful at determining bone disease. The authors believe that routine bone scintigraphy is not indicated in ovarian carcinoma and, rather, should be reserved for patients with symptoms. Harbert et al.[15] reported radionuclide scans performed in patients with gynecologic cancer from 1978 to 1980. None of the 40 patients with ovarian cancer who underwent bone scintigraphy had positive results. Karkavitsas[16] performed bone scintigraphy on 37 patients with ovarian carcinoma and observed no findings consistent with bone metastases.

A review by Simon and Bartucci[17] detailed their experience with 46 patients examined for skeletal metastases of unknown origin. Only 1 of the 46 patients was proved to have ovarian carcinoma as the primary tumor. The authors recommended the following diagnostic study for patients with skeletal metastases at presentation: medical history and physical examination, routine laboratory studies, chest radiograph, bone scintigraphy, CT of the abdomen and pelvis, and mammography in women.

An indirect but important topic pertaining to ovarian cancer is the long-term consequences of being treated for and surviving ovarian cancer. Douchi et al.[18] examined, for bone mineral loss, some young Japanese women undergoing chemotherapy for ovarian cancer. The authors studied 15 women (mean age, 38 years; range, 30 to 46) with ovarian cancer who were treated with a standard 6-month regimen of cisplatin, doxorubicin, and cyclophosphamide. Fifteen age-matched women whose ovaries had been surgically removed for other reasons served as control subjects. None of the women received hormonal treatment. Bone mineral density (BMD) of the lumbar spine (L2 to L4) was measured by dual-energy x-ray absorptiometry before and after chemotherapy. The two groups were compared for percentage change of BMD for the same period. Measurement of fat and lean mass was also performed and considered in the comparisons. The mean BMD decreased to 87% ± 2% after 6 cycles of chemotherapy and to 98% ± 0.4% after 6 months in the control subjects. Low lean mass was an independent predictor of BMD loss during chemotherapy. This study adds support to the concept that chemotherapy-induced BMD loss is more than just hormonal manipulation.

Selected Case Reports

Noguchi and Mori[19] described a patient who underwent tumor debulking and irradiation for ovarian carcinoma; 7 years later, isolated metastasis to the sternum and costae was found. After resection of the bone metastasis, adjuvant chemotherapy and a radioimmunoconjugate were administered. The patient has been disease free for 4 years after the surgery. Dinh et al.[20] described two patients with ovarian carcinoma and symptomatic bone metastases and also reviewed the medical literature. Ontell and Greenspan[21] presented a case of a 75-year-old patient with ovarian carcinoma without obvious dissemination elsewhere and diffuse blastic metastases to bone. Patient survival was 28 months after the diagnosis of bone metastases. Two separate investigators reported on observed bone metastases in patients with endometrioid carcinoma of the ovary.[22,23] Den Boon et al.[24] reported on a case of a 46-year-old woman in whom conus-cauda syndrome was the initial presenting symptom of an endodermal sinus tumor of the ovary.

Related Diseases

A review of musculoskeletal syndromes and malignancy notes a likely association between dermatomyositis or inflammatory myopathies and ovarian cancer.[25] In a series of 140 cases of inflammatory myopathies, seven patients developed ovarian cancer. Young and Scully[26] reported on 21 cases of sarcomas metastasizing to the ovary. The primary lesions were predominantly uterine sarcomas (3 leiomyosarcomas, 8 stromal sarcomas) and soft tissue sarcomas arising in or near the gastrointestinal system. Exceptions were a hemangiosarcoma of the heart, osteosarcoma of the maxilla, chondrosarcoma of the rib, and Ewing's sarcoma. In 3 cases the ovarian tumor(s) preceded detection of the primary tumor by 4 to 10 months. Regarding metastatic disease to the ovary, there also was a case report of a sacral chordoma's metastasizing to the ovary 3½ years after initial resection.[27] A somewhat similar case report describes the presumed finding of the ovary as a primary site for osteosarcoma.[28]

CERVICAL CANCER

Cervical cancer is the third most common malignancy in the United States, occurring in approximately 17,000 women each year and resulting in about 6000 deaths per year. The widespread use of the Papanicolaou test in developed countries has markedly lowered the incidence of this cancer, but it remains the leading cause of cancer death of women in many underdeveloped countries. In the United States the majority of women dying of cervical cancer have not had a Papanicolaou test in the preceding 5 years. Unfortunately, several studies have documented that women dying of cervical cancer without having had a Papanicolaou test have had encounters with the health care system during the preceding years but were not screened. The median age at onset of cervical cancer is only 45 years, so the number of years of life lost to this disease and the impact on families is great.

The risk factors for cervical cancer include early age at intercourse, multiple sexual partners, and partners with multiple sexual partners, all of which point to a component of sexually transmitted disease. The human papillomavirus has been implicated as a significant etiologic factor in the development of cervical cancer. Other cofactors, such as cigarette smoking, also appear to play a significant role.

The presenting symptoms of cervical carcinoma are generally vaginal bleeding or profuse, watery vaginal discharge. Occasionally, vaginal bleeding is associated with intercourse (postcoital bleeding), which is characteristic of significant cervical pathologic changes. Early cervical cancer, either microinvasive or stage IB, may be identified on a Papanicolaou test. The more advanced cervical carcinomas generally occur in women who have not had a Papanicolaou test, and the disease tends to spread throughout the pelvis before symptoms become so dominant that the disease is identified. These symptoms include pelvic pain, low back pain, leg swelling, and malodorous vaginal discharge. In rare cases, patients will have copious vaginal bleeding at presentation and will require emergency embolization or radiotherapy.

The treatment of cervical carcinoma has developed into a multimodality approach. Small or microinvasive tumors can be managed with radical hysterectomy and pelvic lymphadenectomy. However, in more advanced disease the combination of radiotherapy and concurrent chemotherapy has become the standard of care. Concurrent radiation therapy and chemotherapy using either cisplatin, 5-fluorouracil (5-FU), or cisplatin with 5-FU has been shown in several phase III trials to provide better pelvic control and better survival for women with all stages of cervical cancer. The cure rate for stage I cervical cancer is a similar 85% whether surgery or radiotherapy has been used. Surgery allows preservation of ovarian function and avoids late radiation complications such as vaginal stenosis and radiation enteritis. For women with large stage IB tumors, tumors >6 cm, or stage II and III tumors, radiation therapy appears to be a more effective treatment as measured by pelvic control and survival.

The musculoskeletal complications associated with direct extension of this disease are similar to those described for endometrial cancer. Cervical tumors, however, tend to spread directly into the parametrial tissues adjacent to the cervix and bladder and may directly invade the pelvic musculature, including the pelvic floor and the pelvic bones. The sacrum is the most commonly involved of these structures. Direct extension to the obturator internus muscle is also occasionally seen in stage III disease. This disease also spreads by lymphatic or hematogenous metastasis. Hematogenous metastasis is more common in cervical cancer than in endometrial carcinoma.

The musculoskeletal manifestations of metastatic disease include the consequences of obturator lymph node metastasis leading to an obturator neuropathy. In addition, widespread pelvic node metastasis can lead to obstruction of the pelvic lymphatic vessels or pelvic vasculature, causing chronically edematous lower extremities. Metastasis to the vertebral column is also seen in advanced cervical cancer and is hypothesized to occur from spread via Batson's plexus. If bone metastases are isolated, a directed combination of radiotherapy and chemotherapy is the preferred treatment, with possible surgical stabilization if necessary (Fig. 17-4).

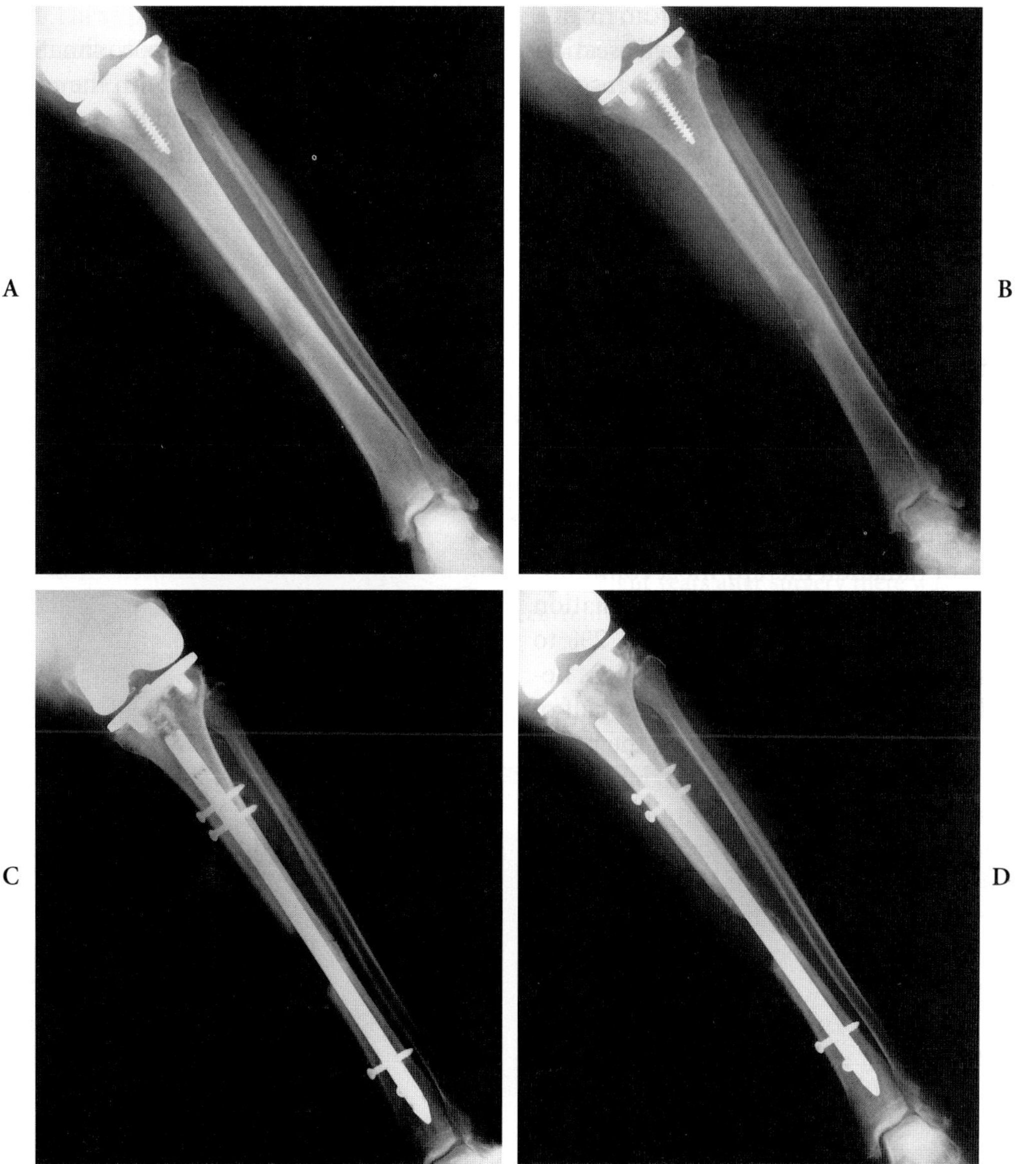

Fig. 17-4 **A,** Anteroposterior radiograph of the tibia, demonstrating a mid-shaft lytic lesion in a patient with a history of metastatic cervical carcinoma. A prior total knee replacement is seen. **B,** The tumor progressed despite radiation therapy. The patient had increasing pain. **C,** Operative stabilization was performed with curettage of the metastatic lesion. A locked intramedullary nail was used. **D,** The tumor continues to destroy increasing amounts of tibia. The patient eventually succumbed to her widespread metastatic disease.

lymph nodes by embolization rather than direct extension, wide radical excision of the vulvar lesion has evolved to become the most common surgical approach to vulvar lesions. The wide radical excision allows preservation of adjacent structures and some of the cosmetic appearance of the vulva. Furthermore, wound healing problems are considerably improved with the less radical procedure. Management of the groin nodes by using separate incisions has also significantly decreased the incidence of wound breakdown. With the traditional en bloc procedure, between 50% and 75% of women had significant wound infections. The inguinal-femoral lymph node dissection continues to carry with it the most significant long-term complications. However, lower extremity edema as a result of either lymphedema or chronic lymphangitis continues to be a problem for approximately 15% of patients. It should be noted that exacerbation of lymphedema or lymphangitis may occur in women who have a history of vulvar cancer and who subsequently undergo orthopedic procedures to the lower extremities or hip.

The musculoskeletal complications associated with vulvar cancer occur primarily in women who receive adjuvant inguinofemoral radiation therapy. Because this radiotherapy is often delivered with a two-field anteroposterior-posteroanterior port, a significant dose of radiation may be delivered to the femoral head. This radiotherapy, when delivered to elderly women with osteopenia, can result in radiation necrosis or an insufficiency fracture of the femoral head or neck (Fig. 17-5). In women who have extensive inguinal node metastasis or difficult groin dissections, injury to the femoral nerve may occur. The femoral neuropathy that develops from groin dissection is usually only partial and generally resolves with time.

GESTATIONAL TROPHOBLASTIC DISEASE: CHORIOCARCINOMA

Choriocarcinoma is a malignancy that arises from trophoblasts, usually in association with a live birth, miscarriage, abortion, ectopic pregnancy, or hydatidiform mole. This malignancy is rare, occurring in association with only 1 in 40,000 pregnancy events. Unfortunately, when this cancer does develop, it is generally in young women of reproductive age and can present a confusing picture.

Choriocarcinoma is characterized by its production of human chorionic gonadotropin (hCG). This tumor marker is an invaluable tool in the monitoring of treatment for choriocarcinoma, but it can also lead to a confusing picture before the initial diagnosis. It is not uncommon for a woman to have evidence of metastatic disease and a positive hCG pregnancy test result, leading to a confusing and difficult moral dilemma. It is not until ultrasonography establishes that a patient is not pregnant that clinicians begin to consider choriocarcinoma as a diagnosis. Choriocarcinoma metastasizes by hematogenous spread and is commonly seen with lung metastases, but it also can be found with vaginal lesions, hepatic lesions, brain metastases, or bone metastases.

Choriocarcinoma is highly sensitive to chemotherapy, and now 85% of women with metastatic disease are ultimately cured. Fortunately, because of its excellent responsiveness to chemotherapy, it is rare that patients require any other type of intervention for choriocarcinoma. This uncommon cancer can be difficult to manage, however; a series of gestational trophoblastic disease centers have therefore been established throughout the United States. It is generally wise to refer any patient with choriocarcinoma to a gestational trophoblastic disease center for the development of appropriate management guidelines, because the experience base in most communities is small.

CONCLUSION

Fortunately the musculoskeletal manifestations of gynecologic malignancy are rare. The majority of these complications are associated with the direct invasion of nodal metastasis into adjacent structures. The most common of these structures include the obturator nerve, the obturator internus muscle, the psoas muscle, the femoral nerve, and the lumbosacral vertebrae. In each case it is imperative that a thorough survey for metastatic disease be carried out because ultimately the best palliative therapy can be designed only with thorough consideration of all the disease sites. Most sites of bone metastasis in gynecologic cancer are responsive to directed radiotherapy and can be managed in a palliative mode in concert with the radiotherapists. In a small number of women, unstable fractures of either the vertebrae or extremities require surgical intervention and stabilization. Generally speaking, the majority of women with gynecologic malignancy are cured. However, women with metastatic gynecologic cancers that have spread to the point of musculoskeletal involvement have a much more dismal prognosis. Gynecologic oncologists embrace the multispecialty approach to these cancers and will actively work with orthopedic colleagues to design the most individualized treatment possible.

REFERENCES

 1. Petereit DG. Complete surgical staging in endometrial cancer provides prognostic information only. Semin Radiat Oncol 10(1):8-14, 2000.
 2. Malicky ES, Kostic KJ, Jacob JH, Allen WC. Endometrial carcinoma presenting with an isolated osseous metastasis: A case report and review of the literature. Eur J Gynaecol Oncol 18:492-494, 1997.
 3. Petru E, Malleier M, Lax S, Lahousen M, Ehall R, Pickel H, Winter R. Solitary metastasis in the tarsus preceding the diagnosis of primary endometrial cancer: A case report. Eur J Gynaecol Oncol 16:387-390, 1995.
 4. Ozols RF, Rubin SC, Thomas GM, Robboy SJ. Epithelial ovarian cancer. In Hoskins WJ, Perez CA, Young RC, eds. Principles and Practice of Gynecologic Oncology, 2nd ed. Philadelphia: Lippincott-Raven, 1997, pp 919-986.
 5. Evans AC, Berchuck A. Tumor markers. In Hoskins WJ, Perez CA, Young RC, eds. Principles and Practice of Gynecologic Oncology, 2nd ed. Philadelphia: Lippincott-Raven, 1997, pp 177-196.
 6. McGuire WP, Hoskins WJ, Brady WF, et al. Cyclophosphamide and cisplatin compared with paclitaxel and cisplatin in patients with stage III and stage IV ovarian cancer. N Engl J Med 334:1-6, 1996.
 7. Julian CG, Goss J, Blanchard K, Woodruff JD. Biologic behavior of primary ovarian malignancy. Obstet Gynecol 44:873-874, 1974.
 8. Abdul-Karim F, Kida M, Wentz B, Carter JR, Sorensen K, Macfee M, Zika J, Makley J. Bone metastasis from gynecologic carcinomas: A clinicopathologic study. Gynecol Oncol 39:108-114, 1990.
 9. Dauplat J, Hacker N, Nieberg R, Berek J, Rose T, Sagae S. Distant metastases in epithelial ovarian carcinoma. Cancer 60:1561-1566, 1987.
10. Kumar L, Bhargava VL, Rao RC, Rath GK, Katarina SP. Bone metastasis in ovarian cancer. Asia Oceania J Obstet Gynaecol 18:309-313, 1992.
11. Bader D. Colon visualization on a bone scan from metastatic ovarian carcinoma: SPECT correlation. Clin Nucl Med 22:52-54, 1997.
12. Uysal U, Kostakoglu L, Elahi N, Aydingoz U, Firat D, Bedik C. Can bone scintigraphy detect additional metastatic sites unrevealed by CT in patients with recurrent ovarian carcinoma? Radiat Med 15:55-58, 1997.
13. Ranner G, Ebner F, Fueger GF, Kullnig P, Tamussino K. Abdominal metastases of an ovarian cancer demonstrated on bone imaging. Clin Nucl Med 14:124-126, 1989.
14. Mettler FA Jr, Christie JH, Crow NE Jr, Garcia JF, Wicks JD, Bartow SA. Radionuclide bone scan, radiographic bone survey, and alkaline phosphatase: Studies of limited value in asymptomatic patients with ovarian carcinoma. Cancer 50:1483-1485, 1982.
15. Harbert JC, Rocha L, Smith FP, Delgado G. The efficacy of radionuclide liver and bone scans in the evaluation of gynecologic cancers. Cancer 49:1040-1042, 1982.
16. Karkavitsas N. Bone and liver metastases in uterine, cervical and ovarian cancer. Rontgenblatter 41:326-328, 1988.
17. Simon MA, Bartucci EJ. The search for the primary tumor in patients with skeletal metastases of unknown origin. Cancer 58:1088-1095, 1986.
18. Douchi T, Kosha S, Kan R, Nakamura S, Oki T, Nagata Y. Predictors of bone mineral loss in patients with ovarian cancer treated with anticancer agents. Obstet Gynecol 90:12-15, 1997.
19. Noguchi H, Mori A. Case report: A case of ovarian cancer with metastasis to the sternum and costae. Gynecol Oncol 52:416-419, 1994.
20. Dinh TV, Liebowitz BL, Hannigan EV, Schnadig VJ, Doherty MG. Bone metastasis in epithelial ovarian carcinoma. Int J Gynaecol Obstet 52:173-176, 1996.
21. Ontell FK, Greenspan A. Blastic osseous metastases in ovarian carcinoma. Can Assoc Radiol J 46:231-234, 1995.
22. Turan I, Sjoden GO, Kalen A. Ovarian carcinoma metastasis to the little finger: A case report. Acta Orthop Scand 61:185-186, 1990.
23. Sansom HE, Fisher C, King DM. Isolated bone metastasis from an endometrioid ovarian carcinoma. Clin Radiol 54:135-137, 1999.
24. den Boon J, Avezaat C, van der Gaast A, Koops W, Huikeshoven FJ. Conus-cauda syndrome as a presenting symptom of endodermal sinus tumor of the ovary. Gynecol Oncol 57:121-125, 1995.
25. Seda H, Alarcon G. Musculoskeletal syndromes associated with malignancies. Curr Opin Rheumatol 7:48-53, 1995.
26. Young R, Scully R. Sarcomas metastatic to the ovary: A report of 21 cases. Int Soc Gynecol Pathol 9:231-252, 1990.
27. Zukerberg LR, Young RH. Chordoma metastatic to the ovary. Arch Pathol Lab Med 114:208-210, 1990.
28. Sakata H, Hirahara T, Ryu A, Sawada T, Yamamoto M, Sakurai I. Primary osteosarcoma of the ovary: A case report. Acta Pathol Jpn 41:311-317, 1991.

Multiple Myeloma

Walter L. Longo, M.D., *Steven P. Howard,* M.D., Ph.D., *and John P. Heiner,* M.D.

Multiple Myeloma

Multiple myeloma is a disease of the bone marrow that can affect the structural integrity of bones. The disease is characterized by abnormal growth and accumulation of a population of malignant cells (monoclonal plasma cells) that produce abnormal immunoglobulins known as monoclonal proteins. These malignant cells are B lymphocytes, and there are consistent chromosomal translocations that frequently involve the immunoglobulin gene locus, which has led to the identification of potential oncogenes that may also play a role in the development of this disease.

These malignant B lymphocytes reside in the bone marrow and are supported by a nonmalignant population of stromal cells, which may also produce cytokines that enhance the growth of these B cells and prevent apoptosis.[1] The infiltration of the bones with these malignant cells leads to osteolysis, which affects the structural integrity of the bone.[2] Lytic lesions that have a typical punched-out appearance on plain radiographs are formed. The bone scan is often normal because osteoblast stimulation is minimal.

INCIDENCE

Multiple myeloma accounts for about 1% of all cancers and about 10% of the hematologic cancers. Multiple myeloma has been identified in a skeleton from the late Middle Ages.[3] The incidence of multiple myeloma is approximately 4 per 100,000 cases

---

Table 18-1   Diagnostic criteria for multiple myeloma, myeloma variants, and monoclonal gammopathy of unknown significance

Multiple myeloma

Major criteria

Plasmacytoma on tissue biopsy
Bone marrow plasmacytosis with >30% plasma cells
Monoclonal globulin spike on serum electrophoresis exceeding 3.5 g/dl for G peaks or 2 g/dl for A peaks, ≥1 g/24 h of κ- or λ-light chain excretion on urine electrophoresis in the presence of amyloidosis

Minor criteria

Bone marrow plasmacytosis 10% to 30% plasma cells
Monoclonal globulin spike present but less than the level defined above
Lytic bone lesions
Residual normal IgM <50 mg/dl, IgA <100 mg/dl, or IgG <600 mg/dl
Diagnosis is confirmed when any of the following features are documented in symptomatic patients with clearly progressive disease. The diagnosis of myeloma requires a minimum of one major + one minor criterion or three minor criteria that must include a + b, i.e.,
   I + b, I + c, I + d (I + a not sufficient)
   II + b, II + c, II + d
   III + a, III + c, III + d
   a + b + c, a + b + d

Indolent myeloma (same as myeloma except)

No bone lesions or only limited bone lesions (≤3 lytic lesions): no compression fractures
M-component levels: (a) IgG <7 g/dl; (b) IgG <5/dl
No symptoms or associated disease features, i.e.:
   Performance status >70%
   Hemoglobin >10 g/dl
   Serum calcium normal
   Serum creatinine <2 mg/dl
   No infections

Smoldering myeloma (same as indolent myeloma except)

No bone lesions
Bone marrow plasma cells ≤30%

Monoclonal gammopathy of unknown significance

Monoclonal gammopathy
M-component level
   IgG ≤3.5 g/dl
   IgA ≤2 g/dl
   BJ protein ≤1 g/24 h
Bone marrow plasma cells <10%
No bone lesions
No symptoms

From Salmon SE, Cassady JR. Plasma cell neoplasms. In De Vita VT Jr, Hellman S, Rosenberg SA, eds. Cancer: Principles and Practice of Oncology, 4th ed. Philadelphia: JB Lippincott, 1993, p 1984.
IgA, immunoglobulin A; IgG, immunoglobulin G; IgM, immunoglobulin M; BJ, Bence Jones light chain.

per year and is twice as high in African Americans as in white persons. Median age at diagnosis is approximately 65 years, with fewer than 3% of all patients being less than 40 years of age.

Other factors associated with risk of development of this disease include tobacco abuse and exposure to asbestos, benzene, and industrial and agricultural toxins. There appears to be a slight trend toward increased incidence in the midwestern agricultural states. Multiple myeloma has been reported in familial clusters of two or more first-degree relatives and in an identical twin. This supports its genetic elements in some patients, but as yet no specific inherited gene is known to put a person at high risk.

DIAGNOSTIC EVALUATION

If multiple myeloma is the suspected diagnosis, the patient should have a complete blood cell count, including hemoglobin, white cell count with differential, and platelet count, in addition to routine history and physical examination. Serum chemistry levels should be studied, including the serum calcium, creatinine, BUN, and serum uric acid values (Table 18-1).

The radiologic workup for multiple myeloma includes what is commonly referred to as a skeletal survey. This includes radiographs of bone marrow–making bones including the skull (Fig. 18-1), anteroposterior (AP) and lateral films of the entire spine, and radiographs of the pelvis and long bones. Technetium bone scans may be performed for myeloma, but many lesions may have minimal uptake of the technetium (Fig. 18-2). The standard radiograph will often show a sharply demarcated lytic lesion with lytic reactive bone around it (Fig. 18-3).

The laboratory workup must also include a serum electrophoresis with serum immunophoresis. Quantitation of serum immunoglobulins is indicated. Patients often are noted to have very high monoclonal protein levels but markedly low and abnormal levels of healthy serum immunoglobulin. A routine urinalysis and urine immunophoresis are indicated if proteinuria is present. It is also helpful at the baseline to obtain a 24-hour urine collection, which would include study of the urine protein excretion and creatinine clearance.

Ancillary laboratory studies include determination of the serum β_2-microglobulin, serum lactate

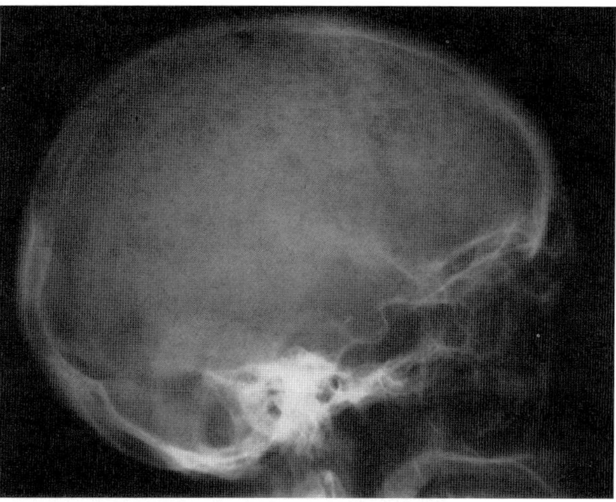

Fig. 18-1 Lateral radiograph of the skull demonstrating the multiple lytic lesions typical of myeloma. The lesions were asymptomatic and were found on a skeletal survey.

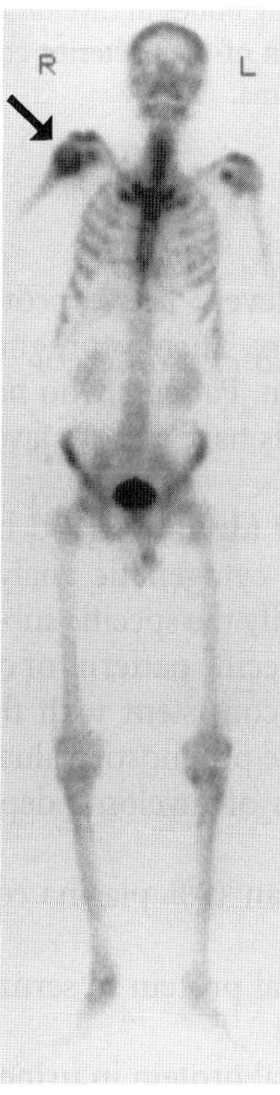

Fig. 18-2 A technetium bone scan reveals an area of increased uptake of a lytic lesion in the right proximal humerus. A bone scan may still be a useful tool in evaluating patients with myeloma. Some lesions may not be seen on a bone scan but are picked up on the skeletal survey.

MANAGEMENT

When one is making decisions about treatment of multiple myeloma, all symptoms, physical findings, and laboratory data must be considered. All patients who have anemia, hypercalcemia, or renal insufficiency should be considered candidates for chemotherapy. Patients with lytic bone lesions or extramedullary plasmacytomas are also in need of treatment, either radiotherapy or chemotherapy.

Chemotherapy

The most common drugs used to treat older patients (usually patients over 70 years of age) are melphalan and prednisone. Administration of melphalan (usually 8 mg/m^2 for 4 days) and prednisone (40 mg/m^2 for 4 days) is repeated every 4 to 6 weeks, with monthly pamidronate (90 mg intravenously) to help maintain bone integrity.[9] Pamidronate is a bisphosphonate that helps to decrease skeletal pain and fractures in patients with multiple myeloma.[10-12]

Many times patients will tolerate the oral chemotherapy agents with very few side effects. There are various schedules for administering various combinations of alkylating agents with steroids in the treatment of this disease. The primary consideration in multiple myeloma is that standard chemotherapy is not curative; if pain is alleviated and laboratory parameters return to normal, many patients are considered at a plateau phase of the disease and chemotherapy can be withheld.

One other common combination of drugs is often referred to as the M2 protocol, which includes vincristine, carmustine (BCNU), melphalan, cyclophosphamide, and prednisone. In a randomized trial done by the Eastern Cooperative Oncology Group with 222 patients randomly assigned to BVMCP and 221 randomly assigned to melphalan and prednisone, the response rate was approximately 72% for the five-drug combination and only 51% for standard melphalan and prednisone. A difference in survival was not statistically significant between these 2 groups.[13] Both regimens have a high subjective response rate and are effective in providing symptomatic improvement in patients.

In general, chemotherapy should be continued for at least 1 year until a documented plateau has occurred. Continued chemotherapy with these alkylating agents for more than 2 or 3 years can lead

to the development of myelodysplastic syndrome or acute leukemias.[14] Patients, therefore, should be followed up closely for changes in blood cell counts during chemotherapy, which could reveal a myelodysplastic syndrome. A second-line chemotherapy regimen is referred to as VAD (vincristine, doxorubicin [Adriamycin], dexamethasone).[15] These drugs are given by intravenous infusions with doxorubicin and vincristine infusing continuously over 96 hours. Doses commonly used for doxorubicin are 12 mg/m^2 per day and for vincristine a total of 2 mg given over the 96-hour infusion. The dexamethasone is administered in oral form, with 40 mg given daily through days 1 to 4, 9 to 12, and 17 to 20. This cycle is repeated every 28 days, and many times the dexamethasone is given for only 4 days on an alternating cycle because of the toxicity of the steroid. This regimen, which was developed as a salvage regimen for patients in whom standard alkylating agent–containing therapies had failed, is now commonly used for induction therapy to obtain the plateau phase. Stem cells can then be collected, as this chemotherapy is not very damaging to the bone marrow. Once stem cells have been collected, an autologous stem cell transplant is used to consolidate the remission.

Radiotherapy

With the exception of solitary plasmacytoma of bone and extramedullary plasmacytoma, for which localized radiation therapy is the primary treatment of choice, local radiation therapy has more of a palliative or adjunctive role in the management of multiple myeloma. Historically, before the development of effective systemic chemotherapy in the late 1960s, total-body irradiation (TBI) techniques were developed as primary therapy for untreated multiple myeloma at presentation and in later years to treat chemotherapy-refractory disease.[16-18] Responses were observed and reasonable palliation of bone symptoms was achieved, but because of the toxic effects of TBI,[19] hemibody irradiation (HBI) soon replaced TBI as a treatment modality and continued as a therapeutic option, either as a single agent or in combination systemic chemotherapy throughout the 1970s and mid 1980s.[20-22] The toxic effects associated with HBI for patients with multiple myeloma have placed serious limitations on its use in the nontransplant setting. These are primarily hematologic in nature and can be attributed to characteristics relatively common to this patient population, including increased patient age, heavy prior treatment, and poor performance status.[23] The Southwest Oncology Group has evaluated HBI used for consolidation after chemotherapy with a randomized clinical trial. Although feasibility could be demonstrated, the investigators found that additional chemotherapy was superior to sequential HBI for consolidation. As a result of this and other smaller clinical trials the use of HBI as a component of primary therapy for untreated or refractory multiple myeloma has declined substantially.[24] However, in the past decade the use of TBI as component of the preparatory regimen for bone marrow transplant in patients with multiple myeloma has been increasing. In this instance, myeloablative doses of chemotherapy with or without TBI are followed by infusion of hematopoietic stem cells derived from blood or bone marrow.[25,26]

Skeletal complications associated with progressive bone disease are a common clinical management issue in multiple myeloma. Radiologic evaluation of the majority of patients with multiple myeloma reveals a mixture of lytic disease and osteoporosis. The indications for radiotherapy include impending spinal cord or nerve compression, prevention of impending pathologic fracture in weightbearing bones, and palliation of bone pain. The efficacy of conventional megavoltage radiotherapy for these indications is well documented.[27-29] The mechanism of bone destruction characteristic of multiple myeloma is primarily osteoclastic, resulting from the activation of latent osteoclast-activating factor by the plasma cell, which in turn stimulates osteoclastic bone absorption. Theoretically, the pain relief and the resolution of the osteoclastic processes observed after local radiotherapy in multiple myeloma results from a reduction in the number of plasma cells locally, which directly decreases the magnitude of the destructive interaction between the bone osteoclast and myeloma cells.[30]

Radiation therapy is an established treatment modality in the management of multiple myeloma and is used in the setting of curative treatment as a component of the conditioning regimen (TBI) in preparation for bone marrow transplant and in a palliative setting to reduce local symptoms result-

ing from progressive bone disease.[25,26] The efficacy of radiotherapy in the palliation of lytic bone lesions as well as the prevention of progression of spinal cord and nerve route compression is well documented.[27,28] For the usual axial skeleton presentations of patients with multiple myeloma with or without spinal cord or nerve compression, most centers deliver 30 Gy in 10 fractions with generous margins. For vertebral body presentations, treatment of one or two vertebral bodies above and below the involved vertebrae with inclusion of the transverse process of the vertebral body is required[29,30] (Fig. 18-4). Appropriate determination of the extraosseous extension is critical, and computed tomography (CT) or magnetic resonance imaging (MRI) can substantially increase the accuracy of the fields to encompass all disease, including subclinical disease. Careful documentation of treatment fields with simulation radiographs is an essential component of a long-term management plan for patients with multiple myeloma. Future treatment of adjacent vertebral bodies and possibly re-treatment of previously irradiated regions may be required, and special attention to details matching radiotherapy fields is required to avoid exceeding spinal cord or nerve root tolerance. There is some debate concerning the role of surgery in the management of multiple myeloma presenting with spinal cord compression.[31-34] Surgical decompression has been evaluated, and if this is the first site of disease there is some clinical evidence to indicate that these patients have a superior outcome with surgical decompression before the initiation of radiotherapy.[35] In a much larger study, however, no added efficacy for surgical decompression was noted.[36] This issue has not been resolved. In addition, there is also some controversy concerning what the total dose should be in the palliation of bone metastasis from multiple myeloma. Leigh et al.[37] have suggested that a total dose of 10 Gy with a mean fraction size of 3 to 4 Gy provides durable symptom relief in the majority of patients.[37,38] In addition, they also demonstrated that no increase in response frequency occurred with doses greater than 15 Gy. The rationale for proceeding with these low-dose initial treatments is that it allows later re-treatment at similar doses and decreases the toxicity. This view was challenged by Adamietz and colleagues,[29] who evaluated symp-

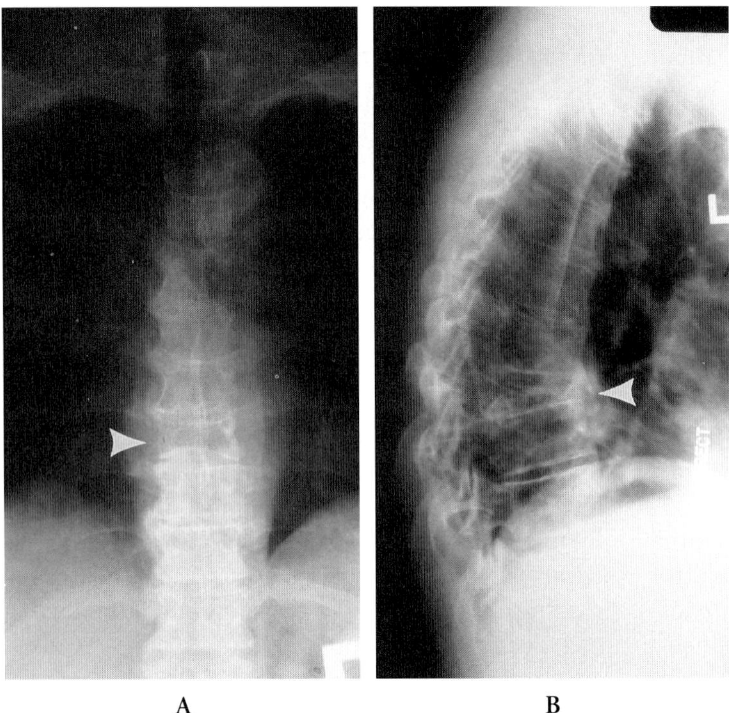

A   B

Fig. 18-4 Anteroposterior (**A**) and lateral (**B**) radiographs of the thoracic spine reveal a compression fracture of the eighth thoracic vertebra in a male patient with multiple myeloma. There was no neural deficit caudal to the fracture. The patient was treated with bracing and radiation. Over several weeks he became minimally symptomatic.

tom relief in multiple myeloma patients treated with chemotherapy combined with or followed by local radiotherapy for painful lesions. These investigators noted a decrease in pain relief at the irradiated site with subsequent treatments; this was especially prominent in the patients in whom the low-dose strategy was used. The role of bone marrow transplant remains controversial in the management of multiple myeloma. The use of lower-dose palliative radiation therapy, however, would be preferable in these patients because it does not prohibit the later use of TBI as part of the preparative regimen for bone marrow transplant.

Surgical Therapy

Myeloma often presents with severe bone pain and a large lytic lesion in the involved bone. In many cases the bone may already have a pathologic fracture. The orthopedic surgeon needs to decide whether surgery or immobilization is the most appropriate treatment strategy for any given lesion.[39] The treating physician must remember that fractures in persons with multiple myeloma can heal with adequate immobilization. This is especially true in the upper extremity and in the spine. The other unique aspect of treating fractures and im-

pending fractures in myeloma is the diffuse osteopenia seen in this disease. In many cases, especially in the spine, the osteopenia may preclude surgical stabilization. Osteoclast inhibitors are frequently used to try to prevent the osteopenia and to decrease the incidence of fracture in these patients. The initial studies with bisphosphonate therapy revealed a decrease in adverse skeletal events with osteoclast inhibitor therapy.[10,12,40]

Fracture immobilization without surgery is most commonly performed in the treatment of myeloma of the spine. In many cases the involvement of the spine is multilevel, and it can be difficult to find healthy vertebrae for any type of fixation.[41,42] In most cases bracing and radiation therapy can be used, with a decrease in back pain, and will provide adequate structural support. Even in cases of vertebral fracture collapse and neurologic involvement, bracing and radiation can produce reasonable results.[43] The bracing may have to be continued for an extended period of time, depending on the level of involvement in the spine and the number of involved vertebrae. The limiting factor in brace management is patient compliance with use of the brace. Many patients who start to improve clinically will often discontinue the brace

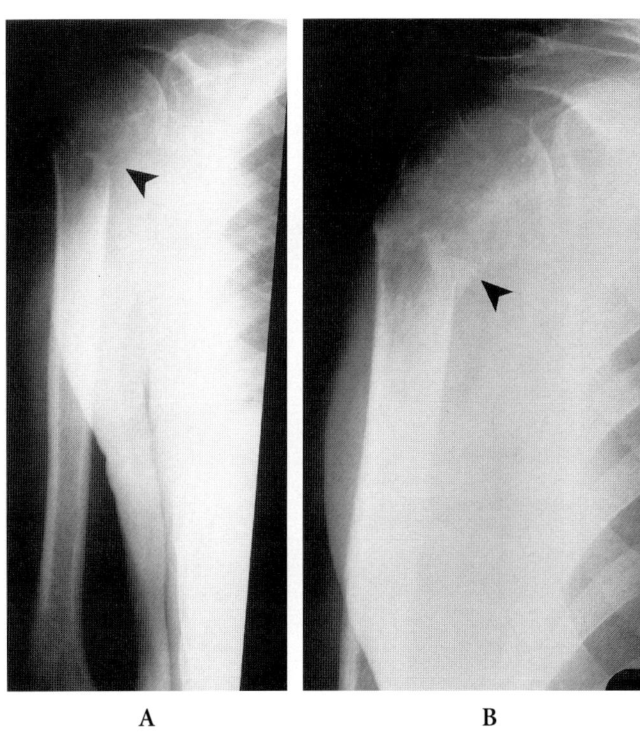

Fig. 18-5   **A,** Anteroposterior radiograph of the right humerus reveals a pathologic fracture of the base of the surgical neck. The patient had multiple myeloma and was treated with chemotherapy and a sling. **B,** A follow-up radiograph at 8 weeks reveals new bone formation and healing of the fracture. The humerus went on to heal uneventfully with good recovery of function by the patient.

because it can feel confining. Patients who are overweight may not adequately fit into a prefabricated brace, and a custom-molded brace may be required. If surgical intervention is required, the spine fixation must be adequate to prevent further vertebral collapse. Because of the severe osteopenia, methylmethacrylate augmentation of the surgical construct may be needed to prevent failure of the fixation. Bone densitometry is a useful preoperative test before surgical fixation is attempted.[44]

The upper extremity is a common site of pathologic fracture in persons with multiple myeloma. The surgical neck of the humerus can often be injured with minor trauma. If the fracture fragments are well aligned, treatment may be initiated with a brace and sling (Fig. 18-5). In many cases, immobilization along with chemotherapy will allow the fracture to heal. If the fracture of the humerus is unstable and displaced, surgical intervention may be needed (Fig. 18-6). With adequate operative stabilization, the bone may unite to allow return of excellent function.

The pelvis and femur often require more aggressive surgical intervention for focal destructive lesions. The loss of ambulatory capability in affected patients is devastating, and every effort should be made to keep the patients ambulatory and independent. The exception to intervention in this area is widespread pelvic disease. With diffuse pelvic disease, operative intervention may not be possible and the patient may need a wheelchair for mobility. In the proximal femur, evaluation of the lesion may require MRI to rule out more extensive bone involvement that cannot be seen on the conventional radiograph. If the femoral head is involved in the disease, prosthetic replacement of the femoral head will give an excellent clinical result.[45] In the shaft of the femur and the tibia, intramedullary nails can be used as in other metastatic tumors. Rarely does myeloma require massive bone resection for local control of the disease. Curettage of localized lytic lesions and postoperative chemotherapy and radiation will usually give local control and pain relief.

Because of its response to chemotherapy and radiation, multiple myeloma does not require surgical intervention as frequently as other metastatic tumors. The osteopenia should be treated with osteoclast inhibitors to decrease pathologic fractures. Surgical intervention should be reserved for focal lytic lesions at risk of fracture where nonsurgical alternatives will not give a satisfactory result. Extramedullary disease may also be encountered in

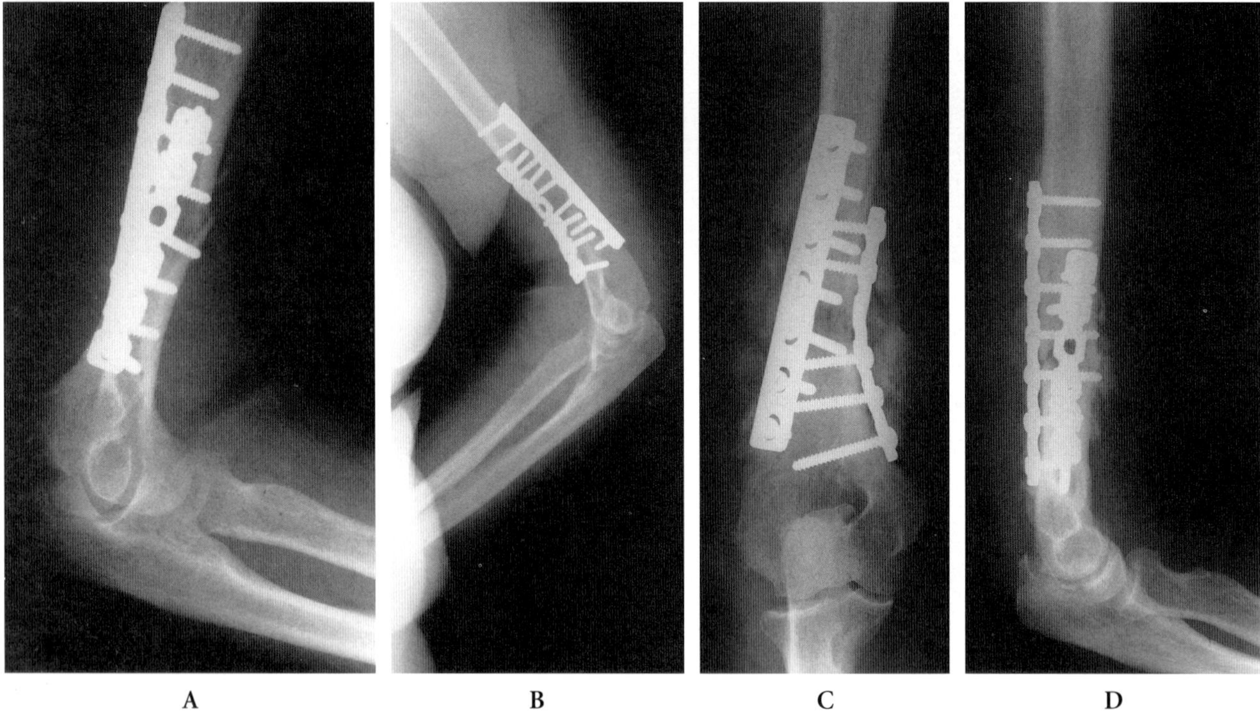

Fig. 18-6   Oblique (**A**) and lateral (**B**) radiographs of the right distal humerus show a pathologic fracture fixed with two plates. Curettage was performed along with humeral shortening. The biopsy was consistent with a plasmacytoma. Anteroposterior (**C**) and lateral (**D**) radiographs 6 weeks after surgery show new bone formation with bridging callus across the fracture site. The patient did well and the fracture healed, but widespread myeloma eventually developed.

the soft tissue. The involvement may be diffuse, and unless it is a solitary lesion the prognosis is usually poor.[46]

Complications

Hypercalcemia occurs in almost one third of patients with multiple myeloma and is often associated with such symptoms as loss of appetite, nausea, vomiting, urinary frequency, and constipation. It is most commonly treated with bisphosphonates such as pamidronate (Aredia) and forced hydration with steroids. Pamidronate is also used to prevent skeletal events and has been shown to reduce pathologic fractures, spinal cord compression, and vertebra fractures.[47]

Widespread myeloma is also associated with anemia, and the chemotherapy for this disease can lead to chronic anemia. The anemia leads to a loss of energy and causes a change in lifestyle for patients with multiple myeloma. Anemia associated with chemotherapy and renal failure responds to treatment with erythropoietin.[48] This drug can be administered on a weekly basis to patients in the range of 30,000 to 40,000 units per week. The goal is to maintain hemoglobin values at greater than 10 g.

Because the malignant population of cells leads to a decline in healthy immunoglobulin levels, patients with myeloma are often susceptible to recurrent streptococcal infections and infections with other common bacterial organisms. Pneumococcal and influenza vaccine should be given to all patients with this diagnosis; if recurrent infections become a problem, prophylactic use of penicillin and infusions of gamma globulin have been helpful. Since abnormal production of immunoglobulin is a part of this disease, patients with multiple myeloma are susceptible to recurrent infections, and many patients do require prophylaxis with antibiotics such as penicillin to prevent infections with encapsulated bacterial organisms such as streptococcal pneumonia. Immunoglobulin infusions are also sometimes needed.

Hyperviscosity syndrome occurs in less than 5% of patients with myeloma. The syndrome is due to protein interactions in large molecules with high intrinsic viscosity. It is most commonly seen in IgM variants of myeloma or in IgG or IgA myeloma, in which multimolecular aggregation occurs. The symptoms of hyperviscosity include bleeding disorders, retinal changes, and various neurologic symptoms (up to and including coma). Hypervolemia may result, requiring plasmapheresis. The hyperviscosity syndrome should be treated with chemotherapeutic agents to decrease the tumor burden and immunoglobulin production.

Amyloid fibril deposition also occurs frequently with myeloma. This occurs in approximately 15% of the patients. Amyloid fibrils in myeloma contain immunoglobulin light chains similar to those of primary amyloidosis. Symptoms often include ankle edema, weakness, weight loss, and neurologic symptoms. Carpal tunnel syndrome with night pain can be caused by amyloid infiltration. Physical examination often reveals macroglossia (20%), ankle edema, and splenomegaly. Besides carpal tunnel syndrome, other musculoskeletal complications include joint involvement. The radiographs can have an appearance similar to that of rheumatoid arthritis. Skin nodules and plaques may also be seen. Rectal biopsy or abdominal fat aspiration may lead to the diagnosis of amyloidosis. For any patient with myeloma and carpal tunnel syndrome, the transverse carpal ligament should be sent to the pathology laboratory to be examined for amyloid. The treatment for amyloid secondary to myeloma should be aimed at controlling the immunoglobulin secretion by aggressive treatment of the myeloma.

Renal failure is a problem in multiple myeloma. An assay to evaluate the effect of Bence Jones proteins on the kidney has been developed.[49] Dense tubular casts are often seen in the urine of patients with myeloma involving the kidney. If the bone marrow response is stable, renal transplantation has even been considered and does prolong survival in patients who have multiple myeloma that is responsive to chemotherapy.

Many patients with multiple myeloma will respond to chemotherapy, and many investigations are being conducted worldwide to assess the role of high-dose chemotherapies with stem cell transplant and the possible role of allogeneic or donor transplant, which may have curative potential for this disease. Needless to say these aggressive forms of therapy have a higher incidence of associated morbidity than some of the currently accepted standard outpatient chemotherapies. Encouraging data is emerging on the use of stem cell rescue after high-dose therapy leading to extension of life and clearly allowing patients to have an increased treatment-free survival, which affects the quality of life.

Autologous Stem Cell Transplantation

Although multiple myeloma is a disease that by its nature involves the bone marrow, peripheral blood stem cells can be acquired by mobilizing these cells through the use of high-dose chemotherapy with specific growth factors. With the acquisition of peripheral blood stem cells, patients who have attained the plateau phase as a result of standard therapies can then undergo courses of high-dose, marrow-ablative chemotherapy.[50]

These patients have been shown to benefit in the short term by the extended treatment-free survival that they experience after undergoing the high dose transplant therapies. Randomized trials looking at patients with newly diagnosed disease and comparing the usual courses of standard chemotherapy followed by autologous stem cell transplant vs. maintenance with standard chemotherapy have also shown long-term survival of the transplant patients.[51] Many trials are ongoing and will help establish the role of stem cell transplants and possibly the benefits of multiple stem cell transplants in patients with this diagnosis.[52]

Allogeneic Transplants

Allogeneic bone marrow transplantation requires the identification of an HLA (human leukocyte antigen)–matched donor. This form of transplantation has a much higher treatment-related mortality rate than autologous transplantation. (The autologous transplant treatment–related mortality rate is less than 5% and the allogeneic transplant treatment–related mortality rate may be as high as 30%.) The advantage of the acquisition of allogeneic immunity is a graft vs. myeloma effect, which as a selected series has been purported to lead to cure of the cancer.[53] To date, allogeneic transplant is the only curative option for patients with multiple myeloma, but again ongoing studies are needed. As with this approach, the treatment-related mortality rate remains high. Unfortunately the complications of allogeneic transplant are greater in older populations and since a majority of patients with this diagnosis are over 60 years of age, the allogeneic approach with its associated morbid-

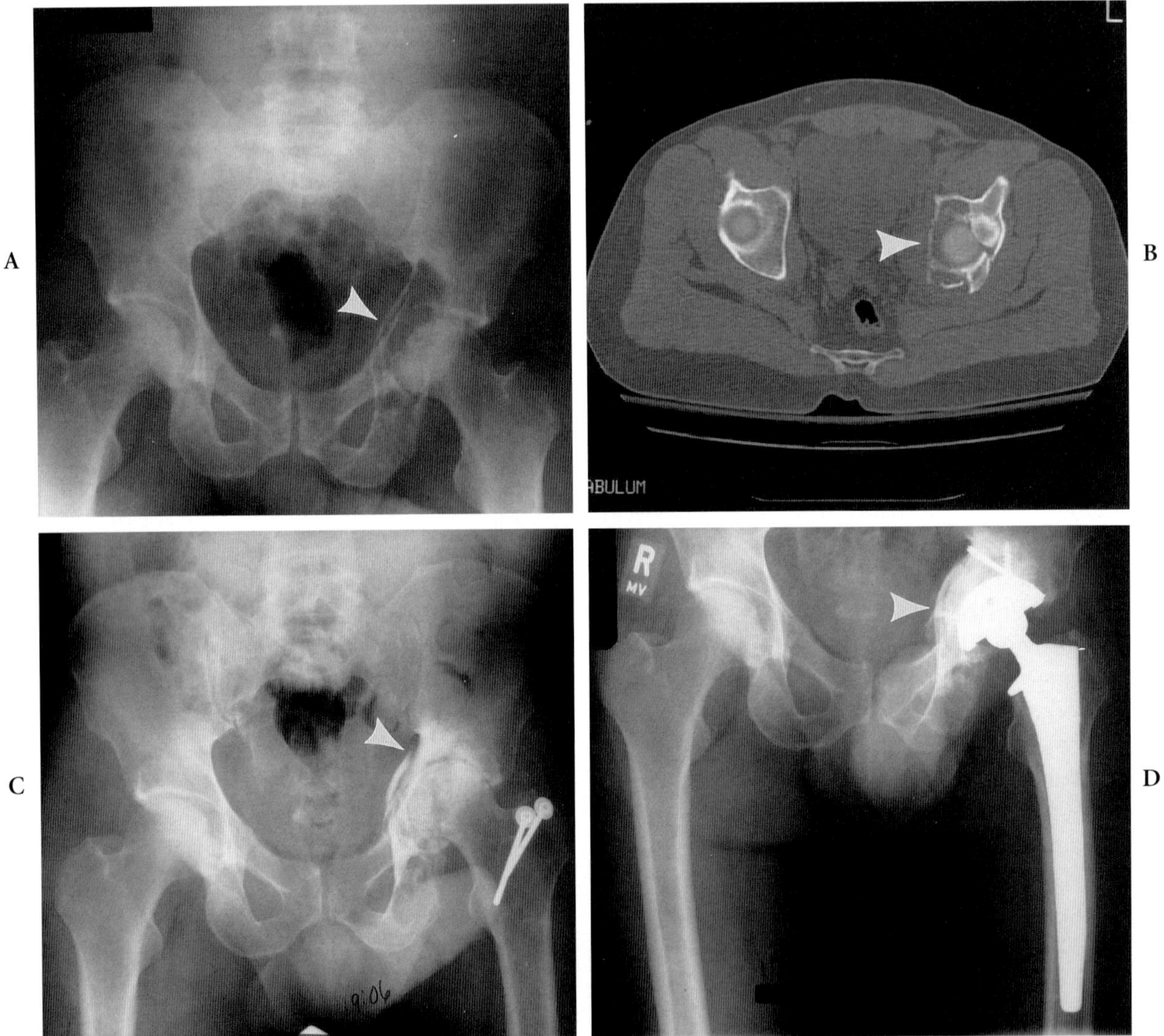

Fig. 18-7 A, Anteroposterior radiograph of the pelvis reveals a large lytic lesion of the left acetabulum in a 37-year-old man. **B,** The patient fell during the evaluation process and sustained a pathologic fracture of the acetabulum. A CT scan reveals the fractures of the medial wall of the acetabulum with the surrounding destructive lytic process. **C,** An open biopsy was required to obtain diagnostic tissue. The pathologic findings were consistent with multiple myeloma. The patient had radiation therapy. Local control of the tumor was excellent, but posttraumatic arthritis developed in the involved acetabulum *(arrow)*. The two screws are from a trochanteric osteotomy at the time of biopsy. **D,** The patient had a bone marrow transplant, and later a total hip replacement was performed with bone grafting of the acetabulum. Currently the patient has been free of disease for 5 years, with excellent function of his total hip.

ity and mortality may prove unacceptable to most patients with the diagnosis (Fig. 18-7).

Advances in Molecular Biology and Future Treatment Directions

Continued studies are being done to clarify the final event that leads to the propagation of the monoclonal B cell malignancy. The recent studies in molecular biology indicate that the final event leading to the differentiation of the malignant B cell in multiple myeloma is associated with a common chromosomal abnormality involving the immunoglobulin heavy chain switch region.[54] Recent studies also suggest a potential role for human herpesvirus 8 (HHV-8) in the pathogenesis of this abnormality.[55] Continued work directed at this common chromosomal abnormality might allow identification of potential new genetic targets for therapy in this disease.

Resistance to chemotherapeutic agents remains a significant obstacle to improving therapeutic outcome in patients with multiple myeloma. There are purported mechanisms of drug resistance that reduce intracellular concentrations of chemotherapy, and clinical studies are being conducted to determine ways to overcome this drug resistance. Future approaches by which we can enhance drug treatment and focus on signal transduction pathways that appear to govern the response of chemotherapy in the myeloma cells are being studied. This work in overcoming drug resistance may be the basis for future therapies that would include multiple courses of high-dose chemotherapy with stem cell rescue to obtain and maintain a prolonged plateau phase in patients with myeloma.

Important to this effort will be the continued pursuit of techniques to detect residual multiple myeloma after aggressive therapy and to develop non-bone-marrow-suppressive therapy. Strategies include drugs such as thalidomide, which has a noncytotoxic immunomodulatory effect on the disease and has an established role in treatment of refractory patients, with further studies needed to establish its role as a possible drug for maintenance therapy.

To date, the management of patients with multiple myeloma is proving to be a rewarding yet challenging proposition. Appropriate use of currently known effective chemotherapeutic agents, the judi-

cious use of radiation therapy for palliation, and the need to pursue surgical options for stabilization and management of weightbearing bone lesions have led to extended survival and improved quality of life for these patients.

Solitary Plasmacytoma

A related problem, which is managed somewhat differently than the systemic B cell malignancy of multiple myeloma, involves the plasmacytomas. The diagnosis of a solitary plasmacytoma is based on histologic specimens showing plasma cells, which are monoclonal and identical to cell populations seen in multiple myeloma. Skeletal radiographs do not show other lytic lesions, and bone marrow does not show infiltration with these malignant cells. In solitary plasmacytoma the serum does not show infiltration with these malignant cells and serum immunofixation does not show a monoclonal protein. Occasionally patients with solitary lesions will have detectable monoclonal protein. When patients present with solitary lesions, they are managed with surgical excision and often with involved-field radiation therapy (Fig. 18-8). Ten-year survival data ranged from 15% to 20% to as high as 50% in patients who truly had solitary lesions and underwent aggressive local management. Unfortunately, multiple myeloma and progression of the solitary lesions to systemic involvement occur within 3 years of the initial problem in approximately 50% to 60% of patients who initially present with solitary plasmacytoma.

Extramedullary plasmacytoma is the term used to describe plasma cell tumor that arises outside the bone marrow. These are more frequently found in the upper respiratory tract, nasal cavity and sinuses, nasopharynx, and larynx. They may also occur in the gastrointestinal tract, central nervous system, urinary bladder, thyroid, breast, parotid gland lymph nodes, and gonadal tissue. Again, these extramedullary sites warrant screening for the systemic disease of multiple myeloma; screening should include examination of the bone marrow and blood marrow and blood and urine for immunofixation and identification of monoclonal protein. If there is no identification of systemic involvement, local therapy is often surgical in combination with potentially curative doses of local ra-

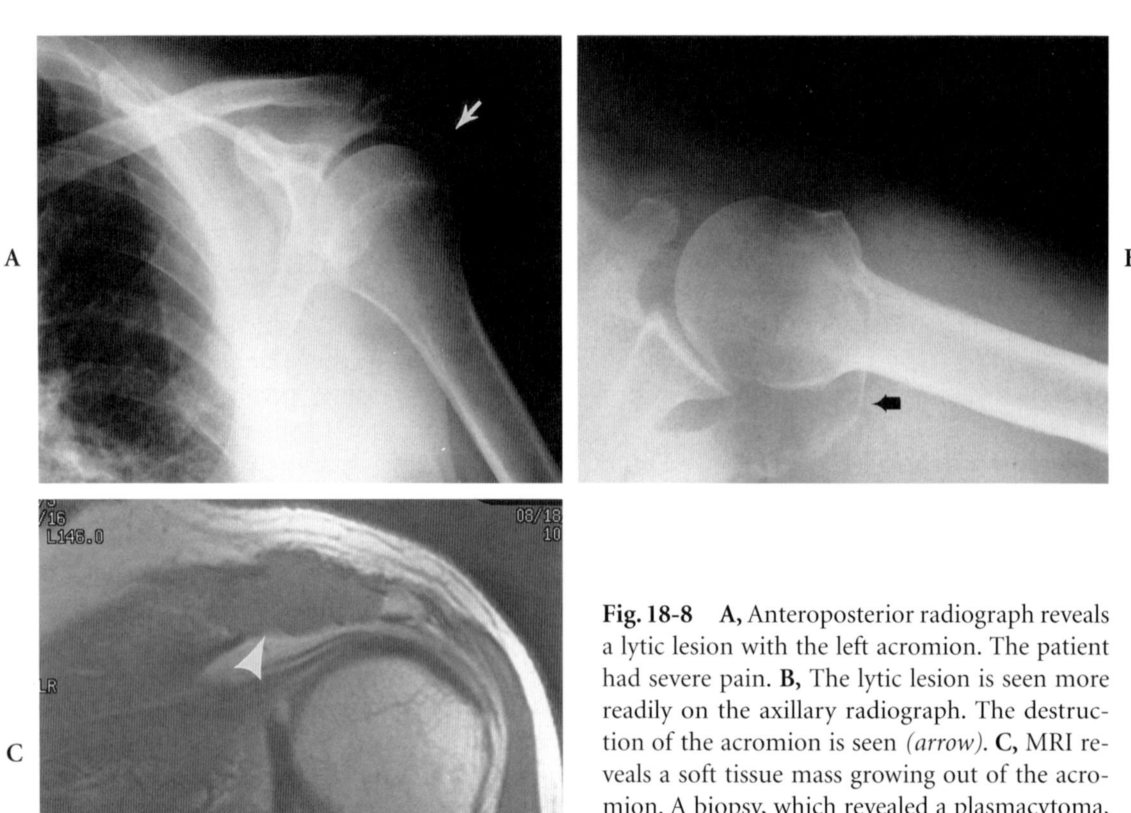

Fig. 18-8   **A,** Anteroposterior radiograph reveals a lytic lesion with the left acromion. The patient had severe pain. **B,** The lytic lesion is seen more readily on the axillary radiograph. The destruction of the acromion is seen *(arrow)*. **C,** MRI reveals a soft tissue mass growing out of the acromion. A biopsy, which revealed a plasmacytoma, and a partial acromionectomy were performed, with excellent clinical relief of pain.

diation therapy. These solitary and extramedullary presentations are rare. They may precede the development of multiple myeloma in as many as 50% to 60% of patients, but if truly isolated and if stage I is potentially curative, they are treated by an aggressive surgical approach in combination with radiation therapy. The role of chemotherapy in these patients is not well established, and there are no large series to show that chemotherapy prevents the eventual development of systemic multiple myeloma.

Solitary plasmacytomas comprise only 2% of plasma cell dyscrasias and may arise in the bone or soft tissues. Plasmacytomas arising inside the bone marrow are classified as solitary plasmacytoma of bone (SPB). Some controversy exists as to what the actual treatment volume should be for SPB. Some authors have recommended that treatment portals should include the entire involved bone and medullary cavity with 2 to 3 cm margins encompassing the entire bone. The rationale for this approach has been that plasmacytomas can both spread freely throughout the medullary cavity and extend directly into the adjacent soft tissue. Opponents of this rationale contend that local fields with generous margins encompassing the osseous primary lesion and any soft tissue extensions are sufficient if an adequate radiological evaluation to determine the true tumor extent has been performed. Both CT and MRI are specifically helpful in delineating the extraosseous extensions into soft tissue, particularly in vertebral body and pelvic bone locations.

Numerous clinical studies from multiple institutions documenting the natural history of SPB have suggested that higher doses and treatment with a curative intent can lead to a cure[56] (Fig. 18-9).

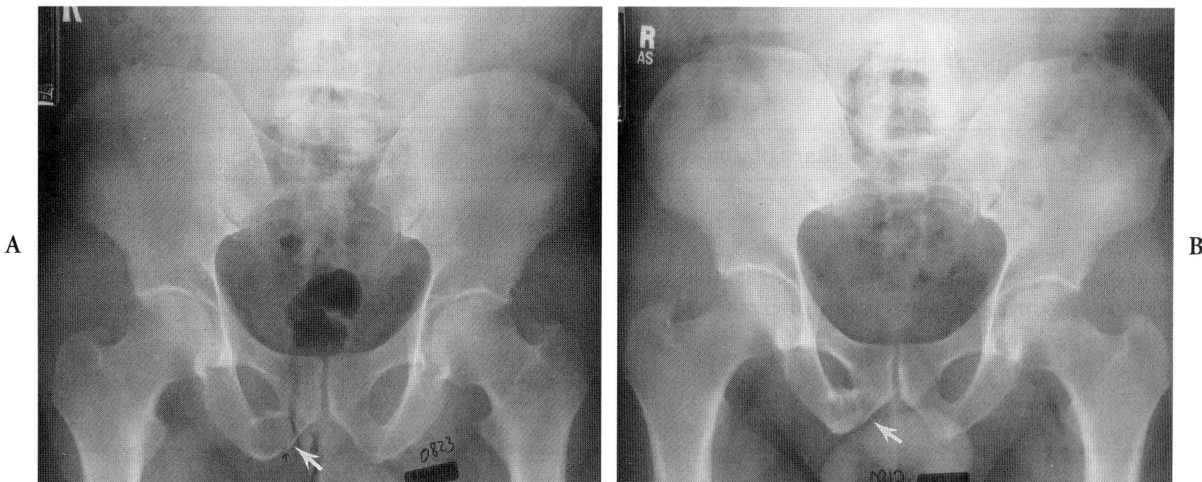

Fig. 18-9   A, Anteroposterior radiograph of the pelvis reveals a lytic right ischial lesion with a pathologic fracture *(arrow)*. The results of an open biopsy were consistent with a plasmacytoma. **B,** Radiograph taken 6 months after 30 Gy of radiation shows that the fracture has healed and much of the ischium has been filled in.

Modern series evaluating the role of radiotherapy in the management of SPB have demonstrated that doses of radiation in the range of 40 to 50 Gy, if normal tissue tolerances permit, delivered over a 4- to 5-week time period, offer probabilities of local control in the range of 95%.[57-59] Of interest, in the largest clinical series reported by Frassica et al.[60] from the Mayo Clinic, in which patients with SPB received doses of 45 Gy or more of conventionally fractionated radiotherapy, no local recurrences were noted. This dose-response relationship has been confirmed in numerous smaller clinical trials by other investigators. Of patients presenting with SPB, the literature suggests that after 10 years approximately 50% and after 15 years more than 90% will ultimately progress to multiple myeloma, illustrating the long natural history of this disease.[61,62] Although the pretreatment evaluation is not reliable enough to distinguish at presentation those patients in whom SPB will not progress, several reports have suggested a higher rate of progression in those patients who have the myeloma protein at presentation. A substantial uncertainty exists in estimating the risk of progression resulting from the wide range of diagnostic criteria used by different authors to define SPB. Some authors consider less than 10% circulating plasma cells, minor serum protein abnormalities, or even the presence of

Bence Jones proteins acceptable criteria for a diagnosis of SPB. Other investigators would exclude these patients from the diagnosis of SPB and consider them to have frank multiple myeloma, thus making the exact incidence of progression difficult to extract from the literature.[62,63] However, it is recommended that all patients with apparent SPB receive potentially curative local radiation therapy.

Plasmacytomas arising outside the bone marrow are classified as extramedullary plasmacytomas (EMP). These lesions have a predilection for the upper aerodigestive tract and are commonly located in the head and neck region. Frequent sites of EMP are the nasopharynx, tonsil, maxillary sinus, nasal vestibule, and trachea. In addition, 10% to 15% of the patients will present with cervical lymph node involvement. Given the propensity for these lesions to metastasize to local regional lymph nodes, the treatment volume should include the draining regional lymph nodes.[56] EMP treated with local fields to the primary lesion have only an 8% to 15% risk of regional failure. In comparison, in patients with SPB treated with local fields local regional lymph node failure is not observed. No apparent differences in the radiotherapy dose-response relationships have been noted for EMP or SPB, and they are treated with similar total doses and fractionation schemes. A somewhat smaller

melphalan and ABMT in myeloma. Proc Am Soc Clin Oncol 12:364, 1993.

52. Attal M, Payen C, Facon T, Michaux JL, Guilhot F, Moconduit M, Fuzibet JG, Caillot D, Corvaux V, Harousseau JL, Cahn JY, Grobois B, Stoppa AM, Ifrah N, Sotto JJ, Pignon B, Bataille R. Single versus double transplant in myeloma: A randomized trial of the Inter Groupe Fracais du Myelome (IFM). Blood 90(Suppl):418a (abstr), 1997.

53. Lokhorst HM, Schattenberg A, Cornelissen JJ, Thomas LL, Verdonck LF. Donor leukocyte infusions are effective in relapsed multiple myeloma after allogeneic bone marrow transplantation. Blood 90:4206-4211, 1997.

54. Alsina M, Boyce B, Devlin RD, Anderson JL, Craig F, Mundy GR, Roodman GD. Development of an in vivo model of human multiple myeloma bone disease. Blood 87(4):1495-1501, 1996.

55. Marcelin AG, Dupin N, Bouscary D, Bossi P, Cacoub P, Ravaud P, Calvez V. HHV-8 and multiple myeloma in France. Lancet 350:1144, 1997.

56. Mayr NA, Wen BC, Hussey DH, Burns CP, Staples JJ, Doornbos JF, Vigliotti AP. The role of radiation therapy in the treatment of solitary plasmacytomas. Radiother Oncol 17:293-303, 1990.

57. Corwin J, Lindberg RD. Solitary plasmacytoma of bone vs. extramedullary plasmacytoma and their relationship to multiple myeloma. Cancer 43:1007-1013, 1979.

58. Mill WB, Griffith R. The role of radiation therapy in the management of plasma cell tumors. Cancer 45:647-652, 1980.

59. Bataille R, Sany J. Solitary myeloma: Clinical and prognostic features of a review of 114 cases. Cancer 48:845-851, 1981.

60. Frassica DA, Frassica FJ, Schray MF, Sim FH, Kyle RA. Solitary plasmacytoma of bone: Mayo Clinic experience. Int J Radiat Oncol Biol Phys 16:43-48, 1989.

61. Dimopoulos MA, Goldstein J, Fuller L, Delasalle K, Alexanian R. Curability of solitary bone plasmacytoma. J Clin Oncol 10:587-590, 1992.

62. Bolek TW, Marcus RB, Mendenhall NP. Solitary plasmacytoma of bone and soft tissue. Int J Radiat Biol Phys 36:329-333, 1996.

63. Holland J, Trenkner DA, Wasserman TH, Fineberg B. Plasmacytoma: Treatment results and conversion to myeloma. Cancer 69:1513-1517, 1992.

64. Knowling MA, Harwood AR, Bergsagel DE. Comparison of extramedullary plasmacytomas with solitary and multiple plasma cell tumors of bone. J Clin Oncol 1:255-262, 1983.

Lung Cancer

Todd E. Williams, M.D., *Charles R. Thomas, Jr.,* M.D.,
John L. Eady, M.D., *and Andrew T. Turrisi III,* M.D.

INCIDENCE AND PATTERNS OF SPREAD

Lung cancer is the deadliest malignant disease in the United States, with an estimated annual incidence of more than 178,000 and deaths exceeding 160,000.[1] The majority of patients do not have early warning signs and present with locally advanced or even metastatic disease. Even among the minority who present with early-stage disease, approximately 50% eventually will succumb and will require palliative therapy. Hence most therapy directed at patients with lung cancer is palliative. The musculoskeletal system serves as one of the most common sites of distant spread, with the incidence of osseous metastases ranging from 20% to 40%.[2,3] Soft tissue metastases are less common, but lung cancer is one of the most common causes of soft tissue metastases.

Older reports of the metastatic process[4,5] suggest that tumor cells directly degrade bone, but growing evidence shows that metastatic cells do not engage in osteoclastic activity. Instead, they release a variety of bone remodeling substances, such as interleukin-6, prostaglandin E2, transforming growth factor-α, and parathyroid hormone–related peptide, nitric oxide, tumor necrosis factor, and interleukin-1β.[6] These substances stimulate osteoclasts and suppress osteoblastic activity. The net effect of these cytokines around a nidus of tumor cells is destruction of bone matrix. Paraneoplastic syndromes may develop in all types of lung cancer (see Chapter 42).

Breast and prostate cancer account for roughly 80% of skeletal metastases, yet prostate cancer, with its propensity to develop blastic metastases, has a much lower incidence of pathologic fracture.[7] Unlike patients with breast and prostate cancer, who have median survivals of 2 to 4 years after the development of bone metastases, patients with lung cancer have a poor prognosis, with a median survival of only 3 to 6 months.[7,8] The odds that symptomatic spinal cord compression will develop are therefore less. In lung cancer the most common sites of pathologic fracture are the femur and the humerus.[9] Metastases to weightbearing bones constitute the greatest concern, because these are more likely to fracture with normal weightbearing and cause the most disability.

TREATMENT OPTIONS

The treatment of bone metastases, including those from lung cancer, is similar regardless of the primary site. Any therapy will be palliative in nature, so it is important to keep in mind the expected median survival when determining aggressiveness and length of treatment. The primary goal is alleviation of symptoms in an efficient manner so that the patient can maintain as normal and functional a lifestyle as possible. Treatment options are varied and include radiation therapy, bisphosphonates, surgery, and systemic radiopharmaceuticals.

Radiation Therapy

Radiation therapy has long been offered as an effective treatment for symptomatic bone metastases. Although numerous phase III, prospective, randomized trials (Table 19-1) have attempted to define the optimal treatment schedule, there is no one regimen that will fit every patient. To some extent this is due to the heterogeneous patient population presenting with malignant diseases that demonstrate varying natural histories as well as patients with different performance statuses. These trials, however, do shed light on various schedules, which prove effective. One of the largest was executed by the Radiation Therapy Oncology Group (RTOG) and reported by Tong et al. in 1982.[10] Of the 1016 patients who were randomized, 759 were evaluable. Patients with solitary metastases received either 40.5 Gy for 3 weeks or 20 Gy for 1 week. Those with multiple metastases were randomly assigned to four groups: 30 Gy for 2 weeks, 15 Gy for 1 week, 20 Gy for 1 week, or 25 Gy for 1 week. Additional stratification was performed by primary site, site of metastasis, use of internal fixation, and institution. The primary objective was frequency and degree of pain relief. An instrument incorporating both a pain and a narcotic use "score" measured initial pain level and response to therapy. A minimal response was defined as a drop in the initial score; a partial response was the pain score dropping below 4; and complete response was a score of 0. The investigators found no statistically significant benefit between the various treatment schedules for either the solitary or the multiple metastases groups. Patients with breast and prostate cancer did experience pain relief more frequently than those with

Table 19-1   Phase III prospective randomized trials of palliative radiotherapy for osseous metastases

Reference	No. of patients	Treatment schedule	Pain palliation (%)		Duration of response (wk)
Tong et al.[10]	266 sm	40.5 Gy/15 fx (3 wk)	61 (CR)	P = NS	16
		vs.			
		20 Gy/5 fx (1 wk)	53 (CR)		14
	750 mm	15 Gy/5 fx (1 wk)	49 (CR)	P = NS	12
		vs.			
		20 Gy/5 fx (1 wk)	56 (CR)		12
		vs.			
		25 Gy/5 fx (1 wk)	49 (CR)		13
		vs.			
		30 Gy/10 fx (2 wk)	57 (CR)		12
Nielsen et al.[11]	241	8 Gy/1 fx	62 (CR and PR)	P = NS	65% experienced no pain progression during the 6-month follow-up period in both arms
		vs.			
		20 Gy/5 fx (1 wk)	71 (CR and PR)		
Gaze et al.[12]	280	10 Gy/1 fx	39 (CR)	P = NS	13.5
		vs.			
		22.5 Gy/5 fx (1 wk)	42 (CR)		14
Niewald et al.[13]	100	20 Gy/5 fx (1 wk)	77 (CR and PR)	P = NS	35
		vs.			
		30 Gy/15 fx (3 wk)	86 (CR and PR)		35
Price et al.[14]	288	8 Gy/1 fx	45 (CR)	P = NS	24
		vs.			
		30 Gy/10 fx (2 wk)	28 (CR)		12
Hoskin et al.[15]	270	4 Gy/1 fx	44 (CR and PR)	P < 0.01	60%-70% maintained pain control for the 12-week follow-up period in both arms
		vs.			
		8 Gy/1 fx	69 (CR and PR)		
Okawa et al.[16]	80	30 Gy/15 fx (3 wk)	76 (CR and PR)	P = NS	Not reported
		vs.			
		22.5 Gy/5 fx (2.5 wk)	75 (CR and PR)		
		vs.			
		20 Gy/10 fx (b.i.d., 1.5 wk)	78 (CR and PR)		
Madsen[17]	57	24 Gy/6 fx (3 wk)	47 (CR and PR)	P = NS	Not reported
		vs.			
		20 Gy/2 fx (1 wk)	48 (CR and PR)		

sm, Single metastases; mm, multiple metastases; fx, fractions; NS, not significant; CR, complete relief; PR, partial relief.

lung cancer did ($P < 0.001$), but the site of metastasis did not matter. Pain relief for responders was not immediate, but most attained at least minimal relief within 2 weeks of initiating therapy, and almost 50% of those who achieved complete relief required more than 4 weeks to achieve maximal benefit. The onset of complete pain relief in the multiple cohort was shortest, with the 15 Gy/5 fractions regimen at 3 weeks ($P < 0.01$). No significant difference was seen between the two arms of the solitary groups. Overall, most patients (89%) experienced at least "minimal" relief, whereas 83% progressed to "partial" relief, and 53% eventually enjoyed "complete" relief from pain. The median duration of minimal response was 20 weeks, whereas that of complete response was 12 weeks. Unfortunately the patients who endured the worst pain exhibited the lowest response rate for partial (79%) and complete (49%) relief, yet of the responders the majority did not experience relapse before death.

Blitzer incorporated several different approaches to perform a reanalysis of the RTOG data.[18] He analyzed the data from the solitary and multiple cohorts together, assuming that they represent a spectrum of the same disease instead of different entities. He gave greater weight to end points that could cloak results such as re-treatment and the use of narcotics. Applying stepwise logistical regression, he suggested that treatment regimens with longer fractionation schemes resulted in superior pain control.

Bisphosphonates

Although bisphosphonates initially were developed to combat hypercalcemia, they have shown significant utility in the palliation of pain in patients with lytic bone metastases. The majority of information involves patients with breast cancer, but data on other primary sites are accruing. These agents likely will become an integral part of the management of this patient population.

Bisphosphonates are a class of drugs that inhibit resorption of bone through several mechanisms. They are characterized by a phosphate-carbonphosphate bond that facilitates their preferential attraction to mineralized bone matrix.[19] They hinder osteoclasts not only directly by reducing H^+ and Ca^{2+} removal and affecting enzymatic action but also indirectly through osteoblasts by reducing secretion of osteoclast recruitment factors.[20] Bisphosphonates have been the treatment of choice for cancer-related hypercalcemia. They have also been found to be efficacious in palliating painful osseous metastases and improving quality of life. Their use reduces the frequency of radiotherapy and pain medications, the incidence of pathologic fractures, and the costs associated with palliative care.[21-25]

Most of the data on the use of bisphosphonates for the palliation of bone metastases involve breast cancer patients with lytic disease. One of the largest studies was reported by Hortobagyi et al., who randomly assigned 382 participants with stage IV breast cancer undergoing systemic chemotherapy to receive pamidronate vs. placebo.[21] The pamidronate (90 mg) was delivered monthly over a 2-hour intravenous infusion for a total of 12 cycles. Patients were stratified according to Eastern Cooperative Oncology Group (ECOG) performance status. There were 185 patients who received pamidronate and 195 who received placebo. They were evaluated at 3- to 4-week intervals for development of skeletal complications, which included hypercalcemia, the need for surgical intervention or radiation therapy, pathologic fractures, and spinal cord compression. At regular intervals during the investigation, pain and analgesic use were assessed, as was performance status. Forty-eight percent of the participants completed all 12 cycles. The median duration of follow-up was 11.9 months for the pamidronate cohort and 10.2 months for the placebo cohort. In all evaluated areas, patients receiving pamidronate fared better than those receiving placebo. The incidence of skeletal complications was statistically lower, 43% vs. 56% ($P = 0.008$), and the time to first complication was longer, 13.1 vs. 7 months ($P = 0.005$). The pamidronate group also experienced superior pain control, with 44% having decreased pain scores compared with 32% in the placebo group ($P = 0.03$). Although palliation was greater in the pamidronate group, survival was not different (14.8 vs. 14.2 months median survival). It is not certain whether bisphosphonates exhibit antitumor activity. The authors believed that because the survival time was similar, they likely do not. Other investigators, however, although not demonstrating improved survival, have demonstrated reductions in certain tumor markers, suggesting antitumoral activity.[26]

Systemic Radiopharmaceuticals

The systemic administration of radiopharmaceuticals has been shown to be effective in the treatment of painful bone metastases. Numerous agents, including phosphorus 32, iodine 131, strontium 89, yttrium 90, samarium 153, and rhenium 186, have been evaluated and used clinically. These have been administered as either ligands (HEDP, EDTMP) or anionic phosphates.[27] Phosphorus 32 and iodine 131 have been used for decades but have limited usefulness in the treatment of bone lesions because of the unacceptably high radiation doses delivered to bone marrow.[28] Most clinical experience with the use of the newer isotopes has been with strontium 89,[29-34] a pure beta emitter with a maximum energy of 1.4 MV and a physical half-life of 50.6 days. It is used in the form of a chloride salt and acts as a calcium analog with preferential attraction to sites of growing bone. It has been shown to be superior to placebo[33,34]; it is a useful adjunct to local radiotherapy[29]; and it compares favorably with radiotherapy alone (both local field and hemibody) in a phase III trial.[30]

A large trial reported by Bolger et al. randomly assigned 305 participants with metastatic prostate cancer to receive either radiotherapy or strontium 89.[30] The radiotherapy was delivered as local field therapy in 148 patients and as hemibody therapy in 157 patients. The extent of osseous involvement determined the treatment. Local radiotherapy consisted of either 20 Gy in 1 week or 8 Gy in 1 fraction. The hemibody regimen delivered a single fraction of either 6 Gy to the upper body or 8 Gy to the lower body. The dose of strontium 89 was 5.4 mCi. Response and toxicity were assessed at regular intervals until 12 weeks after therapy. The patients who received strontium 89 experienced a statistically nonsignificant improvement in "dramatic" pain relief compared with those who underwent local radiotherapy (44.1% vs. 36.4%). Those who received the hemibody therapy had responses similar to those of the strontium group (43.2% vs. 42.4%, respectively). An important observation was a statistically significant reduction in the development of new painful sites in the strontium group as compared with both the local therapy and hemibody

groups (P <0.01 and <0.05, respectively). Survival was comparable in all cohorts, with a median of 30 weeks. Thrombocytopenia and myelosuppression are the major toxic effects of radiopharmaceutical therapy, yet with strontium 89 they are infrequently clinically significant. Radiotherapy was associated with much more gastrointestinal toxicity, with 43% of the hemibody group experiencing side effects as compared with 10% of the strontium 89 patients.

The use of strontium 89 as an adjunct to standard local field radiation therapy was studied by Porter et al. in a phase III trial.[29] One hundred twenty-six patients with hormone-refractory metastatic adenocarcinoma of the prostate were randomly assigned to receive either placebo or 10.8 mCi of strontium 89 after completing a course of local radiation therapy. The radiotherapy schedules were similar to those of the Bolger study: 30 Gy over 2 weeks and 20 Gy in 1 week (rib lesions could be treated with one fraction of up to 10 Gy). Again, pain palliation, analgesic requirements, and quality-of-life measurements were assessed. No statistically significant improvement in pain control at the index sites was demonstrated with the addition of strontium 89. However, the reduction in the use of analgesics, the reduction in the development of new painful sites, and the improvement in quality of life were all statistically superior in the participants who received strontium 89. Toxicity was minimal. An economic analysis performed on a small number of these patients treated at the Cross Cancer Institute in Edmonton, Alberta, indicated that the use of strontium 89 may decrease the overall costs associated with management of this patient population.[35]

Other radiopharmaceutical agents, including rhenium 186 and samarium 153, have also shown utility in clinical trials for bone metastases not only from prostate but also from breast and lung cancer.[36-39] A new isotope of rhenium ([188]Re) may prove to be effective and economical as compared with currently used agents. One advantage that rhenium 186 and samarium 153 have over strontium 89 is that they produce low-energy photons that can be used for imaging and accurate dosimetry. They are expensive, however, being produced in nuclear reactors that use neutron irradiation.

Rhenium 188 may prove more cost-effective because, similar to technetium 99m, it can be made in hospital nuclear medicine departments. It has a short physical half-life of 16.9 hours, is excreted rapidly, and demonstrates good preferential uptake in bone in animal studies.[40]

Surgical Therapy

Surgery plays an important role in the management of patients with fractures resulting from metastatic osseous disease. Although the majority of patients who present with symptomatic bone metastases will not require surgical intervention and can be managed with one or more of the less invasive modalities, surgery is best used in patients with impending or actual pathologic fractures and in selected cases of spinal cord compression. The indications for surgical treatment depend on several factors, including location and size of the metastatic focus, predictability of the involved segment, performance status of the patient, and expected survival. The choice of surgical technique must be individualized and rests heavily on the location and amount of involved bone and soft tissue.[41]

Depending on location, long bone fractures of the lower extremity are often managed differently from those of the arm because of anatomic and functional differences. Because of the weightbearing demands across the anatomic shape of the proximal femur, pathologic fractures in this area of bone rarely heal. Therefore, fractures in this area are better treated with prosthetic replacement (femoral endoprosthesis) if the goals of quality-of-life preservation, prompt return of maximum function, and limitation of associated side effects are to be realized.[41,42] Humeral fractures undergo surgical stabilization to relieve pain, stabilize the fracture, and allow prompt return of the use of the hand. Humeral endoprostheses are an appropriate choice for proximal humeral pathologic fractures, but midshaft fractures are best treated with an intramedullary rod, either with or without adjunctive methyl methacrylate stabilization (Fig. 19-1).

Pelvic and acetabular metastases are common and can generate significant pain and debilitation by the destruction of bone. The goal of managing acetabular lesions surgically is to prevent protrusion of the femoral head into the weakened surrounding bone tissue and dislocation of the femoral head, both of which would severely limit func-

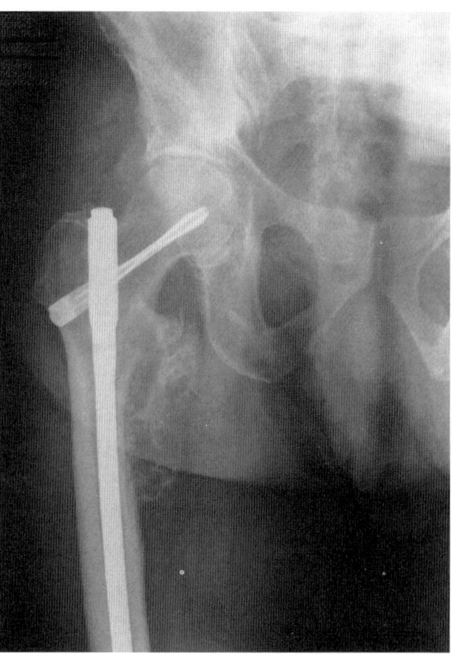

Fig. 19-1 Placement of an intramedullary rod and interlocking pins for stabilization.

tion of the involved limbs. Reconstructive techniques that require bone union for stability are to be avoided; if a total hip replacement is required, the acetabular component should be fixed with methyl methacrylate.[43]

Spinal metastases are common, and the vertebral body is the site most frequently involved. The indications for surgery include spinal instability with or without cord compression, unknown diagnosis (if less invasive biopsy techniques are unsuccessful), and vertebral body collapse with resultant spinal cord or nerve root compression by bone. The preferred surgical approach will depend heavily on the location of the tumor. Posterior approaches with laminectomy are less commonly used because most spinal metastases involve the vertebral bodies. Anterior approaches with removal of involved vertebral bodies and stabilization of adjacent spinal segments have been shown to be effective in relieving pain and compression[44,45] and in providing spinal stability.

SPINAL CORD COMPRESSION

Approximately 20,000 patients per year have spinal cord compressions from neoplastic causes. The thoracic spine is the most common site of compression (70%), followed by the lumbar region (20%) and the cervical vertebrae (10%).[46-48] The incidence of spinal cord compression in patients with lung cancer is approximately 5% and accounts for 15% of all cord compressions, or about 3000 new patients per year.[47,48] Spinal cord compression is a true oncologic emergency, but if it is detected and treated before complete paralysis develops, the odds of retaining good neurologic function are improved. The majority of metastases that cause spinal cord damage do so from an epidural location instead of an intramedullary location. The spread of paraspinal tumor through the intervertebral foramina is also prevalent. Damage to the cord is usually inflicted not by direct invasion but by vascular compromise, and several investigators have demonstrated in animal models that the edema and infarction seen in severe compression most often are due to impairment of the blood flow to and from the spinal cord.[49-51]

The histologic variant of lung cancer most associated with spinal cord compression is small cell carcinoma. It also tends to develop early with small cell cancer. Bach and colleagues found cord compression developing in more than 85% of their patients within 3 months of the initial diagnosis of lung cancer. In most patients with squamous cell cancer, however, compressions did not develop before 30 months after initial diagnosis.[48]

Pain is the most common presenting symptom in patients with spinal cord compression. As the neurologic damage worsens, it usually progresses to paresthesias, extremity weakness, and bowel or bladder incontinence. Because of its insidious onset, more than half the patients with spinal cord compression are unable to ambulate at the time of diagnosis.[52] Having a high index of suspicion for a patient with a known malignant disease in whom back pain develops can help the clinician potentially confine the morbidity.

Both the neurologic functional status at the time of diagnosis and the duration of onset have been shown to be crucial factors in predicting recovery after treatment.[46-48,52] With minimal or no impairment in mobility, most patients (80%) will maintain the ability to ambulate. With worsening paraparesis, only 20% to 60% will regain function, and a mere 15% of those with complete paralysis will regain function. Neurologic deficits with gradual onset are more often reversible than rapidly progressing weakness.[53-56]

MRI of the spine is the study of choice to accompany thorough neurologic examination of the patient with new-onset back pain.[56] It is minimally invasive and delivers more comprehensive information about spinal and paravertebral tissue involvement than CT myelography and plain radiographs.

Treatment of spinal cord compression with surgery, radiotherapy, or both remains controversial because there are no phase III prospective, randomized trials with adequate numbers to guide therapy. Steroid use in the form of dexamethasone is recommended from the time of diagnosis. A common regimen is 6 to 10 mg given intravenously followed by 4 mg given orally or intravenously. The use of higher doses has been shown to expedite pain control, but did not significantly improve neurologic deficits.[57,58]

Radiation therapy remains the primary treatment for the majority of patients with this condition, but surgical decompression and systemic chemotherapy play important roles in selected patients. Young et al.[59] reported a small phase III trial of 29 patients randomly assigned to radiation alone vs. laminectomy plus radiation. There was no statistically significant difference in the rate of ambulation between the two groups. One third of the patients in both groups were walking 4 months after treatment.[59] Although this study, as well as several retrospective reviews, does not find surgical decompression a necessary adjunct, it plays a critical role when (1) a diagnosis is not known, (2) the cord compression is due to mechanical problems caused either by retropulsed bone particles from vertebral body collapse or by spinal instability, (3) the tumor is resistant to radiotherapy, or (4) there is a history of previous radiation that precludes re-treatment.[60,61]

CONCLUSION

Several tools are available for the palliation of bone and soft tissue metastases. Each is effective in its own setting, and care must be exercised in combining them. Lung cancer continues to be the cause of most cancer deaths in the United States and therefore of much of the palliative care given. The actual techniques used to palliate metastases from lung cancer do not differ from those used for metastases originating from other sites, but the natural history of lung cancer is often swift once it is clinically detected. For that reason, symptomatic metastases should be dealt with in a way that will minimize the patients' time under treatment and yet improve their quality of life.

REFERENCES

1. Parker SL, Tong T, Bolden S, Wingo PA. Cancer statistics, 1997. CA Cancer J Clin 47:5-27, 1997.
2. Napoli LD, Hansen HH, Muggia FM, Twigg HL. The incidence of osseous involvement in lung cancer, with special reference to the development of osteoblastic changes. Radiology 108:17-21, 1973.
3. Yoneda T. Cellular and molecular mechanisms of breast and prostate cancer metastasis to bone. Eur J Cancer 34:240-245, 1998.
4. Eilon G, Mundy GR. Direct resorption of bone by human breast cancer cells in vitro. Nature 276:726-728, 1978.
5. Galasko CSB. Mechanisms of bone destruction in the development of skeletal metastasis. Nature 263:507-508, 1976.
6. Hiraga T, Tanaka S, Ikegame M, Koizumi M, Iguchi H, Nakajima T, Ozawa H. Morphology of bone metastasis. Eur J Cancer 34:230-239, 1998.
7. Coleman RE. Skeletal complications of malignancy. Cancer 80(Suppl):1588-1594, 1997.
8. Rubens RD. Bone metastases—The clinical problem. Eur J Cancer 34:210-213, 1998.
9. Sullivan FJ. Palliative radiotherapy for lung cancer. In Pass HI, Mitchel JB, Johnson DH, Turrisi AT, eds. Lung Cancer: Principles and Practices. Philadelphia: Lippincott-Raven, 1996, pp 775-789.
10. Tong D, Gillick L, Hendrickson FR. The palliation of symptomatic osseous metastases. Cancer 50:893-899, 1982.
11. Nielsen O, Bentzen SM, Sandberg E, Gadeberg CC, Timothy AR. Randomized trial of single dose versus fractionated palliative radiotherapy of bone metastases. Radiother Oncol 47:233-240, 1998.
12. Gaze MN, Kelly CG, Kerr GR, Cull A, Cowie VJ, Gregor A, Howard GC, Rodger A. Pain relief and quality of life following radiotherapy for bone metastases: A randomised trial of two fractionation schedules. Radiother Oncol 45:109-116, 1997.
13. Niewald M, Tkocz H-J, Abel U, Scheib T, Walter K, Nieder C, Schnabel K, Berberich W, Kubale R, Fuchs M. Rapid course radiation therapy vs. more standard treatment: A randomized trial for bone metastases. Int J Radiat Oncol Biol Phys 36:1085-1089, 1996.
14. Price P, Hoskin PJ, Easton D, Austin D, Palmer SG, Yarnold JR. Prospective randomized trial of single and multifraction radiotherapy schedules in the treatment of painful bony metastases. Radiother Oncol 6:247-255, 1986.
15. Hoskin PJ, Price P, Easton D, Regan J, Austin D, Palmer S, Yarnold JR. A prospective randomized trial of 4 Gy or 8 Gy single doses in the treatment of metastatic bone pain. Radiother Oncol 23:74-78, 1992.
16. Okawa T, Kita M, Goto M, Nishijima H, Miyaji N. Randomized prospective clinical study of small, large and twice-a-day fraction radiotherapy for painful bone metastases. Radiother Oncol 13:99-104, 1988.
17. Madsen LE. Painful bone metastasis: Efficacy of radiotherapy assessed by the patients: A randomized trial comparing 4 Gy × 6 versus 10 Gy × 2. Int J Radiat Oncol Biol Phys 9:1775-1779, 1983.
18. Blitzer PH. Reanalysis of the RTOG study of the palliation of symptomatic osseous metastasis. Cancer 55:1468-1472, 1985.
19. Body JJ. Bisphosphonates. Eur J Cancer 34:263-269, 1998.
20. Rogers MJ, Watts DJ, Russell RGG. Overview of bisphosphonates. Cancer 80(Suppl):1652-1660, 1997.
21. Hortobagyi GN, Theriault RL, Porter L, Blayney D, Lipton A, Sinoff C, Wheeler H, Simeone JF, Seaman J, Knight RD, Heffernan M, Reitsma DJ. Efficacy of pamidronate in reducing skeletal complications in patients with breast cancer and lytic bone metastases. N Engl J Med 335:1785-1791, 1996.
22. Conte PF, Latreille J, Mauriac L, Calabresi F, Santos R, Campos D, Bonneterre J, Francini G, Ford JM. Delay in progression of bone metastases in breast cancer patients treated with intravenous pamidronate: Results from a multinational randomized controlled trial. J Clin Oncol 14:2552-2559, 1996.
23. Paterson AH, Powles TJ, Kanis JA, McCloskey E, Hanson J, Ashley S. Double-blind controlled trial of oral clodronate in patients with bone metastases from breast cancer. J Clin Oncol 11:59-65, 1993.
24. Ernst DS, Brasher P, Hagen N, Paterson AHG, MacDonald RN, Bruera E. A randomized, controlled trial of intravenous clodronate in patients with metastatic bone disease and pain. J Pain Symptom Manage 13:319-326, 1997.
25. Biermann WA, Cantor RI, Fellin FM, Jakobowski J, Hopkins L, Newbold RC. An evaluation of the potential cost reductions resulting from the use of clodronate in the treatment of metastatic carcinoma of the breast to bone. Bone 12:S37-S42, 1991.
26. Coleman RE, Pruohit OP, Vinholes JJ, Zekri J. High dose pamidronate. Cancer 80(Suppl):1686-1690, 1997.
27. Serafini AN. Current status of systemic intravenous radiopharmaceuticals for the treatment of painful metastatic bone disease. Int J Radiat Oncol Biol Phys 30:1187-1194, 1994.
28. Joshi DP, Seery WH, Goldberg LG. Evaluation of 32-phosphorus for intractable pain secondary to prostatic carcinoma metastasis. JAMA 193:621-623, 1965.
29. Porter AT, McEwan AJB, Powe JE, Reid R, McGowan DG, Lukka H, Sathyanarayana JR, Yakemchuk VN, Thomas GM, Erlich LE, Crook J, Gulenchyn KY, Hong KE, Wesolowski C, Yardley J. Results of a randomized phase III trial to evaluate the efficacy of strontium-89 adjuvant to local field external beam irradiation in the management of endocrine resistant metastatic prostate cancer. Int J Radiat Oncol Biol Phys 25:805-813, 1993.
30. Bolger JJ, Dearnaley DP, Kirk D, Lewington JV, Mason MD, Quilty PM, Reed NSE, Russel JM, Yardley J. Strontium-89 (Metastron) versus external beam radiotherapy in patients

with painful bone metastases secondary to prostatic cancer: Preliminary report of a multicenter trial. Semin Oncol 20:32-33, 1993.

31. Lee CK, Aeppli DM, Unger J, Boudreau RJ, Seymour LH. Strontium-89 chloride (Metastron) for palliative treatment of bony metastases: The University of Minnesota experience. Am J Clin Oncol 19:102-107, 1996.

32. Guerrieri P, Modoni S, Parisi S, Fusco V, Oriolo V, Rendina G, Paleani-Vettori PG. Bone formation markers and pain palliation in bone metastases treated with strontium-89. Am J Clin Oncol 17:77-79, 1994.

33. Lewington VJ, McEwan AJ, Ackery DM, Bayly RJ, Keeling DH, Macleod PM, Porter AT, Zivanovic MA. A prospective, randomized double-blind crossover study to examine the efficacy of strontium-89 in pain palliation in patients with advanced prostate cancer metastatic to bone. Eur J Cancer 27:954-958, 1991.

34. Buchali K, Correns HJ, Schuerer M, Schnorr D, Lips H, Sydow K. Results of a double blind study of 89-strontium therapy of skeletal metastases of prostatic carcinoma. Eur J Nucl Med 14:349-351, 1988.

35. McEwan AJB, Amyotte GA, McGowan DG, MacGillivray JA, Porter AT. A retrospective analysis of the cost effectiveness of treatment with metastron in patients with prostate cancer metastatic to bone. Eur Urol 26:26-31, 1994.

36. Turner JH, Claringbold PG. A phase II study of treatment of painful multifocal skeletal metastases with single and repeated dose samarium-153 ethylenediaminetetramethylene phosphate. Eur J Cancer 27:1084-1086, 1991.

37. Maxon HR, Schroder LE, Hertzberg VS, Thomas SR, Englara EE, Samaratunga R, Smith H, Moulton JS, Williams CC, Ehrhardt GJ, Schneider HJ. Rhenium-186(Sn)HEDP for treatment of painful osseous metastases: Results of a double-blind crossover comparison with placebo. J Nucl Med 32:1877-1881, 1991.

38. Limouris G, Shukla SK, Manetou A, Kouvaris I, Plataniotis G, Triantafyllou N, Rigas AV, Vlahos L. Rhenium-186-HEDP palliative treatment in disseminated bone metastases due to prostate cancer. Anticancer Res 17:1699-1704, 1997.

39. De Klerk JM, van het Schip AD, Zonnenberg BA, van Dijk A, Quirijnen JM, Blijham GH, van Rijk PP. Phase 1 study of rhenium-186-HEDP in patients with bone metastases originating from breast cancer. J Nucl Med 37:244-249, 1996.

40. Lin WY, Lin CP, Yeh SJ, Hsieh BT, Tsai ZT, Ting G, Yen TC, Wang SJ, Knapp FF Jr, Stabin MG. Rhenium-188 hydroxyethylidene disphosphonate: A new generator-produced radiotherapeutic drug of potential value for the treatment of bone metastases. Eur J Nucl Med 24:590-595, 1997.

41. Harrington KD. Orthopedic surgical management of skeletal complications of malignancy. Cancer 80(Suppl):1614-1627, 1997.

42. Finn HA. Hip and proximal femur. In Simon MA, Springfield D, eds. Surgery for Bone and Soft-Tissue Tumors. Philadelphia: Lippincott-Raven, 1998, pp 683-703.

43. Finn HA. Pelvis and acetabulum. In Simon MA, Springfield D, eds. Surgery for Bone and Soft-Tissue Tumors. Philadelphia: Lippincott-Raven, 1998, pp 671-682.

44. Harrington KD. Anterior cord compression and spinal stabilization for patients with metastatic lesions of the spine. J Neurosurg 61:107-117, 1984.

45. Moore AJ, Uttley D. Anterior decompression and stabilization of the spine in malignant disease. Neurosurgery 24:713-717, 1989.

46. Janjan NA. Radiation for bone metastases. Cancer 80(Suppl):1628-1645, 1997.

47. Fuller BG, Heiss J, Oldfield EH. Spinal cord compression. In DeVita VT, Hellman S, Rosenberg SA, eds. Cancer: Principles and Practice of Oncology, 5th ed. Philadelphia: Lippincott-Raven, 1997, pp 2476-2486.

48. Agerlin N, Sorensen JB, Rasmussen TB, Dombernowsky P, Sorensen PS, Hansen HH. Metastatic spinal cord compression secondary to lung cancer. J Clin Oncol 10:1781-1787, 1992.

49. Doppman JL, Girton M. Angiographic study of the effect of laminectomy in the presence of acute anterior epidural masses. J Neurosurg 45:195-202, 1976.

50. Agruello F, Baggs RB, Duerst RE, Johnstone L, McQueen K, Frantz CN. Pathogenesis of vertebral metastasis and epidural spinal cord compression. Cancer 65:98-106, 1990.

51. Ushio Y, Posner R, Posner JB, Shapiro WR. Experimental spinal cord compression by epidural neoplasm. Neurology 27:422-429, 1977.

52. Nielsen OS, Munro AJ, Tannock IF. Bone metastases: Pathophysiology and management policy. J Clin Oncol 9:509-524, 1991.

53. Tarlov IM, Klinger H, Vitale S. Spinal cord compression studies. I. Experimental techniques to produce acute and gradual compression. Arch Neurol Psychiatr 70:813, 1957.

54. Tarlov IM, Klinger H. Spinal cord compression studies. II. Time limits for recovery after acute compression in dogs. Arch Neurol Psychiatr 71:271, 1954.

55. Tarlov IM. Spinal cord compression studies. III. Time limits for recovery after gradual compression in dogs. Arch Neurol Psychiatr 71:588, 1954.

56. Helweg-Larsen S, Rasmusson B, Sorensen PS. Recovery of gait after radiotherapy in paralytic patients with metastatic epidural spinal cord compression. Neurology 40:1234-1236, 1990.

57. Vecht CJ, Haaxma-Reiche H, van Putten WL, de Visser M, Vries EP, Twijnstra A. Initial bolus of conventional versus high-dose dexamethasone in metastatic spinal cord compression. Neurology 39:1255-1257, 1989.

58. Greenberg HS, Kim JH, Posner JB. Epidural spinal cord compression from metastatic tumor: Results of a new treatment protocol. Ann Neurol 8:361-366, 1980.

59. Young RJ, Post EM, King GA. Treatment of spinal epidural metastases: Randomized prospective comparison of laminectomy and radiotherapy. J Neurosurg 61:107, 1984.

60. Byrne TN. Spinal cord compression from epidural metastases. N Engl J Med 327:614-619, 1992.

61. Landmann C, Hunig R, Gratzl O. The role of laminectomy in the combined treatment of metastatic spinal cord compression. Int J Radiat Oncol Biol Phys 24:627-631, 1992.

Malignant Melanoma

Mark R. Albertini, M.D., *Paul M. Harari,* M.D., *and Douglas Reintgen,* M.D.

Malignant melanoma is an increasingly common disease. Recent estimates from the American Cancer Society are that 47,700 new cases of melanoma will be diagnosed in the United States in 2000.[1] Since 7700 cancer deaths due to melanoma are expected to occur this year,[1] this is an important clinical problem. Many of the patients will be quite young, as the average age at diagnosis of melanoma is approximately 50 years.[2] Although melanoma caught early can be cured, the successful treatment of patients with metastatic disease remains elusive. The median survival for patients with metastatic melanoma is about 7 months, and the percentage of metastatic melanoma patients with 5-year survival is approximately 6%.[3] Thus emphasis on prevention and early detection of this disease is appropriate. It is essential that all health care providers recognize the appearance of early melanomas, as early recognition and removal of suspicious pigmented skin lesions can result in long-term survival and cure for the patient. In addition, evolving guidelines for primary management and staging of melanoma need to be recognized to accurately identify patients at risk of recurrent or metastatic disease and to identify candidates for adjuvant therapy.

In the staging of primary melanoma, emphasis is on the depth of the primary melanoma and reflects the importance of microscopic depth of tumor invasion in determining overall prognosis. The vertical depth of the melanoma is referred to as the Breslow depth and is the single most important prognostic factor for a localized melanoma.[3] A commonly used staging system is the American Joint Committee on Cancer (AJCC) staging system for cutaneous melanoma. Stage I melanoma comprises localized melanomas not more than 1.5 mm thick and stage II melanoma comprises localized melanomas deeper than 1.5 mm, either with or without satellite(s) within 2 cm of the primary tumor. Patients with stage III melanoma have either regional lymph node or in-transit metastases, and patients with stage IV disease have distant metastases. Important additional prognostic factors not included in this staging system are ulceration of the primary melanoma and number of positive nodes.[3] A revised staging system is anticipated to be available in the year 2001.[4]

PATTERNS OF SPREAD

The pattern of metastases for metastatic melanoma has been reported from many clinical series and includes skin, subcutaneous tissue, and lymph nodes (42% to 59% of patients), lung (18% to 36% of patients), liver (14% to 20% of patients), brain (12% to 20% of patients), bone (11% to 17% of patients), intestine (1% to 7% of patients), and other sites.[5] Autopsy series report a greater percentage of patients with metastatic disease to these sites, as well as additional patients with further sites of metastatic disease, including heart, pancreas, adrenals, kidney, and thyroid.[5] These studies suggest that clinical evaluation of patients often underestimates the extent of metastatic disease as well as the actual tumor burden. Bone and muscle metastases are uncommonly the initial site of recurrence and are much more commonly involved in patients with diffusely metastatic disease. The axial skeleton is most commonly involved when melanoma is metastatic to bone, and the most common site of metastasis is the spine.[6,7] Although the pathophysiology for bone destruction by metastatic melanoma has not been clearly defined, several preclinical models suggest a role for osteoclasts[8,9] as well as for interleukin-11[10] and matrix metalloproteinases.[11] Because bone and muscle metastases are a significant source of morbidity for many patients with metastatic melanoma, appropriate management guidelines are needed.

INITIAL SURGICAL MANAGEMENT

The appropriate management of patients with melanoma requires an understanding of the indications and techniques of biopsy of skin lesions suspected of being melanoma. Because early melanoma can be cured, the surgical margins of excision needed for a primary melanoma must be recognized to maximize the possibility of cure while also avoiding unnecessary morbidity for the patient. Recent advances in our understanding of the pattern of spread of melanoma have allowed for selected additional surgical staging to stratify patients into better-defined risk groups for systemic relapse. Since effective adjuvant therapy for this disease has now been identified,[12] the understanding of systemic recurrence risk is of major importance in determining which patients should be offered possible adjuvant therapy for their surgically resected melanoma. This discussion will outline the initial considerations in the surgical management of patients with melanoma as well as describe the surgical evaluation of patients for possible regionally metastatic disease.

Indications and Techniques of Biopsy

Biopsies for melanomas can be either excisional or incisional.[13] Whichever technique is used, full-thickness biopsy into the subcutaneous tissue must be performed to permit microstaging of the lesion for thickness and level of invasion. Shave or curette biopsies are absolutely contraindicated for lesions suspected of being melanomas; these biopsy techniques invariably give a positive deep margin, and therefore true tumor thickness cannot be ascertained. Because tumor thickness is the one prognostic variable of primary melanoma that greatly influences treatment decisions, patient care suffers if tumor thickness cannot be ascertained because of inappropriate biopsy techniques. For instance, if a pigmented lesion is suspicious and a shave biopsy is performed that cuts through the melanoma at a depth of 0.60 mm, then the surgeon is left to contemplate whether that melanoma originally had a thickness greater than 0.76 mm, which would make the patient a candidate for regional nodal staging.

Excisional Biopsies

An excisional biopsy is indicated for a suspicious lesion that is not large (<1.5 cm in diameter) and is situated so that the amount of skin excised is not critical (e.g., on the trunk). The lesion should be excised with an elliptical incision that includes a narrow margin (2 mm) of normal-appearing skin. Taking slightly larger margins (e.g., 1 cm) of skin may be insufficient for a malignant lesion and excessive for a benign one.

The direction of the biopsy incision is important because a biopsy that is not properly oriented may necessitate a skin graft when an elliptical incision and primary closure might have been possible. The biopsy incision should be oriented so that the site can be reexcised with optimal skin margins and minimal skin loss if the lesion proves to be malignant. For lesions on an extremity, the recommendation is that the biopsy axis be oriented in the same direction as the axis of the extremity. Punch biopsies may be performed if the entire lesion can be encompassed with the punch, with the largest punch biopsy available being 6 mm. Care should be taken to take this biopsy into the subcutaneous fat, so that the evaluation of tumor thickness is not compromised.

Incisional Biopsies

Incisional biopsies should be performed when the amount of skin removed is critical (e.g., face, hands, or feet). They may also be indicated for large lesions for which an excisional biopsy would be a formidable procedure. An incisional biopsy can be done with a scalpel, but usually a 6 mm punch biopsy is preferred to take a full-thickness core of skin and subcutaneous tissues from the most raised or irregular area of the lesion.

The biopsy specimen should not be taken at the periphery of the lesion unless there are areas of raised nodularity at this location. No decrease in survival rates or increase in local recurrence rates has been observed with the incisional approach.[14] Moreover an incisional biopsy is a simple, expedient office procedure and if performed properly provides representative tissue.

Surgical Margins of Excision

Local control of a primary melanoma requires wide local excision (WLE) of the tumor or biopsy site with a margin of normal-appearing skin. A WLE is recommended because in approximately 5% of the primary melanomas a satellite focus of disease separated from the main lesion will be found. Until recently the routine surgical approach was to excise all primary melanomas with a 3 to 5 cm margin and apply a split-thickness skin graft to the defect. It has become increasingly clear, however, that the risk of local recurrence correlates more with the tumor thickness than with the margins of surgical excision.[15] It therefore seems more rational to excise melanomas with surgical margins that vary according to tumor thickness and ulceration, since these factors correlate best with the risk of local recurrence.

Intraoperative Lymphatic Mapping and Sentinel Lymph Node Biopsy

A new procedure has been developed to assess the status of the regional lymph nodes more accurately and to decrease the morbidity and expense to the

The nervous system can be divided into two major systems: the central nervous system (CNS) and the peripheral nervous system (PNS). This chapter discusses the incidence, mechanisms, sites of involvement, symptoms, diagnostic study, and treatment of extraneural musculoskeletal metastases from primary tumors of the CNS and the PNS.

Neural tumors are relatively rare. Tumors of the nervous system are estimated to have accounted for 17,400 tumors in 1998, or approximately 1.4% of all new cancer cases.[1] Systemic metastases, including osseous metastases, from neural tumors are extremely uncommon.

Tumors of the Central Nervous System

INCIDENCE

Primary tumors of the CNS uncommonly metastasize outside the CNS axis. In 1926 Bailey and Cushing[2] proclaimed that these tumors never give rise to metastases outside the CNS. Davis[3] reported the first case of extraneural metastases from a glioblastoma multiforme in 1928, and since the 1950s there have been an increasing number of case reports.[4-8] In 1963 Glasauer and Yuan[4] found 88 cases reported in the world literature, and in 1977 Pasquier et al.[5] found 248 cases. The incidence of extraneural metastases from primary CNS tumors is estimated to be about 0.4% to 0.5%,[5,6] although one pediatric series found the incidence to be as high as 26%.[9] This increase may be due to improved treatment techniques for the primary tumors, resulting in longer patient survival time, improvement in diagnostic imaging techniques, or a greater recognition that the condition exists.

PATHOLOGIC CRITERIA

In 1955 Weiss[10] set the following strict criteria for the diagnosis of extracranial metastases from primary CNS lesions: the metastatic lesion must be histologically characteristic of a CNS tumor; the clinical history indicates a primary CNS lesion; a complete postmortem examination should be done to exclude peripheral primary lesions; and identical histologic features must be present in both the CNS and the metastatic lesion. Unfortunately the requirement for postmortem verification limits the applicability of these criteria. Yung et al.[7] described a technique permitting premortem diagnosis of bone marrow metastasis from malignant gliomas, using peroxidase-antiperoxidase staining of the marrow specimen for glial fibrillary acidic protein (GFAP), a glia-specific marker. They concluded that a positive result indicates a primary CNS lesion, whereas a negative result cannot exclude this possibility. Thus a premortem diagnosis may be made by using this technique in combination with Weiss's criteria.

TUMOR TYPES AND METASTATIC SITES

Extracranial metastases can occur with a number of intracranial primary tumors. They are most commonly seen with medulloblastoma, high-grade malignant gliomas, and hemangiopericytomas, but there have been reports of extracranial metastases from ependymoblastomas, pineal tumors, sarcomas, melanomas, and endodermal sinus tumors.[4-19]

Medulloblastoma

In a review by Campbell et al.,[8] 21 of 917 children with a primary CNS tumor had extracranial metastases. Medulloblastoma, which comprised only 16.5% of the 917 cases, was the most frequent cause of metastases (71% of the metastatic cases). Extracranial metastatic medulloblastoma most frequently is manifested by skeletal involvement and is usually multifocal in nature. Approximately 3% to 5% of patients with medulloblastoma have systemic metastases. Ninety percent of these patients have radiologic evidence of bone metastases. Skeletal metastases may be either osteoblastic or osteolytic and most commonly involve the pelvis, femur, and vertebrae.[8,11,12] In more than 50% of patients with metastatic disease, medulloblastoma may also metastasize to the bone marrow. Peritoneal metastases are seen in about 30% of patients. In a review by Kleinman et al.,[12] approximately 65% of patients had lymph node metastases, 30% had liver metastases, and 10% to 30% had lung metastases. The median interval to the development of metastases is approximately 18 to 24 months from diagnosis of the original tumor.[8,13]

Malignant Glioma

Although malignant glioma accounts for a higher total number of metastatic cases than medulloblastoma, the percentage of patients with metastases is much lower. This is due to the substantially higher incidence of glioma than of medulloblastoma. Glioblastoma multiforme rarely metastasizes outside the neuraxis, but in the few such reported instances, extracranial metastatic sites included the lungs and lymph nodes. In rare cases, metastases to the bones and liver developed.[5] Pasquier et al.[5] reviewed 72 cases of astrocytoma and glioblastoma with extracranial metastases and found 30.5% of cases had bone involvement. Of these, 73% involved the vertebrae, 23% the ribs, 18% the sternum, 14% the skull, and 9% the acetabulum. In a review by Smith et al.,[6] 26% of cases of glioblastoma multiforme with extraneural metastases involved bone sites. The sites were often isolated, although diffuse disease may occur on occasion. Malignant glioma can also metastasize to a number of other organs and systems, including the lungs (60%), lymph nodes (51%), liver (22%), heart (7%), and, even more rarely, the adrenal glands, kidneys, diaphragm, mediastinum, pancreas, thyroid gland, and peritoneum.[4,5]

Meningeal Hemangiopericytoma

Meningeal hemangiopericytoma (HPC) has the propensity for both local recurrence and extraneural metastases. Although HPC accounts for fewer than 1% of CNS tumors, metastases occur in 12% to 57% of patients.[14] In a review of 169 cases of HPC, Bastin and Mehta[14] found that 21% of patients had metastatic disease at presentation. Metastases may be multiple and can develop in many organs and systems. HPC of the CNS most commonly metastasizes to bone (41%), liver (36%), lungs (36%), CNS and meninges (23%), and abdominal cavity (25%), and, more uncommonly, to lymph nodes, skeletal muscles, kidneys, pancreas, skin, breast, adrenal glands, and gallbladder.[15] Guthrie et al.[16] demonstrated an increasing metastatic frequency from treatment time of 13%, 33%, and 64% at 5, 10, and 15 years, respectively.

MECHANISMS FOR METASTASES

Several mechanisms may be responsible for the development of extraneural metastases in primary brain tumors. Liwnicz and Rubinstein[17] emphasized that surgical procedures play a significant role in the dissemination of disease by enabling tumor cells to escape the confines of the CNS. A surgical procedure may aid in hematogenous tumor spread via the venous system or may result in direct invasion of the scalp and, subsequently, the lymphatic vessels. In Hoffman and Duffner's review[11] of 282 cases of extraneural metastases, 80% of cases had CNS surgery. These procedures included craniotomy, laminectomy, ventricular tap, and intracranial shunt placement.

The use of cerebrospinal fluid (CSF) shunts has also been implicated as a possible route of spread, although this implication remains controversial. Shunts provide a direct channel between the CNS and the abdomen (in ventriculoperitoneal shunts) or between the CNS and the heart (in ventriculoatrial shunts). In a review of 60 patients with medulloblastoma, Park et al.[18] noted that of 49 patients with ventriculoperitoneal shunts, 6 subsequently had extraneural metastases. Of these patients, only one had a Millipore filter inserted. Berger et al.[19] reviewed 415 pediatric cases of primary brain tumors, of which 37% had shunts placed. Metastatic disease developed in only 8 of the 415 patients, and 3 of them had shunts. The authors analyzed a number of factors, including shunt characteristics, and concluded that CSF shunts, regardless of type, location, revision rate, or filter insertion, did not predispose the patients to the development of extraneural metastases.

PRESENTATION

Presenting symptoms in patients with metastatic disease depend on the organs and systems involved. Patients with osseous metastases generally have bone pain, pathologic fractures, or both at presentation. They may also have hypercalcemia or neurologic symptoms related to compression of the spinal cord, peripheral nerves, or cranial nerves from extraosseous extension of tumor or bone collapse. Patients with bone marrow metastases may have hematologic abnormalities when first seen.

STAGING

Staging evaluation should include basic laboratory studies, including a complete blood cell count, liver function tests, and chemical studies. For specific evaluation for skeletal metastases, a bone scan should be obtained, followed by plain radiographs of suspected areas of uptake. Lesions may be osteolytic or osteoblastic. Magnetic resonance imaging (MRI) may be necessary in patients with neurologic symptoms for identification of cord compression or nerve root involvement, if present. MRI is also valuable for detection of marrow involvement. Soft tissue extension of the skeletal metastases is often best defined by computed tomography, which helps to define treatment options and radiation portals. In patients with medulloblastoma, a bone marrow biopsy should be considered.

MANAGEMENT

Because there are only a limited number of cases of skeletal metastases from primary brain tumors, no major clinical trials are feasible and management decisions are extrapolated from trials of other skeletal metastases. Management options include supportive care, surgery, radiation therapy, and chemotherapy. Supportive care measures are aimed at managing pain and decreasing the risk of further injury to the patient. These measures include pain medications, ambulatory aids, and education regarding decreased activity during the course of treatment and recovery. Hospice or nursing care may also be necessary, depending on the patient's social situation.

The goals of surgical procedures for bone metastases from CNS tumors include pain control, stabilization of impending or pathologic fractures of bones, and ambulatory assistance. Decompression of the spinal cord with spinal stabilization may be indicated in acute cord compression. Internal fixation is most often used for metastases to the long bones, and prosthetic joint replacement may be considered in selected situations.

External beam radiotherapy is used to aid in pain relief and decrease the need for pain medications, as well as to increase ambulation. Radiation also works to control local tumor growth to prevent spinal cord or nerve root compression or pathologic fracture. Radiation can be given by using multiple techniques, including involved-field radiation, wide-field radiation, hemibody radiation, and systemic radiation. Involved-field radiation is by far the most commonly employed method of palliation. Radiation fields should cover the affected bone with a margin of several centimeters. For vertebral bodies the affected body plus one or two adjacent vertebral bodies should be included. Field size may be limited by normal tissue tolerance, chemotherapy, or prior radiotherapy.

A randomized study by the Radiation Therapy Oncology Group evaluated multiple-dose fractionation schedules (2.7 Gy × 15; 3 Gy × 10; 3 Gy × 5; 4 Gy × 5; 5 Gy × 5) and found no difference in response between the different groups.[20] A reanalysis by Blitzer[21] revealed that the more protracted schedules of 2.7 Gy × 15 and 3 Gy × 10 were more effective than the shorter courses. Several other studies comparing the efficacy of shorter courses of therapy with longer courses have not shown any significant differences.[22-25] In a review of the literature, Madsen[24] found that an optimal schedule or dose did not exist. The Patterns of Care Study Survey, reported by Coia et al.,[26] showed that the most common fractionation schedule used in practice is 3 Gy × 10 fractions. Rose and Kagan[27] reported the recommendations of a panel of experts for the treatment of bone metastases. They found that 4 Gy × 5, 3 Gy × 10, and 2.5 Gy × 14 were acceptable dose-fractionation schemes for the majority of patients and that a more rapid course of therapy may be acceptable in patients with a life expectancy of less than 3 months.

Chemotherapy has been used in medulloblastoma metastatic to bone. Dramatic responses of extraneural lesions have been seen with a variety of single and combination chemotherapy programs, including adriamycin alone; methyl lomustine alone; and vincristine, actinomycin D (dactinomycin), and cyclophosphamide in combination.[28] Chamberlain et al.[13] reported on seven patients with metastatic medulloblastoma who received cyclophosphamide, doxorubicin, and vincristine. All seven patients had both a decrease in their bone pain and improvement on their bone scans. The median duration of response was 18 months, with a range of 4 to 65 months. Lundberg et al.[29] described a case of recurrent metastatic medulloblastoma involving lymph nodes, bone, and bone marrow. The patient was treated with multiagent cytoreductive salvage chemotherapy, followed by an allogeneic bone marrow transplant, and was alive and well at 28 months.

OUTCOME

Extraneural metastases from primary CNS tumors are almost universally fatal. Hoffman and Duffner[11] found the median survival time in such cases to be 2 years. Pasquier et al.[5] found the median survival time in metastatic gliomas to be 18.2 months and found that almost 83% of the patients had died within the first 2 years. Guthrie et al.[16] also found the median survival time in HPC of the CNS to be 24 months.

Tumors of the Peripheral Nervous System

INCIDENCE

Neuroblastoma is the fourth most common pediatric malignancy and accounts for approximately 500 new cases of cancer per year. It is a tumor that can occur anywhere along the sympathetic nervous system. Most commonly it occurs first in the adrenal medulla and the paraspinal sympathetic ganglia. Approximately 60% of patients have metastatic disease at presentation, and 47% of patients with relapse of stage I, II, or III disease will later have distant disease.[30]

METASTATIC SITES

The most common sites of metastasis from neuroblastoma are the lymph nodes, bone marrow, bone, liver, and subcutaneous tissue. Berthold et al.[30] reviewed 381 cases of stage I-III neuroblastoma and found 77 cases of relapse. Of the patients with systemic relapse, 41% had bone marrow metastases, 39% had lymph node metastases, and 37% had bone metastases. The median time for the development of metastatic disease in these patients was 13 months from initial diagnosis.

PRESENTATION

Presenting symptoms in patients with metastatic neuroblastoma depend on the sites of metastatic involvement. Pain is the most common presenting symptom in neuroblastoma metastatic to bone and bone marrow. Although more common from the primary tumor than from bone metastases, spinal cord compression with paralysis may occur. Patients may also have hematologic abnormalities at presentation.

STAGING

In patients with neuroblastoma the staging evaluation for bone and bone marrow metastases should include a bone scan, a skeletal survey, and a bone marrow biopsy and aspiration. A scan with iodine 131–labeled meta-iodobenzylguanidine (MIBG) can also be obtained. MIBG is preferentially taken up by cells with adrenergic secretory vesicles and thus allows for the imaging of most neuroblastomas.[31]

MANAGEMENT

Chemotherapy is the main therapeutic modality in treating metastatic neuroblastoma. The most commonly used agents include cyclophosphamide, cisplatin, doxorubicin, and teniposide.[32,33] It appears that intensive high-dose chemotherapy is superior to less intensive regimens.[33] There is some evidence that myeloablative therapy followed by bone marrow transplantation may be more effective than conventional chemotherapy.[34] Patients who undergo bone marrow transplantation tend to have relapse in the site of previous disease, which suggests that additional localized therapies may improve local control and decrease the frequency of relapse.[35,36]

Radiation therapy may be used for consolidation, palliation, or myeloablation before bone marrow transplantation. Bone metastases are often more extensive than is apparent on plain films, and thus portals should include a generous margin. Field design and fractionation schedule should take into account the patient's life expectancy. In patients with a poor prognosis, large fields and hypofractionated schedules should be employed to allow for less time spent in treatment. In patients with a good prognosis, special attention must be given to decrease the amount of normal tissue treated and to treat bones symmetrically to decrease late radiation effects, including spinal deformities and limb shortening. For patients in the good prognosis group, fraction size should be 1.2 to 1.5 Gy, given twice daily. Total doses for metastatic disease (9 to 36 Gy) are similar to those for curative treatment and are age dependent.

OUTCOME

In patients with metastatic disease at presentation the case is staged according to the sites of metastasis and the patient's age at diagnosis. Bone metastases confer a worse prognosis as does age greater than 1 year. Those patients who are less than 1 year of age and whose metastases are limited to the liver, bone marrow, or skin (stage IV-S) have a high rate of spontaneous regression and a survival rate as high as 90%.[37] Those patients with stage IV disease (age >1 year, distant metastases to sites other than those listed here) have a 3-year survival rate of 10% to 40%.[32,37]

Conclusion

Neural tumors of the central and the peripheral nervous systems are relatively uncommon malignancies and rarely metastasize outside the neuraxis. Because of the small number of cases of osseous metastases in neural tumors, there is a lack of specific clinical trials to define management of these patients. Treatment recommendations are based on principles defined for other skeletal metastases and integrate radiation therapy, chemotherapy, and surgery.

REFERENCES

1. Landis SH, Murray T, Bolden S, Wingo PA. Cancer statistics, 1998. CA Cancer J Clin 48:6-29, 1998.
2. Bailey P, Cushing P. A Classification of the Tumors of the Glioma Group on a Histogenetic Basis With a Correlated Study of Prognosis. Philadelphia: JB Lippincott, 1926, p 175.
3. Davis L. Spongioblastoma multiforme of the brain. Ann Surg 87:8-14, 1928.
4. Glasauer FE, Yuan RHP. Intracranial tumors with extracranial metastases: Case report and review of the literature. J Neurosurg 20:474-493, 1963.
5. Pasquier B, Pasquier D, N'Golet A, Panh MH, Couderc P. Extraneural metastases of astrocytomas and glioblastomas: Clinicopathological study of two cases and review of literature. Cancer 45:112-125, 1980.
6. Smith DR, Hardman JM, Earle KM. Metastasizing neuroectodermal tumors of the central nervous system. J Neurosurg 31:50-58, 1969.
7. Yung WK, Tepper SJ, Young DF. Diffuse bone marrow metastasis by glioblastoma: Premortem diagnosis by peroxidase-antiperoxidase staining for glial fibrillary acidic protein. Ann Neurol 14:581-585, 1983.
8. Campbell AN, Chan HSL, Becker LE, Daneman A, Park TS, Hoffman HJ. Extracranial metastases in childhood primary intracranial tumors: A report of 21 cases and review of the literature. Cancer 53:974-981, 1984.
9. Duffner PK, Cohen ME. Extraneural metastases in childhood brain tumors. Ann Neurol 10:261-265, 1981.
10. Weiss L. A metastasizing ependymoma of the cauda equina. Cancer 8:161-171, 1955.
11. Hoffman HJ, Duffner PK. Extraneural metastases of central nervous system tumors. Cancer 56:1778-1782, 1985.
12. Kleinman GM, Hochberg FH, Richardson EP Jr. Systemic metastases from medulloblastoma: Report of two cases and review of the literature. Cancer 48:2296-2309, 1981.
13. Chamberlain MC, Silver P, Edwards MS, Levin VA. Treatment of extraneural metastatic medulloblastoma with a combination of cyclophosphamide, adriamycin, and vincristine. Neurosurgery 23:476-479, 1988.
14. Bastin KT, Mehta MP. Meningeal hemangiopericytoma: Defining the role for radiation therapy. J Neuro Oncol 14:277-287, 1992.
15. Mena H, Ribas JL, Pezeshkpour GH, Cowan DN, Parisi JE. Hemangiopericytoma of the central nervous system: A review of 94 cases. Hum Pathol 22:84-91, 1991.
16. Guthrie BL, Ebersold MJ, Scheithauer BW, Shaw EG. Meningeal hemangiopericytoma: Histopathological features, treatment, and long-term follow-up of 44 cases. Neurosurgery 25:514-522, 1989.
17. Liwnicz BH, Rubinstein LJ. The pathways of extraneural spread in metastasizing gliomas: A report of three cases and critical review of the literature. Hum Pathol 10:453-467, 1979.
18. Park TS, Hoffman HJ, Hendrick EB, Humphreys RP, Becker LE. Clinical presentation and management: Experience at the Hospital for Sick Children, Toronto 1950-1980. J Neurosurg 58:543-552, 1983.
19. Berger MS, Baumeister JR, Geyer JR, Milstein J, Kanev PM, LeRoux PD. The risks of metastases from shunting in children with primary central nervous system tumors. J Neurosurg 74:872-877, 1991.
20. Tong D, Gillick L, Hendrickson FR. The palliation of symptomatic osseous metastases: Final results of the Study by the Radiation Therapy Oncology Group. Cancer 50:893-899, 1982.
21. Blitzer PH. Reanalysis of the RTOG study of the palliation of symptomatic osseous metastasis. Cancer 55:1468-1472, 1985.
22. Okawa T, Kita M, Goto M, Nishijima H, Miyaji N. Randomized prospective clinical study of small, large and twice-a-day fraction radiotherapy for painful bone metastases. Radiother Oncol 13:99-104, 1988.
23. Price P, Hoskin PJ, Easton D, Austin D, Palmer SG, Yarnold JR. Prospective randomized trial of single and multifraction radiotherapy schedules in the treatment of painful bony metastases. Radiother Oncol 6:247-255, 1986.
24. Madsen EL. Painful bone metastasis: Efficacy of radiotherapy assessed by the patients—a randomized trial comparing 4 Gy × 6 versus 10 Gy × 2. Int J Radiat Oncol Biol Phys 9:1775-1779, 1983.
25. Cole DJ. A randomized trial of a single treatment versus conventional fractionation in the palliative radiotherapy of painful bone metastases. Clin Oncol 1:59-62, 1989.
26. Coia LR, Hanks GE, Martz K, Steinfeld A, Diamond JJ, Kramer S. Practice patterns of palliative care for the United States, 1984-1985. Int J Radiat Oncol Biol Phys 14:1261-1269, 1988.
27. Rose CM, Kagan AR. The final report of the expert panel for the radiation oncology bone metastasis work group of the American College of Radiology. Int J Radiat Oncol Biol Phys 40:1117-1124, 1998.
28. Nathanson L, Kovacs SG. Chemotherapeutic response in metastatic medulloblastoma: Report of two cases and a review of the literature. Med Pediatr Oncol 4:105-110, 1978.

29. Lundberg JH, Weissman DE, Beatty PA, Ash RC. Treatment of recurrent metastatic medulloblastoma with intensive chemotherapy and allogeneic bone marrow transplantation. J Neuro Oncol 13:151-155, 1992.

30. Berthold F, Hero B, Breu H. The recurrence patterns of stage I, II and III neuroblastoma: Experience with 77 relapsing patients. Ann Oncol 7:183-187, 1996.

31. Shapiro B. Imaging of catecholamine-secreting tumors: Uses of MIBG in diagnosis and treatment. Baillieres Clin Endocrinol Metab 7:491-507, 1993.

32. Bowman LC, Hancock ML, Santana VM, Hayes FA, Kun L, Parham DM. Impact of intensified therapy on clinical outcome in infants and children with neuroblastoma: The St. Jude Children's Research Hospital experience, 1962 to 1988. J Clin Oncol 9:1599-1608, 1991.

33. Cheung NV, Heller G. Chemotherapy dose intensity correlates strongly with response, median survival, and median progression-free survival in metastatic neuroblastoma. J Clin Oncol 9:1050-1058, 1991.

34. Kai T, Ishii E, Matsuzaki A, Inaba S, Suita S, Ueda K. High-dose chemotherapy and autologous blood stem cell transplantation in children with metastatic neuroblastoma. Acta Paediatr Japonica 39:54-60, 1997.

35. Matthay KK, Atkinson JB, Stram DO, Selch M, Reynolds CP, Seeger RC. Patterns of relapse after autologous purged bone marrow transplantation for neuroblastoma: A Childrens Cancer Group pilot study. J Clin Oncol 11:2226-2233, 1993.

36. Sibley GS, Mundt AJ, Goldman S, Nachman J, Reft C, Weichselbaum RR, Hallahan DE, Johnson L. Patterns of failure following total body irradiation and bone marrow transplantation with or without a radiotherapy boost for advanced neuroblastoma. Int J Radiat Oncol Biol Phys 32:1127-1135, 1995.

37. Nickerson HJ, Nesbit ME, Grosfeld JL, Baehner RL, Sather H, Hammond D. Comparison of stage IV and IV-S neuroblastoma in the first year of life. Med Pediatr Oncol 13:261-268, 1985.

Prostate Cancer

Arthur T. Porter, M.D., Edgar Ben-Josef, M.D.,
Wilson C. Mertens, M.D., and James R. Ryan, M.D.

Much of the clinical practice of oncology involves palliative care. Palliation, simply defined, is the alleviation of symptoms in a patient with active disease, for whom the prognosis is limited and the focus of care is preservation of quality of life. The basic tenets of palliation are to do good, minimize harm, and foster patient autonomy. Due consideration is given to the condition of the patient, to the chances of effecting palliation, and to the patient's wishes. Palliative radiotherapy can effectively relieve pain, prevent hemorrhage and obstruction, and improve organ function. It can be delivered in a relatively short time frame and with few side effects when the tolerance of normal tissues is respected.

Effective palliation requires thorough knowledge of the natural history of the disease. A key consideration is the patient's overall prognosis and life expectancy. Although the survival of patients with bone metastases is generally poor, potential long-term survivors must be identified. Not only would they require a more durable relief, but they are also more at risk of having a late treatment-related complication. In a Radiation Therapy Oncology Group (RTOG) trial,[1] median survival in patients with solitary and multiple bone metastases was 36 and 24 weeks, respectively. Patients with breast and prostate primary tumors survived significantly longer (30 to 73 weeks), whereas patients with lung cancer died within a median of 12 to 14 weeks. Other factors that affect survival include hormone responsiveness and performance status.

The American Cancer Society estimates that 184,500 new cases of prostate cancer will be diagnosed during 1998 in the United States and that 39,200 patients will die of prostate cancer, making this disease the second leading cause of cancer death in men.[2] Prostate cancer spreads by local extension, via lymph and blood vessels. At diagnosis the disease is confined locally in 50% of patients. Lymph node and distant metastases occur in 20% and 30% of patients, respectively.[3] Regional lymph node involvement follows a predictable pattern: periprostatic and obturator nodes are involved first, followed by internal and external iliac, common iliac, and periaortic nodes.[4] Spread to supradiaphragmatic nodes is less common.[5] Distant spread occurs most commonly to the bone. Visceral metastases are usually a feature of advanced disease and involve lungs, liver, adrenal glands, kidneys, and the epidural space.[6,7] Rare instances of spread to the testis,[8] male breast,[9] and brain[10] have also been reported.

PATTERNS OF SPREAD

The spine is the most frequently involved skeletal structure, followed by the femur, pelvis, rib cage, skull, and humerus. It has been postulated that this predilection is the result of communication of the venous drainage of the primary site with Batson's presacral plexus.[11] More recently this concept has been challenged by reports describing prostate cancer skeletal metastases distributed in a manner similar to that seen in nonprostatic malignancies.[12,13] It is now thought that skeletal dissemination is dependent on the regional arterial blood supply, rather than the venous drainage,[13] and on interactions between prostatic epithelial cells and bone stroma. It is increasingly recognized that the interaction of metastatic cells with host tissues is modulated by stimulatory and inhibitory signals from a variety of autocrine and paracrine pathways, with the eventual outcome dependent on the net balance of these regulators. Therefore the site-specific pattern of metastasis is, at least in part, dependent on the existence of a favorable microenvironment in the target organ. Prostate cancer growth-stimulating factors have been identified in human bone-marrow stroma.[14,15]

MANAGEMENT OF BONE METASTASES
Diagnosis

Osseous metastasis is the most common cause of intractable pain in patients with cancer.[16] Bone pain results in immobility, anxiety, and depression and severely diminishes a patient's quality of life. In autopsy series the prevalence of skeletal metastases in patients who died of prostate cancer is 46% to 85%.[17] In a prospective longitudinal series of hospital patients,[18] prostate cancer carried the highest risk of resulting in bone metastases (32%).

Most bone metastases can be diagnosed by physical examination, plain radiographs, and bone scan. Plain radiographs are highly accurate in detecting metastatic lesions, particularly in association with pain, but have a low degree of sensitivity. This is directly related to the pathogenesis of bone metastases.[19] Because the cortical bone is affected relatively late, large metastatic deposits in the intramedullary canal may go unrecognized. Within the spine, although the vertebral body is affected first, the first noted radiologic findings are those of pedicle destruction. Radiographs of a painful lesion may show a pathologic fracture or an impending fracture. Two views are recommended to diagnose the latter. The radiographic pattern of prostate cancer metastasis is typically blastic.

Bone scanning is a useful adjunct to plain films. Technetium Tc 99m diphosphonate is taken up in areas of osteoblastic activity and can be used for detection of bone metastases and after response to therapy. Bone scintigraphy is more sensitive than plain radiographs.[20] It can frequently show metastatic lesions long before changes on plain films are appreciated.[21]

Computed tomography (CT) can differentiate between metastases and degenerative changes, even when the two conditions coexist and even though the latter is a common cause of increased uptake on a bone scan.[22] CT is also valuable in evaluating soft tissue involvement and can be combined with myelography for detecting extradural tumor spread in patients unable to undergo magnetic resonance imaging (MRI).

More recently, MRI has been described as the method of choice for examining the spine. It is more sensitive than a bone scan for detecting early metastases within the medulla, but both T1- and T2-weighted images are required. It is the procedure of choice when neural compression is suspected.[23] When cord impingement is suspected, imaging of the entire spine should be considered because approximately 10% of patients have multiple levels of cord impingement.[24] MRI is also used in discriminating between benign and malignant vertebral collapse. Disadvantages of MRI include its high cost, exclusion of patients with metal implants, severe claustrophobia, and inferior visualization of the cortex in comparison with a CT scan.

Bone biopsy is not required routinely. It is helpful in patients with no history of malignancy, in patients with a solitary lesion, and in patients with more than one suspected primary lesion. In the latter situation it may make a difference in the systemic therapy.

Pharmacologic Therapy

Pharmacologic therapy for bone metastases encompasses analgesics (aspirin, acetaminophen, nonsteroidal anti-inflammatory agents, steroids, opiates, and others), bisphosphonates, and specific antitumoral therapy.

Prostate cancer is sensitive to hormonal manipulation, with as many as 80% of patients showing some degree of response.[25] Androgen suppression can be achieved by orchiectomy, or it can be achieved chemically with luteinizing hormone-releasing hormone (LHRH) agonists, exogenous estrogens, progesterones, antiandrogens, or adrenal enzyme synthesis inhibitors. Controversies remain regarding the optimal form of hormonal manipulation. A flare response is noted in 8% to 30% of patients treated with an LHRH agonist. This response can be avoided by the use of an antiandrogen during the first weeks of therapy. The National Cancer Institute trial[26] comparing leuprolide with or without flutamide showed a significant advantage of total androgen blockade in patients with low-burden disease. The 303 patients receiving the combination therapy had a longer progression-free survival (16.5 vs. 13.9 months, $P = 0.039$) and a longer median survival (35.6 vs. 28.3 months, $P = 0.035$) than the 300 patients receiving leuprolide with a placebo.[26] Similar results were seen in a phase III EORTC trial.[27]

The bisphosphonates have a phosphate-carbon-phosphate backbone that binds tightly to calcified bone matrix and inhibits osteoclast-mediated bone resorption. The exact mechanism is unclear, but postulated mechanisms include direct biochemical effects on the osteoclast, prevention of osteoclast attachment to the bone matrix, and inhibition of differentiation of osteoclast precursors and recruitment.

Data on the efficacy of bisphosphonates have been collected primarily in patients with breast cancer.[28-32] Relief of pain with intravenously administered pamidronate was noted in approximately 50% of patients, and approximately 25% showed radiographic evidence of bone healing. Paterson et al.[30] reported a significant reduction in the

phosphate (EDTMP), to produce a bone-seeking complex. About 50% of an intravenously administered dose is retained in bone.[58,59] The absorbed doses in bone and red marrow have been estimated at 2.5 cGy/MBq and 0.57 cGy/MBq, respectively.[59]

The maximal tolerated dose of [153]Sm was determined to be 2.5 mCi/kg.[60] The principal toxic effect observed was hematologic, with maximal myelosuppression occurring at 3 to 4 weeks. A flare of bone pain occurred in 12% of patients. The overall pain relief rate was 74%, with a median duration of palliation of 2.6 months. In responders, relief was obtained promptly, within 7 to 14 days of treatment. Response rates were significantly higher with 2.5 mCi/kg than with 1 mCi/kg. Two phase-III studies comparing 0.5 mCi/kg, 1 mCi/kg, and placebo were recently reported.[61,62] In both studies, 60% to 72% of patients had some pain relief within 4 weeks.

Rhenium 186 emits beta-particles of 1.07 MeV and a 137 keV gamma ray and has a short half-life of 3.8 days. Like [153]Sm, it has been complexed to a bone-seeking phosphonate, hydroxyethylenediphosphonic acid (HEDP). Retention in bone is about 50% of the injected dose, with the rest excreted through the kidneys into the urine.[63] Rhenium 186 has been studied in a small number of patients with metastatic cancer of the prostate, breast, colon, and lung.[64] After administration of 33 to 35 mCi, 75% to 80% of patients had pain relief, most often within 2 weeks.[55-57] The average duration of palliation was 5 weeks. The therapeutic efficacy of [186]Re has been confirmed in a double-blind crossover comparison with placebo.[65] Myelosuppression begins 2 weeks after treatment, peaks at 4 to 6 weeks, and resolves by 8 weeks.[64] A pain flare occurs in 10% of patients 2 to 3 days after treatment and resolves within 1 week.

In summary, in addition to external beam radiotherapy, SRs have proved useful in the treatment of widely metastatic disease. They are most useful in patients without a predominantly painful site, as a first-line therapy, and when options for external beam therapy have been exhausted and normal tissue tolerance has been reached. Patients should have a life expectancy of at least 3 months and a good marrow reserve. There should be no evidence of imminent epidural cord compression, pathologic fracture, or mechanical instability.

In 1998 the membership of the American Society for Therapeutic Radiology and Oncology were surveyed regarding the management of painful osseous metastases.[66] The survey consisted of 30 multiple-choice questions regarding four hypothetical clinical scenarios likely to be encountered in daily practice. Questions related to the technique of choice (LFI vs. HBI), the use of SRs, fractionation schemes, dose, the integration of modalities, and follow-up.

Of 3268 cases, 817 (33%) responses have been received and analyzed. The results indicated that LFI is the most common form of therapy. It was used alone or in combination with other forms of therapy in 54% and 74% of patients, respectively. LFI was used more frequently in patients with breast cancer than in patients with prostate cancer (79% vs. 45%; $P = 0.0001$). Long fractionation schemes were used by 90% of physicians in 96% of cases. Short fractionation schemes were used by 7% of physicians in 4% of cases. This tendency was more pronounced in private practice than in university or government multidisciplinary settings ($P = 0.008$) or in the private practice of physicians starting their practice before 1982 ($P = 0.05$). The most common schedule was 30 Gy in 10 fractions, used by 77% of physicians in 64% of cases. HBI was used alone or in combination with other forms of therapy in 1% and 2% of patients, respectively. It was used more frequently in patients with prostate cancer than in patients with breast cancer (1.2% vs. 0.1%, respectively; $P < 0.0001$). SRs were used alone or in combination with LFI in 21% and 40% of cases, respectively. SRs were used more frequently in patients with prostate cancer than in those with breast cancer (28% vs. 0.2%, respectively; $P < 0.00001$). The most common radionuclide in use is [89]Sr (99%) at a dose of 4 mCi (73%) or 10.8 mCi (26%). These results demonstrate the emergence of a new pattern of practice: LFI to the painful site in combination with SRs for clinically occult metastases.

Radiotherapy

The majority of patients can be managed successfully with external-beam radiotherapy. Although a large body of clinical evidence documents the effectiveness of LFI, the optimal dose and fractionation schedule have not yet been determined. A summary of the major prospective clinical trials that addressed these issues is provided in Table 22-1.

Between 1974 and 1980 the RTOG conducted a large national study to determine the effectiveness of five different dose fractionation schedules.[1] A total of 1016 patients were entered, 266 into a "solitary metastasis" stratum and 750 into a "multiple metastases" stratum. The former were randomly assigned to treatment with 40.5 Gy in 15 fractions or 20 Gy in 5 fractions. The latter were assigned to 30 Gy in 10 fractions, 15 Gy in 5 fractions, 20 Gy in 5 fractions, or 25 Gy in 5 fractions. A quantitative measure of pain, based on severity and frequency of pain and on the type and frequency of pain medications used, was devised to evaluate response. Overall, 89% of patients had minimal relief, whereas 83% achieved partial relief and 54% obtained complete relief. There were no significant differences between the treatment arms in both strata. The initial pain score was found to be a useful predictor; patients with high scores were less likely to respond and were less likely to have a complete response. Patients with breast and prostate cancer were significantly more likely to respond than patients with lung or other primary lesions. Patients completing their treatment as planned had a significantly higher rate of complete response than those who did not. Although some relief was achieved almost invariably within the first 4 weeks, complete relief was first reported later than 4 weeks after the start of treatment in about 50% of patients. The median duration of minimal and complete pain relief was 20 and 12 weeks, respectively. There were no significant differences in the duration of pain relief between the different arms. It was concluded that all treatment dose schedules were equally effective.

A reanalysis of the RTOG study was reported by Blitzer.[67] Using a stepwise logistic regression, he examined the effect of the number of fractions, the dose per fraction, and solitary vs. multiple metastases on the probability of attaining complete pain relief and the need for retreatment. This multivariate technique allowed patients with solitary and multiple metastases to be analyzed together. By in-

Table 22-1   Summary of prospective clinical trials of radiotherapy for painful osseous metastases

Reference	Patients (no.)	Total dose (Gy)	Fractions (no.)	Overall response (%)	Complete response (%)
Tong et al.[1]	759	40.5	15	85*	61*
		20	5	82*	53*
		30	10	87	57
		15	5	85	49
		20	5	83	56
		25	5	78	49
Hoskin et al.[70]	270	4	1	44	36
		8	1	69	39
Price et al.[69]	288	8	1	82	45
		30	10	71	28
Okawa et al.[71]	92	30	15	76	—
		22.5	5	75	—
		20	10†	78	—
Madsen[72]	57	24	6	47	—
		20	2	48	—

*Patients with solitary metastases.
†Twice a day.

creasing the number of subjects and events, the statistical power of the analysis was increased. The number of fractions was the only variable that was significantly associated with outcome. There was no correlation of the time-dose factor[68] with outcome. It was concluded that the more protracted schedules resulted in improved pain relief.

Price et al.[69] randomly selected 288 patients to receive either 8 Gy in one fraction or 30 Gy in 10 daily fractions. Pain was assessed with a questionnaire completed by the patient at home on a daily basis. No differences were found in the probability of attaining pain relief, the speed of onset, or the duration of relief between the two arms.

Hoskin et al.[70] randomly selected 270 patients to receive either 4 Gy or 8 Gy in one fraction. Pain (assessed by the patient) and analgesic use were recorded before treatment and at 2, 4, 8, and 12 weeks. At 4 weeks the response rates were 69% for 8 Gy and 44% for 4 Gy ($P < 0.001$). The duration of the effect was independent of dose.

Two other randomized trials have been reported.[71,72] Given the small difference in the biologic effective dose between the arms[71] and the small number of patients accrued,[71,72] it is not surprising that no differences between the treatment arms were detected.

Although the studies noted here failed to demonstrate a clear dose-response analysis of pain relief, the relief of pain continues to be an important clinical issue, with potential impact on the quality of life of the dying patient and with major financial implications. Recently we conducted a dose-response analysis using pooled data from published phase III clinical trials. The end point selected for the analysis was complete response. It was thought that this end point was more likely than partial or minimal response to be evaluated consistently across the studies. One study[72] was excluded from the analysis because outcome was not reported by means of conventional definitions of complete and partial response. The biologic effective dose was calculated for each schedule by using the linear-quadratic model and an α/β value of 10, and the data were fitted to a logistic dose-response model. The analysis demonstrated a highly significant dose-response effect for complete relief of pain at 13 weeks.

Most patients with bone metastases have multiple sites of involvement. As many as 76% of patients receiving therapy to a local field require additional treatment for pain at other sites within 1 year.[73] Wide-field radiotherapy has been used to address this problem. A summary of results of this form of therapy is provided in Table 22-2. Response rates are similar to those observed with LFI, but the onset of relief is more rapid, occurring often within 24 hours of treatment. HBI may require hospitalization for hydration and premedication with steroids and antiemetics and tends to be associated with substantial morbidity. Most patients have acute gastrointestinal toxic effects, with nausea, vomiting, and diarrhea that persist for 24 to 48 hours. Myelosuppression is commonly observed but is rarely of clinical significance. Radiation pneumonitis is rare at doses of less than 7 Gy to the lungs.

The RTOG conducted a phase III study to evalu-

Table 22-2   Wide-field radiotherapy for painful osseous metastases

| Reference | Field treated (no.) | Dose (Gy) | | Response (%) |
		Upper	Lower	
Fitzpatrick[75]	570	3-6	10	55-72
Rowland et al.[76]	96	7.5	10	80
Qasim[77]	129	7-8*	7-8*	76
Salazar et al.[74]	168	6	8	73
Wilkins and Keen[78]	141	6	8	82
Poulter et al.[73]	229	8	8	93

*A dose of 3 to 4 Gy in patients with multiple myeloma.

ate the efficacy of HBI in addition to LFI.[73] A total of 499 patients were randomly assigned to receive either HBI or no further therapy after completion of LFI to a symptomatic site. Entry was stratified by the extent of metastatic disease (solitary or multiple) and the targeted hemibody area (upper, middle, or lower). LFI consisted of 30 Gy in 10 fractions; HBI consisted of 8 Gy in one fraction given within 7 days of completion of LFI. Partial transmission blocks were used to reduce the dose to the lungs to 7 Gy. Time to disease progression, time to new disease, and time to a new course of therapy were significantly longer in the HBI arm. Progression of disease was faster in patients with involvement of the upper and middle hemibody (compared with the lower hemibody) and in patients with multiple metastases (compared with a solitary metastasis). As expected, toxic effects were significantly higher in the HBI arm, but there were no fatalities and no occurrences of radiation pneumonitis. Although the impact of HBI on clinically occult metastatic disease was demonstrated unequivocally, the absolute benefit was relatively small. The ultimate progression rates were not significantly different between the arms, and at 1 year, 60% of the HBI group had to undergo additional treatment.

Surgery

Surgery should be considered for patients with pathologic fractures or impending fractures. In the former situation, fixation can reduce pain and expedite healing. In the latter, prophylactic fixation may prevent a fracture, thereby eliminating functional loss and reducing the risk of nonunion of a fracture.

There are no good methods to predict the risk of a pathologic fracture. Factors that have been examined as potential predictors include site, level of pain, radiographic appearance, and size of the lesion.[79-82] Pathologic fractures most often involve weightbearing regions (femoral neck, peritrochanteric, subtrochanteric) and the humerus. Lesions in these locations should be regarded as high risk, particularly if they are osteolytic, are associated with intense pain, involve a length of cortex equal to or greater than the cross-sectional diameter of the bone or greater than 2.5 cm in axial length, or cause destruction of 50% or more of the cortex.[81,82] In general, patients considered for prophylactic fixation should have a life expectancy longer than 3 months and should be medically fit to tolerate major surgery. The quality of bone proximal and distal to the lesion must be adequate to support a fixation device.

SPECIAL PROBLEMS
Management of Spinal Cord Compression

Malignant spinal cord compression occurs in 5% of all patients with malignant disease and in approximately 20% of patients with metastases to the vertebral column.[83] More than 95% of spinal cord compressions are due to extramedullary malignancy, most commonly because of involvement of the vertebral column anterior to the spinal cord, less frequently by tumors posterior to the spinal cord, and occasionally by invasion of the epidural space.

Any metastasis to the bone can eventually result in a cord compression. Most commonly seen primary tumors include those of lung, breast, prostate, and kidney. The majority of patients have pain, motor loss, autonomic dysfunction, and sensory loss at presentation.[84] Pain is often radicular for weeks or months before onset of the neurologic symptoms. Autonomic dysfunction may occur early and be manifested as hesitancy and urgency. Weakness usually precedes sensory loss, with incontinence, paraplegia, and paralysis being late effects. Pain was the initial symptom in 96% of the patients but is a poor indicator of spinal-epidural involvement.[85] On the other hand, 75% of patients with major neurologic involvement also have involvement of the epidural space.

Early diagnosis is essential because recovery of neurologic function is related to the degree of loss. A careful history and physical examination focusing on neurologic examination, with a high index of suspicion in patients with known malignancy, are the key to early diagnosis. Diagnostic investigations varying from plain spinal x-ray films to myelograms have been used in the past. MRI is now the diagnostic study of choice. The entire length of the spinal cord and its relationship with surrounding structures can be visualized without the use of intrathecal contrast medium.[86,87] Distortion of the theca by extradural lesions and soft tissue abnormalities can be easily identified.[87,88] In case of compression fracture, protrusion of the vertebral body or tumor into the spinal canal is seen clearly, as is the impingement of nerve roots and neural foramina.[86] Approximately 10% of patients have multiple sites of cord compression and perhaps benefit from imaging of the entire spine.

A multidisciplinary approach is recommended for management of spinal cord compression. High-dose steroid therapy should be administered after a clinical diagnosis, and doses should then be tapered rapidly as tolerated. A surgical approach should be considered in a patient without a histologic diagnosis of the primary tumor or in a patient who has received the maximal tolerable dose to the region. A randomized trial comparing laminectomy followed by radiation vs. radiation alone in the treatment of spinal epidural metastasis showed no significant difference in the effectiveness of treatment in regard to pain relief, improved ambulation, or improved sphincter function.[89]

Treatment outcome is dependent on pretreatment function. In a study of 137 patients with malignant spinal cord compression, 81% of patients who were ambulatory before treatment remained so afterward, whereas only 16.5% of those who were nonambulatory before treatment became ambulatory afterward. Pain abated after treatment in 73% of the patients regardless of ambulatory status.[83]

Palliative Therapy for Local Symptoms of Advanced Disease

Genitourinary hemorrhage may occur in patients with locally advanced, uncontrolled prostate cancer. Irradiation is the treatment of choice in these cases. A variety of regimens have been studied.[90,91] A common regimen of 30 Gy in 10 fractions stops macroscopic hematuria in more than 80% of patients within 4 weeks.

Pelvic pain and obstructive uropathy resulting from local extension can also be treated with radiation therapy. Higher doses (40 to 50 Gy in 20 to 25 fractions) are recommended. Kraus et al.[92] described satisfactory palliation in patients treated with doses of 22.5 to 66 Gy. Rectal symptoms were alleviated in 5 of 5 patients, gross hematuria cleared in 13 of 13 patients, and urethral obstruction responded in 4 of 5 patients. Kynaston et al.[93] reported useful palliation in 24 of 26 patients treated for bleeding or lower urinary outflow tract obstruction. Wells et al.[94] reported alleviation of obstruction (removal of an indwelling catheter) in 17 of 19 patients. The median time from completion

of radiotherapy to catheter removal was 10 weeks. Surgical intervention is usually reserved for nonresponsive patients or when immediate relief is required.

CONCLUSION

Metastatic disease to the skeleton is extremely common in prostate carcinoma. Hormonal therapy, chemotherapy, and radiation therapy are first-line treatments for the skeletal disease. Surgical intervention is only occasionally indicated, usually in osteolytic disease. Many patients live a number of productive years with metastatic prostate carcinoma.

REFERENCES

1. Tong D, Gillick L, Hendrickson FR. The palliation of symptomatic osseous metastases: The results of the Radiation Therapy Oncology Group. Cancer 50:893-899, 1982.
2. Cancer Facts and Figures—1998. Atlanta: The American Cancer Society Inc., 1998.
3. Scardino PT, Weaver R, Hudson MA. Early detection of prostate cancer. Hum Pathol 23:211-222, 1992.
4. Narayan P. Neoplasms of the prostate gland. In Tanagho EA, McAninch JW, eds. Smith's General Urology, 14th ed. Norwalk, Conn.: Appleton & Lange, 1995, p 392.
5. Cho KR, Epstein JI. Metastatic prostate carcinoma to supradiaphragmatic lymph nodes: A clinicopathologic and immunohistochemical study. Am J Surg Pathol 11:457-463, 1987.
6. Abrams HL, Spiro R, Goldstein N. Metastases in carcinoma: Analysis of 1000 autopsied cases. Cancer 3:74-75, 1950.
7. Saitoh H, Hida M, Shimbo T, Nakamura K, Yamagata J, Satoh T. Metastatic patterns of prostate cancer: Correlation between sites and number of organs involved. Cancer 54:3078-3084, 1984.
8. Tiltman AJ. Metastatic tumours in the testis. Histopathology 3(1):31-37, 1979.
9. Lo MC, Chomet B, Rubenstone AI. Metastatic prostatic adenocarcinoma of male breast. Urology 11:641-646, 1978.
10. Catane R, Kaufman J, West C, Tsukada Y, Murphy GP. Brain metastasis from prostatic carcinoma. Cancer 38:2583-2587, 1976.
11. Batson OV. The function of vertebral veins and their role in the spread of metastasis. Ann Surg 112:138, 1940.
12. Dodds PR, Caride VJ, Lytton B. The role of vertebral veins in the dissemination of prostatic carcinoma. J Urol 126:753-755, 1981.
13. Morgan JWM, Adcock LA, Donohue RE. Distribution of skeletal metastases in prostatic and lung cancer. Urology 36:31-34, 1990.
14. Chackal-Roy M, Niemeyer C, Moore M, Zetter BR. Stimulation of human prostatic carcinoma cell growth by factors present in human bone-marrow. J Clin Invest 84(1):43-50, 1989.
15. Lang SH, Clarke NW, George NJ, Allen TD, Testa NG. Inter-

action of prostate epithelial cells from benign and malignant tumor tissue with bone-marrow stroma. Prostate 34:203-213, 1998.

16. Foley KM. The treatment of cancer pain. N Engl J Med 313: 84-94, 1985.

17. Tubiana-Hulin M. Incidence, prevalence and distribution of bone metastases. Bone 12(Suppl 1):S9-S10, 1991.

18. Galasko CSB. Incidence and distribution of skeletal metastases. Clin Orthop 210:14-22, 1986.

19. Johnston AD. Pathology of metastatic tumors in bone. Clin Orthop 73:8-32, 1970.

20. Pagani JJ, Libshitz HI. Imaging in bone metastases. Radiol Clin North Am 20:545-560, 1982.

21. Glasko CSB. Skeletal metastases. Clin Orthop 210:18-30, 1986.

22. Muindi J, Coombes RC, Golding S, Powles TJ, Khan O, Husband J. The role of computed tomography in the detection of bone metastases in breast cancer patients. Br J Radiol 56:233-236, 1983.

23. Daffner RH, Lupetin AR, Dash N, Deeb ZL, Sefczek RJ, Schapiro RL. MRI in the detection of malignant infiltration of bone marrow. AJR Am J Roentgenol 146:353-358, 1986.

24. Bonner JA, Lichter AS. A caution about the use of MRI to diagnose spinal cord compression. N Engl J Med 322:556-557, 1990.

25. Huggins C. Endocrine-induced regression of cancers. Cancer Res 27:1925-1930, 1967.

26. Crawford ED, Eisenberger MA, McLeod DG, Spaulding JT, Benson R, Dorr FA, Blumenstein BA, Davis MA, Goodman PJ. A controlled trial of leuprolide with and without flutamide in prostatic carcinoma. N Engl J Med 321:419-424, 1989.

27. Denis LJ, Carnelro de Moura JL, Bono A, Sylvester R, Whelan P, Newling D, Depauw M. Goserelin acetate and flutamide versus bilateral orchidectomy: A phase III EORTC trial (30853). Urology 42(2):119-129, 1993.

28. Coleman RE, Woll PJ, Miles M, Scrivener W, Rubens RD. Treatment of bone metastases from breast cancer with (3-amino-1-hydroxypropylidene)-1,1-bisphosphonate (APD). Br J Cancer 58:621-625, 1988.

29. Morton AR, Cantrill JA, Pillai GV, McMahon A, Anderson DC, Howell A. Sclerosis of lytic bone metastases after disodium aminohydroxypropylidene bisphosphonate (APD) in patients with breast cancer. BMJ 297:772-773, 1988.

30. Paterson AH, Powles TJ, Kanis JA, McCloskey E, Hanson J, Ashley S. Double-blind controlled trial of oral clodronate in patients with bone metastases from breast cancer. J Clin Oncol 11:59-65, 1993.

31. Van-Holten–Verzantvoort AT, Kroon HM, Bijvoet OL, Cleton FJ, Beex LV, Blijham G, Hermans J, Neijt JP, Papapoulos SE, Sleeboom HP. Palliative pamidronate treatment in patients with bone metastases from breast cancer. J Clin Oncol 11: 491-498, 1993.

32. Hortobagyi GN, Thieriault RL, Porter L, Blayney D, Lipton A, Sinoff C, Wheeler H, Simeone JF, Seaman J, Knight RD, Heffernan M, Reitsma DJ. Efficacy of pamidronate in reducing skeletal complications in patients with breast cancer and lytic bone metastases. N Engl J Med 335:1785-1791, 1996.

33. Lipton A, Glover D, Harvey H, Grabelsky S, Zelenakas K, Macerata R, Seaman J. Pamidronate in the treatment of bone metastases: Results of 2 dose-ranging trials in patients with breast or prostate cancer. Ann Oncol 5(Suppl 7):S31-S35, 1994.

34. Tannock IF, Osoba D, Stockler MR, Ernst DS, Neville AJ, Moore MJ, Armitage GR, Wilson JJ, Venner PM, Coppin CM, Murphy KC. Chemotherapy with mitoxantrone plus prednisone or prednisone alone for symptomatic hormone-resistant prostate cancer: A Canadian randomized trial with palliative end points. J Clin Oncol 14:1756-1764, 1996.

35. Sella A, Kilbourn R, Amato R, Bui C, Zukiwski AA, Ellerhorst J, Logothetis CJ. Phase II study of ketoconazole combined with weekly doxorubicin in patients with androgen-independent prostate cancer. J Clin Oncol 12:683-688, 1994.

36. Seidman AD, Scher HI, Petrylak D, Dershaw DD, Curley T. Estramustine and vinblastine: Use of prostate-specific antigen as a clinical trial end point for hormone refractory prostatic cancer. J Urol 147(3 Pt 2):931-934, 1992.

37. Hudes GR, Greenberg R, Krigel RL, Fox S, Scher R, Litwin S, Watts P, Speicher L, Tew K, Comis R. Phase II study of estramustine and vinblastine, two microtubule inhibitors, in hormone-refractory prostate cancer. J Clin Oncol 10:1754-1761, 1992.

38. Amato RJ, Ellerhorst J, Bui C, et al. Estramustine and vinblastine for patients with progressive androgen-independent adenocarcinoma of the prostate. Urol Oncol 1:168, 1995.

39. Pienta KJ, Redman B, Hussain M, Cummings G, Esper PS, Appel C, Flaherty LE. Phase II evaluation of oral estramustine and oral etoposide in hormone-refractory adenocarcinoma of the prostate. J Clin Oncol 12:2005-2012, 1994.

40. Hudes GR, Nathan F, Khater C, Haas N, Cornfield M, Giantonio B, Greenberg R, Gomella L, Litwin S, Ross E, Roethke S, McAleer C. Phase II trial of 96-hour paclitaxel plus oral estramustine phosphate in metastatic hormone-refractory prostate cancer. J Clin Oncol 15:3156-3163, 1997.

41. Pecher C. Biological investigations with radioactive calcium and strontium: Preliminary report on the use of radioactive strontium in treatment of metastatic bone cancer. University of California Publications Pharmacology 11:117-149, 1942.

42. Silberstein EB. The treatment of painful osseous metastases with phosphorus-32 labeled phosphates. Semin Oncol 20(3 Suppl 2):10-21, 1993.

43. Landaw SA. Acute leukemia in polycythemia vera. Semin Hematol 23:156-165, 1986.

44. Blake GM, Zivanovic MA, McEwan AJ, Ackery DM. Sr-89 therapy: Strontium kinetics in disseminated carcinoma of the prostate. Eur J Nucl Med 12:447-454, 1986.

45. Breen SL, Powe JE, Porter AT. Dose estimation in strontium-89 radiotherapy of metastatic prostatic carcinoma. J Nucl Med 33:1316-1323, 1992.

46. Ben-Josef E, Lucas RD, Vasan S, Porter AT. Selective accumulation of strontium-89 in metastatic deposits in bone: Radio-histological correlation. Nucl Med Commun 16:457-463, 1995.

47. Blake GM, Zivanovic MA, Blaquiere RM, Fine DR, McEwan AJ, Ackery DM. Strontium-89 therapy: Measurement of absorbed dose to skeletal metastases. J Nucl Med 29:549-557, 1988.

48. Ben-Josef E, Maughan RL, Vasan S, Porter AT. A direct measurement of ^{89}Sr activity in bone metastases. Nucl Med Commun 16:452-456, 1995.

49. Tennvall J, Darte L, Lindgren R, El Hassan AM. Palliation of multiple bony metastases from prostatic carcinoma with strontium-89. Acta Oncol 27:365-369, 1988.

50. Silberstein EB, Williams C. Strontium-89 therapy for the pain of osseous metastases. J Nucl Med 26:345-348, 1985.

51. Laing AH, Ackery DM, Bayly RJ, Buchanan RB, Lewington VJ, McEwan AJ, Macleod PM, Zivanovic MA. Strontium-89 chloride for pain palliation in prostatic skeletal malignancy. Br J Radiol 64:816-822, 1991.

52. Robinson RG, Spicer JA, Preston DF, Wegst AV, Martin NL. Treatment of metastatic bone pain with strontium-89. Nucl Med Biol 14:219-222, 1987.

53. Correns HJ, Mebel M, Buchali K, Schnorr D, Seidel C, Mitterlechner E. Strontium-89 therapy of bone metastases of carcinoma of the prostate gland. Eur J Nucl Med 4:33-35, 1979.

54. Firusian N, Mellin P, Schmidt CG. Results of strontium-89 therapy in patients with carcinoma of the prostate and incurable pain from bone metastases: A preliminary report. J Urol 116:764-798, 1976.

55. Lewington VJ, McEwan AJ, Ackery DM, Bayly RJ, Keeling DH, Macleod PM, Porter AT, Zivanovic MA. A prospective randomized double-blind crossover study to examine the efficacy of strontium-89 in pain palliation in patients with advanced prostate cancer metastatic to bone. Eur J Cancer 27: 954-958, 1991.

56. Porter AT, McEwan AJB, Powe JE, Reid R, McGowan DG, Lukka H, Sathyanarayana JR, Yakemchuk VN, Thomas GM, Erlich LE, et al. Results of a randomized phase-III trial to evaluate the efficacy of strontium-89 adjuvant to local field external beam irradiation in the management of endocrine resistant metastatic prostate cancer. Int J Radiat Oncol Biol Phys 25:805-813, 1993.

57. Quilty PM, Kirk D, Bolger JJ, Dearnaley DP, Lewington VJ, Mason MD, Reed NS, Russell JM, Yardely J. A comparison of the palliative effects of strontium-89 and external beam radiotherapy in metastatic prostate cancer. Radiother Oncol 31:33-40, 1994.

58. Bayouth JE, Macey DJ, Kasi LP, Fossella FV. Dosimetry and toxicity of samarium-153–EDTMP administered for bone pain due to skeletal metastases. J Nucl Med 35:63-69, 1994.

59. Eary JF, Collins C, Stabin M, Vernon C, Petersdorf S, Baker M, Hartnett S, Ferency S, Addison SJ, Appelbaum FR, et al. Samarium-153–EDTMP biodistribution and dosimetry estimation. J Nucl Med 34:1031-1036, 1993.

60. Collins C, Eary JF, Donaldson G, Vernon C, Bush NE, Petersdorf S, Livingston RB, Gordon EE, Chapman CR, Appelbaum FR. Samarium-153–EDTMP in bone metastases of hormone refractory prostate carcinoma: A phase I/II trial. J Nucl Med 34:1839-1844, 1993.

61. Serafini AN, Houston SJ, Resche I, Quick DP, Grund FM, Ell PJ, Bertrand A, Ahmann FR, Orihuela E, Reid RH, Lerski RA, Collier BD, McKillop JH, Purnell GL, Pecking AP, Thomas FD, Harrison KA. Palliation of pain associated with metastatic bone cancer using samarium-153 lexidronam: A double-blind placebo-controlled clinical trial. J Clin Oncol 16:1574-1581, 1998.

62. Resche I, Chatal JF, Pecking A, Ell P, Duchesne G, Rubens R, Fogelman I, Houston S, Fauser A, Fischer M, Wilkins D. A dose-controlled study of [153]Sm-ethylenediaminetetramethylenephosphonate (EDTMP) in the treatment of patients with painful bone metastases. Eur J Cancer 33:1583-1591, 1997.

63. Maxon HR III, Schroder LE, Thomas SR, Hertzberg VS, Deutsch EA, Scher HI, Samaratunga RC, Libson KF, Williams CC, Moulton JS, et al. Re-186(Sn) HEDP for treatment of painful osseous metastases: Initial clinical experience in 20 patients with hormone-resistant prostate cancer. Radiology 176:155-159, 1990.

64. Maxon HR III, Thomas SR, Hertzberg VS, Schroder LE, Englaro EE, Samaratunga R, Scher HI, Moulton JS, Deutsch EA, Deutsch KF, et al. Rhenium-186 hydroxyethylidene diphosphonate for the treatment of painful osseous metastases. Semin Nucl Med 22:33-40, 1992.

65. Maxon HR III, Schroder LE, Hertzberg VS, Thomas SR, Englaro EE, Samaratunga R, Smith H, Moulton JS, Williams CC, Ehrhardt GJ, et al. Re-186(Sn) HEDP for treatment of painful osseous metastases: Results of a double-blind crossover comparison with placebo. J Nucl Med 32:1877-1881, 1991.

66. Ben-Josef E, Shamsa F, Williams AO, Porter AT. Radiotherapeutic management of osseous metastases: A survey of current patterns of care. Int J Radiat Oncol Biol Phys 40:915-921, 1998.

67. Blitzer PH. Reanalysis of the RTOG study of the palliation of symptomatic osseous metastasis. Cancer 55:1468-1472, 1985.

68. Orton CG, Ellis F. A simplification in the use of the NSD concept in practical radiotherapy. Br J Radiol 46:529-537, 1973.

69. Price P, Hoskin PJ, Easton D, Palmer SG, Yarnold JR. Prospective randomized trial of single and multifraction radiotherapy schedules in the treatment of painful bony metastases. Radiother Oncol 6:247-255, 1986.

70. Hoskin PJ, Price P, Easton D, Regan J, Austin D, Palmer S, Yarnold JR. A prospective randomized trial of 4 Gy or 8 Gy single doses in the treatment of metastatic bone pain. Radiother Oncol 23:74-78, 1992.

71. Okawa T, Kita M, Goto M, Nishijima H, Miyaji N. Randomized prospective clinical study of small, large and twice-a-day fraction radiotherapy for painful bone metastases. Radiother Oncol 13(2):99-104, 1988.

72. Madsen EL. Painful bone metastases: Efficacy of radiotherapy assessed by the patients: A randomized trial comparing 4 Gy × 6 versus 10 Gy × 2. Int J Radiat Oncol Biol Phys 9:1775-1779, 1983.

73. Poulter CA, Cosmatos D, Rubin P, Urtasun R, Cooper JS, Kuske RR, Hornback N, Coughlin C, Weigensberg I, Rotman M. A report of RTOG 8206: A phase III study of whether the addition of single dose hemibody irradiation to standard fractionated local field irradiation is more effective than local field irradiation alone in the treatment of symptomatic osseous metastases. Int J Radiat Oncol Biol Phys 23:207-214, 1992.

74. Salazar OM, Rubin P, Hendrikson FR, Komaki R, Poulter C, Newall J, Asbell SO, Mohiuddin M, Van Ess J. Single-dose half-body irradiation for palliation of multiple bone metastases from solid tumors: Final Radiation Therapy Oncology Group report. Cancer 58:29-36, 1986.

75. Fitzpatrick PJ. Wide-field irradiation of bone metastases. In Weiss L, Gilbert HA, eds. Bone Metastases. Boston: GK Hall, 1981, pp 83-113.

76. Rowland CG, Bullimore JA, Smith PJB, Roberts JBM. Half body irradiation in the treatment of metastatic prostatic carcinoma. Br J Urol 53:628-629, 1981.

77. Qasim MM. Half body irradiation in the treatment of metastatic carcinomas. Clin Radiol 32:215-219, 1981.

78. Wilkins MF, Keen CW. Hemibody radiotherapy in the management of metastatic carcinoma. Clin Radiol 38:267-268, 1987.

79. Keene JS, Sellinger DS, McBeath AA, Engber WD. Metastatic breast cancer in the femur: A search for the lesion at risk of fracture. Clin Orthop 203:282-288, 1986.

80. Hipp JA, Springfield DS, Hayes WC. Predicting pathological fracture risk in the management of metastatic bone defects. Clin Orthop 312:120-135, 1995.

81. Mirels H. Metastatic disease in long bones: A proposed scoring system. Clin Orthop 249:256-264, 1989.

82. Lane JM, Sculo TP, Zolan S. Treatment of pathologic fractures of the hip by endoprosthetic replacement. J Bone Joint Surg Am 62:954-959, 1980.

83. Turner S, Marosszeky B, Timms I, Boyages J. Malignant spinal cord compression: A prospective evaluation. Int J Radiat Oncol Biol Phys 26:141-146, 1993.

84. Gilbert RW, Kim JH, Posner JB. Epidural spinal cord compression from metastatic tumor: Diagnosis and treatment. Ann Neurol 3:40-51, 1978.

85. Graus F, Krol G, Foley K. Early diagnosis of spinal epidural metastases: Correlation with clinical and radiological findings. Proc Am Soc Clin Oncol 4:269, 1985.

86. Han JS, Benson JE, Yoon YS. Magnetic resonance imaging in the spinal column and craniovertebral junction. Radiol Clin North Am 22:805-827, 1984.

87. Modic MT, Weinstein MA, Pavlicek W, Starnes DL, Duchesneau PM, Boumphrey F, Hardy RJ Jr. Nuclear magnetic resonance imaging of the spine. Radiology 148:757-762, 1983.

88. Paushter DM, Modic MT. Magnetic resonance imaging of the spine. Appl Radiol 13:61-68, 1984.

89. Young RF, Post EM, King GA. Treatment of spinal epidural metastases. Randomized prospective comparison of laminectomy and radiotherapy. J Neurosurg 53:741-748, 1980.

90. Spanos WJ, Wasserman T, Meoz R, Sala J, Kong J, Stezt J. Palliation of advanced pelvic malignant disease with large fraction pelvic radiation and misonidazole: Final report of RTOG phase I/II study. Int J Radiat Oncol Biol Phys 13:1479-1482, 1987.

91. Spanos WJ, Clery M, Perez C, Grisby PW, Scotte Doggett RL, Poulter CA, Steinfeld AD. Late effect of multiple daily fraction palliation schedule for advanced pelvic malignancies (RTOG 8502). Int J Radiat Oncol Biol Phys 29:961-967, 1994.

92. Kraus PA, Lytton B, Weiss RM, Prosnitz LR. Radiation therapy for local palliative treatment of prostatic cancer. J Urol 108:612-614, 1972.

93. Kynaston HG, Keen CW, Matthews PN. Radiotherapy for palliation of locally advanced prostatic carcinoma. Br J Urol 66: 515-517, 1990

94. Wells P, Hoskin PJ, Towler J, Saunders MI, Dische S. The effect of radiotherapy on urethral obstruction from carcinoma of the prostate. Br J Urol 78:752-755, 1996.

Renal and Bladder Tumors

Kurt R. Oettel, M.D., *Lynn Van Ummersen*, M.D.,
Gregory H. Ripple, M.D., *John P. Heiner*, M.D.,
and George Wilding, M.D.

Neoplasms of the kidney, ureter, and bladder account for 10% of all tumors in male patients and 4% of all tumors in female patients. In 2000 it was estimated that 86,700 people would be diagnosed with a urologic malignancy and that 24,600 people would die of the disease.[1] Urologic malignancies can vary widely in their histologic characteristics and overall behavior, but this group of cancers share a common presenting sign of hematuria. A clear understanding of the evaluation of patients with hematuria at presentation is crucial in discussing urologic malignancies.[2] In this chapter we will discuss urologic malignancies in the context of metastatic bone disease. We will evaluate bladder and renal cancers individually, looking at incidence, presenting signs and symptoms, diagnostic tests, and operative and nonoperative management. We will then focus on issues common to both renal and bladder cancers with metastatic bone involvement, such as pain control, complications such as hypercalcemia, and the role of new agents such as osteoclast inhibitors. We will conclude with a summary of renal and bladder cancers separately, including prognosis.

METASTATIC RENAL CELL CARCINOMA
Incidence and Patterns of Spread

Renal cell carcinoma, the most common designation, is also called renal adenocarcinoma, nephrocarcinoma, hypernephroma, alveolar carcinoma, clear cell renal carcinoma (associated with von Hippel–Lindau disease), or Grawitz tumor, reflecting the historical controversy regarding histologic origin of this cancer.[3] Renal cell cancer arises from the proximal renal tubular epithelium, with three histologic types seen: the classic "clear cell" cancer, characterized by small nuclei with abundant cytoplasm containing cholesterol, triglycerides, and glycogen; a granular cell type, with cytoplasm containing a large number of mitochondria and cytosomes; and a rare spindle cell variety, characterized by a fusiform cell type with multiple cell sizes, often seen in combination with the granular or clear cell type.[4] The most common risk factors associated with renal cell carcinoma are smoking, obesity (particularly in women), and a familial multiple cancer syndrome, von Hippel–Lindau disease.[5-7] Renal cell carcinoma is the most common renal

malignancy, accounting for 80% to 85% of malignant kidney tumors. In 2000 it was estimated that there would be more than 31,200 new cases diagnosed and 11,900 deaths from renal cell carcinoma in the United States. Worldwide, the incidence has been increasing by about 2% per year.[1] The disease most typically occurs in adults 50 to 70 years of age, although it has been seen in children as young as 6 months. Unfortunately, because of the lack of early warning signs, up to one third of patients with renal cell carcinoma will have metastatic disease at the time of diagnosis and an additional 40% will have metastases at some point during the course of their disease.[8] Renal cell carcinoma often metastasizes in a rather poorly understood and unusual pattern. Metastases are commonly seen in the lung (36%), soft tissues (20%), and bone (18%), with a widespread pattern of bone metastases that will be discussed further.[9] With the increase in the incidence of this disease, there has also been an improvement in survival. This may be due to improved diagnostic capabilities: the more widespread use of abdominal computed tomography (CT) and ultrasonography has resulted in an increase in the number of smaller, more localized lesions that potentially can be resected for a cure.[10]

Presenting Signs and Symptoms

The most common presenting symptom in renal cell cancer is hematuria, which occurs in 50% to 60% of patients. Evaluation of hematuria should include a thorough history and physical examination, with attention to any history of previous urologic disease, history of urinary tract infections, calculus disease, or previous neoplasms. Hematuria can be macroscopic, which occurs in fewer than 15% of symptom-free patients.[11] Gross hematuria requires further evaluation with either fiber-optic instrumentation or excretory urography.[12,13] In addition to hematuria, abdominal pain occurs in about 40% of patients and a palpable flank mass in about 38% of patients. The combination of these three constitutes the "classic triad," which is seen in only about 10% of patients at presentation.[14] Patients who do have this "classic triad" are much more likely to have bone metastases.[15] A wide range of paraneoplastic syndromes can accompany renal cell cancer, including erythrocytosis, hypercalcemia (which may be a result of tumor-produced hormonelike substances), hepatic dysfunction, and amyloidosis.[16,17] The presence of a paraneoplastic syndrome does not necessarily imply metastatic bone disease, nor does it contraindicate resection of a localized renal primary neoplasm or an isolated bone metastasis.[18]

Bone metastases from renal cell carcinoma are osteolytic in nature and are often associated with pain on presentation, pathologic fractures, and a generally poor survival rate. Osteolytic metastases may be accompanied by a large soft tissue mass (Fig. 23-1). This is in contrast to osteoblastic bone lesions, which generally are not as painful and cause pathologic fractures less frequently. Almost 20% of patients who have metastatic renal cancer at presentation will have bone metastases.[19] Bone metastases occurring in renal cancer are characterized by the often unusual pattern of metastases, although the bones most commonly involved are the ribs, vertebrae, ilium, femur, humerus, skull, and scapula[20] (Fig. 23-2). When metastases are limited to one organ, the most common site is the lung (40%) or bone (22%).[21] In patients with a solitary metastatic lesion at diagnosis, the metastatic site is

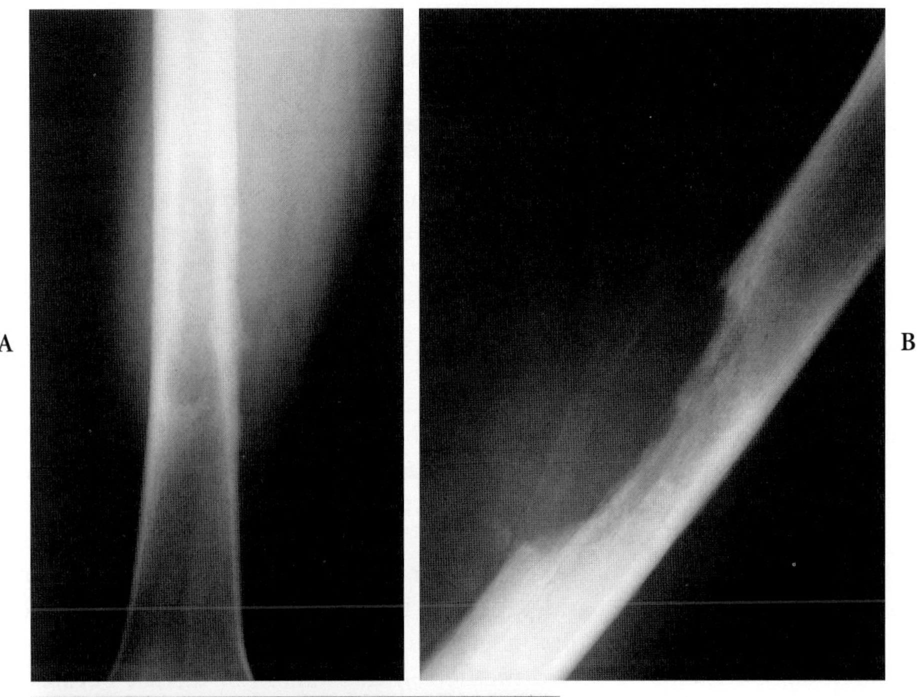

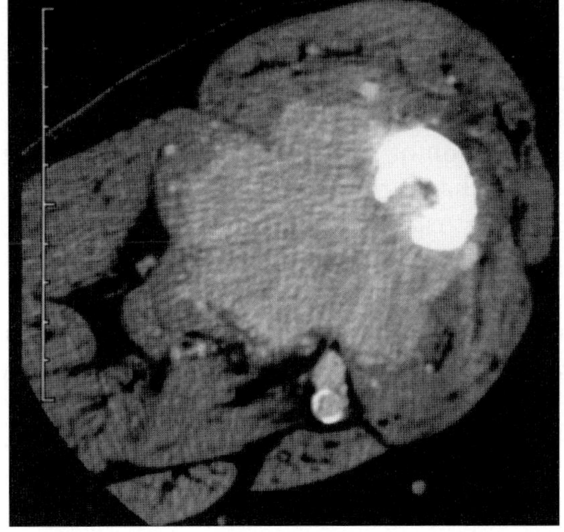

Fig. 23-1   **A,** Anteroposterior x-ray film of femur, demonstrating osteolytic metastatic renal cell carcinoma. **B,** Lateral x-ray film of femur, with large osteolytic deficit in the femur and cortical destruction. A soft tissue mass can be seen along with the calcified femoral artery. **C,** CT showing extent of soft tissue mass at the time of embolization. It is crucial to debulk the soft tissue masses when one is surgically treating metastatic renal cell carcinoma.

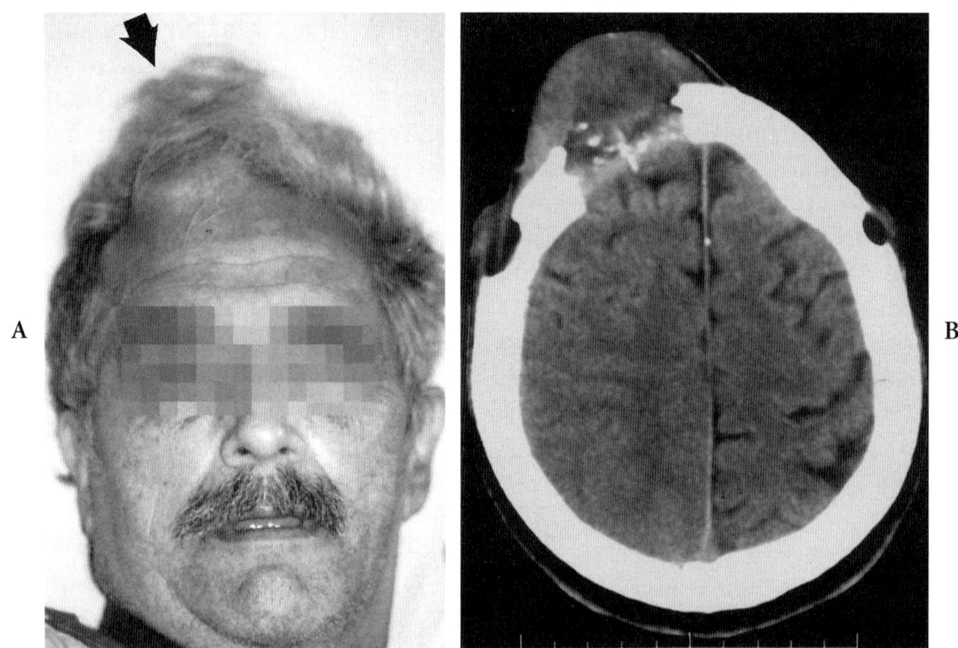

Fig. 23-2 **A,** Clinical presentation of a patient with renal cell carcinoma metastatic to the skeleton. He has a pathologic fracture of the left humerus and a large lytic lesion of the skull with a secondary soft tissue mass *(arrow)*. **B,** CT showing destructive osteolytic skull lesion. A large soft tissue mass can be seen. The patient underwent palliative radiation but soon died.

usually cerebral or bone. However, a solitary metastatic lesion that develops after the initial diagnosis is usually found in the lung or brain.[22]

Evaluation

The most appropriate diagnostic test in the initial diagnostic study is dictated to some extent by the presentation of each patient individually. Patients who have hematuria at presentation should undergo intravenous urography, whereas patients who have a suspicious renal mass demonstrated by ultrasonography or intravenous urography should undergo CT scanning. Intravenous urography as a sole technique in evaluating renal masses is only about 75% sensitive; however, if calcification is also seen, the probability of a malignant mass is increased. In a study by Daniel et al.,[23] 87% of renal masses with central calcification and 20% of those with peripheral calcification were malignant. Thus any calcium-containing mass seen on urography needs further imaging, the most helpful being a CT scan. Ultrasonography is a less invasive and inexpensive test for further evaluation of renal masses. It can be a valuable tool in defining renal cysts and

can spare patients a needle biopsy. The sensitivity for diagnosing a renal mass is slightly greater than that of intravenous urography when tumors are small (<3 cm).[24] CT for detection of renal masses has been shown to be more sensitive than ultrasonography or intravenous urography.[25] In addition to identifying renal masses, CT is also the preferred method in the staging of disease because it includes the renal vein, inferior vena cava, adrenal glands, and regional lymph nodes, as well as adjacent organs. CT usefulness is limited in the evaluation of tumor progression in the vena cava and in the evaluation of regional lymph nodes, especially those less than 2 cm in diameter, which may represent either reactive hyperplasia or metastases.[26,27] Magnetic resonance imaging (MRI) is superior to CT scanning for the evaluation of inferior vena caval involvement. MRI is also helpful for staging renal tumors when the intravenous contrast medium used in CT scanning cannot be given.[28,29]

Routine bone scans of all patients with newly diagnosed renal cell cancer have been controversial. Because of the high morbidity associated with bone fractures, which could be missed on the initial diagnostic study, some clinicians advocate bone scans for all patients with newly diagnosed renal cell cancer. At this time it is thought that in patients with no bone pain and a normal alkaline phosphatase value, a bone scan can safely be omitted from the initial diagnostic study.[30] When viewed by plain films, osteolytic lesions can be seen as bubbly, highly explosive, so-called "blow out" lesions. This is in contrast to osteoblastic lesions, which appear sclerotic. Large soft tissue masses may accompany the lesions. It should be noted, however, that after treatment with radiation therapy, chemotherapy, or hormonal therapy, purely lytic lesions can look sclerotic. Bone destruction in this lytic appearance is always mediated by tumor-induced osteoclast bone resorption.[31]

Management
Nonoperative Therapy

Chemotherapy. Overall, standard chemotherapeutic agents have shown little activity in this disease and are not thought to be warranted for the treatment of advanced renal cell carcinoma, particularly as single agents.[32] Currently a number of clinical trials are attempting to use chemotherapeutic agents such as gemcitabine, but to date there have been no sustained or reproducible results with response rates greater than 20%.[33] It is believed that a multi-drug-resistant gene *(mdr1)* may play a role in the overall poor response rates seen in this cancer.[34] Current strategies are employing chemotherapeutic agents in combination with biologic response modifiers. Several studies have combined 5-fluorouracil (5-FU) with interleukin 2 (IL-2) and interferon, but the toxic effects of these regimens can be severe (vascular leak syndrome requiring pressor support), and the response rates are not significantly greater than when IL-2 or interferon is given alone.[35,36]

Immunotherapy. The observations of rare spontaneous regressions and occasional prolonged disease stabilization in the absence of active treatment have suggested that the immune system is important in spontaneous remissions.[37] Interleukins and interferons have been the most heavily studied in this area and today, despite the rather poor response rates, are considered the "gold standard" in systemic therapy for this disease. A recent study by a French group (Negrier et al.[38]) compared patients with metastatic renal cell cancer by randomly as-

signing them to therapy with IL-2, interferon alfa-2a, or the combination of both. Response rates among the three groups were significantly different in the group receiving the combination of interferon and IL-2 (18.6% for the combination vs. 6.5% for IL-2 alone and 7.5% for interferon alfa alone), but overall survival rates among the three groups did not differ significantly.[39] Toxic effects were substantially worse in those patients receiving IL-2. It was suggested that patients being considered for cytokine treatment be carefully selected and have no major organ failure. This study was also able to identify a group of patients for which no cytokine therapy should be considered: patients with more than one metastatic site, with liver involvement, or with metastatic disease that developed within 1 year of diagnosis. More sobering are results reported by Bajamonde's Canadian group (Gleave et al.[39]), which conducted a phase III randomized, masked, placebo-controlled trial designed to determine whether interferon gamma prolongs the time to disease progression and prolongs survival. This trial showed no difference in outcome in the treatment vs. the placebo group.[39] At this time it is unclear whether immunomodulators produce more responses or more-durable responses than those in patients who are not treated, but clearly this is a cancer in search of better treatment options.

Radiation Therapy. Radiation treatment for bone metastatic cancer of any origin is most often done with palliative intent. The aggressiveness of radiation therapy is generally based on the patient's overall health status, life expectancy, ability to commute to and from a radiation therapy center, and the site and extent of the disease. There are multiple schedules for delivering radiation therapy to patients with bone metastatic disease. Treatment is generally given for a number of fractions (10 to 15), for a total of 30 to 40 Gy. Pain relief, for which radiation therapy is most often given in this setting, can be expected in 50% of patients, with another 35% expected to have partial relief.[40]

Radiation therapy for renal cell carcinoma may have different goals from those of therapy for other cancers with bone metastases.[41] In patients with solitary metastases, particularly in the lungs and bones, data indicate that aggressive treatment of the metastatic lesion, in conjunction with resection of the primary lesion in patients with synchronous metastases, improves 5-year survival rates and per-

some cases, if surgical access is difficult, arterial embolization may be warranted. Arterial embolization decreases the blood supply to the tumor, thereby facilitating resection and decreasing the incidence of serious intraoperative hemorrhage (Fig. 23-4). Arterial embolization does not appear to affect fracture healing as measured by callus formation and resolution of pain.[50]

METASTATIC BLADDER CARCINOMA
Incidence and Patterns of Spread

Bladder cancer is the fourth most common cancer in men and the ninth most common cancer in women. It was estimated that this cancer would be diagnosed in 53,200 patients in 2000 and that 12,200 patients would die of it. Men are almost three times as likely to have this disease as women.[51] The average age at diagnosis is 65 years, with few patients receiving a diagnosis before the age of 40 years. At the time of diagnosis, approximately 85% of tumors are localized and 15% are metastatic. Ninety-eight percent of all bladder cancers are epithelial in origin, with the vast majority of those being transitional cell. About 15% of patients with bladder cancer have metastatic disease at presentation, and approximately 30% to 40% with invasive

disease will subsequently have distant metastases despite radical cystectomy.[1] *It is estimated that 50% of patients with invasive bladder cancer have distant metastases at the time of diagnosis and that the incurability of this disease represents microscopic and macroscopic metastases rather than local treatment failures.*[52] *Bone has been shown to be the most frequent site of metastases outside the pelvis, followed by lymph nodes and lung*[53] (Fig. 23-5).

Presenting Signs and Symptoms

The most common presentation of bladder cancer is hematuria. Hematuria may be gross or microscopic and often is intermittent rather than constant. Other signs include urinary tract infections, symptoms of urinary frequency, or flank pain resulting from obstruction.[54] The majority of patients, however, have no physical signs or symptoms of bladder cancer. In contrast to patients with local disease, patients with invasive disease may be found to have a palpable mass or bladder wall thickening, signs that may be detected by careful bimanual examination with the patient under anesthesia. Invasive or metastatic disease may also be accompanied by hepatomegaly, splenomegaly, or lymphedema from occlusive pelvic lymphad-

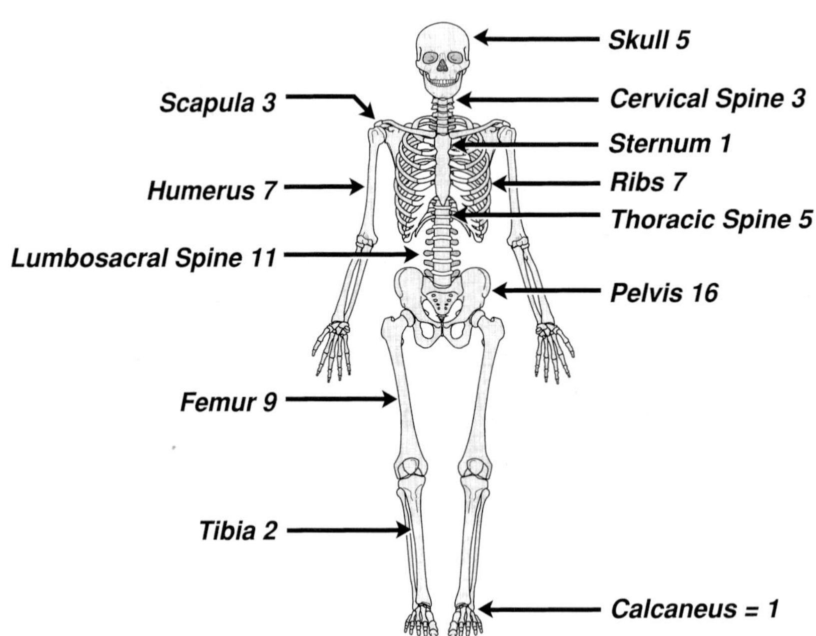

Fig. 23-5   Distribution of skeletal metastases in 24 patients with metastatic bladder cancer. The pelvis, lumbar spine, and femur were the three most common locations.

enopathy.[55] Other symptoms of diffuse disease may be bone pain from metastases or flank pain and azotemia resulting from ureteral obstruction or retroperitoneal masses. Another presenting symptom of metastatic disease may be anemia, which is often due to bone marrow replacement with metastatic disease, blood loss, or a combination of both.[56]

Evaluation

Diagnosis often begins with a thorough physical examination and urinalysis if a bladder tumor is suspected. After a complete history and physical examination an excretory urogram (intravenous pyelogram) is often used to evaluate both the upper urinary tract and bladder filling. This diagnostic study is often followed by cystoscopy, by which the bladder can be visually inspected for evaluation of lesions for size, shape, location, and growth pattern (papillary, solid). Any visualized lesions can then have biopsy specimens removed or can be resected for pathologic evaluation. To help diagnose metastatic disease and prevent unnecessary surgery, preoperative bone scans have been suggested for all patients undergoing a cystectomy (similar to the argument for diagnostic study of patients undergoing a nephrectomy). In several studies addressing this question, it has been shown that the preoperative use of bone scans, even in patients with an elevated serum alkaline phosphatase value, did not justify the routine use of this diagnostic tool because it rarely changed disease management.[57] In a recent study, however, there does appear to be a statistically significant relation between an elevated alkaline phosphatase value or the degree of change on a precystectomy bone scan and the final outcome.[58]

Management
Nonoperative Therapy

Chemotherapy. Chemotherapy has become standard treatment for nonoperable bladder cancer. Results with single-agent drugs or in combination show significant partial and complete response rates in metastatic bladder cancers.[59] The single most active agent evaluated to date is cisplatin, which when used alone shows response rates in the 30% range.[60] Improved response rates have been seen when cisplatin is used in combination with several other agents. Currently the two most commonly used chemotherapy regimens are a combination of methotrexate, vinblastine, doxorubicin, and cisplatin (M-VAC) and a combination of cisplatin, methotrexate, and vinblastine (CMV).[61] Approximately 15% to 35% of patients receiving these regimens will go on to have a complete response; however, the median survival time is only 12 months for patients with visceral or bone metastatic disease, with the majority of patients ultimately having a relapse and succumbing to the cancer.[56] Because of the poor survival time in patients with transitional cell carcinoma, a number of other agents have been tried in this area.[62-65] Toxicity of either single-agent therapy or the more standard combination therapies is significant. Neutropenia and complications of fever, in combination with impaired renal function, are the most common toxic effects of cisplatin-based therapies. Other common toxic effects are mucositis, nausea, and vomiting.

Radiation Therapy. For patients with muscle-invasive carcinoma of the bladder, radical cystectomy is considered to be the standard of care. Bladder sparing to maintain quality of life is thought to be secondary to the primary treatment goal of curing the patient. Radiation therapy is often used in combination with cystectomy and cisplatin-based chemotherapy regimens for local control.[66,67] For many patients in whom local control fails and whose disease is incurable, the role of radiation therapy is primarily palliative. Radiation in the setting of advanced bladder cancer metastatic to bone is generally given in the range of 30 Gy for 10 fractions; however, this "recipe" is often altered, with each institution's having its own slight variation.[68] The results of radiation therapy in this setting are encouraging, with high response rates (>90%) to local metastatic disease control and response rates nearly that high in pain control[69,70] (Fig. 23-6). Patients with bone metastatic bladder disease, however, do poorly, with median survival rates around 12 months despite aggressive radiation or other treatment.[71]

Operative Therapy

Surgery for bladder cancer, cystectomy, is the standard of care in localized disease; however, for patients with metastatic disease there is no role for

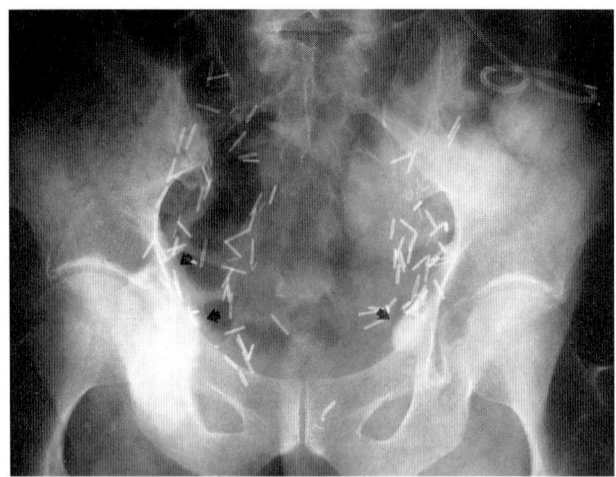

Fig. 23-6 Osteoblastic bladder cancer of the acetabulum of the pelvis, with extension to the ischium. The patient was treated with radiation. No surgery was required.

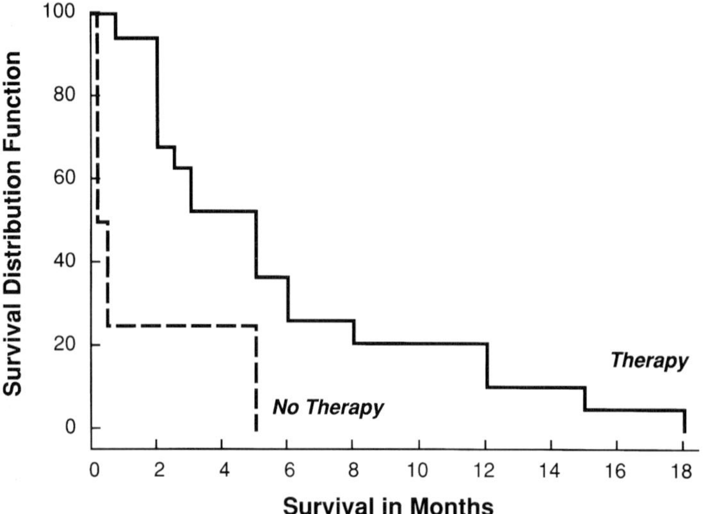

Fig. 23-7 Survival of patients at the University of Wisconsin with skeletal metastases from bladder cancer. Time zero is the point when metastatic skeletal disease was recognized. As the graph shows, the prognosis is grim.

cystectomy. For patients with metastatic bladder cancer and bone metastases, there is also probably no role for wide resection of the primary tumor or for surgery to treat any metastatic disease, as there may be in cases of renal cancer. In an unpublished evaluation of patients with bladder cancer with metastatic disease at the University of Wisconsin from 1982 to 1990, it was seen that 24 of 115 patients with metastatic disease had bone involvement and that the average time of survival from diagnosis of bone metastatic disease was only 6 months (Fig. 23-7). Patients were identified with both osteolytic and osteoblastic disease (Fig. 23-8).

There was no apparent survival advantage to patients who were treated with radiation, or chemotherapy, or both. The conclusion of this evaluation was that although the goal of surgery is to restore weightbearing capacity, optimal function, and comfort, in some situations the usual pathologic fracture management may not be indicated when predicted survival is extremely short (Fig. 23-9). Given this information, surgical intervention in bladder cancer with bone metastases should be reserved for stabilization of impending fractures or reduction of pathologic fractures that have already occurred.

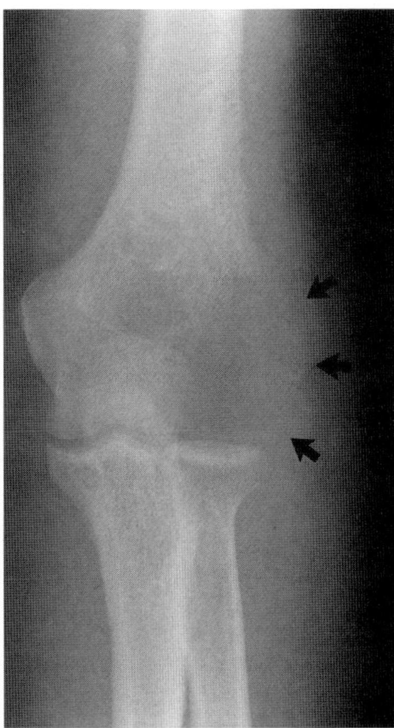

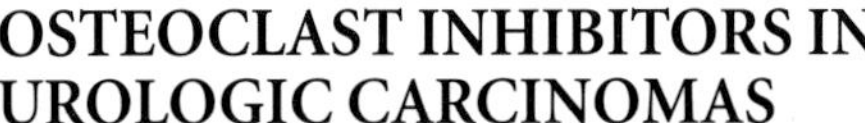

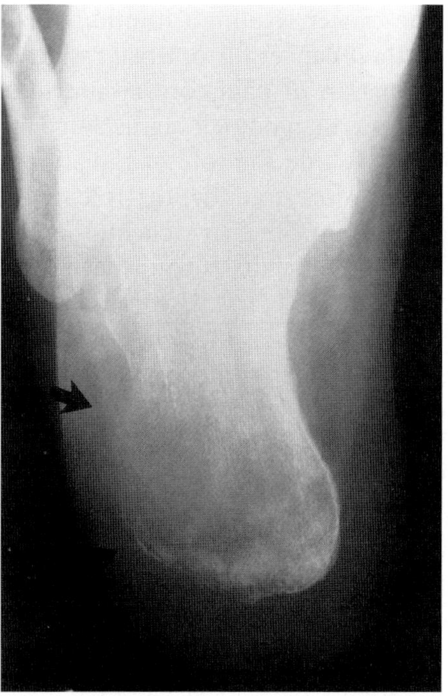

Fig. 23-8 Osteolytic invasive bladder cancer affecting the lateral condyle and capitulum of the distal portion of the humerus.

Fig. 23-9 Osteolytic bladder cancer affecting the calcaneus. The patient had severe heel pain at presentation. During the staging evaluation, the primary bladder cancer was discovered. The patient died 4 months after diagnosis.

OSTEOCLAST INHIBITORS IN UROLOGIC CARCINOMAS

Bisphosphonates are pyrophosphate analogs that inhibit the formation of calcium phosphate crystals. When used in vivo, bisphosphonates inhibit osteoclast-mediated bone resorption.[72] This group of drugs has been used primarily in the treatment of osteoporosis and in the management of hypercalcemia, but more recently it has been used in cancer-related bone metastases.[73] Several clinical trials have demonstrated the antiosteolytic effect of bisphosphonates, primarily in bone metastatic breast cancer and in multiple myeloma.[74] It is thought that the mechanism of action is direct inhibition of the osteoclast-mediated bone resorption.[75] What is more intriguing is that in a recent study by Diel et al.[76] there was not only a reduction in the number of bone metastases but also a reduction in the tumor burden of nonskeletal disease, suggesting an alternative mechanism of inhibition. This alternative mechanism may be an alteration of the microenvironment in which tumor cells grow, perhaps by inhibiting the release of bone-derived tumor growth factors, such as transforming growth factor beta, insulin-like growth factor I, and tumor-derived parathyroid hormone–related peptide. This inhibition could lessen the proliferative stimulus to tumor cells and decrease growth in both bone and soft tissue disease.[77] Nearly all of the work involving cancer and bisphosphonates has been done in breast cancer and multiple myeloma, with little information regarding renal or bladder cancer.[78,79] Whatever the mechanism, this therapy is still in its infancy in cancer treatment and has yet to be proved for renal cell or bladder cancer.

OUTCOMES OF RENAL CELL AND BLADDER CARCINOMAS

In general, therapy for bone disease from urologic cancer is palliative and aimed at (1) control of symptoms such as pain, (2) maintenance of bone integrity and stabilization to avoid pathologic fractures, and (3) treatment of complications such as hypercalcemia.[47] Attempts at overall tumor control are poor at best when either renal cell or bladder cancer has metastasized.[39,80] Patients with metastatic bone cancer require a multidisciplinary approach to their cancer for optimal results. This requires evaluation of pain control and nutritional, electrolyte, and hematologic status. Further evaluation should include the role of radiation therapy, surgery, and, more recently, the role of osteoclast inhibitors. Systemic therapy (chemotherapy or immunotherapy), which has already been discussed in both renal and bladder cancer, also plays a large role in management of metastatic disease but not specifically in management of bone metastatic disease.

Renal Cell Carcinoma

The prognosis for patients with metastatic renal cell carcinoma remains poor.[81] As with other malignancies, prognosis is highly dependent on stage. For patients with early-stage, resectable cancers (stages I and II), the 5-year survival rate is 50% to 80%. Patients with local vascular involvement (stage IIIA) have 5-year survival rates of around 50% with aggressive surgical resection, compared with <30% for those with regional lymph node involvement (stage IIIB), presumably reflecting a difference in the biology of the disease.[15] For patients with distant metastases (stage IV), the 5-year survival rate is ≤10%, reflecting the lack of effective systemic therapy options in this disease. In a recent study evaluating prognostic factors in patients treated with biologic response modifiers (the treatment of choice for the majority of patients who receive treatment), it was shown that Eastern Cooperative Oncology Group (ECOG) performance status (1 vs. 0), presence of bone metastases, recent history of weight loss, no history of nephrectomy, recurrence at the renal bed, and sarcomatoid histologic findings were statistically important prognostic indicators of survival. This same analysis was able to show that stratification of patients based only on ECOG performance status, presence of bone metastases, and presence of sarcomatoid histologic findings was able to identify three groups of patients. These three groups' overall survival time ranged from 18.6 months (ECOG performance status 0, no bone metastases, and nonsarcomatoid histologic findings) in the best group to 3.8 months (sarcomatoid histologic findings regardless of performance status or bone metastases) in the worst group.[82] Other prognostic factors that have been identified include time to development of metas-

tases, the number of metastatic sites, the presence of hypercalcemia at presentation, and the erythrocyte sedimentation rate.[8,9,83] Althausen et al.[84] assessed prognostic factors specifically in patients with bone involvement. They found improved survival in patients with solitary metastases, increased time from diagnosis to the development of metastatic disease, and metastases to the appendicular as opposed to the axial skeleton. They concluded that aggressive treatment, including complex orthopedic procedures, may be warranted in patients meeting these characteristics.[84] Despite the numerous prognostic risk factors identified and the significance of each, what remains clear is that renal cell cancer, like other bone metastatic cancer, requires a multifocal approach for optimal outcome.

Bladder Carcinoma

The prognosis of bladder cancer, like that of renal cell cancer, is highly dependent on the stage of disease. Patients with superficial bladder cancer currently have an excellent prognosis. Survival at 5 years currently approaches 85% to 90%, with roughly a 10% chance of progression overall. This outcome appears to be particularly influenced by tumor grade.[56] As the tumor stage progresses from T2 to T4, the prognosis worsens, and treatment plans tend to become more multifocal and less controlled. When disease is systemic and metastases are identified, the prognosis is grim, with few patients surviving 5 years.[65] For localized tumors the largest predictors of treatment failure are tumor size, number of tumors, tumor grade, histologic stage, time of disease recurrence, and presence of carcinoma in situ. For patients with metastatic disease the Karnofsky performance status and alkaline phosphatase value were particularly useful in predicting prolonged survival.[85,86] In patients with bladder cancer and bone metastases the prognosis is grim; surgical intervention should therefore be limited to completed pathologic fractures and impending fracture. Chemotherapy and radiation therapy play a far more important role in the management of the disease.

CONCLUSION

Urologic malignancies are especially common in men. Renal carcinoma commonly metastasizes to bones, often with large lytic defects and pathologic fractures. Surgery frequently is required to resect the tumor and stabilize the spine and long bones. Bladder carcinoma much less frequently involves the skeleton, and skeletal metastatic lesions are seen late in the illness.

REFERENCES

1. Greenlee RT, Murray T, Bolden S, Wingo PA. Cancer statistics, 2000. CA Cancer J Clin 50:7-33, 2000.
2. See W, Williams RD. Tumors of the kidney, ureter and bladder. West J Med 156:523-534, 1992.
3. Dreicer R, Williams RD. Renal parenchymal neoplasms. In Tanagho EA, McAninch JW, eds. Smith's General Urology, 14th ed. Norwalk, Conn.: Appleton & Lange, 1995, p 372.
4. Presti J, Rao P, Chen Q, Reuter V, Li F, Fair W, Jhanwar S. Histopathologic, cytogenetic, and molecular characterization of renal cortical tumors. Cancer Res 51:1544-1552, 1991.
5. Yu M, Mack T, Hanisch R, Cicioni C, Henderson B. Cigarette smoking, obesity, diuretic use, and coffee consumption as risk factors for renal carcinoma. J Natl Cancer Inst 77:351-356, 1986.
6. Cohen A, Li F, Berg S, Marchetto D, Tsai S, Jacobs S, Brown R. Hereditary renal-cell carcinoma associated with a chromosomal translocation. N Engl J Med 301:592-595, 1979.
7. Linehan W, Lerman M, Zbar B. Identification of the *VHL* gene: Its role in renal carcinoma. JAMA 273:564-570, 1995.
8. Stenzl A, deKernion JB. Pathobiology, biology, and clinical staging of renal cell carcinoma. Semin Oncol 16:3-11, 1989.
9. Maldazys JD, deKernion JB. Prognostic factors in metastatic renal carcinoma. J Urol 136:376-379, 1986.
10. Porena M, Vespasiani G, Rosi P, Costantini E, Virgili G, Mearini E, Micali F. Incidentally detected renal cell carcinoma: Role of ultrasonography. J Clin Ultrasound 20:395-400, 1992.
11. Mohr D, Offord K, Owen R, Melton L. Asymptomatic microhematuria and urologic disease: A population-based study. JAMA 256:224-229, 1986.
12. Kumon H, Tsugawa M, Matsumura Y, Ohmori H. Endoscopic diagnosis and treatment of chronic unilateral hematuria of uncertain etiology. J Urol 143:554-558, 1990.
13. Corwin H, Silverstein M. The diagnosis of neoplasia in patients with asymptomatic microscopic hematuria: A decision analysis. J Urol 139:1002-1006, 1988.
14. Ritchie A, Chisholm G. The natural history of renal carcinoma. Semin Oncol 10:390-400, 1983.
15. Golimbu M, Joshi P, Sperber A, Tessler A, Al-Askari S, Morales P. Renal cell carcinoma: Survival and prognostic factors. Urology 27:291-301, 1986.
16. Nseyo U, Williams P, Murphy G. Clinical significance of erythropoietin levels in renal carcinoma. Urology 28:301-306, 1986.
17. Gotoh A, Kitazawa S, Mizuno Y, Takenaka A, Arakawa S, Matsumoto O, Kitazawa R, Fujimori T, Maeda S, Kamidono S. Common expression of parathyroid hormone–related protein and no correlation of calcium level in renal cell carcinomas. Cancer 71:2803-2806, 1993.
18. Motzer R, Bander N, Nanus D. Renal cell carcinoma. N Engl J Med 335:865-875, 1996.
19. Swanson D, Orovan W, Johnson D, Giacco G. Osseous metastases secondary to renal cell carcinoma. Urology 18:556-561, 1981.
20. Jacobsen K, Folleras G, Fossa S. Metastases from renal cell carcinoma to the humerus or the shoulder girdle. Br J Urol 73:124-128, 1994.
21. Sufrin G. The challenges of renal adenocarcinoma. Surg Clin North Am 62:1101-1118, 1982.
22. O'Dea MJ, Zincke H, Utz DC, Bernatz PE. The treatment of renal cell carcinoma with solitary metastasis. J Urol 120:540-542, 1978.
23. Daniel WW Jr, Hartman GW, Witten DM, Farrow GM, Kelalis PP. Calcified renal mass: A review of ten years' experience at the Mayo Clinic. Radiology 103:503-508, 1972.
24. Amendola M, Bree R, Pollack H, Francis I, Glazer G, Jafri S, Tomaszewski J. Small renal cell carcinomas: Resolving a diagnostic dilemma. Radiology 166:637-641, 1988.
25. Warshauer D, McCarthy S, Street L, Bookbinder M, Glickman M, Richter J, Hammers L, Taylor C, Rosenfield A. Detection of renal masses: Sensitivities and specificities of excretory urography/linear tomography, US, and CT. Radiology 169:363-365, 1988.
26. Johnson C, Dunnick N, Cohan R, Illescas F. Renal adenocarcinoma: CT staging of 100 tumors. AJR Am J Roentgenol 148:59-63, 1987.
27. Studer U, Scherz S, Scheidegger J, Kraft R, Sonntag R, Ackermann D, Zingg E. Enlargement of regional lymph nodes in renal cell carcinoma is often not due to metastases. J Urol 144:243-245, 1990.
28. Semelka R, Shoenut J, Margo C, Kroeker M, MacMahon R, Greenberg H. Renal cancer staging: Comparison of contrast-enhanced CT and gadolinium-enhancing fat-suppressed spin-echo MR imaging. J Magn Reson Imaging 3:597-602, 1993.
29. Rofsky N, Weinreb J, Bosniak M, Libes R, Birnbaum B. Renal lesion characterization with gadolinium-enhanced MR imaging: Efficacy and safety in patients with renal insufficiency. Radiology 180:85-89, 1991.
30. Seaman E, Goluboff E, Ross S, Sawczuk I. Association of radionuclide bone scan and serum alkaline phosphatase in patients with metastatic renal cell carcinoma. Urology 48: 692-695, 1996.
31. Greenspan A, Remagen W, eds. Differential Diagnosis of Tumors and Tumor-Like Lesions of Bones and Joints. Philadelphia: Lippincott-Raven, 1998.
32. Yagoda A, Abi-Rached B, Petrylak D. Chemotherapy for advanced renal-cell carcinoma: 1983-1993. Semin Oncol 22:42-60, 1995.
33. De Mulder PH, Weissbach L, Jakse G, Osieka R, Blatter J. Gemcitabine: A phase II study in patients with advanced renal cancer. Cancer Chemother Pharmacol 37:491-495, 1996.
34. Fojo A, Shen D, Mickley L, Pastan I, Gottesman M. Intrinsic drug resistance in kidney cancers is associated with expression of a human multidrug resistance gene. J Clin Oncol 5:1922-1927, 1987.
35. Savage P, Costelna D, Moore J, Gore M. A phase II study of continuous infusional 5-fluorouracil (5-FU) and subcutaneous interleukin-2 (IL-2) in metastatic renal cancer. Eur J Cancer 33:1149-1151, 1997.

36. Joffe J, Banks R, Forbes M, Hallam S, Jenkins A, Patel P, Hall G, Velikova G, Adams J, Crossley A, Johnson P, Whicher J, Selby P. A phase II study of interferon-alpha, interleukin-2 and 5-fluorouracil in advanced renal carcinoma: Clinical data and laboratory evidence of protease activation. Br J Urol 77:638-649, 1996.

37. Young R. Metastatic renal cell carcinoma: What causes occasional dramatic regressions? N Engl J Med 338:1305-1306, 1998.

38. Negrier S, Escudier B, Lasset C, Douillard JY, Savary J, Chevreau C, Ravaud A, Mercatello A, Peny J, Mousseau M, Philip T, Tursz T. Recombinant human interleukin-2, recombinant human interferon alfa-2a, or both in metastatic renal-cell carcinoma. N Engl J Med 338:1272-1278, 1998.

39. Gleave ME, Elhilali M, Fradet Y, Davis I, Venner P, Saad F, Klotz LH, Moore MJ, Paton V, Bajamonde A, Canadian Urologic Oncology Group. Interferon gamma-1b compared with placebo in metastatic renal-cell carcinoma. N Engl J Med 338:1265-1271, 1998.

40. Frassica D, Frassica F. Nonoperative management. In Simon M, Springfield D, eds. Surgery for Bone and Soft-Tissue Tumors. Philadelphia: Lippincott-Raven, 1998, pp 633-637.

41. Seitz W, Karcher K, Binder W. Radiotherapy of metastatic renal cell carcinoma. Semin Surg Oncol 4:100-102, 1988.

42. Kavolius JP, Mastorakos DP, Pavlovich C, Russo P, Burt ME, Brady MS. Resection of metastatic renal cell carcinoma. J Clin Oncol 16:2261-2266, 1998.

43. Bukowski R, Novick A, Krishnamurthi V. Efficacy of multimodality therapy in advanced renal cell carcinoma. Urology 51:933-937, 1998.

44. Taneja S, Pierce W, Figlin R, Belldegrun A. Management of disseminated kidney cancer. Urol Clin North Am 21:625-637, 1994.

45. Halperin E, Hariadis L. The role of radiation therapy in the management of metastatic renal cell carcinoma. Cancer 51:614-617, 1983.

46. Onufrey V, Mohiuddin M. Radiation therapy in the treatment of metastatic renal cell carcinoma. Intl J Radiat Ther Biol Phys 11:2007-2009, 1985.

47. Finn HA. Carcinoma metastatic to bone: General considerations. In Simon MA, Springfield D, eds. Surgery for Bone and Soft-Tissue Tumors. Philadelphia: Lippincott-Raven, 1998, pp 609-614.

48. Henriksson C, Haraldsson G, Aldenborg F, Lindberg S, Pettersson S. Skeletal metastases in 102 patients evaluated before surgery for renal cell carcinoma. Scand J Urol Nephrol 26:363-366, 1992.

49. Hipp J, Springfield D, Hayes W. Predicting pathologic fracture risk in the management of metastatic bone defects. Clin Orthop 312:120-135, 1995.

50. Braaedel H, Zwergel U, Knopp W. Embolization of pelvic bone metastases from renal cell carcinoma. Eur Urol 10:380-384, 1984.

51. Cohen SM, Johansson SL. Epidemiology and etiology of bladder cancer. Urol Clin North Am 19:421-428, 1992.

52. Prout GR, Griffin PP, Shipley WU. Bladder carcinoma as a systemic disease. Cancer 43:2532-2539, 1979.

53. Sengelov L, Kamby C, Von Der Masse H. Pattern of metastases in relation to characteristics of primary tumor and treatment in patients with disseminated urothelial carcinoma. J Urol 155:111-114, 1996.

54. Badalament RA, Schervish EW. Bladder cancer, current diagnostic and treatment options. Postgrad Med 100:217-230, 1996.

55. Scher H, Shipley W, Herr H. Cancer of the bladder. In Devita V, Hellman S, Rosenberg S, eds. Cancer: Principles and Practice of Oncology, 5th ed. Philadelphia: Lippincott-Raven, 1997.

56. Carroll PR. Urothelial carcinoma cancers of the bladder ureter and renal pelvis. In Tanagho EA, McAninch JW, eds. Smith's General Urology. Norwalk, Conn.: Appleton & Lange, 1995.

57. Brismar J, Gustafson T. Bone scintigraphy in staging of bladder cancer. Acta Radiol 29:251-252, 1988.

58. Braendengen M, Winderen M, Fossa SD. Clinical significance of routine pre-cystectomy bone scans in patients with muscle-invasive bladder cancer. Br J Urol 77:36-40, 1996.

59. Scher H, Sternberg CN. Chemotherapy of urologic malignancies. Semin Urol 3:239-280, 1985.

60. Yagoda A. Chemotherapy for advanced urothelial cancer. Semin Urol 1:60-74, 1983.

61. Donat MS, Herr HW, Bajorin DF, Fair WR, Sogani PC, Russo P, Sheinfeld J, Scherr HI. Methotrexate, vinblastine, doxorubicin and cisplatin chemotherapy and cystectomy for unresectable bladder cancer. J Urol 156:368-371, 1996.

62. McCaffrey JA, Hilton S, Mazumdar M, Sadan S, Heineman M, Hirsch J, Kelly WK, Scher HI, Bajorin DF. Phase II randomized trial of gallium nitrate plus fluorouracil versus methotrexate, vinblastine, doxorubicin, and cisplatin in patients with advanced transitional-cell carcinoma. J Clin Oncol 15:2449-2455, 1997.

63. Roth BJ, Dreicer R, Einhorn LH, Neuberg D, Johnson DH, Smith JL, Hudes GR, Schultz SM, Loehrer PJ. Significant activity of paclitaxel in advanced transitional-cell carcinoma of the urothelium: A phase II trial of the Eastern Cooperative Oncology Group. J Clin Oncol 12:2264-2270, 1994.

64. Einhorn LH, Roth BJ, Ansari R, Dreicer R, Gonin R, Loehrer PJ. Phase II trial of vinblastine, ifosfamide, and gallium combination chemotherapy in metastatic urothelial carcinoma. J Clin Oncol 12:2271-2276, 1994.

65. McCaffrey JA, Hilton S, Mazumdar M, Sadan S, Kelly WK, Scher HI, Bajorin DF. Phase II trial of docetaxel in patients with advanced or metastatic transitional-cell carcinoma. J Clin Oncol 15:1853-1857, 1997.

66. Sauer R, Birkenhake S, Kuhn R, Wittekind C, Schrott KM, Martus P. Efficacy of radiochemotherapy with platin derivatives compared to radiotherapy alone in organ-sparing treatment of bladder cancer. Int J Radiat Oncol Biol Phys 40(1):121-127, 1998.

67. Chauvet B, Brewer Y, Felix-Faure C, Davin JL, Choquenet C, Reboul F. Concurrent cisplatin and radiotherapy for patients with muscle invasive bladder cancer who are not candidates for radical cystectomy. J Urol 156:1258-1262, 1996.

68. Salminen E. Unconventional fractionation for palliative radiotherapy of urinary bladder cancer: A retrospective review of 94 patients. Acta Oncol 31:449-454, 1992.

69. Aass N, Fossa SD. Aims and results of palliative radiotherapy in urologic cancer. Curr Opin Oncol 6:308-312, 1994.

70. Murai N, Koga K, Nagamachi S, Nishikawa K, Matsuki K, Kusumoto S, Watanabe K. Radiotherapy in bone metastases—with special reference to its effect on relieving pain. Gan No Rinsho 35:1149-1152, 1989.

71. Frazier HA, Robertson JE, Dodge RK, Paulson DF. The value of pathologic factors in predicting cancer-specific survival among patients treated with radical cystectomy for transitional cell carcinoma of the bladder and prostate. Cancer 71:3993-4001, 1993.

72. Rogers MJ, Watts DJ, Russell RGG. Overview of bisphosphonates. Cancer 80(Suppl): 1652-1660, 1997.

73. O'Rorke N, McCloskey E, Houghton F, Huss H, Kanis J. Double-blind, placebo-controlled, dose-response trial of oral clodronate in patients with bone metastases. J Clin Oncol 14:929-934, 1995.

74. Hortobagyi GN, Theriault RL, Porter L, Blayney D, Lipton A, Sinoff C, Wheeler H, Simeone J, Seaman J, Knight R, Heffernan M, Reitsma D. Efficacy of pamidronate in reducing skeletal complications in patients with breast cancer and lytic bone metastases. N Engl J Med 335:1785-1791, 1996.

75. Delmas PD. Bisphosphonates in the treatment of bone disease. [Editorial.] N Engl J Med 335:1836-1837, 1996.

76. Diel IJ, Solomayer EF, Costa S, Gollan C, Goerner R, Wallwiener D, Kaufmann M, Bastert G. Reduction in new metastases in breast cancer with adjuvant clodronate treatment. N Engl J Med 339:357-363, 1998.

77. Mundy GR, Yoneda T. Bisphosphonates as anticancer drugs. [Editorial.] N Engl J Med 339:398-400, 1998.

78. Body JJ, Bartl R, Burckhardt P, Delmas PD, Diel IJ, Fleisch H, Kanis JA, Kyle RA, Mundy GR, Paterson AH, Rubens RD. Current use of bisphosphonates in oncology. International Bone and Cancer Study Group. J Clin Oncol 16:3890-3899, 1998.

79. Body JJ, Coleman RE, Piccart M. Use of bisphosphonates in cancer patients. Cancer Treat Rev 22:265-287, 1996.

80. Redman BG, Smith DC, Flaherty L, Du W, Hussain M. Phase II trial of paclitaxel and carboplatin in the treatment of advanced urothelial carcinoma. J Clin Oncol 16:1844-1848, 1998.

81. Kosary C, McLaughlin J. Kidney and renal pelvis. In Miller BA, Ries LAG, Hankey BF, et al., eds. SEER Cancer Statistics Review, 1973-1990. Bethesda, Md.: National Cancer Institute, 1993.

82. Mani S, Todd M, Katz K, Poo W. Prognostic factors for survival in patients with metastatic renal cancer treated with biologic response modifiers. J Urol 154:35-40, 1995.

83. Ljungberg B, Grankvist K, Rasmuson T. Serum acute phase reactants and prognosis in renal cell carcinoma. Cancer 76: 1435-1439, 1995.

84. Althausen P, Althausen A, Jennings L, Mankin H. Prognostic factors and surgical treatment of osseous metastases secondary to renal cell carcinoma. Cancer 80:1103-1109, 1997.

85. Geller N, Strenberg C, Penenberg D, Scher H, Yagoda A. Prognostic factors for survival of patients with advanced urothelial tumors treated with methotrexate, vinblastine, doxorubicin, and cisplatin chemotherapy. Cancer 67:1525-1531, 1991.

86. Sengelov L, Kamby C, Schou G, Van der Masse H. Prognostic factors and significance of chemotherapy in patients with recurrent or metastatic transitional cell cancer of the urinary tract. Cancer 74:123-133, 1994.

Sarcomas

William G. Ward, M.D.

Bone metastases of sarcomas present a potentially devastating problem for afflicted patients. There is little published literature on the subject to guide the practitioner's treatment of these problems. In 1996 approximately 8600 new cases of sarcoma were diagnosed in the United States alone.[1] Considering that roughly 30% to 50% of patients with sarcomas ultimately succumb to their disease, approximately 4000 patients per year will have new metastatic sarcomatous disease. Although the pulmonary system is the most common site of sarcoma metastases, the skeleton is the second most common site.[2-15] Thus in a significant number of patients with sarcomas, metastatic involvement of the skeletal system will develop. The management of these skeletal metastases is not an entirely uncommon problem, especially in the practice of the orthopedic oncologist, and will be the subject of this chapter.

The dearth of literature regarding the proper management of skeletal metastases of sarcomas is understandable in light of the fact that limb salvage surgery for sarcomas has become a widely accepted practice only over the past 10 to 20 years.[11,16-18] The pioneer surgeons developing these techniques have, for the most part, reported on surgery only for the primary tumors.[16-18] Informal discussions with these surgeons have confirmed that these pioneers have tended to employ similar resection tactics for the occasional patient with skeletal metastases but have published few reports on the subject. Routine aggressive management of pulmonary metastases of osteosarcoma began only 20 or so years ago.[3,10,15,19] With the dramatic advances in the chemotherapeutic and surgical management of sarcomas, an increasing number of these patients will be saved, thereby increasing the odds of encountering patients with bone metastases. Because of the absence of published work on the management of skeletal metastases of sarcomas, the practitioner is forced to rely on his knowledge of the individual sarcomas, the needs and desires of the patients, and an extrapolation of experience from the management of bone metastases of carcinomas and other malignant tumors to guide the management of these problems. Such extrapolation may or may not be appropriate in the management of sarcomas metastatic to the skeletal system. This chapter will explore the current state of knowledge regarding metastatic patterns of the sarcomas, will review the available literature regarding the management of sarcoma metastases, and will present my anecdotal experience in treating sarcomas metastatic to the skeletal system.

METASTATIC PATTERNS

Most sarcomas, such as osteosarcoma, metastasize by way of the bloodstream. As a result, 90% of patients with metastatic osteosarcoma have metastases in the pulmonary parenchyma. The high rate of pulmonary spread is presumably because the lungs provide the first capillary bed to filter the blood after it enters the venous circulation at the site of the primary tumor. Roughly 10% to 15% of patients with metastatic sarcomas, such as osteosarcomas or malignant fibrous histiocytoma of bone, have metastases in the bone.[4,7,15] It is uncommon for sarcomas to metastasize to the regional lymphatic system. The overall incidence is estimated to be somewhere in the 2% to 3% range, possibly up to 6% if one relies on autopsy data.[20,21] However, autopsy data are likely to be skewed, as terminal patients develop lymphatic involvement late in their disease. There are several notable exceptions to these generalizations. Epithelioid sarcoma, synovial cell sarcoma, and clear cell sarcoma may metastasize to the lymphatic system in up to 35% of cases.[5] Alveolar rhabdomyosarcoma also has a high predilection for brain and bone metastases.[5] There are occasional metastases of sarcoma to tissues such as the abdominal cavity (liposarcomas have a 10% to 20% propensity to metastasize to the retroperitoneal tissues), liver, subcutaneous tissue, epidural space, heart, mediastinum, adrenal glands, and elsewhere.[5,22]

The propensity for bone and bone marrow metastasis varies among the different sarcomas. Several sarcomas, most notably those that generally fit within the category of small round blue-cell tumors, frequently metastasize to the marrow of other bones. In fact, at my institution and at some others, a standard part of the initial staging workup for both Ewing's sarcoma and rhabdomyosarcoma includes aspiration of bilateral iliac crest bone marrow because of the high propensity for bone marrow spread of these diseases.[23] A positive result places a patient at an Enneking stage III level of disease with a concomitant poor prognosis.[15,24-26] It is considered possible, but difficult, to cure a patient

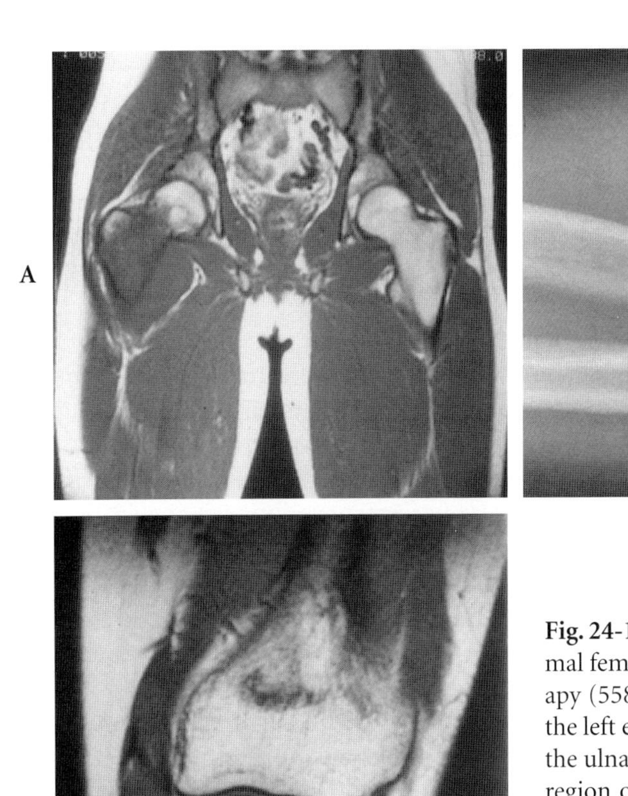

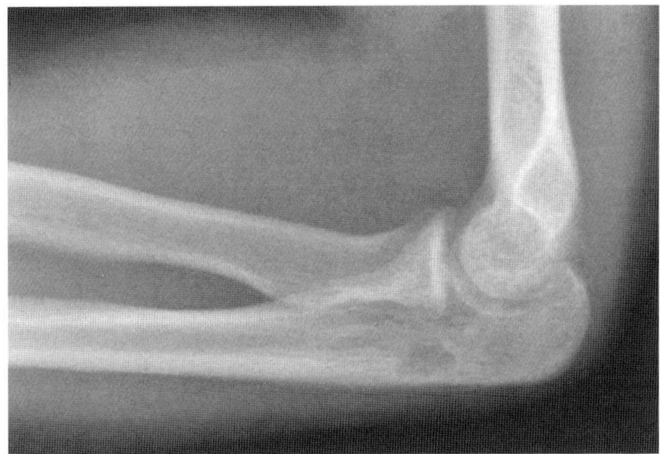

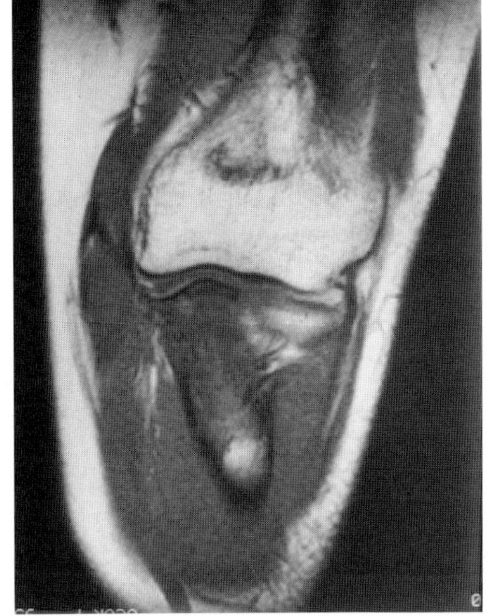

Fig. 24-1 **A,** Coronal MRI of a 19-year-old man with proximal femoral Ewing's sarcoma who underwent radiation therapy (5580 cGy) plus chemotherapy. **B,** Lateral radiograph of the left elbow 20 months later, revealing a metastatic lesion in the ulna. The patient also had a bone metastasis in the L4, L5 region of the spine. **C,** T1-weighted MRI scan of the left elbow revealing decreased signal in the ulna, reflecting the systemic metastasis to the bone. Retreatment with chemotherapy and radiation therapy was planned after complete staging revealed the absence of additional metastatic involvement. (Case courtesy of Dr. Franklin Sim, Mayo Clinic, Rochester, Minn.)

with a small round blue-cell tumor, such as Ewing's sarcoma, that is metastatic to bone marrow. Systemic treatment and perhaps radiation will be required[23,24,26,27] (Fig. 24-1). It is, however, generally considered impossible with current systemic treatment regimens to cure a patient with chondrosarcoma or osteosarcoma that is widely metastatic to the bone marrow without surgical excision of the metastatic lesions. Patients with limited or isolated skeletal metastases of osteosarcoma are generally considered potentially curable with chemotherapy and bone metastasectomy, although long-term survival is unlikely. In one study of 111 patients with osteosarcoma, all who had bone metastases were dead within 48 months.[15] Thus the management of patients with bone metastases of sarcoma differs, depending on both the histologic diagnosis and the location, extent, and number of metastases. Before initiating treatment of bone metastatic disease, the physician must determine whether the treatment goal is palliation or cure. The answer will guide the physician in the selection of the appropriate treatment regimen. To understand the various approaches to the treatment of bone metastases of sarcomas, a brief overview of the major sarcomas relative to metastatic disease is indicated.

Osteosarcoma

Osteosarcoma is usually a monostotic disease that affects teenagers. The most frequent site of metastases at the time of presentation is the lung. An occasional patient will present with synchronous osteosarcoma, i.e., osteosarcoma that appears to originate in two or more primary sites at the same time. In general, this syndrome is associated with a poor prognosis. In a series of 12 cases of synchronous osteosarcoma, eight patients were dead within 3 years and only one had survived more than 3 years at the time of publication.[28] The other variety of multicentric osteosarcoma, metachronous osteosarcoma, refers to patients who have what clinically appear to be individual primary osteosarcomas that have arisen at different times. In a Mayo Clinic review of 962 patients with osteosarcoma, 12 had multiple metachronous lesions without intervening involvement of other organs. Five of these twelve patients survived more than 5 years, and two survived at least 10 years.[29] Because of this potential for long-term survival, treatment of an isolated bone metastasis of an osteosarcoma should be curative in intent. Systemic chemotherapy and resection of the lesion are recommended. Because of the potential for both pulmonary and bone metastases, the initial workup of patients with osteosarcoma usually includes chest radiographs, a chest computed tomography (CT) scan, and a bone scan, in addition to plain radiographs, a magnetic resonance imaging (MRI) scan of the primary tumor, and standard blood tests. A complete restaging at the time of diagnosis of a bone metastasis is indicated.

In patients with widely metastatic disease, such as multiple pulmonary metastases or multiple bone metastases, a radical curative approach would be inappropriate. In patients with limited bone metastases, a curative approach might be indicated.[28,29] In patients with multiple bone metastases, palliative treatment with chemotherapy and radiation might be all that is required. Potentially curative doses of radiation might be selected. In such patients, skeletal surgery should be reserved for skeletal stabilization or reconstruction of actual or impending pathologic fractures that are not amenable to conservative treatment and for resection of symptomatic lesions that are otherwise untreatable. In the patient with an intermediate level of metastatic involvement, such as several pulmonary nodules and one skeletal site of involvement, a reasonable approach would be to administer chemotherapy initially. If the patient's tumors respond, the pulmonary metastases either stabilize or diminish, and no further bone or systemic metastases develop, a

pulmonary metastasectomy and an osseous metastasectomy would be appropriate. Thus treatment must be individualized, and the treating physician must remain cognizant of the potential for cure and must also compare the morbidity of resection and chemotherapy with the morbidity of conservative, palliative efforts.

Ewing's Sarcoma

Ewing's sarcoma is a high-grade sarcoma that usually appears in young persons between the ages of 5 and 20 years. It most commonly originates in the diaphyseal marrow of the long bones or in the flat bones. The patients usually present with large soft tissue masses resulting from the permeative extension through the cortices of the bone. Ewing's sarcoma frequently is metastatic at presentation. Common sites of metastases include bone marrow and lung. In addition to a standard general medical and laboratory evaluation, an appropriate workup at the time of the initial presentation includes radiographs and MRI of the involved bone as well as a systemic bone scan, a chest radiograph, a chest CT scan, and iliac crest bone marrow aspiration.[23,24,26] Patients usually undergo chemotherapy, followed by radiation therapy, surgical excision, or a combination of these latter two modalities.[23,24,26,30] Improved survival has been reported for those patients who are able to undergo successful surgical extirpation of the primary site when compared with those who are treated with radiation therapy.[30] Surgical resection and skeletal reconstruction eliminate the risks of late pathologic fracture and radiation-induced osteosarcoma, which are common complications of radiation treatment. Adequate surgical resection, however, may require complex reconstructive procedures or even amputation. For patients with pelvic tumors in whom an adequate excision can be accomplished, reported survival has been better than for those who do not have adequate excision.[31,33] However, because of the difficulty of achieving a true wide margin, as well as of performing a satisfactory and durable reconstruction, the recommended treatment of pelvic Ewing's sarcoma at this point is still controversial. The late development of bone metastases of Ewing's sarcoma without concomitant systemic involvement is uncommon and has not been encountered by me or by my primary mentor, Dr. Jeffrey J. Eckardt of

UCLA, despite a combined total of 26 years of orthopedic oncology practice. This situation has been occasionally encountered by other orthopedic oncologic surgeons[31] (see Fig. 24-1). If faced with such a patient, I recommend restaging the patient entirely and deciding on whether to treat with a curative intent (i.e., treat a new isolated lesion with chemotherapy and resection or radiation) or with a palliative intent (i.e., treat widespread bone metastases with chemotherapy and radiation, with surgical intervention limited to functional bone reconstruction). When a patient with bone metastasis is encountered, a complete restaging as outlined is appropriate.

Chondrosarcoma

Patients with chondrosarcomas are more heterogeneous. The lesions include low-grade chondrosarcomas with low metastatic potential, high-grade primary and secondary chondrosarcomas with high metastatic potential, and dedifferentiated high-grade chondrosarcoma with very high metastatic potential, as well as several less commonly encountered varieties such as mesenchymal chondrosarcoma and clear cell chondrosarcomas. The initial workup of patients with chondrosarcomas should usually include a chest radiograph and CT scan, bone scan, radiographs and MRI scan of the primary tumor, and basic blood tests. The discussion in this chapter will primarily consider the management of patients with high-grade chondrosarcomas.

Of particular interest with chondrosarcomas is the empirically noted increased susceptibility of cartilage cells to ectopic transplantation or tumor spread. This feature has been clinically confirmed as an increased tendency for chondroid tumors to recur locally after surgery. After incomplete resection or improper biopsy, tumor cells can be spilled and can flourish in ectopic locations. This enhanced transplantability is probably related to the metabolic needs of the malignant cartilage cells. Most tissues require an intact blood supply to provide nutrition for their metabolic needs. Mature cartilage tissue, however, survives by nutrient diffusion, since mature cartilage is normally devoid of circulation. The metabolic demands of chondrocytes can normally be met by nutrient diffusion. Thus malignant cells derived from cartilage can

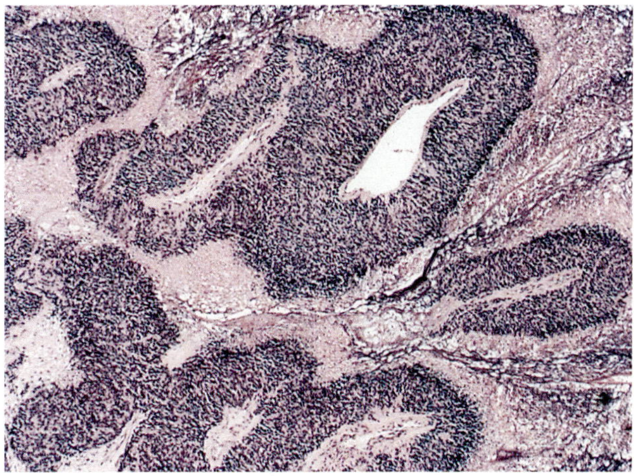

Fig. 24-2 Histologic specimen revealing viable Ewing's sarcoma only in the perivascular areas. This well-vascularized tissue was able to support the metabolic demands of the tumor, but the tissues farther from the blood supply demonstrate only necrotic tumor.

probably survive more readily in an ectopic or transplanted site because of lower nutritional metabolic demands. This is in contradistinction to cell lines, such as Ewing's sarcoma, which derive from the highly vascularized and oxygenated bone marrow. Biopsy specimens of Ewing's sarcoma are frequently noted pathologically to contain viable cells only in perivascular areas, with areas farther from the vascular supply containing only necrotic tumor cells (Fig. 24-2). Chondrosarcomas contain necrotic areas less commonly because these tumors rarely outgrow their blood supply until they are massive in size. This tendency for cartilage transplantability was previously noted in a review of the influence of pathologic fractures and other factors on the incidence of local recurrence after resection of 242 primary sarcomas of bone. In this as yet unpublished study, we noted that of seven high-grade osteosarcomas with pathologic fracture, only one ultimately sustained a local recurrence. This may be related to both the ability of the transplanted osteosarcoma cells to survive in the ectopic position and to their susceptibility to chemotherapy. Conversely, in three cases of chondrosarcoma with pathologic fracture, all developed a local recurrence after resection. This was most likely related to the ability of the transplanted cartilage cells to survive in the ectopic tissues at the time of spread

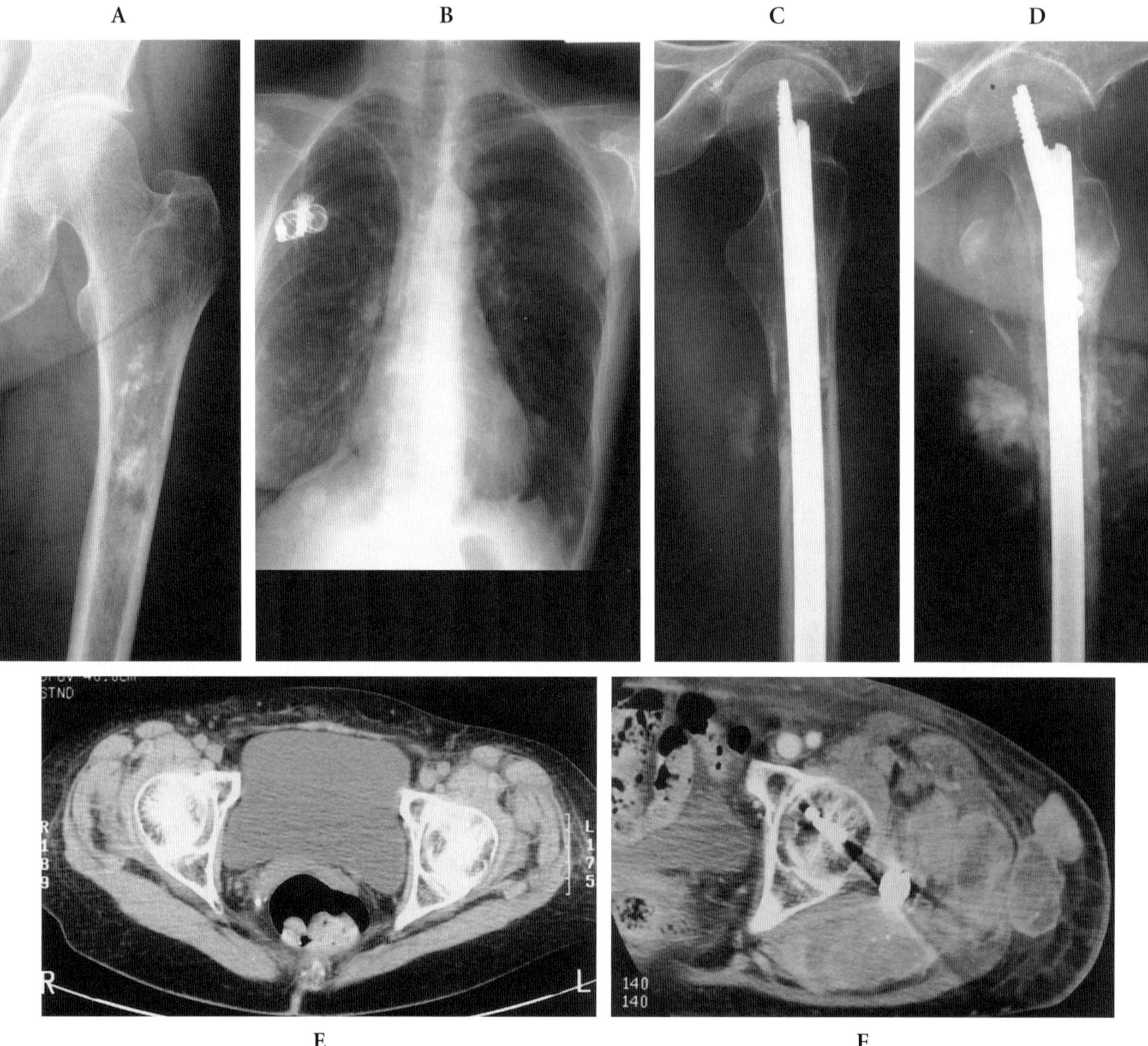

Fig. 24-3 **A,** Anteroposterior radiograph of proximal femur of a 56-year-old woman who presented with thigh pain and a remote history of breast carcinoma 17 years previously with no prior metastatic disease. She was referred for internal fixation. Because of the long disease-free interval, as well as the radiographic appearance suggesting a cartilaginous lesion, an open biopsy was performed and confirmed high-grade primary chondrosarcoma. **B,** Chest radiograph confirmed systemic disease. The patient preferred only internal fixation. **C,** Lateral radiograph in the early postoperative period demonstrating minimal soft tissue involvement. **D,** Similar lateral radiograph 3 months later demonstrating extensive soft tissue involvement and local progression of disease. **E,** CT scan at the level of the middle of the femoral heads performed immediately preoperatively demonstrating the absence of any localized disease in the area. **F,** CT scan of the same hip 3 months later, revealing the tip of the nail with extensive soft tissue implants of chondrosarcoma.

from the hematoma associated with the pathologic fracture. The poor responsiveness of chondrosarcoma to adjuvant treatment, compared with that of osteosarcoma, may also be related to the higher risk of local spread of the tumor from the pathologic fracture. Because of the risk of local tumor spread, it is my recommendation that patients with chondrosarcomas who experience pathologic fractures with any significant hematoma spread at all, if treated with a curative intent, should generally have a primary amputation.

This transplantability of tumor cells has important implications in the treatment of skeletal metastases because of the high likelihood of spreading this tumor locally if one attempts an intralesional procedure. A recently treated 56-year-old woman presented with a painful impending pathologic fracture of the femur from a suspected metastatic breast cancer. Biopsy proved her to have a high-grade primary chondrosarcoma (Fig. 24-3). Work-up confirmed diffuse systemic metastatic disease. After carefully considering all options, she elected palliative treatment with an intramedullary nail fixation. In 3 months widespread local disease developed as a result of local tumor spread from the internal fixation procedure. Local treatment would have required a complicated reverse-flap hemipelvectomy had she not died of pulmonary metastatic disease and pulmonary complications.

Not all cartilage tissue has this high degree of transplantability. Enchondromas are usually resected in intralesional procedures, as are the so-called grade ½ chondrosarcomas, with a virtually nil rate of local recurrence or local spread. Thus this local transplantability of chondrosarcomas may also be determined in part by the histologic grade of the chondrosarcoma, with moderate and high-grade chondrosarcomas having greater transplantability.

Soft Tissue Sarcoma

Tumors of the soft tissue sarcoma category present the greatest diversity in both histologic appearance and biologic behavior.[5] These tumors usually appear as asymptomatic soft tissue masses. They rarely cause symptoms other than the presence of a mass itself, unless they encroach upon surrounding neurovascular or musculoskeletal structures, in which case pain, bone erosion, or restrictions of movement may occur. Soft tissue sarcomas may arise in the deep soft tissues and go undetected un-til they achieve significant size. The more superficial lesions are generally detected earlier and have a better prognosis simply because they tend to be detected when smaller. The prognosis after diagnosis of a soft tissue sarcoma varies greatly between tumor types and depends on the histologic subtype, the aggressiveness and growth rate of the lesion, the extent of the lesion, and the overall stage. As a general rule, most soft tissue sarcomas metastasize primarily to the lung, with bone being the second most common site.[5] As mentioned previously, several soft tissue sarcomas, most notably epithelioid sarcoma and alveolar rhabdomyosarcoma, have a much higher tendency to metastasize to lymphatic tissue. Certain soft tissue sarcomas have been reported to have a 10% or greater incidence of metastases to bone. As mentioned previously, rhabdomyosarcoma metastasizes to the bone marrow in many cases, necessitating bone marrow biopsy as part of the initial staging of rhabdomyosarcoma at our institution. The diagnosis of soft tissue sarcoma is usually made after a mass is evaluated. As with the primary bone sarcomas, workups should generally include an MRI scan of the primary lesion as well as a chest radiograph and a chest CT scan to evaluate for metastatic disease. Bone scan is a baseline screening test that can be employed to evaluate for bone metastases. Bone marrow aspiration is indicated only in those tumors with a predilection for bone marrow spread (i.e., rhabdomyosarcoma).

EVALUATION

The presence of bone metastases of any sarcoma is usually detected in one of five ways. It may be detected because of the presence of pain, mass, or pathologic fracture. The metastasis may be a serendipitous discovery, or it may be discovered on routine postoperative screening of a patient who has been treated for a primary sarcoma.

There are few outcomes-based data to guide the orthopedic surgeon in the appropriate routine follow-up of patients with sarcomas in regard to the development of metastatic disease. My general practice after resection of high-grade bone sarcomas is to obtain a chest radiograph every 3 months for the first 2 years, every 6 to 12 months for 5 years, and at least every other year thereafter. CT scans of the chest may occasionally be obtained at this frequency but usually at a lesser frequency.

Many factors, including cost, inconvenience, and anxiety for the patient, and aggressiveness of the lesion, may influence the selection of the time interval between the various tests. Bone scans in patients with lesions that have a tendency to metastasize to bone are often obtained as part of the initial staging. Routine scheduled bone scans may also be obtained at various stages of postoperative follow-up. In addition, patients are instructed to report any areas of bone or deep pain, which can be further evaluated with bone scans, radiographs, and other tests, depending on the clinical evaluation and presentation of the patient at that time. Any time a patient with a history of a sarcoma has an area of bone pain, especially if it occurs at night and is a nonmechanical type of pain, one must suspect metastatic tumor involvement and evaluate the area appropriately with radiographs, a bone scan, or an MRI scan as indicated. The radiographs will show the characteristics of primary malignant tumors. Blastic lesions may be manifested by osteosarcoma, and occasionally by chondrosarcoma, but the majority of metastatic lesions will present as bone-destructive lytic lesions that have permeative or moth-eaten lytic areas with wide zones of transition. There may be cortical breakthrough, soft tissue extension, and an associated Codman's triangle or other periosteal reaction. The presence of a fracture in association with any of these radiographic features should make one highly suspicious of a pathologic fracture through a metastatic lesion. The bone scan will show increased uptake in metastatic lesions. A CT scan of the bone may also be indicated. This is the best test for assessing bone integrity if the examiner is trying to estimate the risk of pathologic fracture. The CT scan is quite useful in planning bone reconstruction or stabilization. MRI scanning is the best imaging modality to assess the full extent of the lesion to determine the bone marrow extension, the soft tissue extension, and the relationship to surrounding structures, particularly neurovascular bundles. MRI provides an anatomic road map before almost all sarcoma resections in my practice.

It is important to confirm the diagnosis of an initial metastatic lesion histologically, especially if the lesion appears lytic and is the first metastasis. Infections and other processes can have a pseudo-malignant appearance, and one would not want to radiate an area of focal osteomyelitis under the mistaken impression that it represented an initial metastasis of a previous sarcoma. I have treated patients with a variety of benign conditions that masqueraded as metastatic conditions, including an osteoporotic vertebral compression fracture that masqueraded as a metastatic lesion and two osteomyelitic lesions that masqueraded as metastases. One patient presented with a humeral fungal osteomyelitis 4 years after she had been successfully treated for lung cancer elsewhere. On initial presentation, her physicians believed that she had metastatic cancer and chemotherapy had been recommended by the initial physician. Open biopsy confirmed the diagnosis, and appropriate treatment ensued. The patient with the chondrosarcoma presented in Fig. 24-3 was referred to me because of "metastatic breast cancer." She had had 17 disease-free years after her mastectomy for breast cancer. Thus it is important to obtain diagnostic confirmation in these cases, especially when tumors occur many years after an initial cancer resection. In my institution, fine-needle aspiration biopsy (FNAB) is usually performed in these situations and is usually adequate for diagnosis. It must be stated, however, that these biopsies should be performed by or under the direction of the surgeon who may ultimately have to excise the biopsy tract. The pathologic interpretation of the cytologic material should be done by a pathologist (cytopathologist) with experience and expertise in the evaluation of bone and soft tissue tumors. It must be remembered that a negative FNAB does not mean that there is no cancer, only that none was seen on the slides, which can be due to nonrepresentative or inadequate sampling as well as to a benign etiology.

The physician who examines any patient with a presumed metastatic sarcoma should determine that there is not another primary cancer elsewhere and that the lesion does not represent a new cancer. Similarly, for example, the physician who encounters a fibrous sarcoma of bone must always consider that this may be an unusual presentation of a fibroblastic renal cell carcinoma.

MANAGEMENT

A number of treatment options are available to the orthopedic practitioner for treating patients with skeletal metastases of sarcomas. These treatment options include, but are not limited to, chemotherapy, radiation therapy, surgical resection (both wide or intralesional), internal fixation of the lesion, bone reconstruction or replacement with endoprosthesis, allograft, allograft-endoprosthetic composites, amputation, and combinations of these. The treatment plan for any individual patient must be based on the individual goals and needs of the patient with knowledge of the behavior of the underlying individual tumor.

Factors to consider in the selection of treatment include the histologic diagnosis and the overall prognosis, which will be affected not only by the histologic tumor type but also by the number of metastases, extent of metastases elsewhere, and the interval between primary disease and the onset of metastases. It has been shown in prior studies that the greater the time interval between the initial tumor and the appearance of metastatic disease, the better the prognosis.[13] Response to previous treatment is an important factor to consider. If the tumor initially was unresponsive and grew regardless of adjuvant treatments, such as chemotherapy or radiation therapy, then it is unlikely that it will be any more responsive in an ectopic metastatic location. If diffuse metastatic disease has developed, this factor must be taken into consideration. The age and overall health of the patient should also be considered, as well as the symptoms and morbidity that the metastatic lesion is causing or is expected to cause in the near future. In addition, the morbidity of each of the treatment options must be considered. In general terms, the ease and morbidity of resection and reconstruction vs. the ease and morbidity of internal fixation plus radiation treatment vs. the ease and morbidity of conservative treatment with radiation therapy and chemotherapy are factors that must be considered. A tumor in an expendable bone, especially an isolated metastasis in an expendable bone, would almost always warrant a wide excision to totally eliminate the problem. Conversely, a small metastatic lesion in a nonweightbearing bone in a patient with multiple skeletal lesions and innumerable pulmonary metastases would almost always call for conservative management with radiation therapy alone.

When one is confronted with a patient who has a presumed bone sarcoma metastasis, a whole-body bone scan should be obtained to evaluate the entire skeleton. The lungs should be investigated with a CT scan to rule out systemic involvement. If the lesion is a metastatic liposarcoma, an abdominal and pelvic CT scan or an MRI scan will help determine the presence or absence of retroperitoneal disease. If the lesion is known to have a potential for lymphatic spread, such as an epithelioid cell sarcoma, then palpation and possibly an imaging study of the regional lymph nodes may be indicated to provide additional information to be taken into consideration with regard to the treatment. Ultimately the surgeon must decide whether the goal is palliation, in terms of both pain relief and the preservation or restoration of function, or is potential cure, as in the patient with isolated or few metastases in whom resection is indicated. One should also take into consideration the "resectability and reconstructibility" of the lesion. For instance, a spinal, pelvic, or sacral metastatic lesion might simply be treated with radiation therapy because of the need for debilitating or paralyzing nerve resection surgery to get an adequate margin, especially when the likelihood of achieving a well-functioning reconstruction is slim. This is especially true if the likelihood of obtaining a true wide margin is low and the likelihood of truly obtaining a cure is low. Conversely, for example, an isolated distal femoral metastasis would lend itself well to resection and reconstruction with a distal femoral replacement.[34] Thus the treating surgeon would be more likely to recommend a surgical resection for an otherwise similar situation because it is possible to do a well-functioning reconstruction and usually is quite possible to obtain an adequate margin.

Once the extent of disease has been determined with proper staging, then one must select a specific treatment regimen. A general overview follows.

Isolated Metastasis to Bone

In the treatment of isolated metastases, the goal is usually long-term survival of the patient. The surgeon and treating physician's goal is to eliminate any systemic disease. Therefore, in a tumor that is usually responsive to chemotherapy, such as Ewing's sarcoma, osteosarcoma, rhabdomyosarcoma, malignant fibrous histiocytoma, or synovial cell sarcoma, a course of neoadjuvant chemotherapy might be indicated. If the metastatic lesion responds, then resection should be strongly considered. If there is no evidence of pulmonary or other systemic spread, I recommend resection of the lesion. Expendable bones can be simply resected. A critical but relatively reconstructible bone such as the femur, humerus, or proximal tibia should be resected and reconstructed, usually with an endoprosthesis. I recommend against the routine use of allografts in patients with metastatic disease of any type because of the overall dismal prognosis and the desirability of early functional use of the extremity.[34] Endoprosthetic reconstruction allows almost immediate functional use of the extremity, with few early complications. Endoprosthetic complications, primarily loosening, usually occur as late events.[34,35] In contrast, allograft complications, including fracture, infection, and nonunion, are more frequent and occur early.[36-38] After allograft implantation, prolonged immobilization is the norm during the wait for host-allograft union to occur. Thus in these patients with generally grim overall prognoses, despite the optimistic goal of long-term survival, endoprosthetic reconstruction offers the best chance for an early return to function and a low risk of complications in the shortened life span that they usually have remaining.[34,35]

For pelvic sarcoma, one would have to weigh the morbidity of resection against the potential benefit. If the lesion was isolated to the iliac wing, then resection might be quite beneficial. If there was extensive acetabular or sacral involvement, however, I would be somewhat less likely to recommend resection and would more likely opt for radiation and chemotherapy unless the patient was otherwise verifiably free of disease and understood the still grim overall prognosis and the poor function that follows acetabular or sacral resection. For metastatic Ewing's sarcoma, radiation treatment should be strongly considered as an alternative to surgical resection in most anatomic locations.

In some cases an amputation may occasionally be indicated. Amputation is generally a good option for sarcomatous lesions of the foot and ankle region. It is uncommon for bone sarcomas of the foot and ankle to be detected at a stage where they can be widely excised anatomically and still allow for satisfactory function. The same should be true of metastatic sarcoma involvement of the foot and ankle, although I have never encountered such a case. Below-the-knee amputation allows particu-

larly good function with a prosthesis. Amputation certainly is a good option if the metastatic lesion is large and is associated with a pathologic fracture or has failed to respond to radiation therapy. On occasion a major amputation such as a hemipelvectomy may be indicated, but the risks and benefits would have to be carefully weighed and discussed frankly with the patient, who would have to participate in that decision.

Multiple Metastases to Bone

When diffuse or systemic metastases are present, systemic treatment, primarily chemotherapy, is usually indicated, especially in tumors that are thought to be responsive to chemotherapy. Osteosarcoma, Ewing's sarcoma, rhabdomyosarcoma, synovial cell sarcoma, and malignant fibrous histiocytoma are sarcomas in which I have seen excellent responses to chemotherapy (Fig. 24-4). In addition to addressing metastatic disease throughout the body, this modified neoadjuvant chemotherapy may make the bone metastasis more amenable to successful treatment.

Radiation therapy is the mainstay of local therapy for patients with multiple metastases. When there is an impending pathologic fracture, if the tumor responds to the chemotherapy, the lesion might well reossify to the point where surgical stabilization is unnecessary. I have seen cases of primary osteosarcoma ossify on neoadjuvant chemotherapy. In patients with advanced systemic disease, if an impending pathologic fracture develops, then the general guidelines one would employ for metastatic carcinoma often are satisfactory (Fig. 24-5). In these cases, curettage and internal fixation with possible cement augmentation may well preserve skeletal integrity and allow the patient to remain functional. In many cases, intramedullary rod stabilization without cementation will suffice.

A wide excision with a curative intent would rarely be indicated in a patient with multiple metastases. However, a wide excision and endoprosthetic reconstruction may be indicated in an effort to obtain local control and to allow the best local function for destructive lesions that have destroyed the bone beyond simpler repair and for those lesions that fail to respond to chemotherapy or radiation therapy, even in the setting of diffuse metastatic disease.

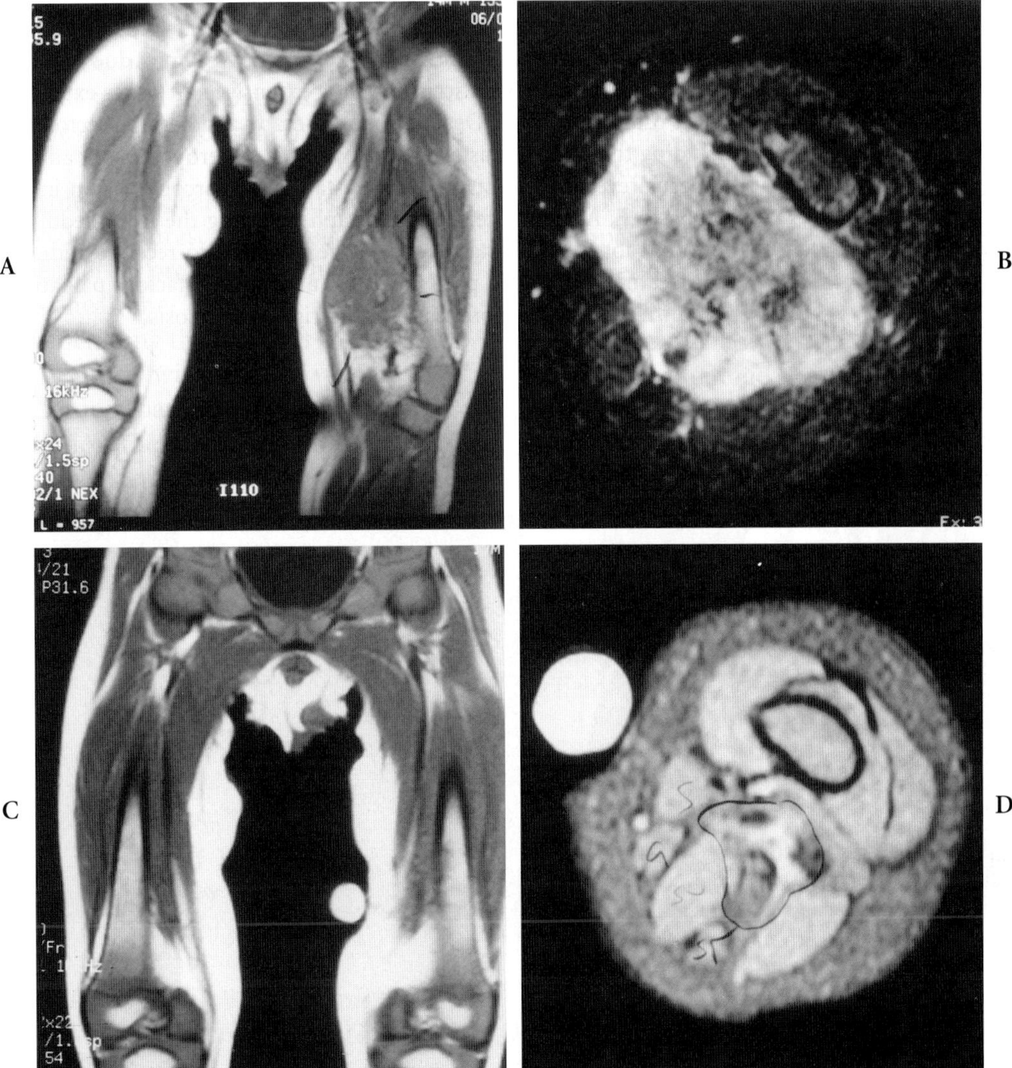

Fig. 24-4   **A,** A coronal MRI demonstrating a large rhabdomyosarcoma of the posterior medial left thigh of a 14-month-old child. **B,** Axial MRI reveals the large extent of the lesion. The patient had a positive bone marrow biopsy at initial presentation. **C,** Postchemotherapy preresection coronal MRI reveals a significant decrease in the size of the lesion as a result of neoadjuvant chemotherapy. Bone marrow biopsy performed after neoadjuvant chemotherapy revealed no detectable tumor. **D,** Axial MRI confirmed the small residual tumor, which was resected. The patient remains free of disease following completion of chemotherapy 1 year after presentation.

Table 25-3 Clinical syndromes of base of skull metastases

Syndrome	Common symptoms	Common clinical findings	Common radiographic findings
Parasellar	Unilateral frontal headache, diplopia, facial numbness	Ophthalmoplegia (CN III, IV, VI), paresthesias of CN V_1,V_2	CT: bone destruction involving petrous apex or sella turcica
Orbital	Periorbital pain, diplopia, dull constant frontal headache	Proptosis, periorbital edema, palpable	CT: orbital mass, orbital wall destruction
Middle fossa	Facial numbness, facial pain, facial palsy, diplopia	CN V_1,V_2, VI, VII dysfunction	Rare radiographic changes
Jugular foramen	Hoarseness, dysphagia, unilateral occipital or postauricular pain	CN IX, X, XI, dysfunction, vocal cord paralysis, tongue/SCM atrophy	Late radiographic changes with bone destruction or mass jugular foramen
Occipital condyle	Severe unrelenting unilateral occipital headache	Headache with neck flexion, unilateral CN XII palsy	CT: destruction of the occipital condyle

Adapted from Greenberg HS, Deck MDF, Vikram B, Chu FCH, Posner JB. Metastasis to the base of the skull: Clinical findings in 43 patients. Neurology 31:530-537, 1981. Used with permission.

Table 25-4 Clinical syndromes of orbital metastases

Syndrome	Symptoms/clinical findings
Mass	Mass effect: proptosis, axial and nonaxial displacement, palpable mass
Infiltrative	Diffuse or localized infiltration of orbital tissues: diplopia, ptosis, enophthalmos, firm orbit, "frozen globe," ocular dysmotility
Functional	Isolated or combined cranial nerve II, III, IV, V, VI dysfunction out of proportion to mass or infiltrative syndromes
Inflammatory	Acute or subacute onset of pain, chemosis, scleral or conjunctival injection, pain with eye movement, erythema, periorbital edema
Silent	No signs or symptoms: detected serendipitously during CT evaluation or other imaging or invasive procedure

Adapted from Goldberg RA, Rootman J, Cline RA. Tumors metastatic to the orbit: A changing picture. Surv Ophthalmol 35:1-24, 1990. Used with permission.

Radiology
Plain Radiographs

For patients in whom there is a symptomatic lesion and in whom metastatic disease is suspected, the plain radiograph remains the most expeditious, least expensive, and most readily available imaging technique to confirm diagnoses. Most lesions will conform to the category of lytic, sclerotic, or mixed. Sclerotic metastatic bone lesions are a common manifestation of cancers of the prostate, breast, gastrointestinal tract, and bladder. Lytic bone lesions can occur with virtually every type of primary tumor, and mixed lesions most commonly arise from breast and prostate cancers.[59] Plain radiographs require an approximately 30% change in bone density for defects to be detected. This degree of insensitivity makes detection of subtle orbital, facial bone, and base-of-skull lesions difficult. However, for instances in which skull and mandibular lesions are clinically evident, this modality is quite accurate, with radiographic abnormalities detected in up to 95% of the cases.[28] Special imaging techniques, such as Water's, Caldwell, lateral, and basal views for paranasal sinus involvement and Panorex studies for mandibular lesions, may demonstrate abnormalities not seen on conventional radiographs. These types of plain films can be rapidly obtained and reviewed and can help guide the selection of additional diagnostic studies.

Bone Scintigraphy

The technetium diphosphonate bone scan represents an optimum method to assess for systemic metastatic disease because of the ability to examine the entire bone skeleton.[60] Bone scans are generally more sensitive than plain radiographs[61-63] because they detect functional rather than structural

changes. A subtle 5% to 10% increase in tracer uptake can be readily detected, compared with at least a 30% change in structural composition required for radiographic delineation.[64] In many instances bone scan abnormalities should be followed by plain radiographs to help assess structural integrity. A limitation of bone scans is that they do not detect all lesions; purely lytic lesions and rapidly growing lesions in which new bone growth is not commensurate with bone destruction are not readily identified.[65]

CT and MRI

The use of more sophisticated imaging modalities (e.g., CT and MRI) to evaluate metastatic disease has become more common in recent years. This is certainly true in the case of craniofacial metastases in which symptoms and clinical findings are complex and frequently require detailed imaging of the

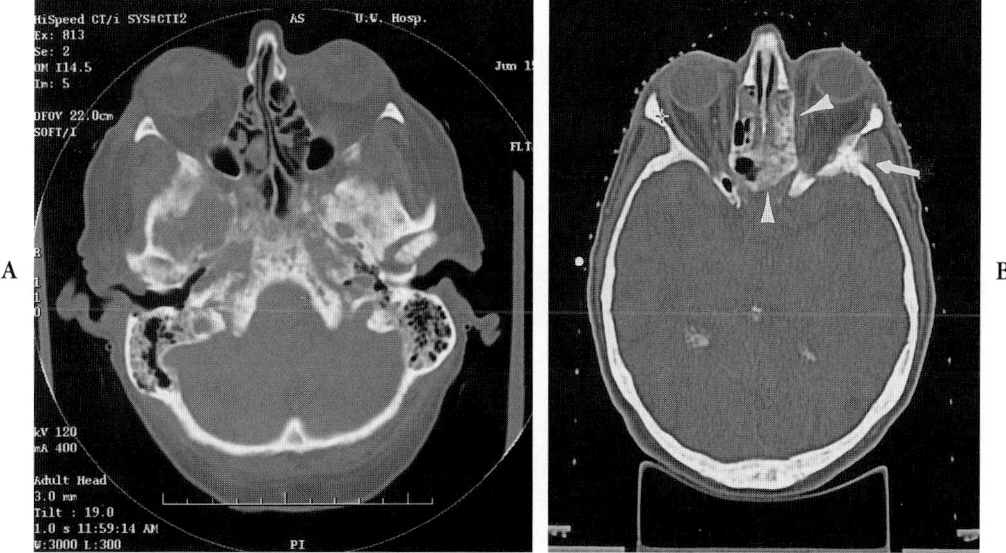

Fig. 25-3   A, CT image of a 67-year-old man with metastatic adenocarcinoma of the prostate presenting with decreased visual acuity in the left eye. Bone windows demonstrate diffuse metastatic involvement of the base of skull. Other findings included multiple dura-based metastases compressing brain parenchyma. Palliative whole-brain radiation therapy to 30 Gy in 10 fractions with an additional 7.5 Gy boost to the base of skull was delivered. The patient achieved improvement in both visual acuity and visual field defect 1 month after completing radiation therapy. **B,** CT image of elderly man with metastatic adenocarcinoma of the prostate presenting with left facial numbness, left periorbital pain, and hyperlacrimation. Bone windows from CT scan demonstrated diffuse metastatic involvement of the base of the skull, bilateral ethmoid sinuses *(arrowheads),* and left orbital bones *(arrow).* The patient underwent palliative radiation therapy to the base of skull and bilateral orbits (30 Gy in 12 fractions). The patient experienced significant resolution of all his presenting symptoms by the completion of treatment.

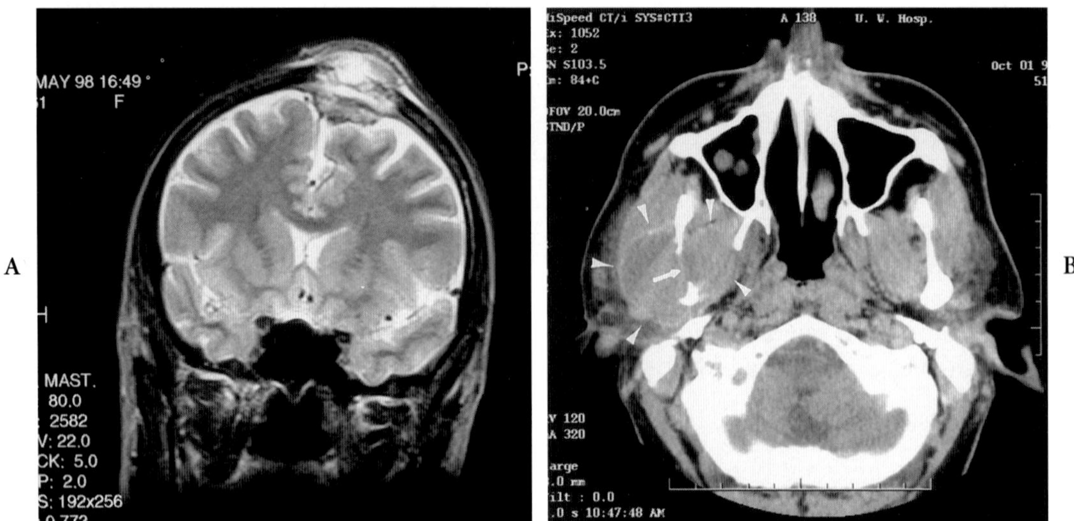

Fig. 25-4 **A,** T2-weighted coronal MRI image of a 60-year-old woman demonstrating a calvarial mass (a left frontal parenchymal metastases is not shown). Fine-needle aspiration biopsy demonstrated squamous cell carcinoma, with subsequent metastatic workup defining a lung primary. The patient underwent a course of palliative whole-brain radiation therapy to 30 Gy in 10 fractions with an additional 9 Gy involved field boost. The patient experienced significant regression in this mass 1 month after completing treatment. **B,** CT image of patient with 1-month history of right periauricular swelling, trismus, and 20-pound weight loss. Study reveals a 3.5 × 5 cm mass *(arrowheads)* originating from the right mandibular condyle *(arrow)*. Fine-needle aspiration biopsy favored carcinoma, with complete metastatic workup negative. The patient was treated with curative intent with resection and postoperative radiation therapy. Several months after completion of therapy, the patient complained of progressive dysphagia and was found to have a primary adenocarcinoma of the distal esophagus.

base of the skull, orbit, or mandible to precisely delineate the location of the causative lesion. Bone structures are best seen with CT bone windows, which can readily identify destructive lesions involving the base of the skull, orbit, and other osseous structures (Fig. 25-3). Likewise, CT and MRI can provide excellent detail of soft tissues, such as cranial nerves, and can identify concomitant brain metastases, leptomeningeal or meningeal involvement, and tumor extension (Figs. 25-4). The information obtained from CT and MRI can often assist in planning approaches for biopsy or resection (if warranted) and in the precise design of radiation treatment portals.

Biopsy

Biopsy to establish the histopathologic identification of cancer is often necessary in the patient with an unknown primary cancer and is sometimes recommended in those with a known or suspected primary tumor from another site. In selected instances, biopsy of the primary tumor site may be more difficult or morbid than biopsy of the metastatic site within the craniofacial region. Biopsies can sometimes be accomplished with fine-needle aspiration biopsy (FNAB). This method can be augmented with CT guidance to approach lesions that are not readily evident on surface topography. FNAB is typically the least morbid biopsy option. However, the diagnostic accuracy of FNAB is more limited than open biopsy, and it is difficult to perform a needle aspiration through bone. As a result, open biopsy is often required. Open biopsy can be performed in most locations within the head and neck with limited morbidity. In most situations, this will be the only surgical procedure indicated in the diagnosis and treatment of the patient with craniofacial bone metastasis.

Biopsy of tumors within the mandible can be readily accomplished through a transoral approach. Infrequently, a lesion may be present within the condyle of the mandible, necessitating an open biopsy through a facial approach. These facial approaches must respect the adjacent facial nerve distribution.

Malignant tumors of the paranasal sinuses are rare (3% to 5% of upper aerodigestive tract cancers), and metastatic lesions are rarer still. Within the paranasal sinuses the maxillary sinus is the most common focus for metastatic lesions and is also the most common site of primary cancers of the sinuses (typically squamous cell carcinoma or adenocarcinoma). The ethmoid sinuses are the next most common site of primary cancer and also of metastatic lesions. In both of these sites a destructive lesion will first be suspected to represent a primary cancer. In contrast, although less common, a destructive lesion of the frontal or sphenoid sinus will have a much greater likelihood of representing a metastatic lesion because primary cancer of these sites is uncommon.

Metastasis to the bones of the paranasal sinuses can usually be accessed from a transnasal endoscopic approach. These transnasal endoscopic approaches also allow access to lesions involving the inferior and medial walls of the orbit and lesions involving the anterior cranial fossa floor. For lesions involving the bone along the superior or lateral walls of the orbit, an external approach is indicated. An external approach is also necessary for access to the frontal sinus. Lesions involving the majority of the calvarium can be accessed for biopsy through direct external approaches.

Metastatic lesions of the temporal bone most commonly involve the petrous apex, tegmen tympani, mastoid bone, and internal auditory canal.[13] Symptoms of these metastasis might include facial paralysis, unilateral sensorineural hearing loss, tinnitus, dizziness, or infection secondary to obstruction of middle ear aeration. Metastatic lesions are occasionally accessible to biopsy through the external auditory canal or through the tympanic membrane. Most other lesions will be accessible from a transmastoid approach. When lesions involve the superior surface of the petrous apex, a small middle fossa craniotomy can be used for biopsy access. Access to the infratemporal fossa floor is more difficult. Lesions in this area usually present with cranial nerve symptoms secondary to involvement of the basal foramina through which the nerves exit.[7]

This bone can be approached from a transzygomatic or transmaxillary approach. Often, in the patient with known cancer, biopsy of the craniofacial metastasis is not necessary to justify palliative treatment.[10]

Histopathology

The majority of patients presenting with craniofacial metastases will have a known history of cancer. For most of these patients, biopsy confirmation is not warranted in light of the overall clinical presentation of the disease. However, there are several clinical scenarios in which it may be important to pursue histopathologic evaluation of craniofacial metastases. The first is that of the patient in whom a long disease-free interval has transpired and there is concern that the metastatic specimen should be compared with the original primary pathologic specimen. The second is that of the patient with a newly discovered cancer in whom a primary tumor is not yet identified. In this case, some tumors are classified as undifferentiated and will require special immunohistochemical and possibly electron microscopic techniques for a diagnosis. Special stains to arrive at a diagnosis may include keratin (squamous cell carcinoma), PSA (prostate), carcinoembryonic antigen (CEA, gastrointestinal tract), S100 (melanoma), and estrogen and progesterone (breast) receptor status. This information is often invaluable because a definitive diagnosis can assist in determining whether specific therapeutic interventions, such as chemotherapy and hormonal ablation or therapy, may be of benefit.

MANAGEMENT
Rationale for Therapy

As an overall group, patients with metastatic disease to bone (including craniofacial sites) generally experience a relatively short subsequent life span (months to a few years). The primary aim of therapeutic interventions in the setting of metastatic disease is therefore to provide relief from troubling symptoms and to encourage an improvement in overall quality of life. This includes relief of pain, bleeding, or ulceration; elimination or reduction of the need for narcotic analgesics; local control of tumor growth that might otherwise lead to a risk of pathologic fracture or infection of ulcerative areas; and reduction of the risk of recurrent or new symptoms. Nonetheless, it should be remembered

The purpose of a classification system is to provide information relevant to diagnosis, prognosis, treatment options, and the results of treating a particular tumor. Classification systems are also useful for unambiguous communication among treating clinicians. Ambiguity persists, however, among classification systems for spinal metastases. There are numerous parameters from which individual classification systems are constructed. This is in addition to the varied interests and goals of the investigators, the lack of consistent and universal terminology, incomplete follow-up and undetermined end points, and the retrospective nature of many studies. Thus classification systems for spinal metastases within the literature today are at best problematic. It is therefore difficult to compare results of one study or series with others in a meaningful way. Thus the concept of a unifying classification for spinal metastases is rather complex and without uniformity. For one thing, each author has different criteria of importance to his or her particular treatment or report.

In the past, classification systems were developed and reported in retrospect. Here the authors' post hoc attempts were to explain their indications and results rather than to provide specific criteria by which decisions regarding treatment options or prognosis were made. More recently, classification systems have been developed for the prospective evaluation of patients with metastatic disease to the spine. Here treatment options are based on presurgical evaluation, with prognosis playing a larger and more important role.

Current classification systems are variable. Most were developed to include one or more parameters, such as anatomic location, neurologic function, deformity, impending or actual neurologic deterioration, pain, extent of tumor load, systemic considerations, and others. Most systems, however, have not been clinically tested, validated, or accepted for widespread use beyond that of the primary author. The ideal classification system for metastatic disease to the spine might include such information as tumor type, the biologic behavior, grade, and stage of the specific tumor, and systemic extent of tumor load. In addition, the assessment of pain, neurologic status, and mechanical stability of the spine would be crucial to the understanding of the impact of the disease on the patient. Specific information regarding tumor location, potential compartments of involvement, appropriate terminology for the description of the tumor location, and the appropriate description of the procedures involved in treatment of the tumor would be advantageous as well. Finally, a prospective multicenter effort to establish the validity of this ideal classification system would be essential. All this information could then be used to help determine appropriate treatment options and strategies, as well as to provide prognostic information to the treating team and the patient. We are not there as yet.

HISTORICAL PERSPECTIVES

Early classification systems were based on gross neurologic function and were developed primarily for use in spinal trauma. The neurologic function recorded was that of ambulation as the index criterion. Often this simply involved the ability or lack of ability to ambulate or the presence and extent of lower extremity muscle function against gravity. The main purpose of these systems was to report clinical results before and after surgical or nonsurgical treatment, rather than to prospectively assist in the determination of appropriate treatment options or provide any prognostic information. They were primarily descriptive in nature, generally retrospective, and thus limited to what had been recorded in the medical record. Although sphincter function was occasionally reported, it was not usually considered a fundamental measure within a classification system. Sensory function was reported in a similar fashion.

Brice and McKissock

One of the first attempts at classification of neurologic deficits in patients with spinal metastatic disease was presented by Brice and McKissock[1] in 1965 (see box on p. 365). They reported on their surgical experience over a 10-year period in the treatment of 145 patients with metastatic disease to the spine. Their classification system was divided into four groups, based on the degree of neurologic deficit present: Group 1 had mild deficits and retained ambulatory capability; group 2 had moderate neurologic deficit and ability to move legs but not against gravity; group 3 had severe deficits, with only slight residual motor and sensory function, with retention of deep pain and sensation; group 4 had complete deficit with no signs of mo-

Classification Systems for Metastatic Disease of the Spine

Brice and McKissock (1965)
I. Mild neurologic deficit—ambulation retained
II. Moderate neurologic deficit—moves legs, not against gravity
III. Severe neurologic deficit—slight residual motor and sensory function; detention of deep pain sensation
IV. Neurologically complete—no motor or sensory function

Frankel (1969)
American Spinal Injury Association (1992)
A. Complete
B. Sensory only
C. Motor useless
D. Motor useful
E. Recovery

White (1971)
I. Ambulatory
II. Nonambulatory—some motor function
III. Paraplegic—no motor function

Gilbert (1978)
I. Ambulatory with or without weakness
II. Nonambulatory—can lift legs when recumbent
III. Paraplegic—unable to move legs against gravity

Constans (1983)
I. Pain, minor neurologic symptoms—normal social and professional activities
II. Mild neurologic symptoms—normal social but interruption of professional activity
III. Moderate neurologic symptoms—sphincter disturbances; active life impossible
IV. Serious neurologic syndrome—paraplegic, complete sphincter deficit
V. Medullary syndrome of cord transection

DeWald (1985)
I. Destruction, no deformity, moderate pain—three subclasses based on degree of bone involvement
II. Moderate deformity and collapse, immune competent
III. Moderate deformity and collapse, immune incompetent
IV. Marked deformity and collapse, paralysis, immune competent
V. Marked deformity and collapse, paralysis, immune suppressed

Harrington (1986)
I. No neurologic involvement or minor sensory impairment
II. Bone involvement with collapse or instability
III. Major neurologic impairment without significant bone involvement
IV. Vertebral collapse, mechanical pain or instability, no significant neurologic impairment
V. Vertebral collapse and instability combined with major neurologic impairment

Brihaye (1988)
(Shaw and Tong classifications)
I. Walks normally
II. Weak legs, walks unaided
III. Walking with aids
IV. Unable to walk, moves legs
V. Paraplegic

Asdourian (1990)
I. Impending axial instability, with (IA) or without (IB) metastatic vertebral involvement
II. Axial instability
III. Axial instability with vertebral deformity
IV. Impending translational instability II; or III deformity with metastasis

WBB (Weinstein, Boriani, Biagini) (1994)
Anatomic zones and layers; helpful in describing tumor location and extent, and preoperative planning; incorporates Enneking's oncologic classification system; validated in primary bone tumors of the spine

Tomita (1994)
Five anatomic zones and 7 lesion types based on location; incorporates the three-column system of Denis, and the classification system of Enneking and the WBB system; useful for preoperative planning, particularly for spondylectomy procedures

Tokuhashi (1990)
Enkaoua (1997)
Prognostic scoring system for systemic extent of tumor load; uses 6 parameters to determine potential life expectancy for decision making about treatment options and surgical procedure considerations

tor, sensory, or normal sphincter function below the lesion in the spine (see box on p. 365). The authors concluded that this classification proved useful for prognostic purposes, noting that success of surgical intervention was greatest in those with the least neurologic involvement at the time of surgery. They also noted that the speed of onset of the neurologic deficit was of prognostic significance. Those with slow progression were noted to have a better recovery than those with a rapid onset of neurologic deficit, in which case the recovery was minimal if it occurred at all. In this series no patient with a complete lesion had recovery of neurologic function. The authors concluded that "early diagnosis and immediate treatment of spinal cord compression appears to offer the only hope of improving the outlook for these unfortunate individuals." Laminectomy was the procedure of choice in this series, being used for the establishment of diagnosis and to "carry out an adequate rapid decompression of the spinal cord." Of the 145 patients, 10 patients deteriorated neurologically on postoperative day 2 or 3, and 7 of these had anterior compression of the thoracic spinal cord. Six patients in this series died within the first 2 weeks after surgery, and 19 remained alive after 1 year. Brice concluded that only one third of the patients in their series benefited from surgical intervention.

Frankel/American Spinal Injury Association

The next major advancement in the classification of spinal cord dysfunction was the system reported by Frankel et al.[2] This classification was originally designed for patients with traumatic injuries to the spine resulting in loss of spinal cord function and treated by closed methods. It was developed to assess "the bony lesions, their management and the results of postural reduction on the bony and spinal cord lesions" in paraplegic and tetraplegic patients. The series included 612 patients admitted to Stokes Mandeville Hospital from 1951 to 1968 with varying degrees of traumatic spinal cord injury. Patients who had undergone surgical treatment were excluded from the "survey." Five different grades were defined. "Complete" (grade A) indicated that the lesion was found to be "complete," both motor and sensory, below the segmental level marked. "Sensory only" (grade B) implied that there was

some sensation present below the level of the lesion but that the motor paralysis was complete below that level. This grade would apply to those with sacral sparing. "Motor useless" (grade C) implied that there was some motor power below the level of the lesion, but it was of no practical use to the patient. "Motor useful" (grade D) implied the presence of useful motor power below the level of the lesion. Patients in this group could move the lower limbs, and many could walk with or without aids. "Recovery" (grade E) implied that the patient was free of neurologic symptoms; abnormal reflexes might be present.

In addition to the development of this system of grades in the classification of neurologic deficits, Frankel et al. also recorded patient-specific clinical, neurologic, and injury-related data on an "Analysis Proforma Sheet." This documented all pertinent data, including mechanism of injury, spinal segment involved, type and grade of the neurologic injury, associated injuries, and neurologic changes with treatment over time. Neurologic change was indicated by a dot placed on the chart at the neurologic grade on admission, with an additional dot connected by an arrow placed on the subsequent neurologic grade on discharge. Frankel et al. noted that "neurologic classification is relatively crude" but that a system was needed "whereby most cases fell clearly into a specific category and which gave results which could be analyzed." They also noted that this system differed from the earlier grading systems of Guttman,[3] Hardy,[4] Geisler et al.,[5] and others in that it provided more specific neurologic detail as well as a mechanism by which neurologic improvement could be documented and analyzed. This advancement was the major difference in the classification system of Frankel. The Frankel system has been modified by the American Spinal Injury Association (A.S.I.A.) as the Standards for Neurological and Functional Classification of Spinal Cord Injury[6] and remains in common use today for the description of the neurologic status of patients with spinal cord involvement regardless of the cause.

White

Additional classification systems were reported in 1971 by White et al.,[7] who reported on 226 patients from New York Hospital who were treated with laminectomy for metastatic disease to the spine. The goal was to "see if the indications for decompression laminectomy could be established more clearly." Patients were divided into three groups, depending on their neurologic evaluation before surgery. Grade I consisted of ambulatory patients, grade II of nonambulatory patients with some preserved motor function, and grade III of paraplegic patients with no motor function. White et al. found that postoperative recovery was clearly dependent on preoperative neurologic function and that a substantial number of patients subsequently lost the ability to walk soon after surgery.

Gilbert

Gilbert et al.[8] used a similar system in 1978. The clinical findings of 130 patients with metastatic extradural compression of the spinal cord treated at Memorial Sloan-Kettering Cancer Center were reviewed. This study provided a comparison of radiation therapy alone vs. surgical treatment by laminectomy followed by radiation therapy. Motor and ambulatory function was the determining factor in dividing the patients into three grades. Grade 1 patients were ambulatory, with or without weakness of the lower extremities or ataxia. Grade 2 patients were not ambulatory but were able to lift their legs when recumbent. Grade 3 patients were paraplegic or were unable to move their legs against gravity. Sphincter function, sensation, and pain were not considered in determining the grade because they were not recorded in the chart, and thus retrospective determination of these factors was not possible. Ambulatory function was more reliably recorded in the medical record and became the determining factor in the classification system. Using this classification system in the evaluation of the treatment by radiotherapy with or without laminectomy, Gilbert et al. concluded that "We doubt that surgical decompression is necessary or desirable as the initial therapy for most patients with epidural spinal cord compression."

Although the White and Gilbert systems classifying neurologic deficits added little to the literature, they helped to clarify these authors' retrospective findings about their methods of treating metastatic disease to the spine. Limitations persist concerning management based on the extent of tumor involvement. It was clear, however, that (1) those patients with a complete neurologic deficit had a dismal prognosis for recovery of function, regardless of treatment, and (2) the rate of progression of the neurologic deficit had a negative prognostic significance.

Constans

Constans et al.,[9] in 1983, expanded upon these types of classification systems, which had been predominantly based on motor function. In reporting on 600 patients treated between 1965 and 1980 with metastatic lesions to the spine, they divided them into five groups, as assessed by neurologic function at the time of admission. This classification also included sphincter function and such patient-centered parameters as social activities and work capabilities. Grade 1 included patients with pain or "minor neurologic symptoms" and normal social and professional activities. Grade 2 consisted of patients with "mild neurologic symptoms" and normal social life but interruption of professional activities. Grade 3 included patients with "moderate neurologic syndromes," including paraparesis and sphincter dysfunction, but maintenance of an "active life" was impossible in this group. Grade 4 involved "serious neurologic syndromes," paraplegia and complete sphincter dysfunction. Grade 5 was defined as a medullary syndrome of spinal cord transection. Constans et al. concluded that "the classification of patients according to neurologic signs and consequent levels of independence is most useful because it allows an immediate judgment to be made of the severity of the disease, it is of prognostic value, and it indicates precisely the need for speedy treatment." They concluded that grade 1 patients could be treated with radiotherapy alone. Surgical treatment was not justified because there was so little neurologic disturbance and often no medullary compression. Radiotherapy was preferable also because it efficiently relieved such symptoms as pain. In grade 2, 3, and 4 patients, surgery for the relief of compression and pain was preparatory to radiotherapy, which could then be undergone in greater comfort, with better functional status, and with less risk of sudden progression of symptoms. Indications for surgical intervention were more restricted for grade 5 patients. Constans et al. noted that there was little hope of improvement in these patients after 24 hours of paraplegia and that surgery at that time was useless unless it was performed for some other purpose. Thus surgery for grade 5 patients was time dependent.

The Constans system added additional complexity to the concept of classification in that it included patient-centered parameters of physical function and professional and social activity in determining the impact of tumor involvement and functional capabilities. Constans et al. noted that "the preoperative neurologic grade is fundamental to the choice of treatment," and thus treatment was grade dependent from the time of admission. However, there were major limitations to this system as well as to those that preceded it. It was highly subjective in the description of each grade and neurologic function, and thus it provided no objective and presumably no reproducible longitudinal information regarding the effects of treatment over time. Similarly, treatment outcome was graded as "improved, unchanged, or worse" and was determined only within a few weeks of treatment intervention.

DeWald

Despite the advancement seen in the classification systems based on neurologic status, combined with additional data on function, social and professional activity, and pain, these classification systems lacked any mention of the significance of the bone involvement of the spine. Issues of stability, deformity, impending neurologic deterioration, and pain were neglected, particularly with regard to the treatment of spinal metastases with impending mechanical or neurologic deterioration in a prophylactic manner. These are particularly crucial concepts because uncontrolled pain, which is often an indication for surgical intervention, may be caused by microfractures and may also be representative of impending or progressive vertebral collapse, deformity, and neurologic impairment.[10,11]

DeWald et al.[12] addressed some of these issues in 1985, when they reported on spinal reconstruction as palliation for metastatic cancers of the spine. They reported on 17 patients with spinal metastases who were treated for pain, deformity, and paralysis. Prophylactic stabilization and correction of the deformity for pain control, preservation of function, and mobilization were the goals. Stability was described as "lack of structural support" and

was qualified by the degree of vertebral body involvement by metastatic disease.

DeWald et al. established a classification of five types for determining the treatment and prognosis of patients with spinal metastases. Neurologic involvement was described in general terms only, without objective criteria for determining the severity of paralysis or for recording objective neurologic changes with treatment. Importance was placed on spinal stability, alignment, impending deformity, and the underlying immune status of the patient. This was in recognition of the risks inherent in those who are immunocompromised by treatment. Class I patients have no deformity, but pain is present. With less than 50% destruction of the vertebral body, radiotherapy and chemotherapy were thought adequate. With 50% or more involvement of the vertebral body, or with involvement of the pedicles, DeWald et al. thought that the spine was at risk of collapse, progressive deformity, and paralysis. Thus surgical reconstruction was recommended with a good prognosis for the spine. Class II patients are those with moderate deformity and collapse who are at risk of neurologic deterioration, with surgical reconstruction recommended for treatment. Many surgical complications in this series were believed to be associated with perioperative chemotherapy or radiotherapy, and thus DeWald et al. recommended that these treatments be delayed or postponed. Prognosis of the spinal metastases in this group was also believed to be satisfactory. Class III patients are those with moderate deformity and collapse who already are receiving chemotherapy and thus are immunocompromised as a result. These patients were recognized as presenting difficult treatment dilemmas. Strong consideration of halting the chemotherapy with surgical reconstruction to follow once the patient recovered from the chemotherapy was recommended. In class IV patients, those with marked spinal deformity, collapse, paralysis, and immune compromise, surgical reconstruction is a relative surgical emergency, with a guarded prognosis at best. Class V patients, those with marked deformity, collapse, paralysis, and immune suppression, present the most difficult problems. The prognosis is poor, and a joint decision between the surgeon and the oncologist concerning the treatment plan is necessary. DeWald et al. concluded that reduction and rigid spine immobilization would provide pain relief and could significantly improve neurologic function. They also noted the importance of prophylactic stabilization of the spine at risk of impending deformity to prevent collapse and paralysis. DeWald's classification system recommends the treatment of spinal metastases regardless of the underlying tumor type and provides information with regard to the concepts of prophylactic stabilization. Criteria of stability, however, were not described.

Harrington

Much of the early work on mechanical stability in the spine with metastatic involvement is borrowed from the literature of traumatic spinal injuries, much as Frankel's classification of spinal cord injury was developed. The three-column system of spinal stability, popularized by Denis[13] and by White and Panjabi,[14] provided a foundation on which stability and deformity criteria were incorporated into the assessment of metastatic disease to the spine. Harrington[10,11] noted that lytic destruction of the anterior half of the vertebral body, the anterior column only, is often the initial manifestation of metastatic involvement. This does not cause spinal instability and progressive deformity unless the posterior half of the body, the middle column, is destroyed as well. If the body begins to collapse, its ability to function as a weightbearing fulcrum decreases, and the bending moment of the spine shifts posteriorly, with compressive loads on the remaining vertebral body increasing geometrically. A progressive kyphosis follows with extrusion of debris of tumor tissue, disc, and bone posteriorly into the spinal canal with resultant spinal cord compression. Thus Harrington viewed as equally important both the mechanical and the neurologic roles of the spine and the implications of metastatic involvement to these functions of the spine.

Harrington[10] divided patients with spinal metastases into five categories, depending on the extent of neurologic compromise or bone destruction. In class I there is no significant neurologic involvement, whereas in class II there is involvement of bone without collapse or instability. In class III there is major neurologic impairment (sensory or motor) without significant involvement of bone. Class IV is defined by vertebral collapse with pain due to mechanical causes or instability but without significant neurologic compromise. In class V ver-

tebral collapse or instability is combined with major neurologic impairment. Harrington's classification system, however, does not take into account the site of primary tumor of origin or the presence of more generalized metastatic disease and thus is reflective only of the metastatic spinal disease rather than of systemic involvement or biologic behavior of the tumor.

Harrington recommended that treatment be based on the class of involvement. Patients in class I or II, with little or no neurologic involvement and without evidence of bone collapse or instability, generally do well with local irradiation alone. Those in class III usually respond well to radiotherapy alone, augmented by systemic corticosteroids when neurologic deterioration is acute or rapidly progressive. Occasionally patients with prolonged survival who have had maximum irradiation may require decompression to reverse progressive paralysis. Patients in class IV or V, with progressive vertebral collapse and kyphotic deformity, generally require an anterior decompression and reconstruction and possibly augmentation posteriorly as well. Harrington used his classification system to determine treatment strategies and Frankel's classification to evaluate and report the neurologic results of treatment intervention.

Kostuik

Kostuik et al.,[15,16] in 1988, provided a concept similar to Harrington's of using a system of columns to reflect spinal stability. This system was devised with anterior, middle, and posterior columns, each column divided into a left and a right side, providing six overall columns. They concluded that if two of six columns were involved with tumor, the spine was probably stable. If three or more columns were destroyed, an unstable lesion was present. In addition, angulation greater than 20 degrees was considered another sign of instability. These definitions of stability did not take into account soft tissue or epidural extension of tumor into the spinal canal.

Brihaye

Brihaye et al.,[17] in 1988, recognized the limitations of any one single classification system and proposed using the functional classification of Shaw et al.[18] in conjunction with the pain scale of Tong et al.[19] in the assessment of the clinical condition of the patient. Brihaye et al. noted that the two factors most important to patients were ambulatory capability and pain control, and thus they used the combination of these scales to evaluate both factors. They also felt that any system must be simple and "convenient for everybody on the medical nursing staff" to use. Shaw's grading system was based primarily on ambulatory function, graded 1 through 5. Patients with grade 1 are able to walk. Those in grade 2 have weak legs but still are able to walk unaided. Patients in grade 3 walk with an aid. Those in grade 4 are unable to walk but can move the legs. Those in grade 5 are paraplegic. The measure of pain by the method of Tong et al. assessed pain by both a pain score and a narcotic score. The pain score combined the pain severity and the pain frequency, whereas the narcotic score combined the type of pain medication used and the frequency of administration. Brihaye et al. believed that combining these two modalities of grading would "provide an objective appreciation of various therapeutic approaches." Although the concept of combining classification scales and using objective measures was an advancement, notably absent from this review were the clinical use and reporting of these scales to determine treatment options and success.

Asdourian

Asdourian et al.,[20] in 1990, described another deformity-based classification system used in 27 patients who were treated for breast cancer. Magnetic resonance imaging (MRI) analysis was performed to determine the extent of metastatic vertebral body involvement and sagittal spinal deformity, the state of hydration of the intervertebral disc, and whether the spinal canal was compromised. This review revealed a consistent pattern of sagittal spinal deformity from which criteria were established, identifying four stages of instability and subgroups of progressive deformity. This MRI-based classification was used as the method of choice because MRI was superior for determining the extent of soft tissue involvement, including the paravertebral region. In addition, MRI more clearly demonstrates the length and extent of metastatic lesions within the spine, unlike myelography, in which a complete block necessitated an additional study above or below the blocked level. MRI was also critical in determining the direction of compression as well as the visualization of the spinal cord without the risks of myelography, particularly in the presence of a complete block. In this classification system the stages of vertebral body collapse and deformity are described, criteria are established for identifying instability, and a protocol is presented for the treatment of metastatic disease to the spine.

In Asdourian's type I a portion of the vertebral body marrow (IA) or the complete vertebral body (IB) marrow is replaced by tumor. Then vertebral body collapse begins with end plate collapse at either one (IIA) or both end plates (IIB), depending on the degree and distribution of tumor replacement of trabecular bone within the vertebral body. With this collapse the vertebral body balloons out circumferentially with the potential for spinal canal encroachment. Increasing collapse and progressive deformity create a fragment of bone that is composed of the posterior wall of the vertebra and a portion of both the superior and inferior end plates. This fragment coalesces to form a triangular appearance on MRI, termed the "delta" sign. This appearance is consistently present when end-stage collapse occurs, as in type IIIA, where a kyphotic deformity is found, and in type IIIB, where a symmetric collapse is identified without kyphosis. More than 94% of cases of identified spinal canal compromise were primarily due to bone encroachment into the canal. Soft tissue encroachment of the canal was rarely identified. Type IV involvement is one in which there is a subluxation that creates a translational deformity.

In this classification, instability is noted to be either present or impending and is identified in two possible forms: axial or translational instability. Axial instability is impending in type IA or IB and is present in type II or type III vertebral involvement. Impending translational instability is found in types II and III when both pedicles and the posterior elements are involved and is present in type IV vertebral deformity. Treatment guidelines are based on this anatomic and deformity-centered classification system and on the implications for mechanical and neurologic stability. In the presence of impending axial instability, radiation, chemotherapy, or hormonal manipulation is recommended. If spinal canal compromise is present, surgical decompression is considered. Axial instability, with or without canal compromise, warrants an anterior surgical approach if one segment is involved, and a posterior approach, if multiple levels are involved. Impending translational instability is approached surgically, either anteriorly or as a combined anterior and posterior procedure. In the presence of translational instability a posterior approach is recommended for stabilization, and either a posterolateral or an anterior approach is performed for decompression and stabilization. The classification system has not been prospectively tested.

Enneking

Another approach in tumor classification is one based on anatomic compartments. Enneking[21] popularized this in his oncologic staging system, first applied to tumors in the long bones and subsequently adapted for the axial skeleton.[22,23] The tumor histologic grade and tumor location, either intracompartmental or extracompartmental location, is used in determining local surgical planning and treatment options. This staging system incorporates the biologic behavior of the tumor regarding aggressiveness and location. Although it is primarily an oncologic classification system and does not use stability, alignment, deformity, pain, prognosis, and neurologic status directly, the Enneking oncologic staging system is critical to the understanding of the principles of oncologic treatment of spinal lesions. This is reflected in the Weinstein-Boriani-Biagini (WBB) system.

CURRENT CLASSIFICATION SYSTEMS
WBB (Weinstein, Boriani, Biagini)

The WBB system was developed by Weinstein[24] in 1989 and subsequently modified in 1994.[25] One goal of the WBB system is to provide a proper, accurate, and complete anatomic description of the vertebral lesion and the anatomic extent of the metastatic vertebral lesion. The system incorporates a uniform and consistent terminology and defines specific terms for surgical procedures. This system also allows for objective and meaningful communication of information among treatment centers for the comparison of diagnostic criteria and treatment results. The WBB system recognizes the unique anatomy of the vertebrae and the difficulty of surgical resection while providing a specific description of the anatomic compartments and the extent of the lesion.[26-28] Tumor type and biologic behavior also play a key role in this classification system.

The WBB surgical staging system begins by describing the anatomy of the metastatic lesion in the transverse plane, where the vertebra is divided in a clockwise fashion into 12 radiating zones. Additional division of layers from the paravertebral extraosseous region to the dura is accomplished by five anatomic layers in the thoracolumbar spine, denoted as layers A through E. In the cervical spine a sixth layer, denoted F, represents the vertebral artery. The longitudinal extent of tumor involvement is obtained by recording the spinal segments involved. MRI, computed tomography (CT) scans, and occasionally angiography are required to determine the full extent of tumor expansion in the transverse and longitudinal planes. With this system of anatomic zones, layers, and vertebral segments, each tumor can be accurately described, recorded, and communicated in three dimensions. This allows proper preoperative planning and intraoperative surgical techniques to maximize the effectiveness of surgical intervention while minimizing the potential for local tumor recurrence. The WBB system, in conjunction with Enneking's oncologic staging system, has been tested and validated in the treatment of primary bone tumors of the spine by Boriani et al.[27] and Hart et al.[28] These principles of describing the anatomic location and of providing information for surgical planning and communication are also pertinent to metastatic disease to the spine.

Tomita

Tomita et al.,[29,30] in 1994, reported on a system that modified the Enneking system into the Primary Surgical Classification of the Vertebral Tumors and also combined elements of Denis's[16] three-column theory, and Weinstein's[25] surgical approach by zones system. Tomita et al. divided the vertebral body into 5 anatomic areas and derived from this a classification of seven types of lesion involvement. The purpose of this system was to determine the best surgical approach to each lesion, with the potential for curative treatment of those lesions remaining intracompartmental, in which case a total spondylectomy could be performed.

The five vertebral anatomic regions include (1) the vertebral body, (2) the pedicle, (3) the lamina, transverse, and spinous processes, (4) the epidural space, and (5) the paraspinal space. Tomita et al. noted that the progression of any solitary vertebral tumor or metastases was determined by the involvement of these five primary sites. The seven types of vertebral tumor involvement are based on the most common patterns of longitudinal and horizontal spread of the tumor and are grouped as intracompartmental, extracompartmental, or multiple or skip lesions. Lesions within the vertebral body, pedicle or lamina, or growth within the epidural space (when growth is negligible or is encapsulated by reactive tissue) is considered intracompartmental. Those lesions extending to the paraspinal area are extracompartmental. On the basis of this classification system, Tomita et al. recommend an en bloc excision for type 1 and type 2 lesions. For types 3 and 4, total spondylectomy by curettage or piecemeal resection through an anterior or posterior approach, either combined or as a two-stage procedure, is acceptable. In type 5 lesions, the tumor has already extended extracompartmentally, and en bloc spondylectomy is no longer indicated. Type 6 and type 7 lesions would warrant palliative procedures only.

Tokuhashi

An entirely different approach to classification systems for spinal metastases is that of Tokuhashi et al.,[31] reported in 1990. Classification based on one specific localized metastatic lesion or based on neurologic function in isolation of systemic factors is abandoned in favor of a systemic approach of tumor load. The concept of considering the extent of tumor load in treatment decisions is not a new one.[32] Tokuhashi et al. refined this concept to assess the prognosis and life expectancy of patients with metastatic disease. This system of tumor load recognizes the choice of treatment as being dependent on several factors, including the primary cancer involved, and on the results of a local and systemic search for systemic tumor lesions.

The Tokuhashi scoring system is composed of six parameters, recognizing that no single parameter can be used to guide the management of patients with vertebral metastases. These parameters include the patient's overall general health condition, the number of extraspinal metastases, the number of vertebral lesions, metastases to major internal organs, the primary site of the tumor, and

the presence of spinal cord palsy. A point system is applied to correlate the extent of the disease with the prognosis. This scoring system is used preoperatively for procedures considered to be elective and not for those surgical procedures performed emergently when all necessary parameters may not be available.

Tokuhashi et al. tested this classification on 64 patients and found that patients with a point score of 9 or higher survived an average of 12 months or longer. Those with a score of less than 8 survived 12 months or less. Patients with a score of 5 or lower survived 3 months or less. With this prognostic information the treating team can base intervention on more reliable and objective information regarding extent of disease and anticipated potential life expectancy and thus tailor the treatment efforts and expectations according to the patient's potential survival. The recommendation was made that those with a score of 9 or greater be considered for an excisional procedure whereas those with a score of 5 or less be considered for a palliative surgical procedure.

Enkaoua

Enkaoua et al.,[33] in 1997, independently verified Tokuhashi's system in a retrospective review of 71 patients. They found this classification system successful as a preoperative prognostic tool and recommended that the scoring system be amended to improve its prognostic capabilities. The major alteration by Enkaoua et al. was to recognize the greater negative impact that tumors of "unknown primary origin" have on overall life expectancy. Enkaoua et al., using the modified Tokuhashi scoring system, found that those with a score of 7 or less had a mean length of survival of 5 ± 1.2 months. Those with a score greater than 7 had a survival length of 24 ± 5.8 months. With the use of multivariate analysis the parameters that were associated with a poorer prognosis included age, type of cancer, and modified Tokuhashi score.

The Karnofsky performance scale[34] was originally developed in 1961 to assess the systemic response to anticancer drugs. Newer scoring assessment tools that incorporate the tumor load concept, such as the ARETAL system, are under development but await clinical verification.[35] The ARETAL system includes parameters such as primary tumor type, neurologic function, spinal stability and tumor location within the vertebrae, systemic tumor load, and the Karnofsky score on which to base a prognosis and thus to contribute to decision making regarding treatment options.

CONCLUSION

The ability to classify spinal metastases has undergone a significant evolution over the past several decades. The initial classification systems, which merely described patients with neurologic involvement and the results of surgical intervention, have given way to new and more enlightening, yet still imperfect, classification systems. Present-day classification systems use technology, such as the MRI, that by noninvasive means identifies vertebral and spinal canal involvement. Newer concepts using a scoring system to assess the systemic effect of tumor load are under development and will help provide prognostic information to both the patient and the treating team about treatment options. A move toward a unifying terminology for describing tumor location and the type of surgical procedure performed should improve communication among treatment centers. A growing awareness of the need for scientifically and prospectively gathered data through studies designed to help guide treatment efforts will bring even greater knowledge about best treatment practices for these difficult issues.

Given these multiple options, where do we stand with regard to the use of these multiple classification systems for metastatic disease to the spine? The ideal system would go beyond being merely a descriptive system and would actually provide prospective and meaningful information in guiding the treatment and providing information about prognosis. This type of system does not yet exist. In fact, it is unlikely that any one system will provide all the information required to treat these difficult problems. Multiple classification systems, each reflecting an important decision tree, may be the optimal situation. The Frankel system, now adopted with modifications by A.S.I.A., is uniformly accepted for the classification of spinal cord dysfunction due to either traumatic origin or metastatic involvement. The Enneking oncologic system has stood the test of time and is commonly cited as the principal source for rational oncologic treatment. Most recently, the classification system of Tomita

and the WBB system have been reported and validated and, though still not in general use, are likely to provide more widely and uniformly accepted methods for determining the anatomic extent of spinal lesions, appropriate preoperative surgical planning, and intraoperative surgical techniques. These systems will help to maximize the outcome of treatment decisions. Scoring systems such as Tokuhashi's, as modified by Enkaoua, reflect the systemic tumor burden, provide information on the general prognosis and life expectancy, and contribute to planning efforts when varying treatment options are to be considered. Thus no one classification system will provide all the answers to the important questions raised by these difficult and complicated patients. The goal, however, must be to prospectively gather data and thus improve upon those efforts already in place, which help identify options best suited for each problem and each patient.

REFERENCES

1. Brice J, McKissock W. Surgical treatment of malignant extradural spinal tumours. Br Med J 5474:1341-1344, 1965.
2. Frankel HL, Hancock DO, Hyslop G, Melzak J, Michaelis LS, et al. The value of postural reduction in the initial management of closed injuries of the spine with paraplegia and tetraplegia. Paraplegia 7(3):179-192, 1969.
3. Gutmann L. Initial treatment of traumatic paraplegia and tetraplegia. In Harris P, ed. Spinal Injuries: Proceedings of a Symposium Held in the Royal College of Surgeons of Edinburgh, 7th and 8th of June, 1963. Edinburgh: Royal College of Surgeons of Edinburgh, 1967, pp 80-92.
4. Hardy AG. The treatment of paraplegia due to fracture-dislocations of the dorso-lumbar spine. Paraplegia 3(2):112-123, 1965.
5. Geisler WO, Wynne-Jones M, Jousse AT. Early management of the patient with trauma to the spinal cord. Med Serv J Can 22(7):512-523, 1966.
6. American Spinal Injury Association, International Medical Society of Paraplegia (1992). International Standards for Neurological and Functional Classification of Spinal Cord Injury. Revised. Chicago: American Spinal Injury Association, 1992.
7. White WA, Patterson RH, Bergland RM. Role of surgery in the treatment of spinal cord compression by metastatic neoplasm. Cancer 27(3):558-561, 1971.
8. Gilbert RW, Kim J-H, Posner JB. Epidural spinal cord compression from metastatic tumor: Diagnosis and treatment. Ann Neurol 3(1):40-51, 1978.
9. Constans JP, de Diviths E, Donzelli R, Spaziante R, Meder JF, Haye C. Spinal metastases with neurological manifestations. J Neurosurg 59:111-118, 1983.

The medical treatment of cancer patients has made great advances over the last 20 years. As a result, these patients are surviving longer and more are requiring treatment for involvement of the spine, which has been reported to be as high as 70% of patients.[1] Surgical treatment for tumors of the spine has also evolved significantly over the last 20 years. With the development of new approaches and fixation techniques, outcomes have improved dramatically and diminished many of the postoperative complications reported by earlier investigators. Because of these advances, the surgical indications have expanded and procedures that were once considered radical are now seen as commonplace.

Because of improved patient survival and the dramatic impact that appropriate surgical treatment can have, it is important for physicians to develop a logical approach when evaluating patients suspected of having a spine tumor. Unfortunately, there is no uniform approach to the evaluation and treatment of patients with spine tumors. The goals of treatment are to provide functional improvement and pain relief. This chapter will outline the principles in the evaluation and management of patients with tumors of the spinal column.

INCIDENCE

The prevalence of spine tumors varies, depending on whether one is looking at an autopsy series[1-4] or a clinical series. Metastatic spine tumors are seen 40 times as frequently as all primary bone tumors combined.[5] Primary tumors of the spine are very rare.[6] Metastatic spine disease is the presenting picture in 40% of new cancer cases.[7] Seventy percent of patients with cancer will exhibit skeletal metastases at autopsy, with most of these involving the spine.[3] Jaffe[1] demonstrated that more than 70% of persons with metastatic cancer examined post mortem had vertebral column metastases. Nearly one half of these patients required treatment of symptomatic pain caused by their spinal bone metastases. In addition, an autopsy study by Barron et al.[2] found that epidural metastasis developed in 5% of all patients with cancer. A more recent study by Wong et al.[4] found that 1 in 3 patients who died of cancer had metastases to the spine.

The clinical behavior of a tumor affects the perceived prevalence of a tumor; patients with more aggressive tumors, such as metastatic lung carcinoma, often succumb before the spine involvement becomes significant.

Weinstein and McLain[8] have demonstrated that age is an important prognostic factor in patients with both primary and metastatic disease of the spine. Nearly 70% of primary bone tumors observed in children are benign. Conversely, 70% of primary tumors in patients older than 21 years are malignant (see box above). Most carcinomas and subsequently most metastatic lesions of the spine demonstrate a peak incidence in the fifth and sixth decades. Systemic related diseases, such as myeloma and lymphoma, also peak in prevalence during the fifth and sixth decades. Therefore the likelihood that an older patient has a metastatic lesion or malignant lesion of the spine is much greater than when a younger patient has a similar clinical picture.

Location of a lesion within a vertebra is another

Diagnosis of Spine Tumors According to Sex and Age

Male	Less than 10 years
Osteoid osteoma	Neuroblastoma
Osteoblastoma	Leukemia
Multiple myeloma	Ewing's sarcoma
Osteogenic sarcoma	**10 to 30 years**
Eosinophilic granu-	Aneurysmal bone
loma	cyst
Chordoma	Giant cell tumor
Female	Osteoid osteoma
Giant cell tumor	Osteoblastoma
Aneurysmal bone cyst	Eosinophilic granu-
Hemangioma	loma
	Ewing's sarcoma
	30 to 50 years
	Chondrosarcoma
	Chordoma
	Lymphoma
	Hemangioma
	Metastatic
	Over 50 years
	Metastatic
	Myeloma
	Chondrosarcoma

Adapted from Parks PF, Herkowitz HN. Spine tumors—Patient evaluation. Semin Spine Surg 2:154, 1990.

Diagnosis of Spine Tumors According to Location

Anterior elements	Adjacent vertebrae
Metastatic disease	Aneurysmal bone
Eosinophilic granu-	cyst
loma	Chordoma
Giant cell tumor	Chondrosarcoma
Hemangioma	**Multiple vertebrae**
Chordoma	Multiple myeloma
Multiple myeloma	Metastatic
Posterior elements	
Osteoblastoma	
Osteoid osteoma	
Osteochondroma	
Aneurysmal bone cyst	

Adapted from Parks PF, Herkowitz HN. Spine tumors—Patient evaluation. Semin Spine Surg 2:154, 1990.

important prognostic factor. Spine lesions that originate anteriorly in the vertebral body are more often malignant, whether they are primary or metastatic, than lesions that involve the posterior elements[8] (see box above). In addition, tumors show a predilection for certain parts of the vertebrae.

PATHOPHYSIOLOGY

Tumors involving the spine may be primary or, more commonly, may have metastasized to the spine by way of the bloodstream or the lymphatic vessels. Tumors arising from local tissue may come from bone, from the spinal cord, or from contiguous spread of tumors from the soft tissues. The spine is the most common site of metastases, and metastases may occur with any malignant tumor.[8]

Tumors metastasize to the spine by way of the bloodstream. This explains the predilection of malignant lesions for various parts of the spine. Breast tumors drain through the azygous venous system and commonly spread to the thoracic spine. The prostate drains through the pelvic venous plexus, and thus metastases from these tumors are more common in the lumbar spine. Tumors of the lung most commonly metastasize to the thoracic spine and may seed the thoracic spinal column directly through segmental arteries.

Batson first described the importance of the paravertebral venous plexus in the pathophysiology of spinal metastases. This plexus consists of small, thin-walled valveless vessels in the sinuses with a low intraluminal pressure. Tumor cells may become implanted in the vertebral column by retrograde flow through Batson's plexus. It has been shown that the Valsalva maneuver allows retrograde flow of cells.[9] Batson's plexus is most significant in tumors of the breast, lung, and prostate.

PATIENT PRESENTATION

Pain is the most common initial complaint of patients presenting with a suspected spine tumor. The history and physical examination findings should narrow the differential diagnosis, help exclude nontumor sources of back pain, and identify any neurologic deficit. In patients who have tumors involving the spine, symptoms develop from expansion of the cortex of the vertebral body, pathologic fracture, spinal instability, or compression of nerve roots or spinal cord.[10] The nature of the back pain can help differentiate between mechanical and nonmechanical pain. Mechanical back pain is usually activity related and is relieved with rest. In contrast, back pain secondary to a tumor is usually not relieved by rest, is often unrelenting, and intensifies at night.

The pain may be focal, referred, or radicular in its distribution. Referred pain often occurs several segments below the level of the lesion. Referred pain in the subscapular or midscapular region suggests irritation or compression in the cervical spine. Referred pain in the thoracic region may result in circumferential pain or dysesthesias about the chest. In the lumbar spine, referred pain often involves the buttocks and the posterior part of the thigh.[11] Radicular pain results from irritation or compression of the dural sack or nerve roots caused by pathologic fracture or tumor mass. Radicular or referred pain is less common than pain localized to the back. Radicular pain may mimic pain seen with a herniated nucleus pulposus.

Most patients with a spinal tumor present with back pain that usually is subacute and that has progressed over several weeks to months. Pain may precede neurologic symptoms by a variable length of time, depending on the growth rate of the tumor. In patients with breast or prostate cancer, this may be as long as 12 months; in patients with lung carcinoma there is a median time delay of 4

Table 27-1 Presenting symptoms in patients with spine tumors

Presenting symptoms	%	
Pain	84	
Back pain		30
Radicular pain		10
Pain and weakness		28
Pain and mass		11
Weakness	42	
Weakness alone		9
Weakness and pain		28
Mass	16	
Mass alone		5
Mass and pain		11
Asymptomatic	3	

months; in patients with lymphoma there is a 3-month time delay; and in patients with renal cell carcinoma there is a delay of less than 2 months.[2] Other studies have reported pain duration ranging from 7 weeks to 3 or more years before neurologic symptoms appear. The most prominent symptoms at presentation are, in descending order of frequency, back pain, radicular pain, weakness in the lower extremities, sensory loss, and loss of sphincter control (Table 27-1).[8]

The patient with a spinal tumor may report a change in gait pattern, a lack of coordination, or stumbling. Autonomic symptoms occur late in cases of neurologic compression. Complaints of constipation and urinary tension are often associated with sacrococcygeal chordomas.[12] Isolated sphincter dysfunction may be the only presenting symptom in approximately 2% of patients with a metastatic spine tumor.[13] Gilbert et al.[14] noted that bowel and bladder dysfunction may develop in as many as half of the patients with spinal cord compression from metastatic disease to the spine.[14]

Timely diagnosis is extremely important because the neurologic status at the time of diagnosis is one of the most important prognostic factors affecting outcome. Of those patients who have the ability to walk at the time of diagnosis, 60% to 90% will retain that ability after treatment. Patients who have significant weakness are much less likely to continue to ambulate after treatment, and only 30% of

patients who are paraplegic will regain the ability to ambulate.[15-18] Prognostically, the ability to walk and the absence of myelopathy before treatment are correlated with preservation of the patient's ability to ambulate after treatment.[19] Other factors affecting prognosis include the rapidity of onset. Those patients experiencing a major neurologic deficit within 24 hours have a much poorer prognosis than those whose deficits occur over a longer period of time.[8,10]

Spinal Cord Compression

Even though the lumbar vertebrae are most commonly affected by tumor metastases, it is in the thoracic spine that spinal cord compression most often occurs. The spinal cord at the thoracic level is largest relative to the space available for the cord and thus is most susceptible to compression by tumor. In Gilbert's series, 68% of the patients with spinal cord compression had tumor involvement of the thoracic spine, 16% had involvement of the lumbar spine, and 15% had involvement of the cervical spine.[14]

Compression of the spinal cord secondary to spinal metastases is a major cause of morbidity in patients with cancer. In some reports, neoplastic spinal cord compression is the most frequent central nervous system complication of cancer.[20]

Studies have found that epidural metastases developed in 5% of all patients with cancer, with one in three patients who died of cancer demonstrating metastases to the epidural space.[2,4] Epidural spinal cord compression may be the initial manifestation of cancer in a high percentage of cases. In one study, 47% of patients with epidural spinal cord compression had not been diagnosed with a primary tumor at initial presentation.[21] When one is evaluating patients with spinal cord compression, it is important to be vigilant for noncontiguous areas of compression. Six of sixty-two patients with myelographic evidence of epidural spinal cord compression had a second area of compression, which was separated by an average of 12 vertebral segments.[22]

Spinal cord compression usually occurs as a result of one of the following mechanisms: compression by a bone or tumor mass after pathologic fracture (Fig. 27-1), direct pressure from extension of tumor into the epidural space either by extension through the vertebral body or from the intraverte-

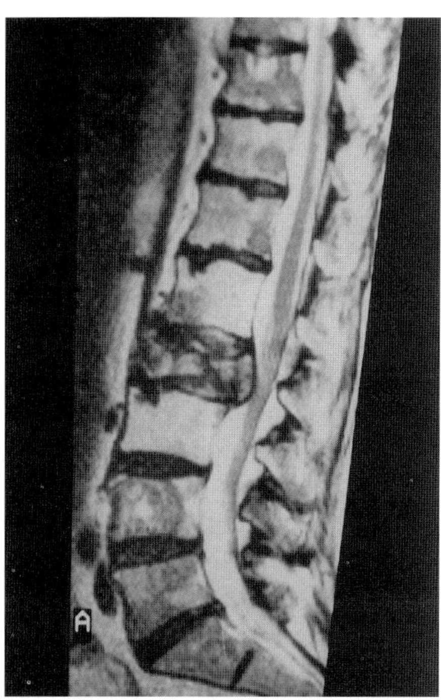

Fig. 27-1 Sagittal MRI scan shows L2 vertebral pathologic fracture secondary to prostate carcinoma. The extent of spinal canal compromise is evident. Marrow infiltration of L4 and L5 is seen as well.

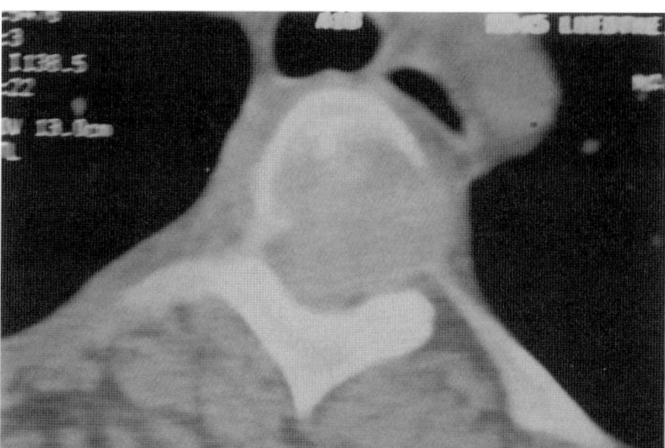

Fig. 27-2 Axial CT scan shows T6 vertebral body involvement from breast carcinoma. The extent of bone destruction is clearly seen.

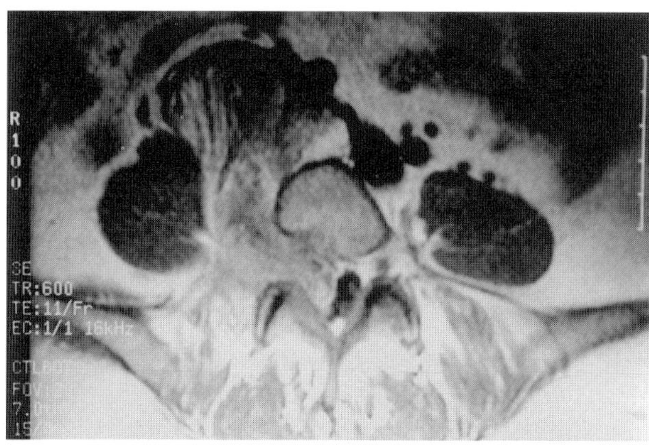

Fig. 27-3 An intraforaminal neurofibroma at the L4 level that had resulted in leg weakness. A complete excision was possible, although a portion of the sciatic nerve was sacrificed.

bral foramen (Fig. 27-2), kyphosis after vertebral collapse, or pressure from intradural metastasis.[3] Several modes of spread to the epidural space have been noted. Most frequently there is a direct extension of tumor into the epidural space from the involved vertebrae. This often occurs with carcinoma of the breast, lung, and prostate. Invasion through the intravertebral foramen into the epidural space is most commonly seen in lymphomas and neuroblastomas (Fig. 27-3). It is rare for the dura or spinal cord to be directly invaded by tumor that has reached the epidural space because the dura forms an effective barrier.

Compression from an epidural mass causes damage to the spinal cord either by a direct mechanical mass effect, with a subsequent demyelination and axonal destruction, or from pressure-induced vascular compromise, which causes venous congestion and edema of the spinal cord.[2]

The pain of epidural spinal cord compression may be accompanied by motor, sensory, and autonomic dysfunction. Because the compression usually occurs anteriorly from the vertebral body, the motor functions of the anterior part of the spinal cord are usually compromised first. Sensory disturbance occurs less frequently, and the level of sensory loss is not a reliable indicator of spinal cord compression. The sensory level is often several segments below the level of the spinal cord lesion. It is unusual for patients with cord compression to present without pain; however, patients with lung lymphoma and renal metastases may present with neurologic deficit in the absence of pain.[2,21]

PHYSICAL EXAMINATION

Physical examination must include an assessment of local tenderness, deformity, range of motion, and neurologic function. Pain on palpation of the spine may be the earliest finding in patients with tumors in the posterior elements. The presence of kyphosis or a gibbus deformity may indicate a pathologic fracture. Painful scoliosis may result from nerve root irritation caused by muscle spasms secondary to an osteoid osteoma or osteoblastoma of the spine. The onset of such a scoliosis may be rapid. Usually the tumor is located within the concavity of the curve.[23,24]

The neurologic examination is the most important part of the physical examination. The neurologic assessment should include testing of muscle function in the upper and lower extremities. Sensory examination should include testing with pin prick and light touch, particularly in the sacral dermatomes, as well as proprioception. Deep tendon reflexes should be tested, and any hyperreflexia or asymmetry should be noted. Pathologic reflexes, including Babinski, Hoffman, and clonus, need to be documented. Rectal examination may disclose a presacral mass indicative of a chordoma or may show a mass or enlarged prostate.

Neurologic deficits are common in patients with spinal tumors. Neurologic deficits occur with rapidly expanding malignant lesions as well as with slowly progressive expansile lesions. Seventy percent of patients with spinal tumors will present with weakness at the time a diagnosis is made.[25] Weinstein and McLain[8] showed that 40% of the patients in their series presented with weakness at the time a diagnosis was made. A painless neurologic deficit may signify intradural tumor. Spasticity and hyperflexia indicate a lesion above the conus medullaris.[26]

IMAGING TECHNIQUES
Plain Films

Plain radiographs of the spine are the initial imaging studies obtained in working up a patient with a spine tumor. Plain radiographs aid in the differential diagnosis of spine tumors, both by the radiographic appearance of the lesion and by the location of the tumor in the spine and in the vertebrae. Primary tumors of the spine are usually localized to single vertebrae. Osteoblastoma and aneurysmal bone cysts are exceptions and may involve multiple contiguous vertebrae. Metastatic lesions of the spine may involve multiple adjacent vertebrae.[13,22,27] Location of a tumor in the vertebrae may help narrow the differential diagnosis (see Fig. 27-1). Weinstein and McLain[8] noted that tumors that arise in

the vertebral body are more often malignant than those that arise in the posterior elements (76% vs. 36%, respectively). Osteoid osteomas, osteoblastomas, and aneurysmal bone cysts occur most frequently in the posterior elements, whereas metastatic disease, Ewing's sarcoma, eosinophilic granuloma, leukemia, and osteosarcoma occur most frequently in the vertebral body (see box on p. 377).[8]

The pattern of bone destruction seen on plain radiographs often gives clues to the benign or malignant nature of the lesion. Lodewick[28] has described three patterns of bone destruction: geographic, moth-eaten, and permeative. Lesions with geographic margins suggest a more benign, slowly growing tumor. A moth-eaten appearance suggests a more rapidly growing tumor. Tumors that have a permeative appearance on plain radiographs are usually highly malignant and aggressive (Fig. 27-4, A).

Plain radiographs of the spine identify 30% to 70% of spine tumors at the time patients begin to experience back pain.[29] Galasko[30] reported a false negative rate of 17% in the ability of plain radiographs to detect skeletal metastasis. Chamberlin noted that up to 60% of patients with lymphoma causing epidural spinal cord compression may have normal plain radiographs. Early lesions are difficult to detect because 30% to 50% of the trabecular bone must be destroyed before they can be seen on plain radiographs.[31] Because of this, often the earliest radiographic sign of vertebral involvement is absence of the pedicle on an anteroposterior (AP) view. The destruction of the cortical bone of the pedicle is much easier to detect than subtle loss of the cancellous bone of the vertebral body.

It is difficult to distinguish between a destructive lesion caused by tumor and one caused by infection. In general, preservation of the intervertebral disc space indicates tumors. Destruction of the intervertebral disc and adjacent end plates suggests an infection. The intervertebral disc is resistant to tumor invasion and usually maintains its height, even in the face of extensive destruction of the vertebral body by tumor.[22]

Bone Scan

Bone scan is a sensitive but nonspecific test for the evaluation of spine tumors. The bone scan is a reflection of the concentration of newly formed osteoid. Bone scans can detect lesions as small as 2

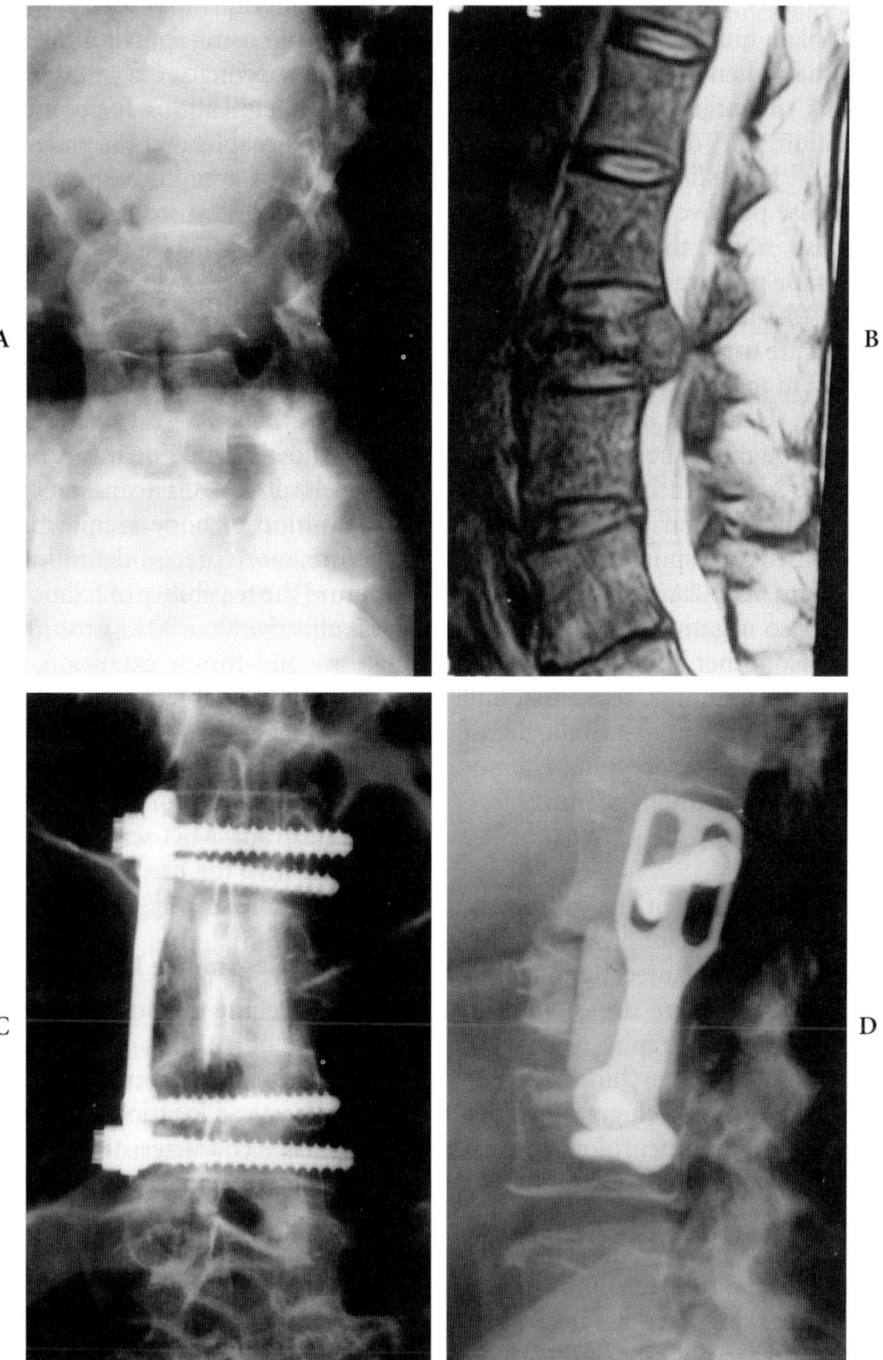

Fig. 27-4   L3 pathologic fracture that resulted from multiple myeloma. The onset of severe paraparesis was acute. **A,** Lateral radiograph demonstrates the pathologic fracture at L3 with compression and retropulsion. **B,** Sagittal MRI scan shows the amount of spinal canal compression secondary to retropulsed bone and tumor. **C,** Lateral flank approach was used to complete an L3 corpectomy and spinal canal decompression. An allograft femoral strut was used in conjunction with a lateral plate. The patient was allowed ad-lib postoperative activity without bracing. **D,** Lateral view shows the reconstruction of sagittal alignment and placement of the strut graft.

mogenous replacement of marrow with a decreased signal intensity on T1 and a high signal intensity on T2, diffuse and irregular borders of marrow involvement, other sites of metastasis, pedicle or posterior element involvement, and a paraspinal mass. They also noted that signal intensity in benign lesions reverts to normal over a 3-month time period.

Other studies have shown a high false positive rate when MRI is used to detect malignant compression fractures, especially at the acute stage, because both malignant and benign compression fractures show a low signal on T1 images.[47] Frager et al.[48] described three patients with false positive MRI scans leading to unnecessary treatment. Tan similarly showed a false positive rate of 20%.[49] An et al.[50] noted that acute healing of benign compression fractures may mimic the findings of compression fractures secondary to metastatic lesions. They noted that use of gadolinium contrast improves the sensitivity in detecting pathologic fractures secondary to cancer. They also noted that the most common error in the use of MRI in differentiating between benign and malignant compression fractures was overinterpretation of benign lesions as malignant (i.e., low specificity). This was most apparent early in the course of healing of benign fractures. The specificity of gadolinium-enhanced MRI scans was 79%. Early in fracture healing the presence of fracture hematoma, paraspinal mass effect, and marrow signal changes had led to the misinterpretation of benign lesions as malignant. Their study showed that when an MRI scan was read as benign, the chance of a false negative scan was low. If a malignant fracture was suggested on MRI scan, they recommended a repeat scan 2 to 3 months later with contrast enhancement; a benign lesion would show diminished contrast enhancement at that time, and metastatic lesions would show progression of tumor involvement of the spine.[50] Therefore it may not be possible to determine at the acute stages whether a compression fracture is a benign osteopenic compression fracture or a pathologic fracture. A reasonable treatment approach to neurologically intact patients presenting with an acute compression fracture is to treat them with an appropriate brace and follow them up radiographically and clinically. Patients with compression fractures due to osteopenia will generally become free of symptoms within 2 to 3 months;

patients with compression fractures secondary to cancer will show progression and should be worked up at that time.

Biopsy

Biopsy represents the final step in the workup of a patient with a spine tumor. There are three types of biopsy: directed needle biopsy, incisional biopsy, and excisional biopsy. The biopsy should be performed at the institution where definitive treatment will be carried out. An ill-planned or poorly performed biopsy can have a significant adverse affect on the patient's care. Mankin et al.[51] found that inadequate or inappropriate biopsies adversely altered patients' care in more than 35% of cases. Once an open biopsy has been performed, the biopsy incision will need to be excised during the definitive procedure.

CT-directed needle biopsy of spine tumors is the method of choice as long as adequate tissue mass is available and the tumor's location is amenable to this technique.[38] Needle biopsy has a low rate of complications and produces little soft tissue contamination. In addition, since there is no surgical wound, chemotherapy or adjunctive radiation therapy can be started early.[52]

Technique

Needle biopsy is performed as an outpatient procedure with the use of local anesthesia. In general, thoracic spine biopsies are performed from the right side to avoid the aorta. Lumbar spine biopsies can be performed from either the left or the right side. Biopsies of thoracic and lumbar spine lesions are performed through a posterior paraspinal approach. Cervical spine lesions are approached anterolaterally. An 18-gauge needle can be used for lytic lesions. Sclerotic or blastic lesions require a thicker needle, such as a Craig needle.

If a needle biopsy either fails to provide enough tissue for diagnosis or is unable to reveal a histologic diagnosis, an open biopsy is required. Lesions of the vertebral body of the cervical spine can be approached through a standard anterolateral approach. Thoracic lesions may be approached anteriorly from a transthoracic or thoracoscopic approach or posterolaterally from a costotransversectomy approach. In the lumbar spine, either a retroperitoneal approach or a posterolateral approach can be used. Another alternative in the lumbar spine is the transpedicular biopsy, which can be performed from a posterior approach.

When an incisional biopsy of the spine is performed, certain basic biopsy principles need to be followed:

1. Transverse incisions should be avoided, flaps should not be created, and the approach should be as direct as possible.
2. Meticulous hemostasis must be achieved.
3. It is preferable to obtain tissue from the periphery or margins of the tumor because the central portions of tumors often are necrotic.
4. All specimens should be sent for a culture as well as for histologic studies.
5. The incision placement should be planned so that the biopsy incision can be removed at the time of tumor excision. Midline posterior incisions should usually be used.
6. Care should be taken to carefully handle the specimen, which should also be large enough for all necessary studies (i.e., immunologic, culture, histologic, and ultrastructural analysis).[53]

PATHOLOGY OF METASTATIC SPINE TUMORS

Metastatic neoplasms are the most common tumors encountered in the adult spine.[54] Breast, lung, and prostate tumors account for the majority of spinal metastases. These three neoplasms give rise to more than 40% of spinal metastases.[55] Tumors of the kidney, thyroid, and gastrointestinal tract account for the majority of the remaining spinal metastases (Table 27-4). Breast cancer is the most common source of bone metastasis, with skeletal disease developing in up to 85% of women who die from breast cancer.[1] Lung and prostate carcinomas are the most common source of metastasis in men. Lymphoreticular cancers, including lymphoma and myeloma, are common sources of spinal involvement; however, they are systemic diseases, do not represent true metastasis, and are not included in many clinical series.

The true incidence of spinal metastases varies from series to series and depends on the type of series reviewed (i.e., autopsy studies or clinical studies). In addition, the primary tumor dictates the overall survival of the patient and, therefore, the clinical significance of the metastatic lesion in the spine (Table 27-5). Patients with either breast or

Table 27-4   Primary site of neoplasm in patients with spinal metastasis in 1432 patients

Primary site	%
Breast	21
Lung	19
Unknown	10
Prostate	10
Lymphoma	8
Kidney	6
Myeloma	5
Gastrointestinal	4

Adapted from Grant R, Papadopoulos SM, Greenberg HS. Metastatic epidural spinal cord compression. Neurol Clin 9(4): 825-841, 1991.

Table 27-5   Mean survival times from time of diagnosis in patients with spine tumors

Site	Survival (months)
Breast	14
Prostate	12
Lymphoma/myeloma	9
Kidney	9
All	8

Adapted from Sorensen PS, Borgesen SE, Rhode K. Metastatic epidural spinal cord compression: Results of treatment and survival. Cancer 65:1502, 1990. Copyright © 1990 American Cancer Society. Reprinted by permission of Wiley-Lios, Inc., a subsidiary of John Wiley & Sons, Inc.

prostate primary tumors who survive for longer periods of time will be more likely to require treatment for their spinal disease, whereas patients with lung primary tumors, whose survival is much more limited, often do not require more than supportive treatment for their spinal lesions. Similarly, patients with gastrointestinal adenocarcinoma often have metastases to the liver and lungs before involvement of the spine.

Lung

Lung carcinoma commonly metastasizes to the liver, skeleton, bone marrow, and brain.[29,56] There are four histologic types of lung cancer: epidermoid, adenocarcinoma, small-cell carcinoma, and large-cell carcinoma. Small-cell carcinoma has the best overall prognosis and longer survival rate, and thus patients with this type of lung cancer have the greatest likelihood of skeletal metastases developing. Treatment of lung carcinoma is dependent on the type of tumor. Small-cell lung carcinoma is more responsive to chemotherapy and radiation therapy. Given the limited survival of patients with lung cancer at the time of diagnosis, they often are not candidates for operative treatment.

Breast

Because the survival time after diagnosis of breast cancer is relatively long, the incidence of skeletal metastases is high.[57] In addition, venous drainage from the breast by the azygous veins and their communication with the paravertebral venous plexus account for the high percentage of thoracic spine metastases in patients with breast cancer. The incidence of women with breast cancer in whom skeletal metastases develop has been estimated as high as 74%.[57] The skeleton is the most common site of metastasis. The metastatic lesions are most commonly osteolytic; however, in 10% to 15% of metastases the lesions are purely blastic.

Metastatic breast cancer often remains confined to the skeleton for a prolonged time. Sherry showed that patients in whom initial metastases of primary breast tumors were to the skeleton had a longer survival than those with extraskeletal metastases. Twenty-one percent developed spinal cord compression.[58] The slow evolution of breast cancer that has metastasized to bone suggests some unique biologic properties of these tumor cells. Breast tumors that metastasize to bone are more frequently estrogen receptor–positive and better differentiated than breast tumors that metastasize to the lungs or liver.[59] It has been shown that patients with bone metastases have a lower rate of response to neoplastic therapy, thereby reflecting a slower rate of growth.[60] Many of these patients require only bracing and radiation.

Prostate

Metastases to the spine are common in prostate cancer. The most common radiographic appearance of prostate lesions is osteoblastic (80%).

Twelve percent present a mixed lytic and blastic appearance, and 4% appear purely lytic.[61] Because these metastatic lesions are usually blastic, pathologic fractures are relatively rare in persons with prostate carcinoma. Likewise, neurologic involvement is uncommon in blastic lesions.[62] Lytic lesions in the spine, however, although rare, can cause neurologic involvement.[62,63]

Treatment of prostate cancer includes hormonal manipulation, radiation, chemotherapy, and surgery. Multiple studies have documented long survival rates in patients with prostate cancer.[10,64-66] Surgery is rarely required for spinal metastases of prostate cancer.

Renal

Patients with renal carcinoma will have metastases to bone in 50% of cases.[67] By the time the primary tumor is diagnosed, it has often reached advanced stages. Eighty percent of patients with renal cell carcinoma eventually will have metastases.[67] Renal cell carcinoma makes up fewer than 10% of all cases of metastatic carcinoma to the spine; however, it is the fourth most common type of metastatic spinal tumor and more commonly causes neurologic deficit.[67,68]

Renal cell carcinoma is commonly hypervascular. The tumors enlarge rapidly. Radiographically, they appear as lytic lesions. The margins are generally indistinct and the often-aggressive lesions expand into the surrounding soft tissues. Pathologic fractures are common.

Chemotherapy and hormonal therapy have been shown to be ineffective in the treatment of renal metastases to the spine.[69] Although radiation treatment is often used, the tumor is relatively radioresistant.[19] Therefore failure to respond to radiation therapy or relapse after radiotherapy is not uncommon. Despite this, the role of surgery in treatment of renal cell metastases to the spine is controversial. Surgical management is indicated in patients with intractable pain or with a neurologic deficit that has not responded to radiotherapy or has relapsed after radiotherapy. Extensive bone destruction of the spinal column will often not improve with radiation therapy alone. Instability should be treated with surgical decompression and stabilization followed by postoperative radiation. Preoperative arteriograms have been recommended to assess the vascularity of the tumor and help plan the surgical approach.[70] Preoperative arterial embolization has also been recommended to diminish intraoperative blood loss, which can be extensive.[67,71] Accurate identification of the spinal cord blood supply is necessary not only to prevent inadvertent embolization but also for surgical planning. In a study by Sundaresan et al.,[71] 90% of patients with neurologic compromise secondary to cord compression showed neurologic improvement after surgery. They noted the significant decrease in intraoperative blood loss with presurgical spinal angiography and embolization.

Surgical management of metastatic renal cell carcinoma of the spine has become more common as surgical techniques have improved. In a study by King et al.,[67] 88% of patients had partial or complete relief of pain, with 64% of the bedridden patients subsequently able to walk. Sixty percent of the patients with a neurologic deficit improved. Compression recurred, however, in 49% of the patients; half of these required repeat decompression, with results similar to those of the primary procedure in terms of pain and neurologic function.

Survival of patients with metastatic renal cell carcinoma is most dependent on the pathologic characterization of the primary tumor. Survival has also been correlated with the severity of the neurologic deficit as well as the presence of other metastases.[67]

Thyroid

Thirty percent of patients with thyroid carcinoma have bone metastases at presentation.[72] The actual prevalence of metastases to the spine from thyroid carcinoma is low because thyroid carcinoma is rare. The risk that a bone metastasis will develop is highest with the follicular type of thyroid carcinoma and lowest with the medullary and papillary forms.[72] Bone metastases are most common in patients older than 50 years and those with tumors larger than 4 cm. In one study,[72] 70% of the patients died within 4 years of discovery of bone metastases. Metastatic lesions are usually lytic. As with renal cell carcinoma, these tumors may be highly vascular. The margins are usually poorly defined, and it is unusual for these lesions to demonstrate a periosteal reaction. Metastatic lesions will usually show increased uptake of nucleotide on bone scan. False negative bone scans due to a low rate of osteoblastic activity have been reported.[73,74]

Multiple Myeloma

Multiple myeloma is most common in patients more than 40 years of age. In 1988 it accounted for 1.6% of cancer deaths.[55] Multiple myeloma and solitary plasmacytoma are considered manifestations of the same lymphoproliferative disease, although the prognosis for patients with plasmacytoma is considerably better. Multiple myeloma involves the uncontrolled proliferation of malignant plasma cells and their products, including immunoglobulins.

The incidence of multiple myeloma is 2 per 100,000. Plasmacytoma is less common, accounting for only 3% of all plasma cell neoplasms.[75] The diagnosis of multiple myeloma is confirmed by the identification of monoclonal proteins in the serum or urine.[76] However, up to 3% of patients may have negative blood and urine electrophoreses. The majority of myeloma lesions in the skeleton are lytic. Bone scans may be negative in a significant number of cases with skeletal involvement.

The prognosis for patients with solitary plasmacytoma and those with multiple myeloma is dramatically different. The course of multiple myeloma is usually rapidly progressive and lethal. By definition, solitary plasmacytoma is an isolated lesion, and the treatment of this lesion may provide long-term disease-free survival or cure. The spinal lesion in multiple myeloma represents a metastasis in a progressive, systemic disease, with a survival of usually less than 2 years despite systemic and local treatment. The 5-year survival rate of patients with disseminated multiple myeloma is 18%, with a median survival of 28 months. With cases involving the spine, the outcome is worse, with 76% of patients dying within 1 year.[75] The 5-year disease-free survival rate for patients with solitary plasmacytoma was 60%, with a median survival of 92 months.

The treatment of choice for both solitary plasmacytoma and multiple myeloma is bisphosphonate therapy, radiation therapy, and bracing. The surgical indications for both multiple myeloma and solitary plasmacytoma are limited, given the radiosensitivity of these tumors. The main surgical indication is spinal instability due to vertebral collapse. However, vertebral collapse and onset or progression of a neurologic deficit are uncommon after the onset of radiotherapy.[8] Surgery is often difficult because of multilevel involvement and the severe osteopenia seen in these patients.

TREATMENT: DECISION MAKING

Decisions that must be made in the treatment of patients with spine tumors include operative vs. nonoperative treatment, an anterior vs. a posterior approach, type of stabilization, and whether to use methylmethacrylate (MMA) cement or bone graft.

The first part of the decision-making process involves a determination of the goals of treatment in a patient with a spine tumor. Is the goal cure, or is it palliation? With slowly growing benign lesions, the goal is often cure, depending on the type of tumor and its location in the spine. With more aggressive malignant primary tumors and metastatic tumors, the goal is usually palliation. Surgery may be considered as primary treatment in selected patients with the goal of early patient mobilization, ambulation, pain reduction, and prolongation and improvement in the quality of life.

When the goal is cure, complete surgical excision, such as en bloc excision of the whole vertebral body, should be performed. The principles of achieving a wide surgical margin are often difficult to achieve in the spine. Usually the best that can be achieved is an intralesional excision or a debulking procedure. Obtaining the widest margin possible is essential and has been shown to improve overall patient survival and provide the greatest return of neurologic function. In the appendicular skeleton, there are anatomic compartments that will contain tumor and are used in determining the type of tumor resection. In the spine, there are no true anatomic compartments. Weinstein[93] divided the vertebral body into four zones to aid in planning tumor resection. Zones 1 and 2 involve the posterior elements; zone 3 is the anterior column; and zone 4 consists of the middle column and the spinal canal. In determining the width of surgical resection, the risk of producing serious neurologic deficits must be weighed against the completeness of tumor excision.

Surgical vs. Nonsurgical Treatment

Until recently, the surgical treatment of spine tumors has been synonymous with laminectomy.

Disappointing results with decompressive laminectomy caused surgical treatment to fall into disfavor, leading many physicians to abandon surgery as the initial treatment in patients with neoplastic spinal cord compression and to use radiation therapy in all patients instead, regardless of the radiosensitivity of the tumor or the location or degree of spinal cord compression.

Numerous investigators have noted a high incidence of neurologic worsening after laminectomy.[12,16,77,78] Several reports comparing radiation with laminectomy plus radiation showed no difference in the results, with only 30% to 50% satisfactory outcomes with either treatment group.

Gilbert et al.,[14] in a widely cited study, concluded that surgery was unnecessary in the treatment of patients with vertebral metastases. In attempting to resolve the medical vs. surgical debate, they compared the results of radiation therapy alone with those of radiation plus laminectomy and noted that fewer than 50% of the patients in either group had a satisfactory outcome. Similarly, Constans et al.[13] found that patients treated with radiotherapy alone experienced neurologic improvement equivalent to that of patients treated with combined laminectomy and radiotherapy. In a prospective study, Yuh et al.[46] also reported equivalent results in patients treated with laminectomy and with radiotherapy. Black[22] reviewed the literature and noted that radiation therapy provided superior results when compared with laminectomy (46% vs. 30% satisfactory results). White and Panjabi[105] presented 226 cases treated with laminectomy and reported a successful outcome in only 36% of his patients; 10% actually had a neurologic worsening following surgery. Hall and McKay[16] noted satisfactory results in only 33% of the reported cases of thoracic metastases. They noted that laminectomy performed for anterior spinal cord compression had only a 9% success rate. Cobb et al.[79] found that 23% of patients treated with laminectomy had a worsening of their neurologic status. Nather and Bose found that the treatment of metastatic spinal disease by laminectomy had a success rate of only 29%.[18]

Although these studies demonstrated that laminectomy is not very effective, studies looking at the efficacy of medical treatment of spine tumors showed that it was not much more successful. In 1966 Mones reported that of 46 patients with metastatic tumors to the vertebral column presenting with severe pain and neurologic deficits, only 31% had a satisfactory short-term outcome when treated medically. In the majority of patients who did respond lymphoma was the primary diagnosis.[80] Schocker and Brady reported better results and noted that, with radiation therapy alone, 72% of their patients improved in the short term; however, 14% worsened over the same 30-day time period.[81]

It takes lamellar bone 6 months to form after radiation. In the presence of a pathologic fracture, the healing process is too slow to prevent further collapse in the neurologic compression. Lord and Herndon reported three cases in which late kyphotic collapse and neurologic deficit occurred after radiation therapy for tumors involving the thoracolumbar spine.[82] These studies indicate that it is not rational to assume that radiation therapy can have any effect on the unstable spine or provide anything more than temporary palliation in patients with radioresistant tumors. In the 1970s, new surgical approaches were developed to better address the anatomic site of involvement in spine tumors; this led to a reexamination of the roles of surgery and radiation therapy in treating these patients.

Because of the poor results with laminectomy, surgery was considered as a "salvage" procedure for those patients who experienced relapse after radiation therapy. Sundaresan et al.[71] demonstrated that patients previously treated with radiation therapy had twice the complication rate. External radiation therapy compromises wound healing and immune function and is associated with an increased breakdown of the surgical wound in 30% of surgically treated patients.[71,83] Sundaresan et al. emphasized that surgery should be considered before radiation therapy in patients with spinal metastases and that major benefits will be reflected in improved neurologic function and a high proportion of long-term survivors. They condemned the practice of considering surgery when patients' conditions deteriorate during radiation therapy because these types of "salvage procedure" are considerably less effective and are associated with much higher morbidity. They also noted that patients who are paraplegic or who have significant weakness rarely benefit from surgery. They performed a prospective study to test the hypothesis that the optimal treatment in patients with neoplastic spinal cord compression would be surgical treatment followed by radiother-

apy. They found that, of the 44% of patients who were nonambulatory before surgery, all became ambulatory after surgery. Their results were clearly superior to those reported for radiation therapy alone. They also noted that compression of the spinal cord recurred after surgery in more than 30% of patients who had been previously irradiated, whereas those patients who underwent repeat surgery often maintained their ambulatory status until death. They recommended that repeat surgery be considered in the majority of patients with spinal cord compression due to neoplasm.[71]

Traditional indications for surgery include the need to establish a histologic diagnosis in cases in which the nature of the primary tumor is not known, recurrence or progression of a tumor after radiation therapy, neurologic compromise caused by pathologic fracture, radioresistant tumors, and progressive deformity secondary to instability.[84,85]

To clarify the surgical indications, Harrington[5] devised a classification system of metastatic tumors. He divided spinal metastases into five categories, depending on the extent of neurologic compromise or bone destruction (see box below). Patients who are in class I or II with no significant neurologic impairment or vertebral collapse or instability are treated with chemotherapy or local ir-

---

Harrington's Five Classification Categories for Metastatic Tumors

Class I	Asymptomatic involvement of bone
Class II	Symptomatic vertebral lesions defined by pain with or without minor neurologic involvement but without collapse or instability
Class III	Major neurologic impairment (motor or sensory) without significant collapse of bone, usually due to epidural extension of tumor
Class IV	Vertebral collapse with pain due to mechanical causes or instability but without significant neurologic compromise
Class V	Vertebral collapse and instability combined with major neurologic impairment

Traditional methods and innovative approaches. J Urol 130: 2-7, 1983.

70. Tomita T, Galicich JH, Sundaresan N. Radiation therapy for spinal epidural metastases with complete block. Acta Radiol Oncol 22:135-143, 1983.

71. Sundaresan N, Digiacinto GV, Hughes JE, Cafferty M, Vallejo A. Treatment of neoplastic spinal cord compression: Results of a prospective study. Neurosurgery 29:645-650, 1991.

72. McConahey WM, Hay ID, Woolner LB, van Heerden JA, Taylor WF. Papillary thyroid cancer treated at the Mayo clinic, 1946 through 1970: Initial manifestations, pathologic findings, therapy, and outcome. Mayo Clin Proc 61:978-996, 1986.

73. Castillo LA, Yeh SD, Leeper RD, Benua RS. Bone scans in bone metastases from functioning thyroid carcinoma. Clin Nucl Med 5:200-209, 1980.

74. Gjorup T, Hartling OJ, Munck-Hansen J, Munck O. Bone-scan "cold" lesion caused by an osteolytic metastasis from an adenocarcinoma of the thyroid. Eur J Nucl Med 10:470-471, 1985.

75. Villas C, Lopez R, Zubieta JL. Osteoid osteoma in the lumbar and sacral regions: Two cases of difficult diagnosis. J Spinal Disord 3:418-422, 1990.

76. Durie BG, Young LA, Salmon SE. Human myeloma in vitro colony growth: Interrelationships between drug sensitivity, cell kinetics and patient survival duration. Blood 61:929-934, 1983.

77. Bell RM. Thyroid carcinoma. Surg Clin North Am 66:13-30, 1986.

78. Whitehill R, Stowers SF, Fechner RE, Ruch WW, Drucker S, Gibson LR, McKernan DJ, Widmeyer JH. Posterior cervical fusions using cerclage wires, methylmethacrylate and autogenous bone graft: An experimental study of a canine model. Spine 12:12-22, 1987.

79. Cobb CA III, Leavens ME, Eckles N. Indications for nonoperative treatment of spinal cord compression due to breast cancer. J Neurosurg 47:653-658, 1977.

80. Muggia FM, Chervu LR. Lung cancer: Diagnosis in metastatic sites. Semin Oncol 1:217-228, 1974.

81. Seagren SL, Herndon, JE, Baeker JR, Boles M, Chung C, Green MR. Alternating irradiation and chemotherapy in stage III A and B nonsmall cell lung cancer: Report of a cancer and leukemia group B phase II study 8636. Int J Radiat Oncol Biol Phys 29:1085-1088, 1994.

82. Levui WJ, Bay J, Dohn D. Spinal cord meningioma. J Neurosurg 57:804-812, 1982.

83. Arbeit JM, Hilaris BS, Brennan MF. Wound complications in the multimodality treatment of extremity and superficial truncal sarcomas. J Clin Oncol 5:480-488, 1987.

84. Welch WC, Jacobs GB. Surgery for metastatic spinal disease. J Neurooncol 23:163-170, 1995.

85. Ratanatharathorn V, Powers WE. Epidural spinal compression from metastatic tumor: Diagnosis and guidelines for management. Cancer Treat Rev 18:55-71, 1991.

86. McAfee PC, Zdeblick TA. Tumors of the thoracic and lumbar spine: Surgical treatment via the anterior approach. J Spinal Disord 2:145-154, 1989.

87. Levine AM. Pathologic fractures. Part 1—Neoplasia. In Browner BD, Jupiter JB, Levine AM, Trafton PG, eds. Skeletal Trauma. Philadelphia: WB Saunders, 1992, pp 401-431.

88. Cahill DW, Kumar R. Palliative subtotal vertebrectomy with anterior and posterior reconstruction via a single posterior approach. J Neurosurg 90(1 Suppl):42-47, 1999.

89. Findlay GF. The role of vertebral body collapse in the management of malignant spinal cord compression. J Neurol Neurosurg Psychiatry 50:151-154, 1987.

90. Solini A, Paschero B, Orsini G, Guercio N. The surgical treatment of metastatic tumors of the lumbar spine. Ital J Orthop Traumatol 11:427-442, 1985.

91. Kostuik JP. Anterior spinal cord decompression for lesions of the thoracic and lumbar spine, techniques, new methods of internal fixation results. Spine 8:512-531, 1983.

92. Martin NS, Williamson J. The role of surgery in the treatment of malignant tumours of the spine. J Bone Joint Surg Br 52:227-237, 1970.

93. Weinstein JN. Surgical approach to spine tumors. Orthopedics 12:897-905, 1989.

94. Sundaresan N, Steinberger AA, Moore F, Sachdev VP, Krol G, Hough L, Kelliher K. Indications and results of combined anterior-posterior approaches for spine tumor surgery. J Neurosurg 85(3):438-446, 1996.

95. Siegal T, Siegal T. Surgical decompression of anterior and posterior malignant epidural tumors compressing the spinal cord: A prospective study. Neurosurgery 17:424-432, 1985.

96. DeWald RL, Bridwell KH, Prodromas C, Rodts MF. Reconstructive spinal surgery as palliation for metastatic malignancies of the spine. Spine 10:21-26, 1985.

97. Rosenthal D, Marquardt G, Lorenz R, Nichtweiss M. Anterior decompression and stabilization using a microsurgical endoscopic technique for metastatic tumors of the thoracic spine. J Neurosurg 84(4):565-572, 1996.

98. Bauer HC. Posterior decompression and stabilization for spinal metastases: Analysis of sixty-seven consecutive patients. J Bone Joint Surg Am 79(4):514-522, 1997.

99. Overby MC, Rothman AS. Anterolateral decompression for metastatic epidural spinal cord tumors: Results of a modified costotransversectomy approach. J Neurosurg 62:344-348, 1985.

100. Sundaresan N, Galicich JH, Lane JM. Harrington rod stabilization for pathological fractures of the spine. J Neurosurg 60:282-286, 1984.

101. Stener B. Total spondylectomy in chondrosarcoma arising from the seventh vertebra. J Bone Joint Surg Br 53:288-295, 1971.

102. Gokaslan ZL, York JE, Walsh GL, McCutcheon IA, Lang FF, Putnam JB, et al. Transthoracic vertebrectomy for metastatic spinal tumors. J Neurosurg 89(4):599-609, 1998.

103. Siegal T, Siegal T. Current considerations in the management of neoplastic spinal cord compression. Spine 14:223-228, 1988.

104. Onimus M, Schraub S, Bertin D, Bosset JF, Guidet M. Surgical treatment of vertebral metastasis. Spine 11:883-891, 1986.

105. White AA III, Panjabi MM. Biomechanical considerations in

the surgical management of the spine. Part 3. Surgical constructs employing methylmethacrylate. In White AA III, Panjabi M, eds. Clinical Biomechanics of the Spine. Philadelphia: JB Lippincott, 1978, pp 424-425.

106. Panjabi MM, Goel VK, Clark CR, Keggi KJ, Southwick WO. Biomechanical study of cervical spine stabilization with methylmethacrylate. Spine 10:198-203, 1985.

107. Wang GJ, Wilson CS, Hubbard SL, Sweet DE, Reger SI, Stamp WG. Safety of anterior cement fixation in the cervical spine: In vivo study of dog spine. South Med J 77:178-179, 1984.

108. Wara WM, Phillips TL, Sheline GE, Schwade JG. Radiation tolerance of the spinal cord. Cancer 35:1558-1562, 1975.

109. Katagiri H, Takahashi N, Inagaki J, Kobayashi H, Sugiura H, Yamamura S, et al. Clinical results of nonsurgical treatment for spinal metastases. Int J Radiat Oncol Biol Phys 42(5): 1127-1132, 1998.

110. Seagren SL, Saunders WM. Radiation therapy of spinal cord tumors. Semin Spine Surg 2:197, 1990.

111. Fletcher GE. Clinical dose-response curves of human malignant epithelial tumors. Br J Radiol 46:1, 1973.

CHAPTER

28

Lesions of the Cervical Spine

Randy F. Davis, M.D., and Santi Rao, M.D.

PATHOLOGY AND NATURAL HISTORY

Although metastatic lesions of the cervical spine account for a relatively small proportion of total spinal metastases, the potential complications of spinal cord impingement from such a lesion are devastating. Cervical spine metastasis certainly occurs less frequently than metastasis to the thoracic or lumbar spine. Various authors have noted an incidence of cervical spine involvement ranging from 8% to 20%.[1-4]

Treatment goals for such patients involve minimizing pain without causing a neurologic deficit and minimizing the use of external bracing so that the patient may sustain an independent lifestyle. Many patients can be treated nonoperatively with radiotherapy or chemotherapy or both. Surgery may not be necessary. The indications for surgery commonly involve progression of pain, development of incipient neurologic compromise, or instability.[5] Metastatic disease to the spine occurs at a rate of 5% per year[6,7] in patients with cancer. The type of primary tumor determines the incidence of bone metastasis; patients with a tumor such as breast carcinoma may have a 70% incidence of vertebral metastasis.[8] Breast, lung, prostate, kidney, lymphoma, and myeloma remain the most common primary tumors.[2,5] Spinal canal compromise from epidural metastasis occurs in 2% to 12% of cases.[9]

As is the case elsewhere in the axial skeleton, metastatic involvement is more often in the vertebral bodies rather than the laminae and pedicles. Compression of the spinal cord usually develops anteriorly rather than posteriorly, as is the case frequently with most pathologic burst fractures. Canal encroachment is therefore more likely to occur anteriorly than posteriorly.[8,10] Only about 15% of cord compression cases occurs posteriorly; it seems to be more common in prostate tumors, and 10% is lateral.[11]

The location of the tumor in the cervical spine has some importance in terms of the clinical presentation. The upper cervical spine has some unusual anatomic features that are distinctly different from those of the lower cervical spine.[10] Unlike the case with metastasis to the lower cervical spine, kyphosis or true flexion instability is a rare sequela of metastatic disease to the upper cervical spine. Frequently local infiltration by the tumor mass is a source of pain and neurologic deficit. It is only with destruction of the facet joints and pedicles that local rotary instability results.[10] This is important, as metastasis of the upper cervical spine most frequently requires a posterior approach for surgical stabilization. Cervical metastatic disease certainly is not always associated with deformity. This may be biomechanically related to the fact that the line of gravity has no anterior lever arm and the weight of the skull is borne by the posterior facets and ligamentous structures.[12] However, once more than 50% of the vertebral body is involved with metastasis, kyphotic deformities frequently ensue with devastating complications.[5]

Because the vertebral body usually is involved, the anterior cord is frequently the site of cord compression. Motor rather than sensory deficits are often the first presenting signs. The incidence of neurologic deficits appears to be lower for the cervical region than for the thoracic or lumbar region, with only 5% to 6% of patients presenting with paraplegia or quadriplegia.[4,7] The prognosis for a high cord compression, however, is poor, as opposed to the partial paraplegia of a lower thoracic or lumbar level lesion.

DIAGNOSIS AND PRESENTATION

Patients with cervical spine metastasis present more often with pain than with a sudden neurologic deficit. Schaberg and Gainor[4] noted that the presentation of cervical spine metastasis differs from that of thoracic or lumbar metastasis. Phillips et al.[10] noted pain in 93% of patients with cervical metastasis and neurologic deficits in 14%, which is less frequent than with thoracic or lumbar metastasis. Localized pain of gradual onset, which is progressive and worse in the evenings, is the most common manifestation of vertebral metastasis. The development of rapidly increasing or crescendo pain is one of the components of the "patient at risk" and deserves early intervention and diagnosis.[5]

It is not uncommon for the diagnosis of cervical spine metastasis to be delayed because of misdiagnosis of degenerative disease. In particular, the upper cervical spine is often difficult to visualize on

Portions of this chapter are modified from Rao S, Davis RF: Cervical spine metastases. In Clark CR, ed.: The Cervical Spine, ed. 3. Philadelphia: Lippincott-Raven Publishers, 1998, pp 603-619. © Lippincott Williams & Wilkins.

plain radiographs, and subtle changes in the bone may be missed. Routine radiographs most commonly will underestimate the presence and extent of metastatic involvement; in fact, 30% to 70% of cancellous bone must be destroyed before they begin to be positive.[13] Unlike the case with the thoracic and lumbar spine, bone changes in the cervical spine are frequently subtle, as the pedicle is not so easy to visualize as it is in the thoracic and lumbar spine.[14]

Bone scintigraphy is a sensitive tool for detecting spinal metastasis but is positive in only half the patients with metastatic cord compression. Primary tumors, such as multiple myeloma and some sarcomas, may not be seen on bone scans. Because scintigraphy lacks specificity, the exact levels of involvement cannot be identified. For specific evaluation of cervical spine metastasis, scintigraphy has been supplanted by cervical magnetic resonance imaging (MRI).[15-17] MRI is the mainstay for the accurate delineation of the spinal lesion, the extent of disease, and the prevalence of epidural metastasis.[18]

Computed tomography (CT) is a useful adjunct for the preoperative determination of the extent of bone destruction. CT reveals bone architecture and the extent of destruction best for the determination of surgical reconstructive procedures. Because some compression fractures in patients with known cancer may not be related to metastasis, the CT scan is helpful in differentiating osteoporosis osteopenia from tumor destruction. With osteoporosis the cortical outline is frequently intact, unlike metastatic disease, in which the cortex is frequently destroyed and the osteolytic areas are larger and irregular.[17,19,20]

Once the diagnosis of a cervical lesion has been made, a tissue diagnosis is mandatory to determine appropriate surgical therapy. This is particularly important in patients with known metastatic disease. Patients with known vertebral metastasis will present with nonmetastatic osteopenic compression fractures, which later are proven by autopsy studies.[21] These lesions obviously should not be immediately treated with radiation or chemotherapy. A tissue diagnosis is imperative even in patients with known vertebral metastatic disease.

Specific histologic diagnosis will assist in establishing the prognosis and will help the surgeon determine the degree of aggressiveness of surgical ablative and reconstructive measures.[22] Although all

regions of the cervical spine are accessible by open surgical techniques or needle biopsy, closed biopsy techniques of the cervical spine are technically demanding and often fraught with potential neurologic and vascular complications, unlike closed biopsy techniques in the thoracic and lumbar spine. It is for this reason that we frequently combine open biopsy with a preplanned definitive surgical procedure. The exception to this rule is the upper cervical spine. It was Ottolenghi who first developed and published the techniques for needle biopsy of the cervical spine.[11] It is helpful to divide the cervical spine into three separate regions: (1) the anterior bodies of the first three cervical vertebrae, (2) the anterior bodies of the fourth through seventh vertebrae, and (3) the posterior elements and posterior epidural space. Our experience with needle biopsy of the upper cervical spine has been through a transoral approach in seven cases to distinguish between infection, pannus, and metastatic tumor. A transoral approach to the bodies of the first three vertebrae can be performed with the patient under general nasotracheal anesthesia and with fiber-optic intubation using a 2 mm biopsy needle and fluorographic control. A diagnosis of vertebral osteomyelitis was made in a patient with a known remote history of breast carcinoma in one instance, and a diagnosis of degenerative pannus was made in a patient with a known remote history of hypernephroma. For lesions in the lower cervical spine with anterior involvement, we have tended to combine the biopsy with a definitive surgical procedure. If the pathologist can establish a diagnosis of metastatic malignant disease via frozen section, then the definitive planned anterior acrylic stabilization can proceed.[23] If, as has happened in two cases, malignant disease cannot be easily established, consideration should be given to the performance of bone grafting and anterior plating rather than introduction of methylmethacrylate.

MANAGEMENT
Nonoperative Therapy

Despite traditional surgical thinking, most cervical metastatic lesions can be treated nonoperatively. The treating physician should consider surgery as only one segment of combination therapy involving radiation, chemotherapy, and bracing. The type of treatment is determined by a complex evaluation of the tumor type, radiosensitivity, history of radiation, patient life expectancy, medical condition, extent of instability, and the presence or absence of neurologic compromise. Different tumor types have different life expectancies and different prognoses from the advent of bone metastasis. Thus lung carcinoma has a mean survival of only 7 to 9 months, whereas breast carcinoma has a survival exceeding 30 months with bone lesions alone.[5] The evaluation of survival, however, frequently does not seem to be as important in determining treatment as development of devastating paraplegia that can end a life. Recently a scoring system was developed to identify patients whose life expectancy may be less than 6 months or more than 12 months with an overall accuracy of 63%.[24] In general, patients can be divided into five categories based on the extent of bone destruction or neurologic compromise[24]:

1. No significant neurologic involvement
2. Involvement of bone but no collapse or instability
3. Major neurologic involvement (sensory or motor) without significant bone involvement
4. Vertebral collapse with pain due to mechanical causes or instability but without significant neurologic impairment
5. Vertebral collapse or instability combined with major neurologic impairment

If the patient has no significant pain or more than 50% involvement of the bone, systemic chemotherapy may be appropriate in a variety of lesions. The patient should then be followed radiographically at a regular interval, usually every 6 weeks. The interval of follow-up should usually be 6 weeks, 3 months, 6 months, and then 1 year from the onset of diagnosis to verify that no kyphosis or progression is developing.

Radiotherapy

Radiation therapy is the mainstay of treatment of spinal metastatic lesions, especially for radiosensitive tumors such as lymphoma, breast cancer, and prostate carcinoma. With early detection, radiation therapy and external mobilization can provide symptomatic and objective relief in most patients. If the patient is going to respond to treatment, it usually will be during the course of treatment or within 2 weeks after completion of treatment.

Radiation therapy may be used as the initial treatment for radiosensitive lesions not causing bone compression.[19] Most patients with lymphoma, carcinoma of the breast, or myeloma will respond well to radiation therapy; however, when compression is anterior and due to a bone fragment or to a slowly progressive radioresistant tumor, radiation therapy should not be used as the primary treatment. Radiculopathy without signs of cord compression may be treated with radiation therapy alone. This was one of the most common presentations at this level in the series of Constans et al.[1]

Asymptomatic upper cervical lesions still may be treated with radiation therapy because of the potential for fracture or dislocation and the disastrous complication of quadriplegia. The usual nonoperative modalities may not be effective with complete destruction of the lateral mass of C1 or C2 or involvement of the dens. Laminectomy and anterior corpectomy are not applicable in the upper cervical spine. Local radiation therapy may be recommended for pain relief. Severe pain, rotary instability, or unresolved block suggest the need for surgery. Patients with minor subluxation may be treated with a collar and radiation. Persistence of pain at the end of radiation therapy suggests instability necessitating surgical stabilization. The most critical feature in patients with posterior C2 arch disease is to institute the radiation therapy early in the pain course so that persistent kyphosis does not develop. Patients with lateral mass destruction of C1 should undergo occiput-to-C3 fusion with adjunctive radiation therapy because rotary instability is common.[10]

The question of compatibility of radiation therapy with the internal fixation devices, methylmethacrylate cement, or the bone graft used invariably arises.[25] Metal does not influence the results of radiation therapy. Supporting bone graft struts may fail because of compromised healing with irradiation. Methylmethacrylate cement does not interfere with any subsequent radiation therapy and is not affected by radiation therapy.[25,26]

Surgical Therapy

Surgery for cervical metastatic disease has undergone a gradual evolution in the last 20 years from primarily decompressive laminectomy to a more direct assault on the location of the lesion. Indeed, anterior vertebral body compression is more common than posterior compression. Improved anterior cervical approaches achieve better results than earlier surgical techniques. Although it referred to spinal metastasis in general, a prospective study of anterior surgery plus radiotherapy reported results superior to those of the historical experience with radiotherapy alone.[27] Comparison of an anterior decompression for anterior disease with a posterior decompression for posterior disease at the same institution has shown twice the rate of improvement after anterior procedures.[28] Indeed, better ambulatory outcome has been described in patients who underwent corpectomy.[29] This would suggest a disproportionate sensitivity of the anterior spinal cord syndromes to anterior surgical decompression. There are, however, certain tumors, such as prostate, that present with a significant posterior component in conjunction with predominantly epidural metastasis. These lesions would not respond to anterior decompression and have to be dealt with posteriorly. Similarly, multiple skip lesions with a predominant epidural component cannot easily be dealt with anteriorly.

The goals of surgery in metastatic disease include (1) prevention or reversal of neurologic deterioration, (2) stabilization of cervical instability, (3) reduction of pain, and (4) potential establishment of a diagnosis. Similarly it has been our experience that surgical stabilization can obviate the use of halos or other orthoses, which we believe significantly affect the quality of life for these patients with already limited life expectancies. Every effort should be made to obtain rigid stabilization at the time of the procedure, so that the patient will not have been subjected to an operation and then still have to use a halo or other sort of uncomfortable and cumbersome brace. It is helpful to establish the concept of the "patient at risk" (Fig. 28-1). Although anecdotal, we have seen 6 patients in whom progressive neurologic deficits developed while they were receiving surgical and medical care. Four of these six patients previously had received radiation therapy and were being followed-up. Two patients had not yet made a decision whether to consent to operative treatment and were being managed medically for pain control. All these patients shared three characteristics:

1. The cervical metastasis showed greater than 50% involvement of the vertebral body as determined by MRI and CT scans.
2. Kyphosis had begun to develop at the involved level and exceeded the White and Panjabi instability criteria established for trauma. Specifically, three of the six had greater than 3.5 mm of subluxation, and all had kyphosis with greater than 11 degrees of adjacent angulation between contiguous vertebral bodies.
3. In all patients crescendo pain developed over a period of weeks prior to the development of progressive neurologic deficits within a 24-hour period that were not reversed with urgent surgical intervention.

Thus we have become more aggressive in recommending earlier surgical intervention in these patients, irrespective of the primary tumor type, once the "patient at risk" signs begin to develop.

Anterior corpectomy and stabilization for lesions from C3 through C7 in one or two vertebrae is almost certainly the procedure of choice. Anterior corpectomy is a relatively simple and quick procedure that provides near-immediate pain relief, in our experience, and can be accomplished with a standard Robinson-Smith approach, which virtually all spinal surgeons are familiar with. Superior results via this anterior approach have been demonstrated by a number of authors.[1,5-7,9-14]

The technique for decompression is similar to that used in trauma. It is important to manage all cervical metastases as you would an unstable cervical spine. This protocol involves (1) fiber-optic intubation to minimize the movement of the neck, (2) application of tongs or a halo ring on an operative wedge frame, and (3) spinal cord monitoring with the patient supine and prone. If there is a change in the monitoring potentials, a wake-up test can be performed. To date, this sequence has en-

---

- **>50% INVOLVEMENT OF THE VERTEBRAL BODY**

- **EXCEEDING WHITE AND PANJABI CRITERIA FOR INSTABILITY**
  >3.5 mm SUBLUXATION
  >11 DEGREES ADJACENT ANGULATION

- **CRESCENDO PAIN**

Fig. 28-1　Patient at risk.

abled us to operate on 32 patients with metastatic cervical spine involvement without any documented evidence of neurologic progression following our surgical procedures.[5]

In anterior cervical decompression the discs and avascular structures should be removed before attention is directed at the corpectomy. Once the corpectomy begins, the surgeon should be prepared to expeditiously remove as much of the cancellous bone as possible and proceed to the epidural space, as brisk bleeding can be encountered. The anesthesiologist should be told that the corpectomy is beginning, as fairly impressive amounts of blood can be lost, and the surgeon should be kept informed, since it is often difficult to estimate the amount of blood loss. Thus, it is our policy to ask the anesthesiologist to notify the surgeon each time 100 ml of blood is lost. We have attempted on several occasions to obtain preoperative embolization of lesions to minimize blood loss, particularly in hypernephroma cases. We believe this has been helpful in hypernephroma cases, but in other metastatic lesions the blood supply seems to be fairly diffuse without a defining vessel. Once the corpectomy is completed, the epidural bleeding can be fairly easily controlled with Avitene, Gelfoam, and light pressure. Inexperienced surgeons should be discouraged from making multiple forays into the corpectomy site, as this tends to potentiate further bleeding, often without making significant gains in decompression. Once the corpectomy is completed, a decision has to be made about the means of stabilization. In the past, bone was used for lesions be-

lieved to be associated with longer life expectancies, such as myeloma or breast cancer. Acceptance of these bone grafts, particularly when radiation is given, has been problematic, and we now almost exclusively use methylmethacrylate for anterior constructs. Scoville introduced the use of methylmethacrylate for dealing with metastatic tumors, and a number of other authors have used this technique successfully.[1,5,23] Subsequent radiotherapy has no effect on the mechanical capacity or resistance of the cement.[25] Although there is often a concern about the heat generated during the polymerization of the cement, it seems not to damage the spinal cord, as the flow of spinal fluid appears to act as a heat sink. Gelfoam is also applied to the spinal cord in a narrow film to provide further protection. Methylmethacrylate reconstruction can be reinforced with a number of materials, as described by various authors.[30] Anterior plate fixation above and below the reconstruction has also been used by a number of authors.[16] As we have personal experience with over 30 cases of methylmethacrylate reconstruction with simple Kirschner wire stabilization, we have found it difficult to justify the additional dissection and expense required for an anterior plate construct. The anterior corpectomy construct involves the insertion of 0.062 mm Kirschner wires bent into an L-configuration. A 5 cc syringe with an attached ureteral catheter adapter is used to fill the corpectomy defect with methylmethacrylate. It is important that the methylmethacrylate be inserted early in a liquid state to maximize fit and fill of the corpectomy defect (see Fig. 28-2 for cor-

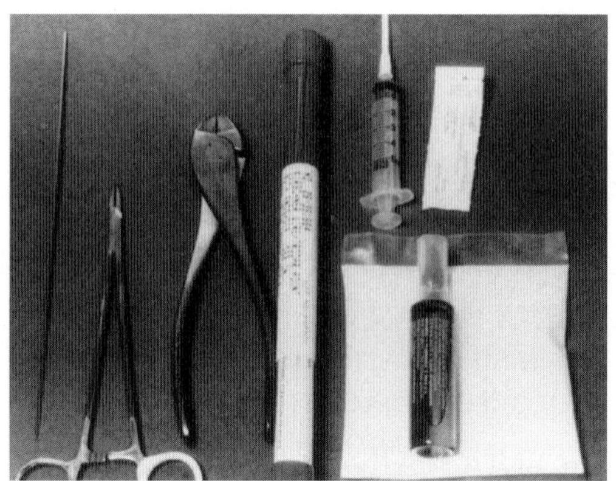

Fig. 28-2   **A** and **B,** Materials needed for corpectomy technique.

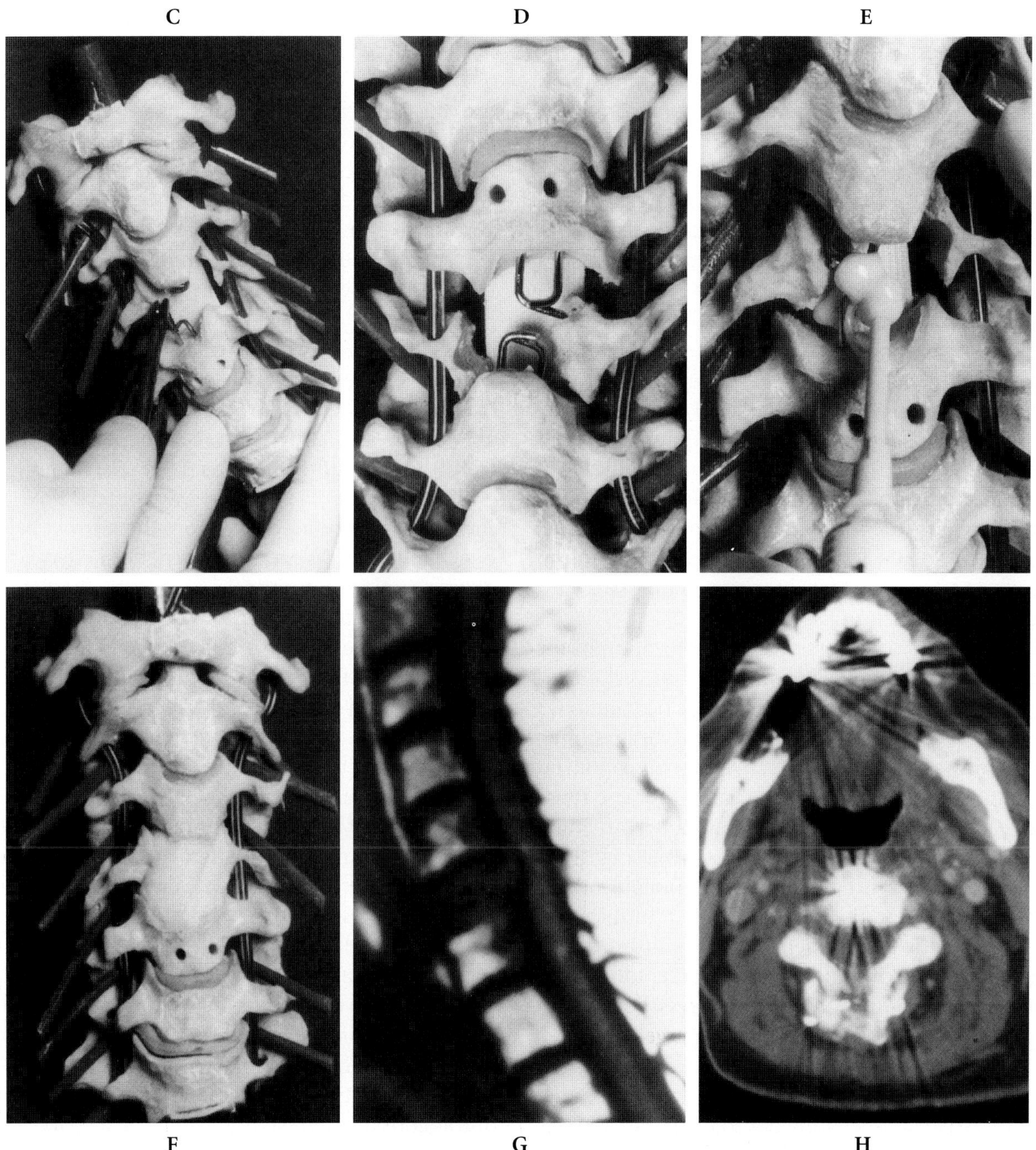

Fig. 28-2, cont'd   C and D, Insertion of 0.062 Kirschner wires. E and F, Filling corpectomy defect and completed construct. G, Single-level breast cancer metastasis to C6. H, Postoperative CT demonstrating good "fit and fill."

pectomy technique). We have used this technique successfully in 18 of 23 patients undergoing operative treatment of cervical metastatic disease. Eight patients improved neurologically, and no patient's condition deteriorated as a direct result of the surgery. Three patients, who were nonambulatory, regained the ability to ambulate postoperatively. The average survival from the time of surgery ranged from 7 weeks to 3 years, with an average survival of 13 months. There were no cases of dislodgement of the acrylic corpectomy mass, although in one patient there was extension of a hypernephroma to the level above the previous cervical corpectomy and a dense neurologic deficit developed that was operated on urgently, but there was no significant return of function.

The economics of medicine today unfortunately is changing some of the directions that therapy has provided. Given that there have been few failures of acrylic with simple Kirschner wire augmentation, it becomes difficult to justify the expense of several thousand dollars for anterior plates and titanium mesh constructs, which has been witnessed on a number of occasions.

Posterior decompression and stabilization of the cervical spine should be considered in certain instances. Lesions that present from the occiput to C3 are often difficult to treat anteriorly. There is often no good way to provide effective anterior stabilization. Similarly, lesions at the cervicothoracic junction are often difficult to address anteriorly, and consideration should be given to treating them posteriorly. Certain other patients, notably those with prostate carcinoma, often have multiple-level vertebral body involvement with a significant component of napkin ring or posterior epidural disease. These patients can also be addressed with posterior procedures. The results of surgery are often not so gratifying as simple one- or two-level anterior corpectomies.[31,32] The decision to perform a decompressive laminectomy has to be made preoperatively and has a significant effect on the type of posterior stabilization that can be used. If posterior elements can be left intact, a standard Rogers or Bohlman triple-wire stabilization procedure with bone graft can be employed posteriorly (Fig. 28-3). Once it has been determined that a laminectomy is necessary, the surgeon must revert to the use of ei-

ther a Southwick type of arthrodesis or posterior cervical plates. The use of methylmethacrylate for posterior stabilization should be viewed with skepticism, as reports of significant failure have been noted.[33] Indeed, the one complication in my series of 23 patients with cervical metastasis involved failure of a posterior acrylic construct with fracture of the spinous processes and wound dehiscence (Fig. 28-4). Laminectomy alone with decompression should be used with caution unless the surgeon is absolutely convinced that there is little anterior involvement and significant amounts of posterior facets can be left to maintain stability and prevent kyphosis.

Posterior stabilization techniques have undergone an evolution over the last 15 years. With the original techniques advocated by Roy-Camille et al.,[34] cervical stabilization can be accomplished from the occiput to the subaxial levels. Plates fixed onto the occiput and the vertebrae below the metastasis can be used to restore the normal height of C1 and C2, thus exerting a beneficial effect by reducing radicular compression.[35] With the Synthes system the plates can be more easily bent to achieve the acute angle necessary for occipital fixation. The best bone on the occiput is more medial, and attempts should be directed at keeping the plates as medial as possible. If the occipital bone is thin and will not hold the screws adequately, wire braided cables can be used to affix the plates to the occiput. The Axis plate by Danek allows more leeway in the placement of medial and lateral subaxial screws, although it is difficult to contour for occipital use. These patients are often elderly and osteopenic, and thus the fixation of screws with lateral mass plates is often less than optimal. Consideration should be given to augmentation with methylmethacrylate in the screwholes to increase the pull out strength. If posterior elements can be left intact, braided titanium cable in conjunction with autologous iliac crest bone graft in a triple-wire configuration is simple and provides good immediate stability with the prospect for long-term stabilization. Titanium enables quite good postoperative MRI and CT visualization of the operative site.

In those instances in which a patient is deemed to have a long life expectancy, usually greater than 2 years, such as in breast carcinoma or myelo-

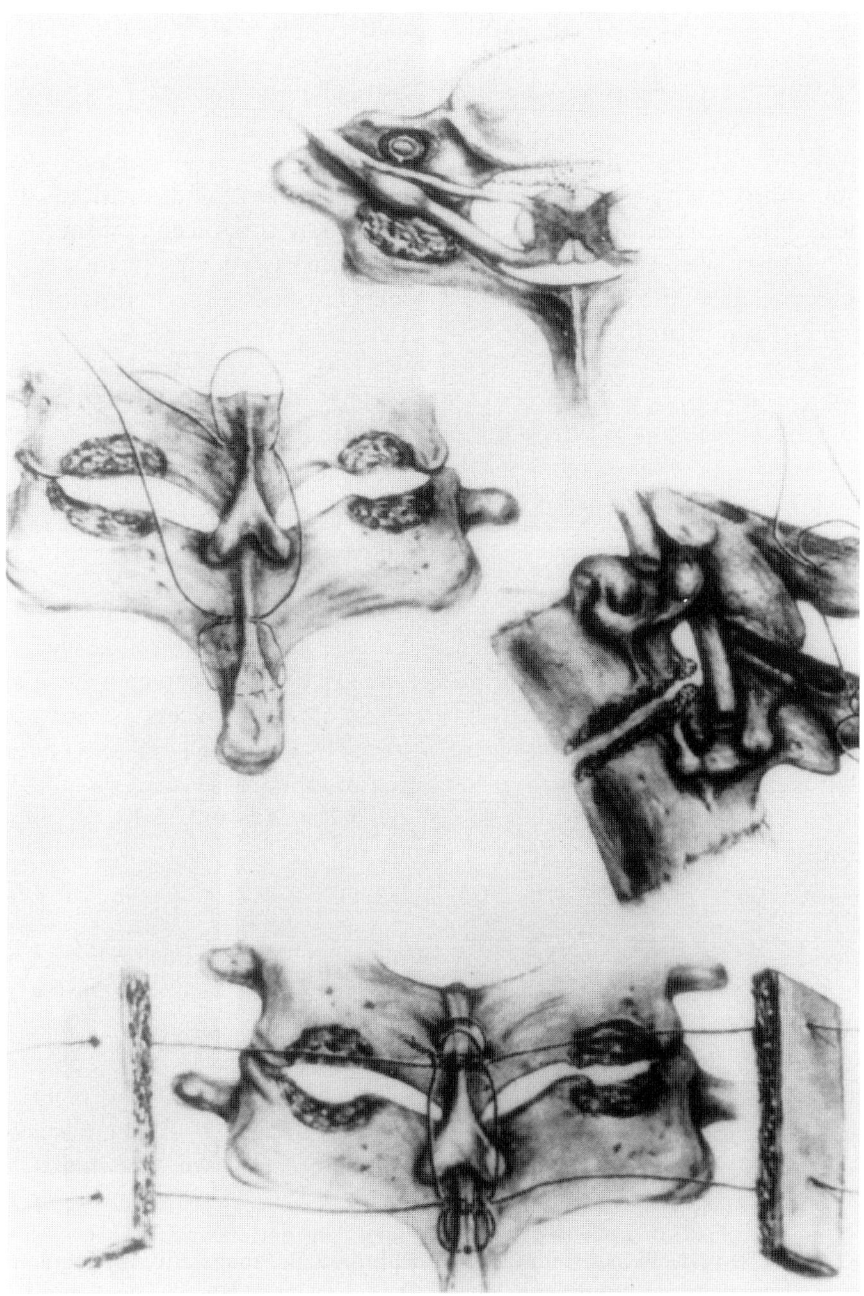

Fig. 28-3 Standard posterior wiring constructs.

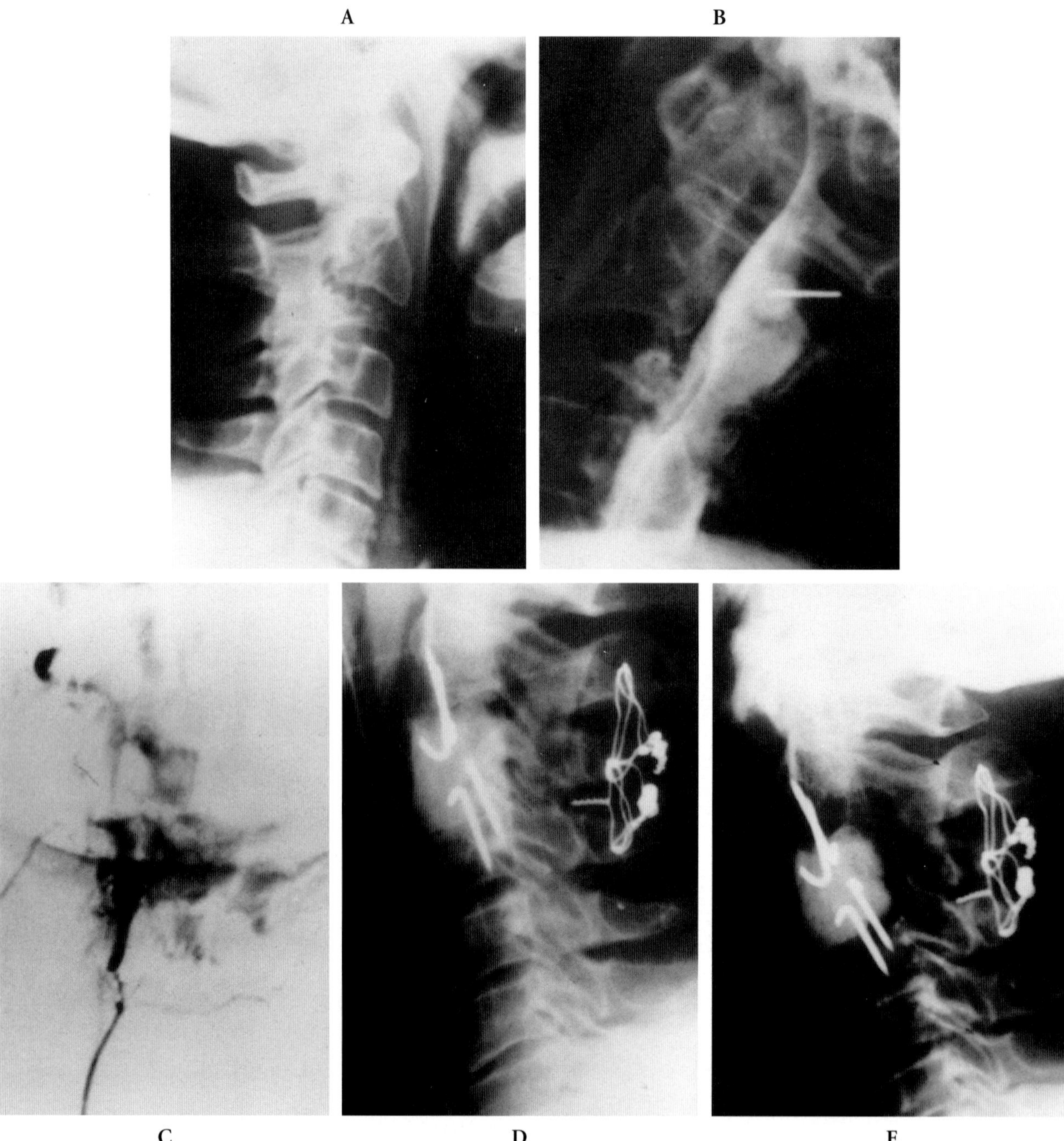

Fig. 28-4 **A,** A 50-year-old man with C3 hypernephroma. **B,** Preoperative myelogram. **C,** Anteroposterior angiogram of tumor with "blush." **D,** Postoperative lateral view. **E** and **F,** An 18-month postoperative plain film and MRI showing extension of the lesion to C2. **G,** Patient subsequently became paraplegic, necessitating emergency laminectomy, revision laminectomy, and extension of fusion.

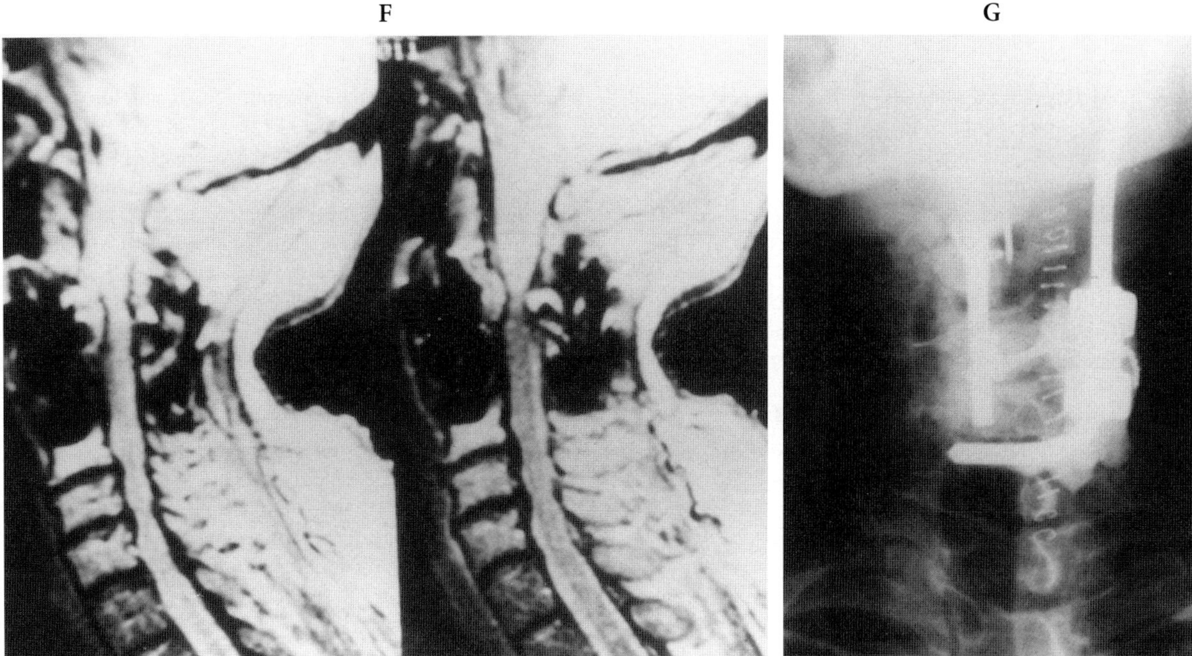

Fig. 28-4   For legend see opposite page.

ma, consideration could be given to a hybrid approach.[5,32] We have used this approach in 8 of 23 patients. The first procedure is the anterior corpectomy with methylmethacrylate stabilization. The patient can then be turned on the operative wedge frame, and a posterior stabilization can be performed with autologous iliac crest bone graft to provide long-term bone stabilization. Initially there were reports of staging the two procedures, but we believe the morbidity and shorter length of hospital stay clearly indicate that the combined procedure is the method of choice.

CONCLUSION

The surgical treatment of metastatic cervical disease is still evolving. Questions that remain involve the longevity of anterior constructs and indeed whether it is necessary to perform posterior stabilization at the same time. Surgical treatment should at all times be directed by a team approach. The ethical and financial considerations involved are beyond the scope of this discussion. The primary goals should be to minimize pain and keep these unfortunate patients ambulatory for the remainder of their life expectancy.

REFERENCES

1. Constans JP, Dedivitiis E, Donzelli R, Spaziante R, Meder JF, Haye C. Spinal metastases with neurological manifestations: A review of 600 cases. J Neurosurg 59:111-118, 1983.
2. Gilbert RW, Kim JH, Posner JB. Epidural spinal cord compression from metastatic tumor: Diagnosis and treatment. Ann Neurol 3:40-51, 1978.
3. Onimus M, Schraub S, Bertin D, Bosset JF, Guidet M. Surgical treatment of vertebral metastases. Spine 11:883-891, 1986.
4. Schaberg J, Gainor BJ. A profile of metastatic carcinoma of the spine. Spine 10:19-20, 1985.
5. Davis RF, Zeidman S. Surgical management of cervical spine metastases. [Abstract.] CSRS, 1990.
6. Black P. Metastatic tumors of the central nervous system: Spinal metastases. In Abeloff MD, ed. Complications of Cancer: Diagnosis and Management. Baltimore: Johns Hopkins University Press, 1979, pp 313-356.
7. O'Connor MI, Currier BL. Metastatic disease of the spine. Orthopaedics 15:611-620, 1992.
8. Sundaresan N, Galicich JH, Bains MS, Martini N, Beattie EJ. Vertebral body resection in the treatment of cancer involving the spine. Cancer 53:1393-1396, 1984.
9. Asdourian PL, Weidenbaum M, Dewald RL, Hammerberg KW, Ramsey RG. The pattern of vertebral involvement in metastatic vertebral breast cancer. Clin Orthop 250:164-170, 1990.
10. Phillips E, Levine AM. Metastatic lesions of the upper cervical spine. Spine 14:1071-1077, 1989.
11. Sundaresan N. Spinal metastasis: Current status and recommended guidelines for management. Neurosurgery 5:726-746, 1979.

12. King GJ, Kostuik JP, McBroom RJ, Richardson W. Surgical management of metastatic renal carcinoma of the spine. Spine 16:265-271, 1991.

13. Levine AM. Operative techniques for treatment of metastatic disease of the spine. Semin Spine Surg 2:210-227, 1990.

14. Nather A, Bose K. The results of decompression of cord or cauda equina compression from metastatic extradural tumors. Clin Orthop 169:103-107, 1982.

15. Lewis DW, Packer RJ, Raney B, Rak IW, Belasco J, Lange B. Incidence, presentation and outcome of spinal cord disease in children with systemic cancer. Pediatrics 78:438-443, 1986.

16. Harrington KD. Current concepts review—metastatic disease of the spine. J Bone Joint Surg Am 68:1110-1115, 1986.

17. Weinstein JN. Surgical approach to spine tumors. Orthopaedics 12:897-905, 1989.

18. Tan SB, Kozak JA, Mawad ME. The limitations of magnetic resonance imaging in the diagnosis of pathologic vertebral fractures. Spine 16:919-923, 1991.

19. Boland PJ, Lane JM, Sundaresan N. Metastatic disease of the spine. Clin Orthop 169:95-102, 1982.

20. Fidler MS. Anterior decompression and stabilization of metastatic spinal fractures. J Bone Joint Surg Br 68:83-89, 1986.

21. Wong DA, Fornasier VL, MacNab I. Spinal metastases: The obvious, the occult, and the impostors. Spine 15:1-4, 1990.

22. Raycroft JF, Hockman RP, Southwick WO. Metastatic tumors involving the cervical spine. J Bone Joint Surg Am 60:763-768, 1978.

23. Harrington KD. The use of methylmethacrylate for vertebral body replacement and anterior stabilization of pathological fracture dislocations of the spine due to metastatic malignant disease. J Bone Joint Surg Am 63:36-46, 1981.

24. Tokuhasi Y, Matsuzaki H. Scoring system for the preoperative evaluation of metastatic spine tumor prognosis. Spine 15:1110-1113, 1990.

25. Eftekhar NS, Thurston CW. Effect of irradiation on acrylic cement with special reference to fixation of pathological fractures. J Biomech 8:53-56, 1975.

26. Spence WT. Internal plastic splint and fusion for stabilization of the spine. Clin Orthop 92:325-329, 1973.

27. Young RF, Post EM, King GA. Treatment of spinal epidural metastases: Randomized prospective comparison of laminectomy and radiotherapy. J Neurosurg 53:741-748, 1980.

28. Smith R. An evaluation of surgical treatment for spinal cord compression due to metastatic carcinoma. J Neurol Neurosurg Psychiatry 28:152-158, 1965.

29. Stark RJ, Henson RA, Evans SJ. Spinal metastases: A retrospective survey from a general hospital. Brain 105:189-213, 1982.

30. Sundaresan N, Bains M, McCormack P. Surgical treatment of spinal cord compression in patients with lung cancer. Neurosurgery 16:350-356, 1985.

31. Tang SG, Byfield JE, Sharp TR, Utley JF, Quinol L, Seagren SL. Prognostic factors in the management of metastatic epidural spinal cord compression. J Neurooncol 1:21-28, 1983.

32. North RB, LaRocca R, North CA, et al. Surgical management of spinal metastases: Analysis of prognostic factors over a ten year experience. Submitted J Neurosurg 1995.

33. McAfee P, Bohlman HH, Ducker T, Eismont FJ. Failure of stabilization of spine with methylmethacrylate: A retrospective analysis of twenty-four cases. J Bone Joint Surg Am 68:1145-1157, 1986.

34. Roy-Camille R, Saillant G, Lapresle P, Mazel C, Mariambourg G. Traitement chirurgical des metastes du rachis par stabilisation a l'aide de plaques posterieures. Rev Chir Orthop 71:483-492, 1985.

35. Dunn EJ, Anas PP. The management of tumors of the upper cervical spine. Orthop Clin North Am 9:1065-1079, 1978.

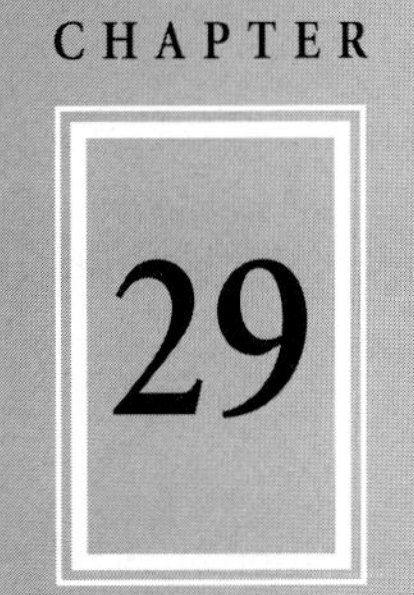

CHAPTER 29

Metastases to the Thoracic Spine and Ribs

Joseph M. Kowalski, M.D., *John G. Heller,* M.D., *and Katsuro Tomita,* M.D., Ph.D.

Advances in cancer awareness, detection, and management have prolonged the life expectancy of patients with a variety of malignant conditions. Patients are living longer and requiring treatment of recurrent disease as well as of metastatic lesions. Of the more than 1 million new cases of cancer diagnosed each year in the United States, approximately one half of the patients will eventually die of their disease. In 50% to 70% of these patients skeletal metastases will develop prior to death, with the spine being the most common site of these deposits (Table 29-1).[1-3]

Spinal metastases may require treatment because of pain, neurologic deficits, mechanical instability, deformity or any combination thereof. Treatment of clinically significant metastases therefore relates to quality of life and function within the patient's remaining life span. Recommendations for any given patient must be tailored to the particular clinical circumstance. The physician must have precise knowledge of the extent of the lesion(s) throughout the spine and within each vertebra, the primary tumor type, and the patient's life expectancy and general medical condition. Above all else, these factors must be weighed along with the patient's wishes regarding the level of intervention desired. Educating the patient and his or her family along these lines will enable them to choose the path of care that they judge most appropriate.

This chapter speaks to the management of metastatic lesions to the thoracic spine. Because each region of the spine differs anatomically, biomechani-cally, and functionally, it is reasonable to expect that there are some subtle differences in both how a lesion can affect different parts of the spine and how one might wish to treat such a lesion. In this chapter we provide a rational method of analyzing lesions to the thoracic spine and a framework for formulating treatment strategies, whether medical, surgical, or a combination of the two.

PATTERNS OF SPREAD

Tumor cells secrete a variety of substances to enhance their ability to survive, proliferate, and spread. Vascular spread is believed to be the most common method of metastasis. Increased porosity in basement membranes is just one known mechanism by which tumors gain access to the vascular system. Other factors secreted by tumor and reactive cells induce tumor angiogenesis. The dysregulation of integrins, immunoglobulins, and other adhesion molecules promote tumor growth and metastases.

Various theories have been proposed to explain the distribution of tumor metastases. The "seed and soil" hypothesis proposed by Paget stated that although the circulating tumor cells could reach all organs, only the organ that offered a cellular environment favorable to the tumor cell would allow a metastatic nidus to be established. In 1928, Ewing attempted to explain metastatic distribution on the basis of circulation. He postulated that a tumor cell would be filtered by the first capillary bed encountered. Batson[4] was the first to demonstrate bidirectional blood flow in the paravertebral venous

Table 29-1   Metastatic disease of the spine (The University of Texas M.D. Anderson Cancer Center)[3]

Primary site	No. of primary tumors	No. with spinal metastasis	% with spinal metastasis	% of total patients with spinal metastasis
Breast	13,977	3,592	25.7	30.2
Lung	10,568	2,410	22.8	20.2
Prostate	6,975	1,137	16.3	9.6
Blood	12,907	1,213	9.4	10.2
Urinary tract	5,692	478	8.4	4.0
Colon	7,107	185	2.6	1.6

plexus in cadaveric specimens. In 1940, he injected dye into the penile dorsal vein in male specimens and breast veins in female specimens and discovered that he could recover dye from the vertebral veins. He postulated that flow of venous blood in this valveless system could be bidirectional and that an increase in intra-abdominal pressure could divert blood to the epidural veins, thus providing a potential pathway of metastatic embolization. In 1951, Coman and Delong,[5] using a rat model, verified this in vivo. The azygous system of veins communicates freely with the lumbar system and provides a potential conduit for metastatic seeding from prostate and renal cell carcinomas. Venous drainage from the breast drains into the azygous system, and the proximity of the two may reflect the propensity of breast carcinoma to metastasize to the thoracic spine.

The gastrointestinal tract drains predominantly via the portal and caval systems, and therefore metastases to the liver and lung are much more common than spinal lesions. Under normal conditions, only 5% to 10% of the blood in the portal and caval systems is shunted into the paravertebral venous plexus and may account for the small number of spinal metastases from gastrointestinal carcinomas.

Once metastatic emboli are within the paravertebral venous system, they primarily seed the osseous structures. Less often, a patient may present with an epidural metastasis and, even more rarely, either subdural or intramedullary metastases.[6]

Metastatic tumors of the pediatric spine are different from those in the adult. Ewing's sarcoma and neuroblastoma are the tumors most commonly causing spinal cord compression in a child.[7] They account for more than 50% of cases, followed by osteogenic sarcoma and rhabdomyosarcoma.[7]

Approximately 85% of metastatic lesions are located within the vertebral body, and the remainder are located within the posterior arch. Local tumor invasion and hypervascularity resulting in periosteal irritation may be responsible for the initial nonmechanical pain. Typically a micro or macrofracture reflects significant vertebral involvement. Many attempts have been made to determine the risk of an impending fracture and the degree of spinal instability. Unlike long bones, the spine may continue to exhibit a degree of load-bearing capacity after fracture, and the concept of being "at risk of pathologic fracture" is not as clearly defined in the spine.

The thoracic spine has additional support provided by the rib cage. The posterior elements act as a tension band to resist kyphosis. To a lesser degree, the bone anatomy also provides a degree of vertical support that resists axial loading. The sternal-rib complex has been referred to as the "fourth column" and acts as a strut, shielding forces from compressing the anterior and middle columns.[8] Therefore the anterior strut of the sternal-rib complex and the posterior strut of an intact posterior arch may protect structural deficiencies of the anterior and middle columns, which are commonly seen in metastatic disease.

Neurologic compromise can result from direct compression by a soft tissue mass. Epidural or intradural seeding may cause neurologic compromise without any evidence of osseous involvement. The mechanism of spinal cord injury caused by tumor compression is one of progressive disturbance of the vascular flow dynamics and the cellular milieu of the spinal cord. Barron and coworkers reported[9] on 127 cases of symptomatic involvement of the spinal cord and cauda equina and observed that paraplegia evolving acutely within 48 hours was most likely to occur with bronchogenic carcinoma, lymphoma, and renal cell carcinoma. In carcinoma of the breast, the neurologic deterioration was always slower. It has been suggested that acute deterioration is the result of disruption of the arterial circulation with spinal cord infarction, whereas slowly evolving neurologic deficits are the result of venous congestion. It is thus important that rapid cord decompression be performed in patients with severe or progressing neurologic deficit that may soon become irreversible.

EVALUATION AND MANAGEMENT

The spine surgeon is only one member of the oncologic team. Treatment options must coincide with the will of the patient, and both the physician and the patient must have realistic expectations. Tumor type and stage, as well as the patient's overall health and nutrition, are factors in determining whether a patient is a surgical candidate. Because it is often difficult to predict life expectancy of any given patient, each needs to be assessed on an individual ba-

Table 29-2 Survival rate from initial accumulation of radioisotope in the spine (%)[10]

Primary site	No. of patients	6 months	12 months	3 years
Pulmonary	149	50	22	3
Breast	114	89	78	48
Prostate	59	98	83	57
Cervical	46	63	45	26
Renal	29	51	51	40
Gastric	28	19	0	0

sis. Generally accepted requirements for surgery are a minimum of 3 to 6 months' life expectancy. Tatsui et al.[10] recently reviewed the survival of patients in whom metastatic spinal column tumors had been diagnosed (Table 29-2). Serial bone scans were performed on 2372 patients, beginning at the time of initial diagnosis. During follow-up, 425 patients were found to have spinal metastases. The 1-year survival rate from the diagnosis of spinal metastasis ranged from 22% for lung cancer to 83% for prostate cancer.

Treatment options may be either curative or palliative. When the goal is curative, complete excision with wide, clean margins is the goal. This is often difficult, if not impossible, in the spine because tissue planes and compartments do not exist as they do in other parts of the body. Palliation is the goal for most tumors in the spine. Maintaining independence and adequate pain control can have a significant impact on the quality of life for a patient with metastatic disease.

The great majority of spinal metastases respond favorably to nonsurgical methods, such as chemotherapy, radiation therapy, and hormonal manipulation. Medical and radiation oncologists are the best resources to identify those patients who are suitable candidates. Edema from spinal cord compression responds favorably to corticosteroids and is commonly employed. Nonsurgical modalities, however, have little or no effect on restoring spinal anatomy once fracture or deformity has occurred. The definitive way to debulk the tumor mass, decompress neural elements, and restore and stabilize the anatomy is through surgical intervention.

Indications for surgical intervention of metastatic spinal disease include the following[11-13]:

1. Intractable pain that is unresponsive to nonoperative measures, such as bracing, chemotherapy and radiation therapy
2. The need to establish a histologic diagnosis
3. A tumor previously irradiated or known to be resistant to chemotherapy or radiation therapy
4. Spinal instability manifested as a pathologic fracture, progressive deformity, or neurologic deficit
5. Clinically significant neural compression, especially by bone or bone debris

There is no consensus regarding how much bone destruction begets spinal instability; however, instability may be presumed if radiographic studies reveal[14-17] translational deformity, vertebral body collapse greater than 50%, three-column involvement (as defined by Denis[17]), or involvement of the same column in two or more adjacent levels. Instability may be present without evidence of neural compromise and, by definition, is aggravated by loads applied to the affected area. The goals of surgical treatment in metastatic spinal disease are as follows[14,15]:

1 Decrease the patient's pain
2. Preserve or improve neurologic function
3. Stabilize the patient's spine to maintain spinal function without the need for an external orthosis

Harrington[18] devised a five-category classification scheme for metastatic spine tumors based on bone destruction and neurologic compromise (see box on p. 415). Harrington recommended that patients with class I or II disease be treated nonoperatively with chemotherapy, hormonal manipulation, or local irradiation. Class IV or V lesions require surgi-

<table>
<tr><td colspan="2">

Harrington's Five Classification Categories for Metastatic Tumors

</td></tr>
<tr><td>Class I</td><td>Asymptomatic involvement of bone</td></tr>
<tr><td>Class II</td><td>Symptomatic vertebral lesions defined by pain with or without minor neurologic involvement but without collapse or instability</td></tr>
<tr><td>Class III</td><td>Major neurologic impairment (motor or sensory) without significant collapse of bone, usually due to epidural extension of tumor</td></tr>
<tr><td>Class IV</td><td>Vertebral collapse with pain due to mechanical causes or instability but without significant neurologic compromise</td></tr>
<tr><td>Class V</td><td>Vertebral collapse and instability combined with major neurologic impairment</td></tr>
</table>

cal intervention, provided that host factors and life expectancy warrant aggressive intervention. They should be treated with surgical decompression and stabilization followed by adjunctive radiation therapy. Although Harrington thought that class III lesions should generally be treated with radiation and chemotherapy, we believe that they represent a gray area where the physician has wide latitude in exercising judgment regarding medical or surgical intervention.[19] Also, lesions unlikely to respond to radiation or chemotherapy, regardless of their Harrington class, are candidates for operative intervention.

Kostuik and coworkers[20] believe that the need for surgical intervention is based on spinal stability. Employing a two-column concept of spinal architecture, they attempted to define stability. This is in contrast to the three-column concept described by Denis[17] for thoracolumbar spine fractures. In the two-column concept, the anterior column consists of the entire vertebral body, including the cortex, while the posterior column consists of the pedicles, laminae, and spinous process. The anterior column is further divided into anterior and posterior halves, as well as left and right sides, which results in four quadrants within the vertebral body. The posterior column is divided into left and right

sides, for a total of six vertebral segments. On the basis of a retrospective study Kostuik et al.[20] believed that the spine was stable if no more than two of the six segments were destroyed. Stability thus determined the need for surgical intervention. McLain and Weinstein[21] proposed a similar but more complicated structural subdivision of vertebral metastases.

Taneichi et al.[22] analyzed the extent of vertebral involvement by metastatic lesions so as to predict the likelihood of pathologic fracture. The fracture risk of a given vertebra was then used to guide the timing and type of intervention. Their work was the first to prove the differences in prognosis for lesions in various regions of the spine. Previously, such differences had been inferred from regional biomechanical differences in the spine. Clear distinctions were reported in the extent of vertebral involvement required for fracture between the thoracic, thoracolumbar, and lumbar spine. As Panjabi and White[23] proposed, the ribs contribute a stabilizing effect on the thoracic spine. Thus an anterior column lesion must involve 50% to 60% of a thoracic (T1 to T10) vertebra vs. 35% to 40% of a thoracolumbar or lumbar vertebra before pathologic fracture is likely. They also noted that destruction of the pedicle has a far more detrimental effect in the thoracolumbar and lumbar spine than in the thoracic spine, again presumably because of the contribution of the rib cage. Because radiation and chemotherapy rely on bone healing to restore spinal integrity, which takes months, the authors implied that the extent of vertebral involvement and fracture risk may be used as guides for surgical intervention.

Spiegel et al.[24] sought to define the surgical indications for spinal metastases among patients with a particular tumor type. They evaluated the clinical course of 114 patients with melanoma metastatic to the spine. Their study is unique in that such studies do not exist for the more prevalent tumors that metastasize to the spine. They found that location and number of nonspinal metastases strongly influenced patient survival and could be used to define a subset of patients who were unlikely to benefit from surgery. Skin or lymph node spread did not affect survival, whereas the number of visceral metastases did. Patients with only one site of visceral metastases survived twice as long as those with two or more sites of visceral lesions (mean,

111 days vs. 57 days). Surgery was therefore not to be recommended for the latter subgroup. The presence of a neurologic deficit did not significantly influence survival among patients with melanoma.

In 1990 Mutsuzaki et al.[25] proposed a scoring system for vertebral metastases that was intended to assist the oncology team in determining the need for and type of surgery required. The scheme takes into account six variables: general medical condition, number of extra-spinal bone metastases, number of vertebral metastases, visceral metastases, primary tumor type, and presence of neurologic deficit. Enkaoua et al.[26] independently evaluated the utility of the Tokuhashi scoring system in the management of patients with three different primary tumors. In reviewing the outcome of vertebral metastases, most of which involved the thoracic spine, from thyroid carcinoma, renal cell carcinoma, and carcinoma of unknown origin, they noted a significant difference in survival as a function of tumor type. The median survival times were 2, 9, and 33 months for unknown primary origin, renal, and thyroid carcinoma, respectively. When the other variables were factored in, patients with a Tokuhashi score greater than 7 had a median survival of 24 months, whereas those with a score less than or equal to 7 survived 5 months. Enkaoua et al.[26] affirmed the prognostic value of the Tokuhashi score, but they did recommend assignment of fewer points for carcinoma of unknown primary origin than originally proposed because of the worse prognosis for this subgroup. The system is of some help in deciding which patients clearly warrant surgery and, to some extent, what type of surgery should be considered. There is still latitude for judgment in the case of patients with a score less than or equal to 7, because quality of remaining life may still be significantly enhanced through palliative techniques with relatively low morbidity.

Tomita and Kawahara (personal communication, April 1998) have tried to take this approach one step further, so that a scoring system might be used not only to determine whether a patient is a candidate for surgical intervention but also to guide the selection of surgery. Their scheme attempts to add metrics to the variables that have been loosely weighed by surgeons struggling to exercise judgment in any given case. Points are assigned for the tissue of tumor origin and the presence of both visceral and bone metastases. Tomita and Kawahara then factor in the general aim of treatment and type or extent of spinal metastases. Thus one has some structure to guide the choice of treatment across the spectrum of potential clinical circumstances. The Tomita system may indicate that wide or marginal excision is indicated to attempt long-term control of an isolated spinal lesion, terminal medical care, or a compromise wherein the goals of surgery are to stabilize the spine, thereby controlling pain and protecting the neural elements. The Tomita scoring system appears to blend in the favorable features of the strategies described here. It then takes us one step further in the thought process of designing the appropriate surgical strategy.

Surgical Treatment

Deciding where to make the incision or incisions to approach a thoracic lesion must take into account the location of the tumor and the oncologic, neurologic, and biomechanical goals of surgery. There are three generic places that a thoracic incision can be made: posterior, lateral and anterior. These incisions, in turn, provide three lines of sight: posterior or posterolateral, lateral, and anterior, respectively. Surgeons' thinking has evolved toward believing that anterior vertebral lesions necessitate anterior solutions and, conversely, that posterior problems beget posterior solutions. To some extent this is both logical and practical. The anatomy of the thoracic region, however, allows a wider latitude in the selection of effective solutions for metastatic problems.

Anterior Approaches

For many years laminectomy was synonymous with surgery for spinal metastases. In the 1970s, studies reporting the results of decompression and reconstruction via anterior approaches began to appear. In 1981, Harrington[27] reported on vertebral body resection and reconstruction with polymethylmethacrylate (PMMA). He noted a greater than 90% improvement in neurologic function and pain relief. Siegal and Siegal prospectively compared patients who underwent surgical decompression of malignant tumors treated through an anterior approach with those treated through a posterior approach.[28] Eighty percent of the patients treated with anterior vertebrectomy maintained the ability to ambulate compared with 40% of the patients treated with laminectomy. Eighty percent of the patients treated from an anterior approach had neurologic improvement, whereas 25% of the patients treated with laminectomy deteriorated. Also, there was a significantly higher rate of complications due to infection and wound healing in the laminectomy group; this was attributed to operating through irradiated tissue. Kostuik et al.,[29] DeWald et al.,[14] McAfee and Zdeblick,[13] and Kaneda and Takeda[15] have reported similar results with excellent pain relief in more than 90% of patients and significant neurologic improvement in the majority of patients with anterior procedures.

A thoracotomy provides access to the thoracic spine from T3 to L1. Unless strongly influenced by the location of the tumor, one generally uses a left-sided approach lower in the thoracic spine. Higher lesions are easier to access from the right because of the position of the aortic arch. A thoracotomy allows for thorough piecemeal resection of one or more involved vertebral bodies, with optimal visualization of the floor of the spinal canal. Direct reconstruction of the anterior column and anterior spinal instrumentation are readily performed through this exposure.

For patients with a single pathologic fracture and a primary goal of palliation, we would consider reconstructing a corpectomy defect with PMMA. The PMMA acts as a grout that should serve to provide clinical stability for at least 1 to 2 years. It should be anchored to the adjacent vertebrae with either an adaptation of distraction instrumentation, as recommended by Harrington, or some variation on the theme. We prefer to use either titanium staples or makeshift "staples" fashioned from Steinmann pins. For patients with a longer anticipated survival, one should consider a biologic union. The options include vertical cages, or diaphyseal allografts supplemented with autogenous bone graft, or a tricortical iliac bone graft (Fig. 29-1). Anterior spinal instrumentation is required under such circumstances. Furthermore, when such a biologic union is sought, postoperative irradiation and chemotherapy are probably best delayed for 6 to 12 weeks to avoid interference with early graft revascularization. If the patient's medical condition warrants early aggressive chemotherapy, or if his or her long-term survival is uncertain, then a compromise approach would be reasonable. This would entail using the PMMA

method initially and then considering a supplemental posterior instrumentation and fusion in 1 to 2 years if the patient has responded well to treatment. Lesions above T4 are more difficult to access and may require a median sternotomy.

A median sternotomy and its various modifications provide excellent, albeit limited, access to the upper thoracic spine or cervicothoracic junction. The exposure is essentially a caudal extension of a left-sided anterior cervical exposure, the lower extent of which is limited by the aortic arch. We favor the left side because of the risk of recurrent laryngeal nerve injury on the right. However, one must be cognizant of the location of the thoracic duct, which may cross from right to left at the inferior extent of the exposure. Ligation of the thoracic duct should be considered if it is at risk of injury, as it is easier to control at this time, rather than risking a chylothorax. Single or multilevel corpectomies and reconstruction can be performed. Anterior spinal plates are difficult to apply through this exposure because of the restricted trajectory available for the instruments. Supplemental posterior instrumentation may be indicated.

Posterior or Posterolateral Approaches

In this day and age a posterior approach should not be misconstrued to imply performance of a laminectomy alone. For the reasons already stated, it would be almost unheard of to perform such an operation in a tumor patient. Granted, a laminectomy for neural decompression may be an essential component of a posterior procedure. However, its destabilizing effect would then be offset by adjunctive posterior segmental instrumentation, with or without fusion. Contemporary modular instrumentation systems allow the surgeon to select a fixation method, depending on local vertebral morphology and bone integrity. Hooks (sublaminar, pedicle, or transverse process), screws (pedicle or transverse process), or cables (sublaminar or transspinous) may be used in any combination to render a rigid construct. Knowledge of all areas of vertebral involvement should be factored into the selection of the instrumented levels, because it is generally wise to extend the purchase two or three levels beyond any known adjacent lesions (Fig. 29-2).

The surgical options with a posterior incision are uniquely broad in the thoracic spine. Because the T2 through L1 nerves can be sacrificed with im-

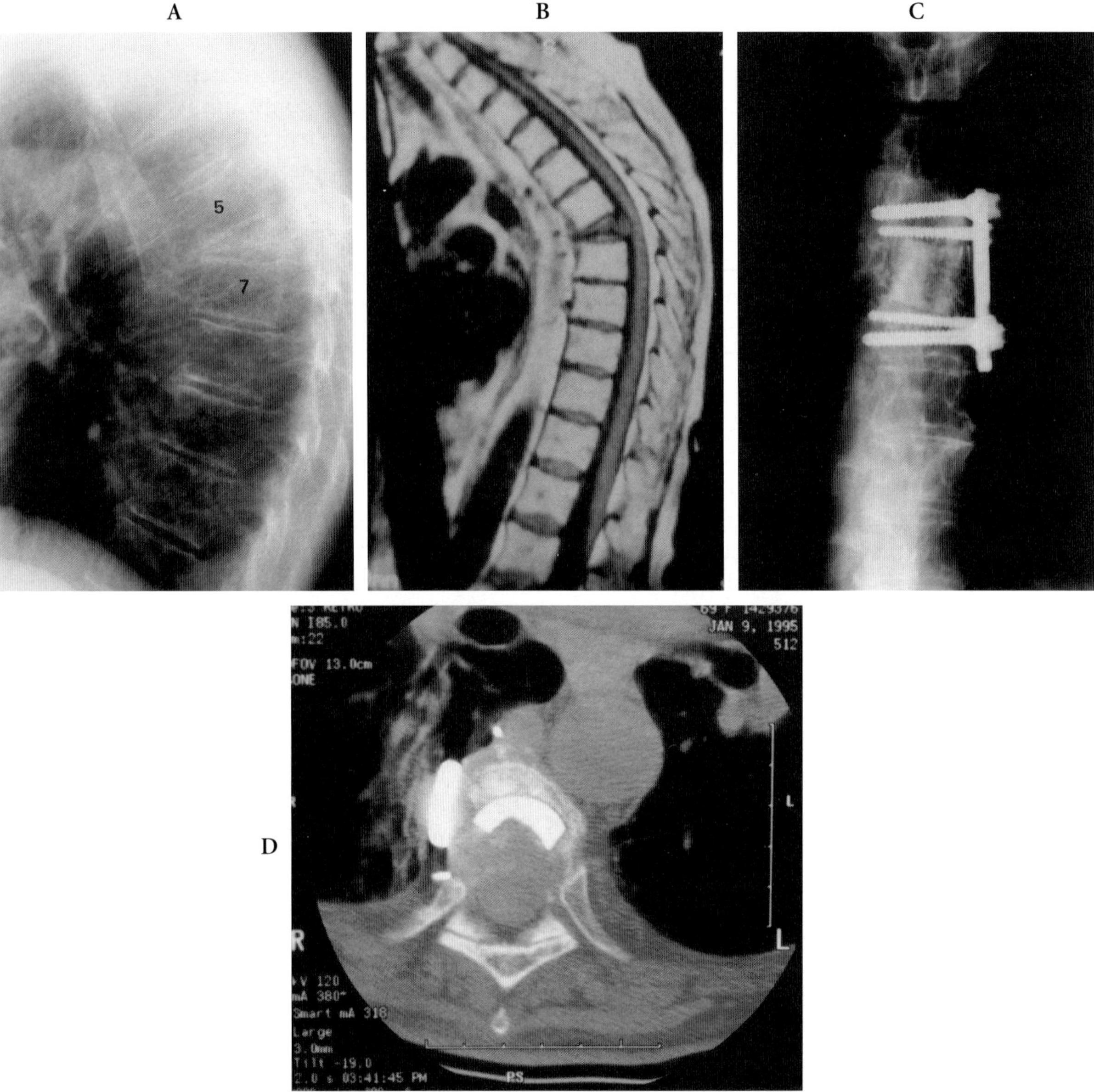

Fig. 29-1   **A,** Lateral radiograph of a 61-year-old patient with myeloma. There has been complete collapse of the T6 vertebra, leaving an angular kyphotic deformity. **B,** Sagittal MRI scan of the same patient shows marked cord compression from retropulsed bone and tumor. The patient presented with paraparesis secondary to this pathologic fracture. When retropulsed bone is the offending material causing cord compression, radiation therapy alone is usually inadequate. **C,** The patient underwent urgent anterior decompression with T6 corpectomy and spinal canal decompression. The vertebral body was reconstructed with a strut graft and an anterior thoracic Z-plate. This anteroposterior radiograph shows the stability obtained with thoracic plating. **D,** Postoperative CT scan demonstrating the adequacy of the spinal canal decompression, the lateral placement of the thoracic plate, and the cortical strut graft.

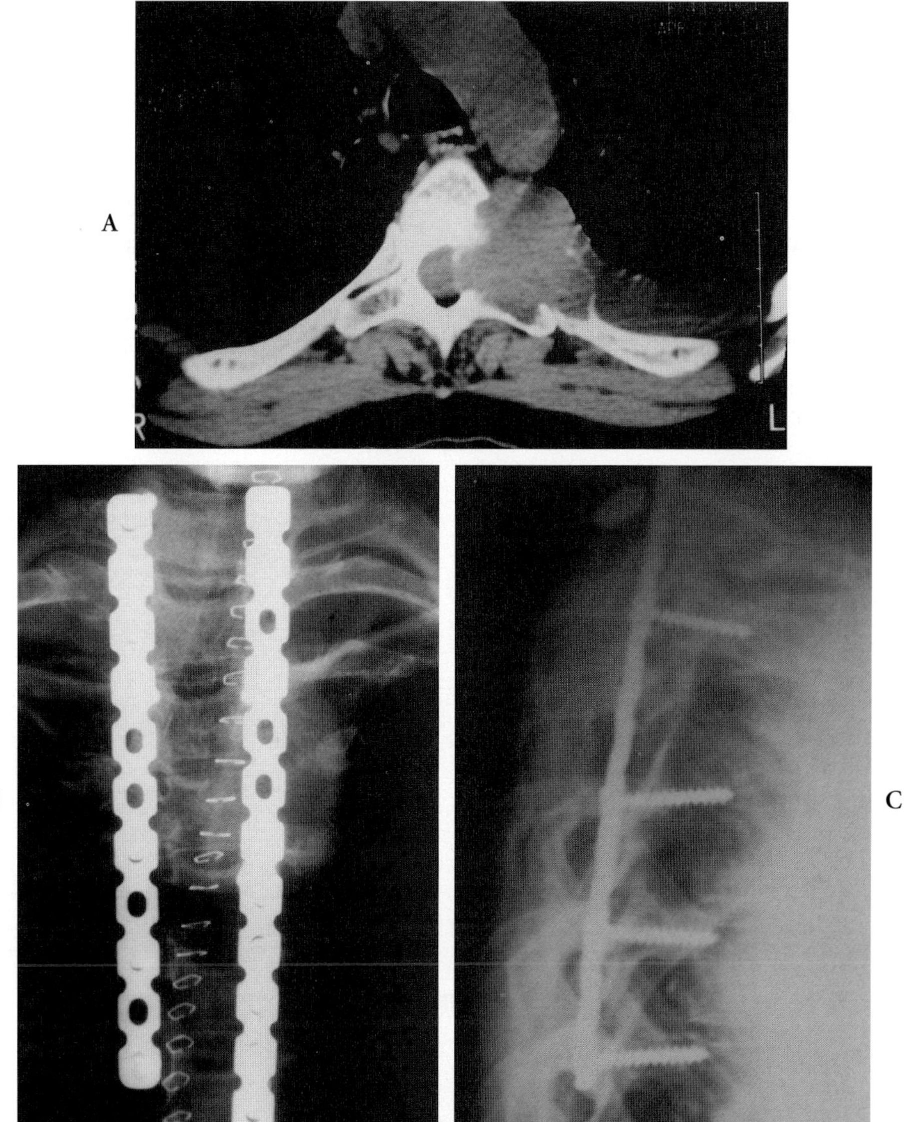

Fig. 29-2 **A,** Thoracic metastases that are posterior or lateral are accessible through a posterior or lateral extracavitary approach. This 61-year-old woman has metastases from a uterine carcinoma involving the pedicle and lateral portions of the vertebral body and transverse process of T3. Unilateral cord compression is present. **B,** A posterior decompression was performed; this involved costotransversectomy, laminectomy, and tumor excision, including a portion of the chest wall. Reconstruction was performed posteriorly with reconstruction plates and pedicle screws. This anteroposterior radiograph shows the postoperative appearance of the reconstruction plates. **C,** Lateral radiograph demonstrates the placement of the pedicle screws in the upper thoracic and lower cervical spine for posterior reconstruction.

punity, it is possible to surgically remove vertebral bodies through such an incision and to reconstruct the anterior column. For surgeons with an anterior bias the visibility is less than optimal, but these options can be of considerable value to patients and surgeons alike. Through removal of the pedicles and rib heads and ligation of the intercostal nerves and vessels, the vertebral bodies can be approached. One can then perform a decompression ranging from a piecemeal intralesional resection, much like what one can accomplish through a thoracotomy, to a total en bloc spondylectomy (TES) as described by Tomita et al.[22,30,31] Total en bloc spondylectomy is an oncologic radical resection of a spinal tumor. The eligibility of a given lesion for this procedure may be determined by Tomita's scoring system for vertebral metastases and by the lesion's classification. A TES is performed through a single posterior exposure and has two principal phases: (1) en bloc laminectomy and provisional posterior instrumentation and (2) en bloc corpectomy and combined reconstruction of the anterior and posterior columns. Use of the novel "T-saw" reduces the risk of nerve root and spinal cord damage during osteotomy of the pedicles and division of the anterior column. Reconstruction of the anterior column defect is also possible through such exposures, but it requires some finesse and attention to detail to avoid spinal cord injury. Such spacers or bone grafts should ultimately be loaded under compression by the posterior instrumentation (Fig. 29-3).

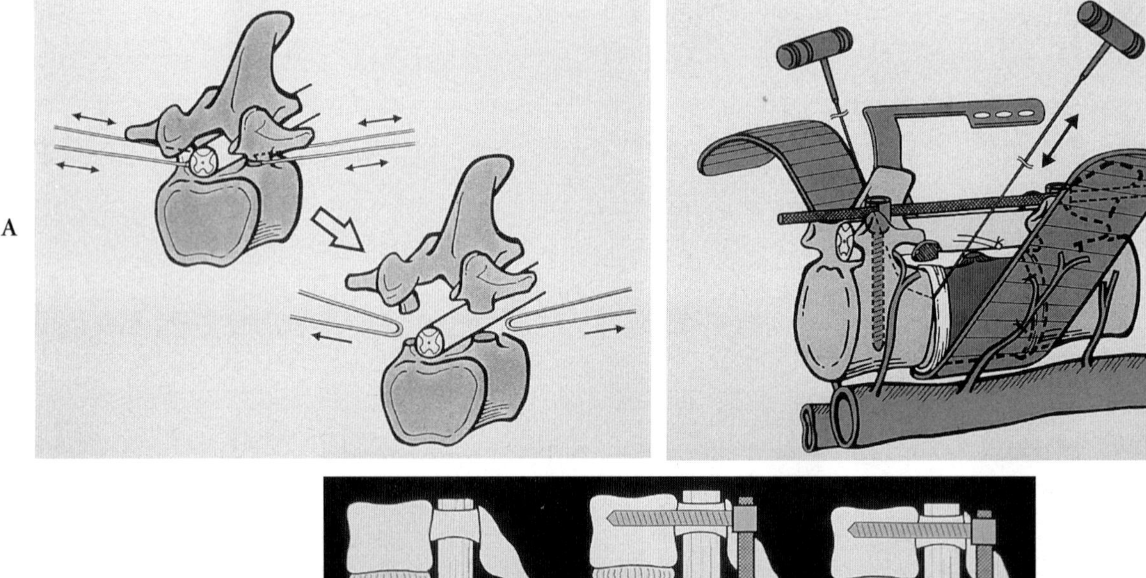

Fig. 29-3 Total en bloc spondylectomy (TES). **A,** A T-saw is passed around each pedicle to perform an osteotomy. **B,** After provisional segmental instrumentation, specialized retractors are used to protect the great vessels and spinal cord as the anterior column is divided with a T-saw. **C,** The area of the anterior defect is reconstructed and placed under compression before bone grafting of the posterior column is done.

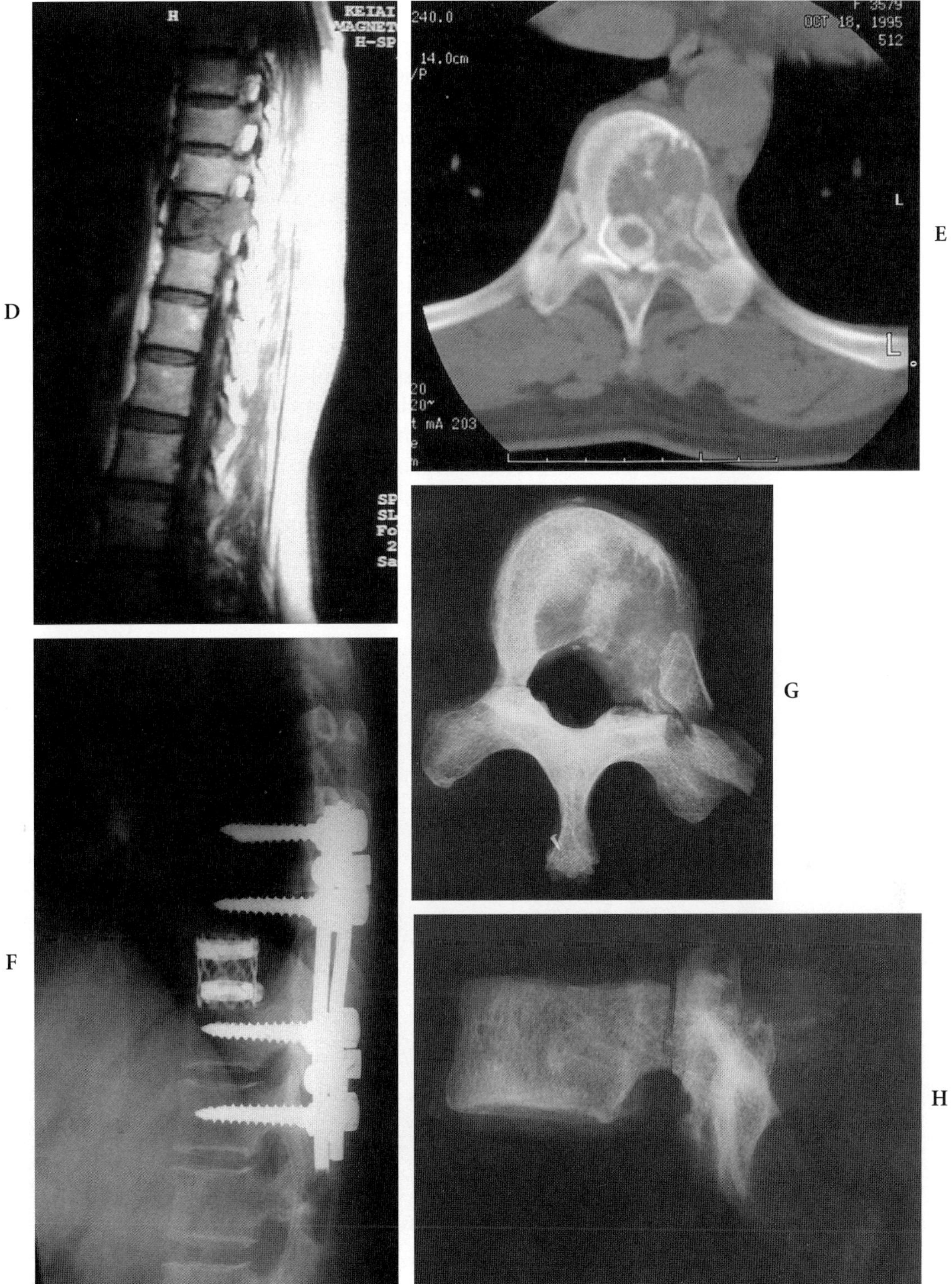

Fig. 29-3, cont'd   Sagittal MRI (**D**) and CT scan (**E**) of a 54-year-old woman with an isolated breast cancer metastasis at T10. Lateral postoperative radiograph following TES (**F**). Axial (**G**) and lateral (**H**) radiographic views of the resected specimen. Note the minimal bone loss at the pedicle osteotomy sites.

A few technical notes are in order to make posterior circumferential thoracic reconstructions easier and safer. Obtaining provisional unilateral segmental fixation before removal of the vertebral body(ies) can lessen the risk of iatrogenic paralysis. This point is especially important near the thoracolumbar and cervicothoracic junctions. As biomechanically transitional regions, they are not as inherently stable as the mid-thoracic spine, and they tend to move with respiration while the patient is prone on the operating table. When one is operating on the high thoracic spine, we recommend immobilization of the head and neck in a neutral position with a Mayfield head fixator or its equivalent.

Combined Approaches

In certain instances it is difficult, if not impossible, to decompress the spinal cord and reconstruct the spinal column through a single approach. Although posterolateral decompression and tumor débridement can be effective, the tumor mass can be located in such a position that an anterior procedure is the only practical option for safely and adequately decompressing the spinal cord. Also, hemorrhage may be easier to control from an anterior exposure. If there is multiple-level disease and instability (≥2 vertebral bodies), however, then posterior instrumentation is required in addition to the anterior reconstruction (Fig. 29-4).

If posterior decompression and resection are necessary, it may be advantageous to begin posteriorly. Instrumentation should be done first to stabilize the spine and should include two to three levels beyond the involved levels as described here. Then spinal cord decompression and tumor resection can be performed. If spinal cord decompression

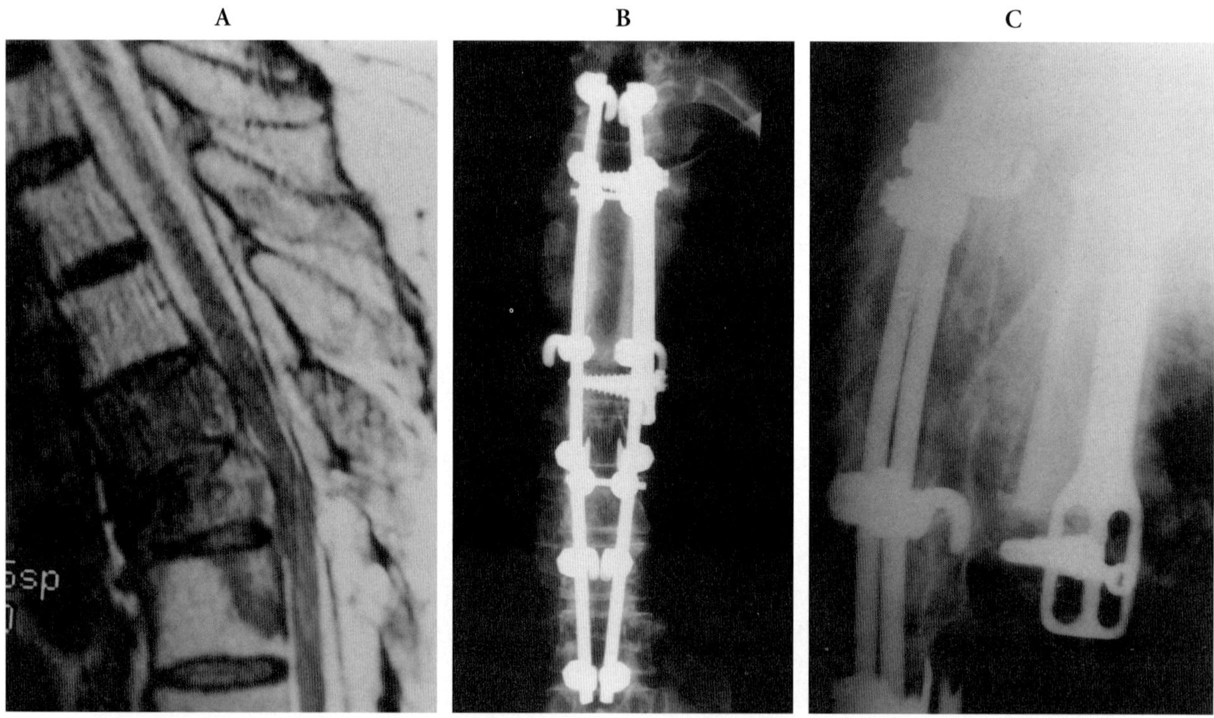

Fig. 29-4 **A,** Metastases in the upper to mid thoracic spine may require extensive reconstruction. This 50-year-old woman with breast carcinoma presented with paraparesis and three-level disease involving the T2, T3, and T4 vertebral bodies. Sagittal MRI scan discloses the amount of spinal canal involvement. **B,** Surgical reconstruction was carried out with both an anterior and a posterior approach. Anteriorly a three-level corpectomy was performed with strut graft placement and a thoracic Z-plate. Posterior stability was obtained with a segmental hook rod construct. For metastatic lesions requiring greater than two-level corpectomy, anterior and posterior reconstruction is recommended. **C,** Lateral radiograph demonstrates the nature of the multilevel strut grafting and plating.

or tumor resection cannot be adequately accomplished from this single posterior approach, then an anterior approach can be used. One advantage of this sequence is that the spine is stabilized first, and then additional tumor resection can be performed as the clinical situation allows. Since the spine is stable, this can be done either immediately after the posterior procedure or in delayed fashion.

Epidural bleeding can be problematic during circumferential posterior procedures. The surgeon commonly agonizes about how much pressure may be safely applied with hemostatic agents (e.g., Gelfoam and thrombin, Surgicel, or Avitene), or how liberal one may be with bipolar coagulation. As for the latter, it may be very helpful to use an angled fine-tipped bipolar forceps to coagulate the epidural vessels adjacent to the zone of resection as the exposure proceeds. This will minimize any retraction of the dura. A thick paste made from powdered Gelfoam and thrombin can be gently packed into the epidural space above and below the intended area of decompression. Finally, Tomita has developed a clever method of infusing fibrin glue under low pressure into the epidural space.[32] This dramatically reduces bleeding by gluing the dura to the walls of the spinal canal, thus imposing tamponade of the epidural vessels. The safety method has been proven in laboratory experiments, and its clinical utility has been validated in our practices.

Ligation of the intercostal nerves warrants comment, too. The length of the thoracic epidural sleeve is generally short but variable. On the one hand, it is desirable to leave a long enough stump to minimize any risk of dural leak, but on the other hand a lengthy stump interferes with visibility and may be inadvertently caught by an instrument (e.g., a curette or power burr), causing a dural tear or spinal cord injury. Some judgment is in order, but we recommend double suture ligation of the proximal stump, regardless of the length. Treating a subarachnoid-pleural fistula can be frustrating. Conventional methods like a diverting lumbar cisternal drain are unlikely to succeed because of the negative intrapleural pressure generated with respiration. In such instances, or in the event that the tumor or fracture has created an irreparable dural tear, an anterior transdiaphragmatic omental pedicle flap can readily seal the leak.

Wound healing complications have been more prevalent with posterior incisions than with thoracotomies, especially if radiation preceded the surgical procedure.[28] There are probably four treatable risk factors for wound dehiscence and the associated risk of secondary infection. First, such patients tend to be relatively inactive and to spend considerable time in bed. Therefore bulky instrumentation or prominent spinous processes can exert undesirable pressure on the incision, interfering with local perfusion and healing. Second, ill-fitting orthoses may exert a similar effect. We recommend using the lowest-profile instrumentation possible, resecting any amount of spinous process that protrudes dorsal to the implants, and designing the operation to leave the patient brace free.

The third risk factor for dehiscence is preoperative radiation therapy. If one chooses to operate through an irradiated posterior field, one should consider enlisting the help of a plastic surgeon to close the wound with local trapezial or latissimus dorsi advancement flaps. Alternatively, one can advise the patient of the potential for such problems, reserving such a plastic procedure for the first sign of failure of wound healing. Persistent or spontaneous wound drainage should be taken as an ominous sign. Early aggressive intervention is easier and more practical at this stage than after a secondary infection is established.

Finally, patient nutrition warrants comment. Anorexia and malnutrition are common among tumor patients, both before and after surgery. This may be due to effects of the tumor itself, medical treatment, depression, or any combination thereof. Rather than fighting an uphill battle trying to convince someone with no appetite to eat, the treating team should have a low threshold for recommending insertion of a percutaneous endoscopic gastrostomy tube (PEG). This is readily accomplished before, during, or after surgery. The PEG is much more convenient for the patient, the family, and the health care team. Adequate nutrition is assured during a critical phase of treatment.

CONCLUSION

In summary, the treatment of thoracic metastases requires knowledge of tumor type, natural history and longevity, and amount of local invasion. Specific surgical therapy is directed toward preservation of spinal cord function and spinal stability, as well as pain reduction and functional improvement.

REFERENCES

1. Boland PJ, Lane JM, Sundaresan N. Metastatic disease of the spine. Clin Orthop 169:95-102, 1982.
2. Jaffe WL. Tumors and Tumorous Conditions of the Bones and Joints. Philadelphia: Lea & Febiger, 1958.
3. York JE, Wildrick DM, Gokaslan ZL. Metastatic Tumors. In Benzel EC, Stillerman CB, eds. The Thoracic Spine. St. Louis: Quality Medical Publishing, 1999, p 393.
4. Batson OV. The function of the vertebral veins and their role in the spread of metastases. Ann Surg 112:138, 1940.
5. Coman DR, Delong RP. The role of the vertebral venous system in the metastasis of cancer to the spinal column. Cancer 4:610, 1951.
6. Brihaye J, Ectors P, Lemort M, Van Houtte P. The management of spinal epidural metastases. Adv Tech Stand Neurosurg 16:121-176, 1988.
7. Klein SL, Sanford RA, Muhlbauer MS. Pediatric spinal epidural metastases. J Neurosurg 74(1):70-75, 1991.
8. Berg EE. The sternal-rib complex: A possible fourth column in thoracic spine fractures. Spine 18(13):1916-1919, 1993.
9. Barron KD, Hirano A, Araki S, Terry RD. Experiences with metastatic neoplasms involving the spinal cord. Neurology 9:91, 1959.
10. Tatsui H, Onomura T, Morishita S, Oketa M, Inoue T. Survival rates of patients with metastatic spinal cancer after scintigraphic detection of abnormal radioactive accumulation. Spine 21:2143-2148, 1996.
11. Asdourian PL. Metastatic disease of the spine. In Bridwell KH, DeWald RL, eds. The Textbook of Spinal Surgery, 2nd ed. Philadelphia: Lippincott-Raven, 1997, pp 2007-2050.
12. Siegal T, Siegal T. Current considerations in the management of neoplastic spinal cord compression. Spine 14(2):223-228, 1989.
13. McAfee PC, Zdeblick TA. Tumors of the thoracic and lumbar spine: Surgical treatment via the anterior approach. J Spinal Disord 2(3):145-154, 1989.
14. DeWald RL, Bridwell KH, Prodromas C, Rodts MF. Reconstructive spinal surgery as palliation for metastatic malignancies of the spine. Spine 10:21-26, 1985.
15. Kaneda K, Takeda N. Reconstruction with a ceramic vertebral prosthesis and Kaneda device following subtotal or total vertebrectomy in metastatic thoracic and lumbar spine. In Bridwell KH, DeWald RL, eds. The Textbook of Spinal Surgery, 2nd ed. Philadelphia: Lippincott-Raven, 1997, pp 2071-2087.
16. Kern MB, Malone DG, Benzel EC. Evaluation and surgical management of thoracic and lumbar instability. Contemp Neurosurg 18:1-8, 1996.
17. Denis F. The three column spine and its significance in the classification of acute thoracolumbar spinal injuries. Spine 8:817-831, 1983.
18. Harrington KD. Current concepts review: Metastatic disease of the spine. J Bone Joint Surg Am 68(7):1110-1115, 1986.
19. Heller JG, Pedlow FX. Tumors of the spine. In Garfin SR, Vaccaro AR, eds. Orthopaedic Knowledge Update: Spine. Chicago: American Academy of Orthopaedic Surgeons, 1997, pp 235-256.
20. Kostuik JP, Errico TJ, Gleason TF, Errico CC. Spinal stabilization of vertebral column tumors. Spine 13(3):250-256, 1988.
21. McClain RF, Weinstein JN. Tumors of the spine. Semin Spine Surg 2:157-180, 1990.
22. Taneichi H, Kaneda K, Abumi K, Satoh S. Risk factors and probability of vertebral body collapse in metastases of the thoracic and lumbar spine. Spine 22:239-245, 1997.
23. Panjabi MM, White AA. Physical properties and functional biomechanics of the spine. In Panjabi MM, White AA, eds. Clinical Biomechanics of the Spine. Philadelphia: JB Lippincott, 1990, pp 1-83.
24. Spiegel DA, Sampson JH, Richardson WJ, Friedman AH, Rossitch E, Hardacker WT, Seigler HF. Metastatic melanoma to the spine: Demographics, risk factors, and prognosis in 114 patients. Spine 20:2141-2146, 1995.
25. Tokuhashi Y, Matsuzaki H, Toriyama S, Kawano H, Ohsaka S. Scoring system for the preoperative evaluation of metastatic spine tumor prognosis. Spine 15:1110-1113, 1990.
26. Enkaoua EA, Doursounian L, Chatellier G, Mabesoone F, Aimard T, Saillant G. Vertebral metastases: A critical appreciation of the preoperative prognostic Tokuhashi score in a series of 71 cases. Spine 22:2293-2298, 1997.
27. Harrington KD. The use of methylmethacrylate for vertebral-body replacement and anterior stabilization of pathologic fracture-dislocations of the spine due to metastatic malignant disease. J Bone Joint Surg Am 63:36-46, 1981.
28. Siegal T, Siegal T. Surgical decompression of anterior and posterior malignant epidural tumors compressing the spinal cord: A prospective study. Neurosurgery 17(3):424, 1985.
29. Kostuik JP. Anterior spinal cord decompression for lesions of the thoracic and lumbar spine: Techniques, new methods of internal fixation results. Spine 8:512-531, 1983.
30. Tomita K, Kawahara N, Baba H, Tsuchiya H, Nagata S, Toribatake Y. Total en bloc spondylectomy for solitary spinal metastases. Int Orthop 18:291-298, 1994.
31. Tomita K, Kawahara N, Baba H, Tsuchiya H, Fujita T, Toribatake Y. Total en bloc spondylectomy; a new surgical technique for primary malignant vertebral tumors. Spine 22:324-333, 1997.
32. Kawahara N, Tomita K, Mizuno K, Toribatake Y, Takino T. Hemostasis in total en bloc spondylectomy—Epidural injection of firin glue. J Jap Orthop Assoc 70:151, 1996.

Metastases to the Lumbar Spine

Thomas A. Zdeblick, M.D.

Metastatic disease affecting the lumbar or lumbosacral spine is much less common than that of the thoracic spine. However, because of the increased loads on the lumbar spine and the lack of additional bone support, such as is provided by the rib cage in the thoracic spine, metastatic lesions to the lumbar spine may result in a higher incidence of instability and subsequent collapse. As in other areas of the spine, metastatic lesions of the breast, prostate, and lung are among the tumors that most commonly metastasize to the lumbar vertebrae.[1] In addition, renal cell carcinoma most often affects the upper lumbar vertebral body by means of direct extension through vascular structures. Certainly, when any patient with a known diagnosis of cancer presents with unremitting low back pain, metastatic lesions should be ruled out.

This chapter will delineate the specific indications for surgery in the lumbar spine. In addition, a variety of surgical approaches that are appropriate in the lumbar and lumbosacral spine will be discussed.

DIAGNOSTIC EVALUATION

The diagnosis of lumbar metastatic disease requires a high degree of suspicion. As in other areas of the spine, radiographic studies are relied upon. Plain radiographs are helpful and should be obtained in all patients with chronic low back pain that is unremitting. On the anteroposterior (AP) view, the absence of a pedicle is often the first harbinger of metastatic disease. In addition, lateral compression fractures or erosions of the transverse process may be seen as well. It is important to obtain an AP radiograph of the sacrum. Sacral lesions are often difficult to diagnose radiographically, but a specific AP x-ray film may show a loss of the sacral foraminal contours. On lateral radiographs, end plate fractures and subtle compression of the vertebral bodies are the earliest findings. In our experience, standing films of the lumbar spine are much more instructive than supine films. Finally, blastic lesions, as can be seen in prostate cancer as well as in breast carcinoma, are best visualized on lateral radiographs.

A bone scan and a lumbar magnetic resonance imaging (MRI) scan should be part of the metastatic workup as well. Bone scanning is effective at ruling out occult metastases and is a screening test. The lumbar MRI is most sensitive at picking up early vertebral metastases. Although there can be confusion between the hematoma from an acute benign compression fracture and a metastatic lesion, most radiographers can differentiate these two with gadolinium contrast. When in doubt, a repeat MRI scan after 3 to 4 weeks of symptoms will help differentiate a compression fracture from a metastatic lesion. The differential diagnosis between metastatic disease and infection may not always be clear. Again, the use of gadolinium contrast should make this differential diagnosis apparent.

Computed tomography (CT) scanning may be helpful in delineating the amount of bone destruction. CT myelography is rarely used. In cases of preexisting lumbar deformity this may be helpful. In general, however, lumbar MRI scanning has replaced CT myelography in the workup of metastatic lesions. MRI scan is more accurate in determining the intradural extent of tumor, the soft tissue extent, and involvement of adjacent vertebrae. When in doubt, the combination of lumbar MRI and plain lumbar CT is excellent.

MANAGEMENT
Nonsurgical Therapy

Most metastatic lesions of the lumbar or lumbosacral spine can be treated without surgery.[2] If they are diagnosed early on the basis of pain and radiographic findings, radiation therapy plus bracing is the treatment of choice. I prefer the use of an antiflexion device, such as the Jewitt brace, for lesions between T7 and L2. For lesions of the lumbar spine, a molded lumbosacral orthosis corset is helpful. Bracing performs two functions. It is helpful in controlling pain while patients are in the early phases of radiation therapy, and it helps prevent a kyphotic collapse during the healing phase. In general, I recommend 10 to 12 weeks of bracing from the onset of radiation therapy. This allows adequate time for tumor destruction and vertebral reossification.

The patient who can be treated with radiation therapy and bracing alone is a patient who has no neurologic deficit, minimal compression fracture, no significant kyphosis, and no bone retropulsion compromising the canal. In addition, the patient who is severely debilitated or has a short life expectancy can be treated nonoperatively. In general, persons with metastatic lesions from the lung to the lumbar spine have a poor prognosis and a short life span. Surgery is rarely indicated in these patients. Also, patients with multiple metastases involving three or more contiguous vertebrae are rarely candidates for surgery.

Surgical Therapy

When a patient has a neurologic deficit, significant bone retropulsion, local kyphosis greater than 20 degrees, or massive bone destruction, surgery can be helpful.[3] Direct consultation with the patient's oncologist, primary care physician, and family is necessary before one embarks on surgical treatment of vertebral body metastases. Rarely is this surgery curative; the patient's longevity and quality of life must be considered in each case.[4] In my experience the patients who do best with surgery for metastatic disease are those who have a diagnosis of either breast cancer, prostate cancer, myeloma, or renal cell carcinoma. If this is the first bone metastasis and is a solitary metastasis, surgery is particularly helpful. In some of these cases the decision needs to be made between en bloc excision and intralesional débridement.

En bloc excision is possible in the lumbar spine because of the mobile nature of the cauda equina.[5] In certain lesions, en bloc excision may be not only helpful but also occasionally curative. For solitary metastases of renal cell carcinoma that have no soft tissue extension, solitary breast carcinoma lesions, and chordoma, I have had success with en bloc excision and spinal stabilization. For the vast majority of lesions, however, intralesional débridement, stabilization, and grafting constitute the procedure of choice. Rarely, stabilization alone is indicated.[6,7]

Surgical Approaches

The level of the lesion in the lumbar and lumbosacral spine dictates the type of surgical approach possible. In the upper lumbar or thoracolumbar spine with a conus medullaris and proximal cauda equina, posterior approaches are less successful than an anterior approach.[8] Most metastatic lesions involve the vertebral body, and neurologic compression is almost always done through an anterior approach. In these patients a retroperitoneal exposure and a vertebral corpectomy provide the best view of the thecal sac for decompression (Fig. 30-1). The approach must be individualized to each patient. Often a lesion will involve one pedicle or the other. The approach should be from the side of the pedicular involvement. This allows a more complete debulking of the tumor. If the tumor is centrally located, I prefer a left-sided retroperitoneal approach. From this approach, it is easier to retract the retroperitoneal structures without having the liver present.

High Lumbar Lesions. In general, for lesions at L1 or L2 the bed of the eleventh or twelfth rib is used for access. Most of the time the diaphragm can be left intact, and the approach can be retroperitoneal or retropleural.[9] Occasionally the diaphragm may need to be detached posteriorly for lesions at L1. Once the retroperitoneal space is entered, blunt dissection exposes the vertebral body as well as the body above and below the diseased area. The segmental vessels at each level are ligated and divided. The psoas muscle must be retracted in an anterior-to-posterior direction to completely expose the lateral margin of each vertebral body. I prefer to expose the lateral aspect of each pedicle and palpate each neuroforamen to maintain orientation to the vertebral body. Anteriorly, exposure should be to the midline of the vertebral body. Retractors should be placed anteriorly to protect the great vessels.

Tumor excision begins with excision of the disc above and below the vertebral body. Once this is performed, the tumor can be rapidly excised with rongeurs and curettes. In cases of highly vascular tumors, preoperative embolization may be necessary. However, when bleeding is encountered during tumor removal, surgeons should work rapidly and use thrombin-soaked Gelfoam or Avitene as necessary for hemostasis. In particular the lumbar epidural tumors may be prone to a great deal of bleeding. Bipolar coagulation may be necessary as well. I tend to remove the posterior longitudinal ligament and visualize the dura across the width of the decompression. All visible tumors should be removed during the débridement.

In general, I leave the end plates above and below the débridement intact. The end plate cartilage can be gently removed with a curette. An allograft humerus or femur strut is preferred for vertebral body reconstruction (Fig. 30-2). These are easily shaped and have a broad weightbearing surface. As an alternative a titanium mesh cage can also be used. Primary anterolateral plate fixation is my stabilization of choice. In most patients, anterolat-

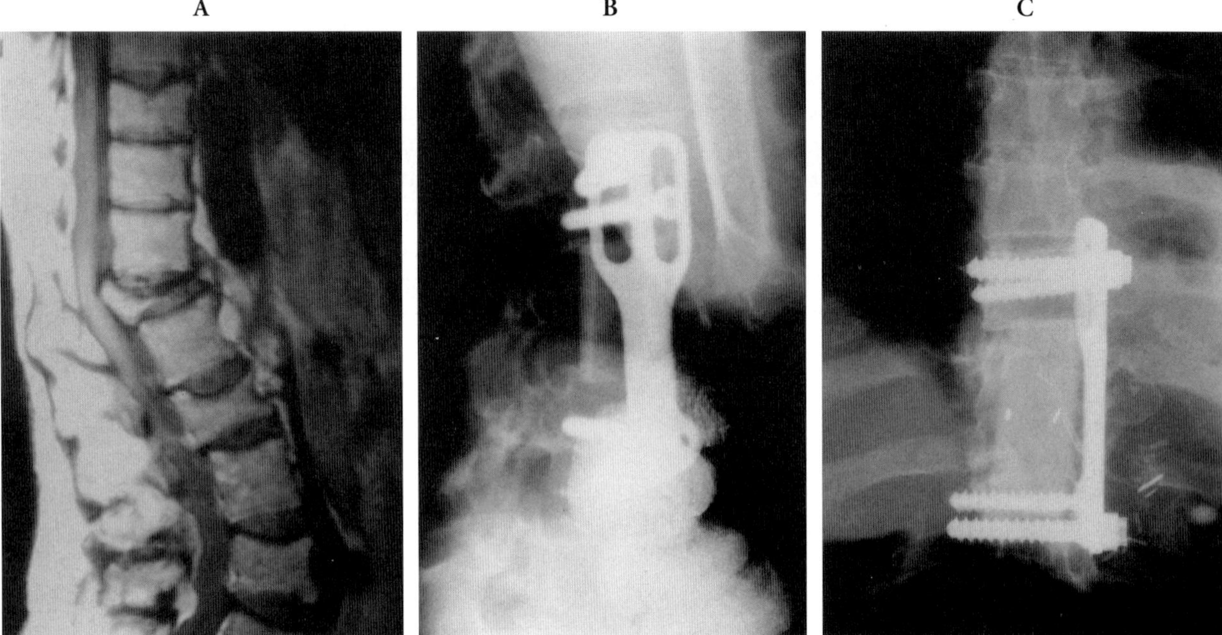

Fig. 30-1 A thoracolumbar pathologic fracture with retropulsion of bone developed in a 70-year-old man with prostate carcinoma. Lower extremity weakness prompted his referral. **A,** Sagittal MRI scan shows the amount of retropulsed bone causing spinal cord compression. The kyphotic deformity is noted. **B,** Surgical treatment was carried out with a thoracolumbar anterior approach, corpectomy, and spinal reconstruction. Allograft humerus bone was used, as well as a lumbar Z-plate. This lateral radiograph shows the restoration of sagittal alignment. **C,** This anteroposterior radiograph shows the strut graft for reconstruction of and the placement of the plate and screws.

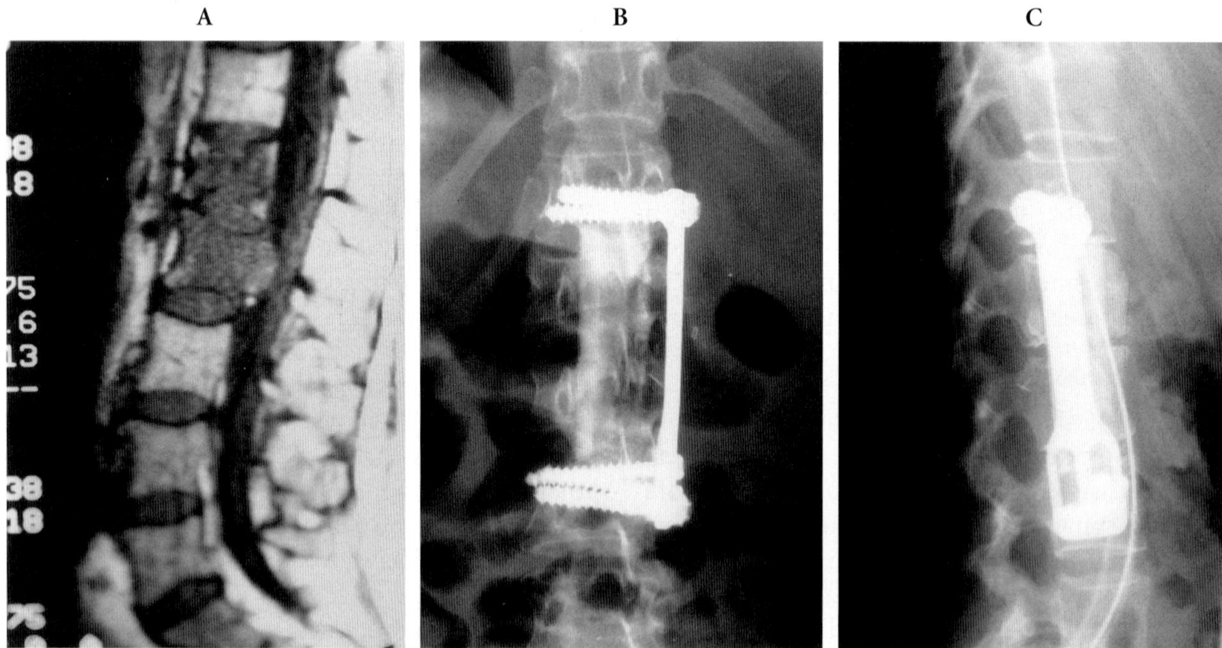

Fig. 30-2 **A,** Two-level reconstruction is possible from an anterolateral approach alone. This 60-year-old woman presented with lower extremity weakness. The sagittal MRI scan shows tumorous replacement of L1 and L2 with a pathologic compression fracture of L2 and tumor causing spinal canal compression. **B,** Surgery was performed with anterolateral decompression of the spinal canal by means of corpectomy of L1 and L2. A femoral shaft was used for a strut graft reconstruction, followed by anterolateral plating. This anteroposterior radiograph demonstrates that the twelfth rib was used for the approach and shows the extent of the strut reconstruction. **C,** This lateral radiograph demonstrates the normal sagittal alignment and the placement of the lateral plate.

eral plate stabilization alone provides stability and allows brace-free recovery postoperatively. In patients with severe osteoporosis, polymethylmethacrylate (PMMA) can be placed into the vertebral bodies, above and below, before bolt and screw placement. This acts as a grout, increasing the purchase power of the bolts and screws. In patients with short life expectancies, methacrylate can also be used as the strut for reconstruction of the vertebral bodies. In most cases in which life expectancy is more than 6 months, however, I prefer allograft reconstruction for long-term stability.

Low Lumbar Lesions. In the low lumbar spine, anterior reconstruction may not be the procedure of choice. Particularly at L4 and L5, exposure of the vertebral bodies is more difficult because of the size of the psoas muscle. In addition, reconstruction options may be limited because of the placement of the iliac vessels. In low lumbar cases the surgeon has two options. One is to perform all surgery from a posterior approach. The other is to provide stabilization through a combined anterior and posterior approach. Because of the mobility of the cauda equina a more aggressive posterior debulking of the tumor can be performed. This requires wide laminectomy and vertebral body debulking from either side of the cauda equina. The difficulty here is control of bleeding. For tumors that involve the pedicle and posterior elements in only a small portion of the vertebral body, however, this approach can be excellent. Stabilization using pedicular fixation is then provided (Fig. 30-3). In those cases in which there is central neurologic compromise and marked collapse of the vertebral body, a combined anterior and posterior approach may be necessary. In these patients débridement and strut grafting are

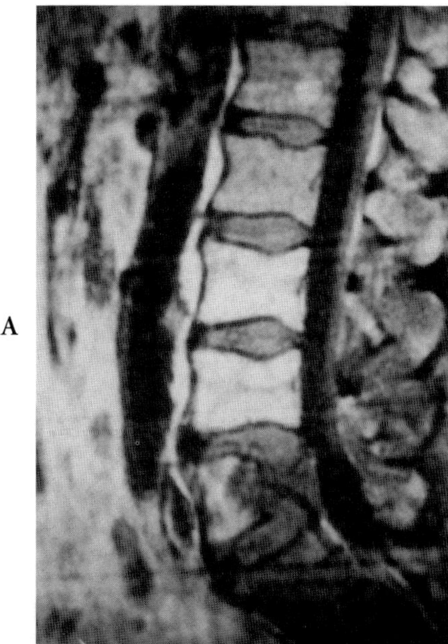

A

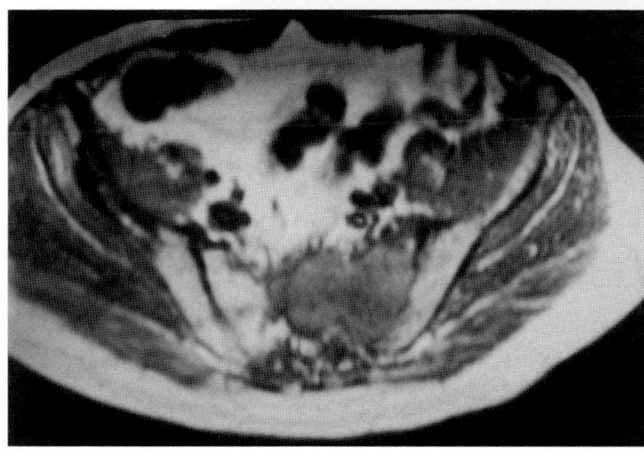

B

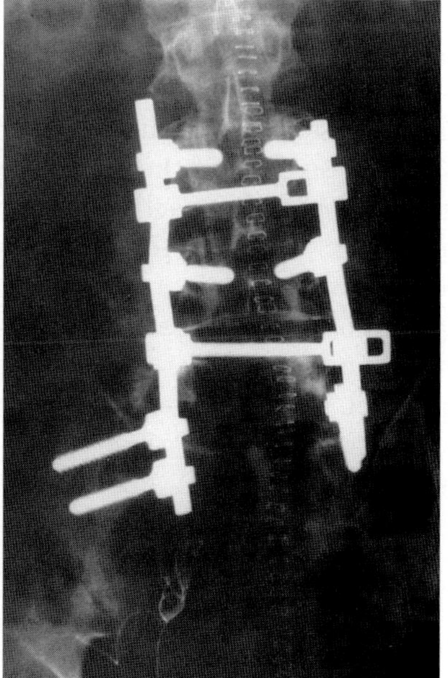

C

Fig. 30-3   A, Lesions of the sacrum and low lumbar spine are usually approached posteriorly. This 68-year-old woman with breast carcinoma presented with loss of bowel and bladder control and increasingly severe pain. This sagittal MRI scan shows pathologic fracture of L5 and involvement of the proximal sacrum. **B,** The axial MRI scan shows the extent of sacral bone destruction. **C,** A posterior approach was used with tumor debulking. Preoperative vessel occlusion was performed radiologically. Posterior reconstruction was performed with the use of pedicle screws in the low lumbar spine and iliac screws in the sacrum.

performed from the anterior approach. Here I usually prefer a direct anterior approach with the patient in the supine position. This allows exposure of the vertebral body without significant retraction of the psoas. Once again, after débridement an allograft strut graft can be placed. Because of the inability to perform anterolateral plate fixation to the sacrum, however, posterior fixation is indicated. In these patients the anterior débridement and strut grafting are performed first, the patient is carefully turned prone, and posterior pedicular fixation is applied. I have found this to be the most common procedure for significant lesions of the low lumbar spine with marked destruction, collapse, or neurologic deficit.

Sacral Lesions. Finally, for lesions that involve the sacrum, a great deal of surgical planning is necessary. If stability is intact and there remains a weightbearing column in the anterior sacrum, then posterior debulking alone is possible. With significant lesions that replace the sacrum or that require sacrectomy, however, more involved surgery is necessary. Often these procedures are performed in conjunction with a general surgeon and an orthopedic oncologic surgeon. Both anterior and posterior exposure of the sacrum is required. Anteriorly the great vessels are controlled and osteotomies are performed just medial to the sacroiliac joints bilaterally. The L5-S1 disc space is incised and removed circumferentially. The patient is then turned into the prone position. Posterior fixation is obtained, with pedicular fixation in the lumbar spine and transiliac fixation into the pelvis. Complete sacrectomy can then be performed by tying off the appropriate level of the dural sac and removing the sacrum en bloc. Stabilization is provided with rods bridging the lumbar pedicular screws and the transiliac screws. I prefer two screws within each ilium and a cross-link between rods. Obviously these are complex cases. Often the assistance of a general surgeon for a diverting colostomy and a plastic surgeon for soft tissue coverage posteriorly is required. Most cases requiring sacral resection should be performed in a tertiary referral center.

Complete Vertebrectomy. In addition, en bloc excision of the lumbar vertebra may be indicated for a curative procedure, as when the diagnosis is a chordoma. For an en bloc excision to be successful, the tumor must be confined within the vertebral margins and limited to one or two levels. The excision is performed from an anterior and a posterior approach. Initially the posterior approach is used. Transpedicular fixation is provided two levels above and two levels below the planned resection. Once all screws are placed, the posterior elements of the affected vertebrae are resected. If the posterior elements are involved with tumor, they need to be removed completely. If they are uninvolved, they may be left in place to provide additional surface area for posterior fusion. The pedicle needs to be transected at the level of the involved vertebrae on either side. I do this with an exposure through a laminectomy as well as a posterolateral approach. Once the pedicle is exposed, a Gigli saw is used to transect the pedicle at its most anterior margin. Retraction of the nerve root and protection with a nerve root retractor are required during this phase. Once the pedicles are divided, the posterior annulus and the posterior longitudinal ligament are divided across each disc space above and below the lesion. This should be done to the midline on either side with protection of the cauda equina. Once this is accomplished, posterior stabilization is finalized with the placement of rods and bone graft. The posterior wound is then closed.

The patient is carefully turned into the lateral position and a retroperitoneal exposure of the vertebral body in question is performed. Segmental vessels are ligated at the level of the involved vertebra, as well as one level above and below. The discectomy is completed above and below the involved vertebra. This discectomy must involve complete division of the annulus circumferentially and the anterior longitudinal ligament. This is done by placing retractors completely around the vertebral body to include the contralateral side. The contralateral segmental vessels must be controlled as well. Once this is accomplished, the vertebral body can be rolled toward the surgeon with division of the remaining posterior epidural adhesions. The vertebral body can then be removed intact. Anterior reconstruction is performed with an anterior allograft strut and, if necessary, an anterolateral plate.

CONCLUSION

In conclusion, metastatic disease of the lumbar spine requires an individualized approach for a successful result. A high degree of suspicion, appropriate radiologic studies, and preoperative planning are all necessary to obtain a successful result. Patient selection is key; the patient must have a tumor diagnosis and life expectancy appropriate for major reconstructive surgery. Attention to detail and the avoidance of complications are necessary to obtain excellent patient results.

REFERENCES

1. Silverberg BS, Lubera BBA. Cancer statistics, 1987. CA Cancer J Clin 37:2-19, 1987.
2. Arcangeli G, Micheli A, Arcangeli GG, Giannarelli D, La Pasta O, Tollis A, Vitullo A, Ghera S, Benassi M. The responsiveness of bone metastases to radiotherapy: The effect of site, histology, and radiation dose on pain relief. Radiother Oncol 14(2):95-101, 1989.
3. Harrington KD. Orthopaedic Management of Metastatic Disease. St. Louis: CV Mosby, 1988, pp 309-338.
4. Tomita K, Kawahara N, Baba H, Tsuchiya H, Nagata S, Toribatake Y. Total en bloc spondylectomy for solitary spinal metastases. Int Orthop 18:291-298, 1994.
5. Bridwell KH, Jenny AB, Saul T, Rich KM, Grubb RL. Posterior segmental spinal instrumentation (PSSI) with posterolateral decompression and debulking for metastatic thoracic and lumbar spine disease: Limitations of the technique. Spine 13:1383-1394, 1988.
6. Zdeblick TA. Z-plate anterior thoracolumbar instrumentation. In Aebi M, Thalgott JS, eds. Manual of Internal Fixation of the Spine: Principles and Techniques in Spine Surgery. Philadelphia: Lippincott-Raven, 1996, pp 77-86.
7. Sundaresan N, Bains M, McCormack P. Surgical treatment of spinal cord compression in patients with lung cancer. Neurosurgery 16(3):350-356, 1985.
8. Kostuik JP, Errico TJ, Gleason TF, Errico CC. Spinal stabilization of vertebral column tumors. Spine 13(3):250-256, 1988.
9. McAfee PC, Zdeblick TA. Tumors of the thoracic and lumbar spine: Surgical treatment via the anterior approach. J Spinal Disord 2(3):145-154, 1989.

Metastatic Lesions of the Pelvis and Acetabulum

Joseph Benevenia, M.D., *Charles S. Cathcart*, M.D., *William M. Parrish*, M.D., *and Juluru P. Rao*, M.D.

Metastatic disease of bone affects the axial skeleton in 80% of patients.[1] Of the axial sites, the spine is most commonly involved, followed by the pelvis, ribs, and scapula.[1,2] Although axial involvement is common, the most symptomatic lesions are in the appendicular skeleton. The femur region most commonly requires surgery (50% to 75%), followed by the humerus (15% to 20%).[3] Pelvic metastases are due to cancers of the breast, lung, prostate, kidney, and thyroid and to multiple myeloma.[2-6] The pelvic lesions that most often require surgery are due to metastatic breast and renal carcinoma.[4,7-11] Pelvic (acetabular) lesions can be extensive, and the orthopedic surgeon must consider several factors before treatment recommendations are made.

BIOMECHANICAL CONSIDERATIONS

The pelvis and acetabulum have a complex musculoskeletal geometry. Bone destruction can be extensive but may spare the weightbearing axis. Lesions that involve the pubis and obturator region cause local pain when they compress the adductor muscles and obturator nerve. Lesions of the ilium also may elicit symptoms because of local involvement of the abductors and iliopsoas. Sacroiliac joint involvement may or may not include sacral alar invasion. In all of these patterns, operative intervention is seldom necessary, and symptomatic treatment with radiation and analgesia is sufficient (Fig. 31-1). Lesions of the acetabulum may compromise bone integrity and lead to pathologic fracture. Lesions presumed to involve the weightbearing regions should be evaluated for pathologic fracture and potential for surgical intervention.

DIAGNOSTIC EVALUATION
Patient Assessment

Patients with presumed or documented metastatic disease of bone should have a complete history and physical examination. Communication with the referring physician is essential to successful management. Patients with a history of head and neck or gastrointestinal malignancy (both of which uncommonly metastasize to bone) should be evaluated for possible secondary carcinomas. (Lung cancer

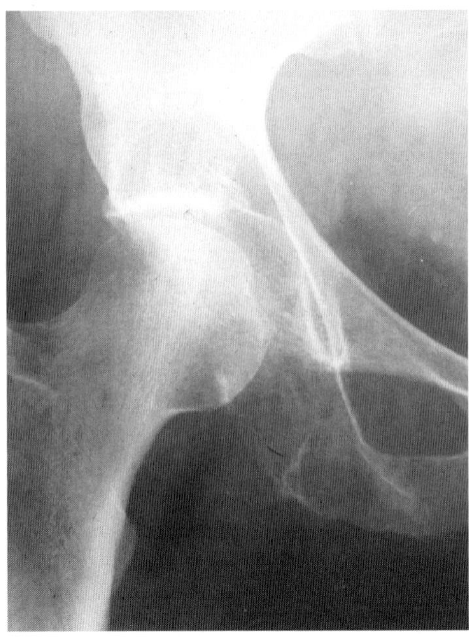

Fig. 31-1 Plain radiograph of 60-year-old woman with stage IV lymphoma. The patient's painful ischial lesion was successfully treated with chemotherapy and radiation.

may occur in 15% to 30% of patients with head and neck carcinomas.) Patients with groin or buttock pain should be examined for spinal or femoral lesions, which are common.[1-3] After a complete physical examination is performed, basic systemic parameters need to be evaluated. A plain chest roentgenogram, complete blood count, calcium and phosphorus levels, and liver function tests may help assess the extent of systemic disease.

Radiographic Assessment

Musculoskeletal imaging should include plain radiographs of the pelvis with Judet views to assess the anterior and posterior columns and medial wall. Magnetic resonance imaging is useful for evaluating soft tissue masses, but computed tomography (CT) is probably the most valuable modality for assessing the osseous pelvis. CT can also help evaluate the soft tissue extent of many tumors. Three-dimensional reconstruction is available to help accurately plan complex reconstructions (Fig. 31-2). Whole-body technetium bone scanning is used to evaluate contiguous bone regions, such as the sacrum, lumbar spine, and femora.

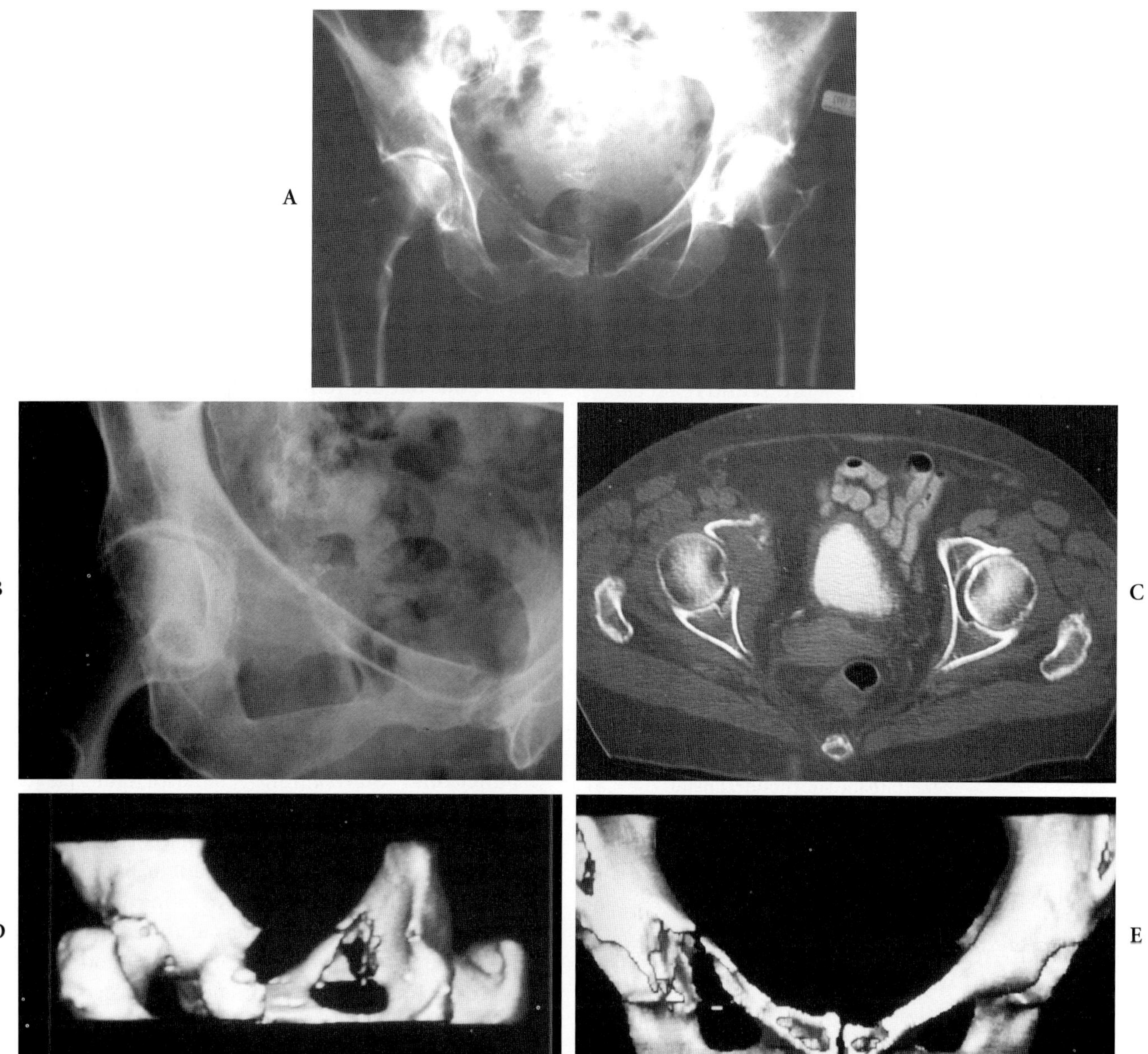

Fig. 31-2   Seventy-eight-year-old woman with metastatic breast carcinoma. **A,** Anteroposterior pelvis. **B,** Judet view. **C,** CT scan. **D** and **E,** 3-dimensional reconstruction.

CLASSIFICATION OF ACETABULAR AND PELVIC INSUFFICIENCY

Pelvic and acetabular insufficiency has been characterized by several authors.[12-14] Despite the descriptive literature on treatment of specific deficiencies, there have been no reports on the natural history of defects of the acetabular bone. Unlike the evaluation systems done in long bones and the spine, there have been no reports indicating the relationship between bone loss and mechanical integrity or fracture risk.

The Harrington system is the most widely used classification of acetabular insufficiency.[12] This system was later modified by Levine to include nonar-

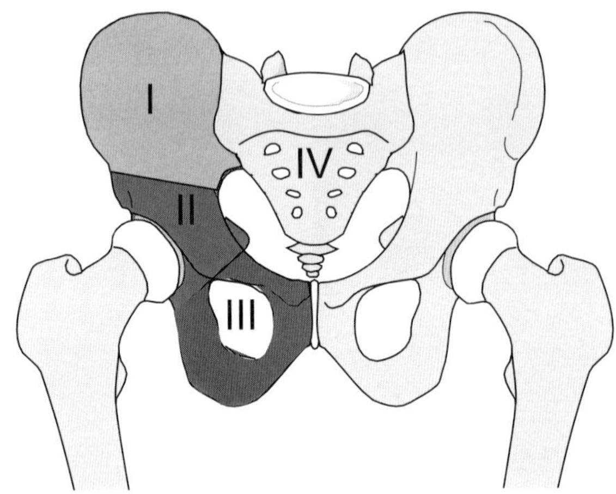

Fig. 31-3 Enneking-Dunham classification of the basic types of pelvic resections: ilium *(I)*, acetabulum *(II)*, ischium-pubis *(III)*, and sacrum *(IV)*. In addition, the classification includes "A," which indicates bone only, and "B," which indicates soft tissue resections.

Harrington Classification (Modified) of Acetabular Insufficiency

Class 0	Supra-acetabular lesion that does not penetrate the subchondral plate
Class I	Contained defect involving the acetabulum with intact lateral cortices, medial wall, and superior dome
Class II	Defect of the medial wall of the acetabulum
Class III	Defect of the lateral cortices, medial wall, and superior dome
Class IV	Resection of lesion is required for cure

---

ticular defects[13] and is based on the anatomic extent of the lesion and necessary treatment (see box above). In addition to the Harrington classification, the system proposed by Enneking and Dunham describes the type of resection necessary and is used for primary tumors and more extensive metastatic lesions[15] (Fig. 31-3).

MANAGEMENT

The treatment of acetabular bone metastases is primarily nonoperative. There have been no data to support prophylactic radiation or surgical treatment in asymptomatic lesions. A painful pelvic acetabular lesion must be evaluated on the basis of several factors: the anatomic location of the pelvic lesion, the histology of the primary tumor, the extent of the patient's systemic disease, the patient's functional status, the presence of a pathologic fracture, and the goals of treatment.

Location of Primary Tumor. Pelvic lesions involving the ilium, ischium, pubis, and sacroiliac joint may constitute a pain problem only. In the event of progression of bone destruction and pathologic fracture, simple rest and radiotherapy may be all that are required. Lesions involving the acetabular weightbearing axis may remain painful and progress to pathologic fracture. There have been no studies to predict fracture risk from extent of bone involvement.

Systemic Disease. Patients with extensive parenchymal involvement, such as lung, liver, bone marrow, and spine, and hypercalcemia can pose challenging perioperative management problems and should be counseled prior to surgery. Patients experience a minimum of 1 L of blood loss during surgery and may require prolonged rehabilitation following reconstruction.

Functional Status. The patient's pain level should be assessed by noting the type of analgesia required for relief of symptoms (narcotic vs. nonnarcotic pain medication). The patient's ambulatory status should be assessed by noting the limitation of walking and use of external assistive devices. Patients requiring nonnarcotic analgesia and using only a cane may not be candidates for surgery.

Primary Tumor. In the event that the patient has responded to a previous course of chemotherapy and radiation, nonoperative management should be considered, especially in breast carcinoma and myeloma. In the case of lesions resistant to chemotherapy and radiotherapy, such as renal carcinoma and hepatoma, operative treatment may be the only option available to maintain ambulatory status and pain relief (Fig. 31-4).

Pathologic Fracture. Patients with pathologic fractures of the ilium and pubic ramus can be managed nonoperatively. Gainor and Buchert showed that the probability of union for a pathologic fracture primarily depends on survival time.[16] In 129 fractures the overall fracture healing rate was 35%. Of patients with fractures due to myeloma, 67%

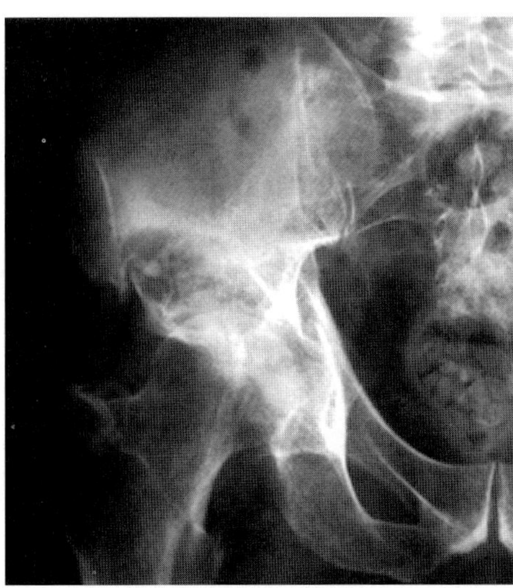

Fig. 31-4 Sixty-five-year-old man with pathologic fracture following radiation therapy for metastatic hepatoma.

healed, whereas no patient with lung carcinoma healed or survived longer than 6 months. In those patients surviving longer than 6 months, 74% of fractures healed. Internal fixation improved fracture healing by 23%, and radiation therapy has not been shown to specifically inhibit pelvic fracture healing.

Goals of Treatment. The goals of treatment in metastatic disease of the pelvis and acetabulum are pain control and maintenance of ambulatory status. The use of nonnarcotic analgesics and limited community ambulation are realistic goals. Advanced recreational activities with impact loading and complete pain relief are unrealistic. When these limitations are clearly outlined for patients, an informed decision can be made.

In a recent study of patients with advanced insufficiency (class III-IV) the average Musculoskeletal Tumor Society–International Society of Limb Salvage (MSTS-ISOLS) score[17] for function, supports, walking ability, and gait was 2.6 out of 5, or 53% maximum.[18]

Radiotherapy

Radiation therapy can be used as a primary treatment modality for pelvic bone metastases. Radiosensitive tumors (e.g., myeloma) that are small or in nonweightbearing areas are best suited for this form of treatment (Fig. 31-5).

Radioresponsive lesions, such as breast carcinoma and myeloma, heal after radiation therapy. Patients with several involved bones and extensive destruction may not be candidates for surgical reconstruction, and radiation may be the best alternative. Patients with lung carcinoma have short survival overall, and lesions almost never heal after radiation. Pain relief, however, can be achieved in the majority of patients, with response rates on the order of 70% at 3 months after completion of radiotherapy.[19] The utility of radiation for asymptomatic metastases is unknown.

Postoperative radiation has been shown to improve survival and function in one series. Townsend et al. found that the addition of radiation to surgery improved the functional status of the extremity from 12% to 53% and survival from 3 to 12 months.[6] Harrington showed that with a combination of surgery and radiation, 80% of patients were ambulatory at 6 months.[12]

The fractionation schedule of radiotherapy to pelvic metastases should be tailored to patients based on their overall performance status and prognosis.[20] The majority of patients should be treated with 10 fractions of 3 Gy to a total dose of 30 Gy. Patients with high performance and expected long-term survival should be treated with 2 Gy fractions on a daily basis to an overall dose of 40 Gy. Poor performance patients, for whom the physical demand of multiple treatments may be burdensome, can be considered for a single high-dose treatment. For selected patients with multiple symptomatic lesions of the pelvic area in whom matching multiple radiation fields might be technically difficult, lower hemibody radiation treatment may be useful but requires hospitalization, hydration, and antiemetics.[21,22]

The technique of radiation should also be customized for individual patients. Most lesions of the acetabular region are safely treated with opposed posteroanterior (APPA) fields. Oblique fields are useful for posterior iliac crest lesions because they limit the dose to the bowel. Lesions of the midline can be treated with APPA fields or with a single field with the patient in the prone position.

Acute complications of radiation therapy to the pelvic region include gastrointestinal disturbances such as diarrhea. Such long-term complications as pathologic fracture (<10%)[19] or small bowel obstruction (<5%)[23] are rare.

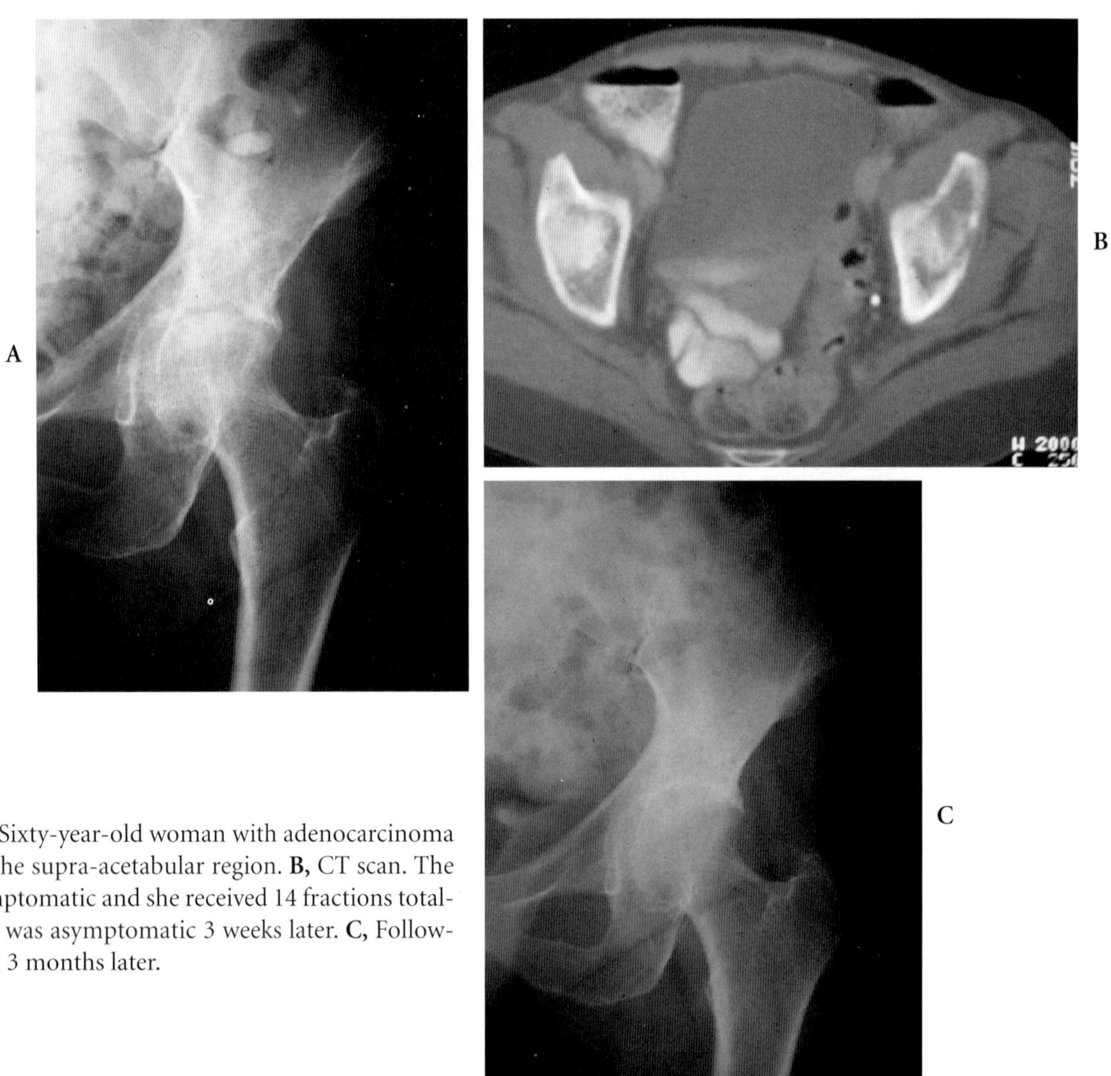

Fig. 31-5   **A,** Sixty-year-old woman with adenocarcinoma metastatic to the supra-acetabular region. **B,** CT scan. The lesion was symptomatic and she received 14 fractions totaling 25 Gy and was asymptomatic 3 weeks later. **C,** Follow-up radiograph 3 months later.

Surgical Therapy
Preoperative Considerations

Most pelvic lesions require preoperative planning using plain radiographs and CT scanning. Pelvic radiographs are used to determine acetabular cup size, and films of the femur determine femoral stems. In most surgeries, 2 to 4 units of blood are required for transfusion. Lesions from myeloma and renal carcinoma are particularly vascular and are prone to intraoperative hemorrhage, and therefore angiography-embolization should be done preoperatively. Maximal effect is obtained when the patient has surgery as soon as embolization is com-

pleted. It has been our practice to obtain embolization in these high-risk patients on the day of surgery (Fig. 31-6).

In addition these patients are at risk for thromboembolic complications, and often the extensive nature of the surgery precludes pharmacologic anticoagulation within the immediate perioperative period. Patients can be considered for vena cava filters (Fig. 31-7).

Epidural catheters may be inserted preoperatively for perioperative pain control. Arterial and central venous lines and Foley catheters are secured before the surgical procedure is begun. Periopera-

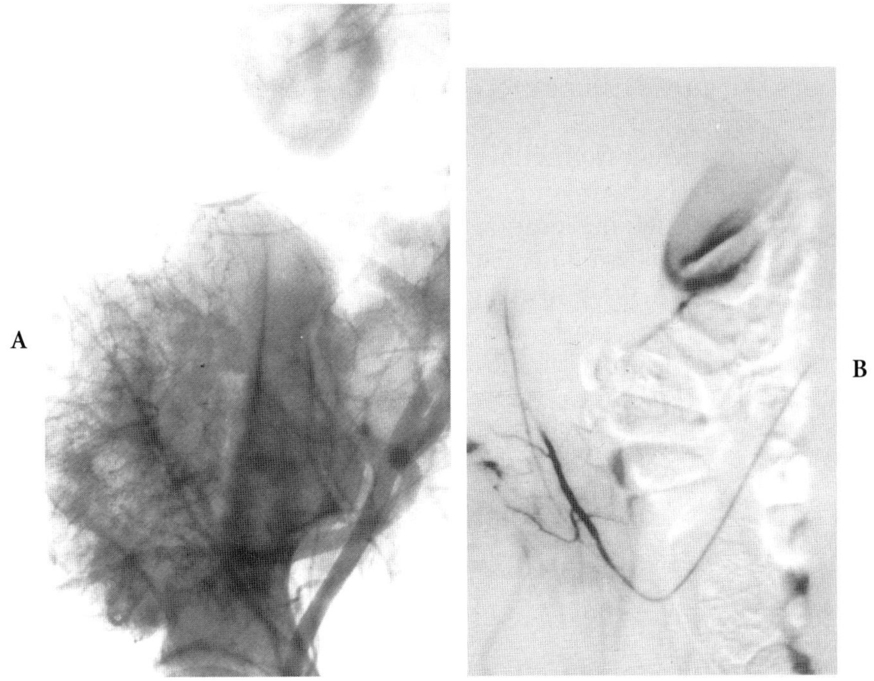

Fig. 31-6   Angiogram showing neovascularization of a painful solitary renal carcinoma metastasis to the ilium prior to (**A**) and following (**B**) embolization.

tive antibiotics are given before the skin incision is made and are repeated every 4 hours during surgery. Patient positioning is done according to the surgeon's preference; the lateral and semilateral ("lazy lateral") positions on a radiolucent table are most versatile.

As in pelvic-acetabular fracture surgery, pelvic clamps and retractors are helpful. Malleable ribbon and abdominal retractors are also required.

Surgical Indications

Indications for the surgical treatment of pelvic-acetabular lesions due to metastatic disease must be individualized. There have been no studies specifically addressing this issue, and general guidelines for the treatment of metastatic bone lesions should be followed. These include functional pain despite radiotherapy and pathologic fracture. The indications for surgical treatment of acetabular lesions are displaced pathologic fractures of the acetabulum, minimally displaced or impending pathologic fracture in solitary and radioresistant metastases, and functional pain despite radiation therapy.

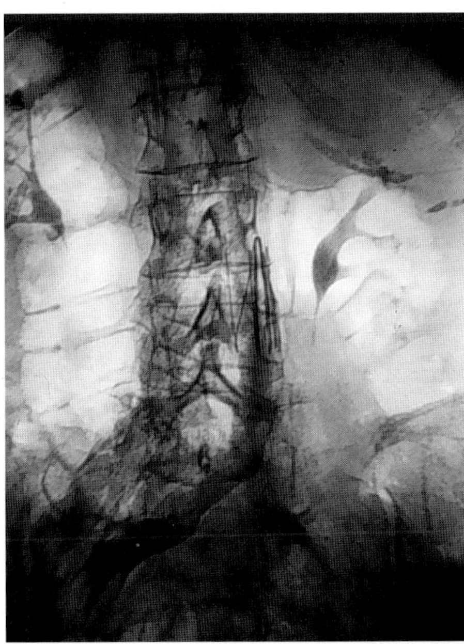

Fig. 31-7   An inferior vena cava filter can be inserted during embolization of the lesion or in the operating suite before surgery.

Operative Approaches

Class 0. Patients in this category have nonarticular, nonacetabular lesions and do not require prosthetic arthroplasty (Fig. 31-8).

Class 0 lesions can be approached from either the anterior (iliofemoral or Smith-Peterson) or posterior exposure. The direction follows the location of the lesion. Iliac and supra-acetabular lesions can be approached anteriorly, and ischial lesions can be exposed posteriorly. Pubic lesions can be best controlled through the medial aspect of the ilioinguinal or Pfannenstiel incision. Since the posterior approach can limit the extent of iliac wing exposure and offer limited access to the iliacus fossa, we prefer the iliofemoral approach, which is extensile. When the lesion is exposed, a combination of curettes and burrs can be used to evacuate the lesion. Steinmann pins, mesh, bone plates, and polymethylmethacrylate (PMMA) are used to reconstruct the defect.

Class I. Class I lesions involve the periacetabular region, but the lateral edges of the acetabulum and medial wall are intact. The insertion of an endoprosthetic acetabular component may be challenging from the iliofemoral approach (Fig. 31-9).

The posterior exposure offers adequate visualization of the lower ilium, acetabulum, and ischium, although anterior approaches are favored for some total hip arthroplasties. With the posterior approach the hip capsule is entered, and the femoral length is determined with the help of a smooth tension wire fashioned as a caliper. The femoral

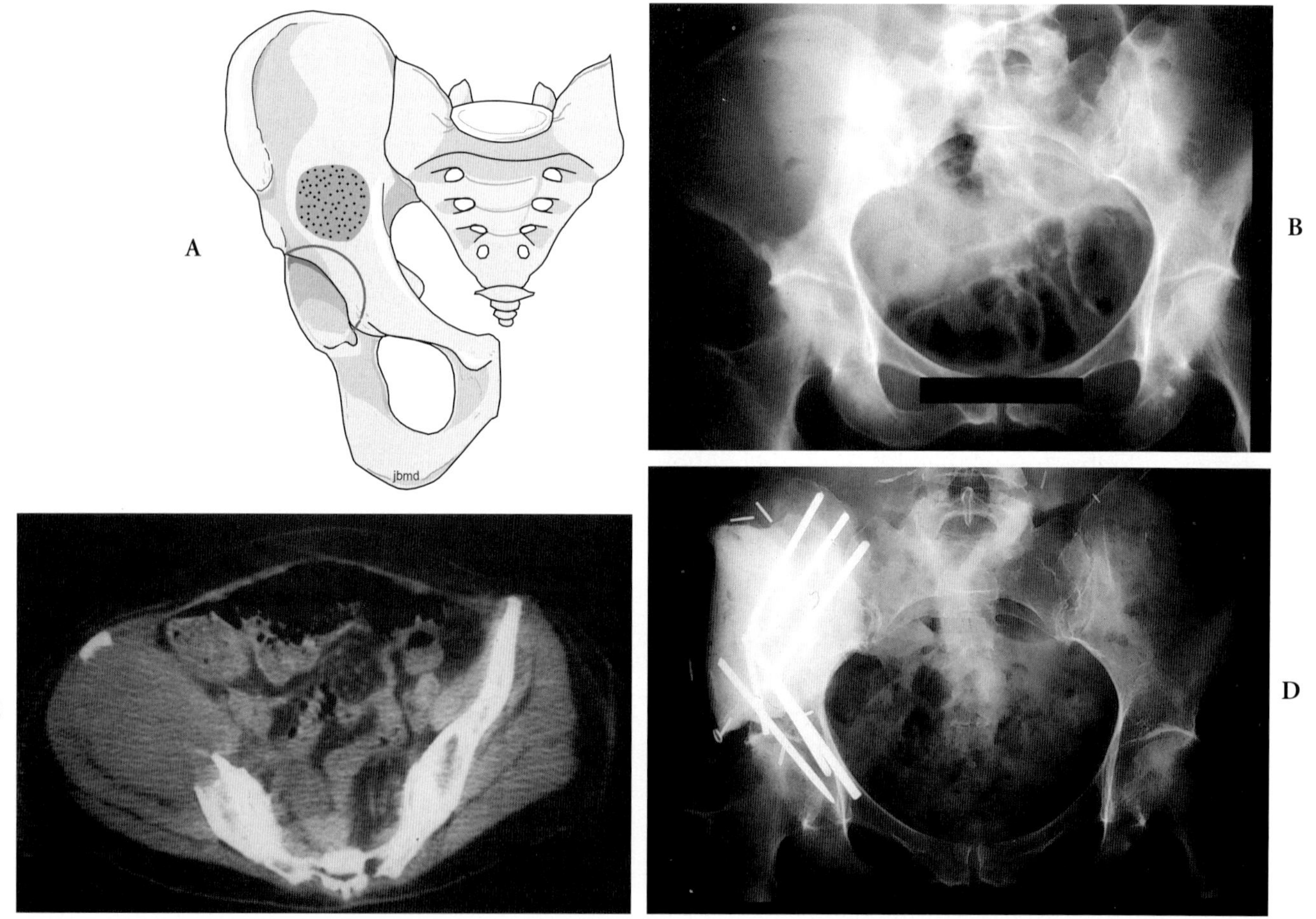

Fig. 31-8   Harrington class 0 lesion (**A**) involving the body of the ilium (**B**) with large soft tissue mass shown on CT scan (**C**). Patient had an anterior approach with curettage of the lesion and cementation (**D**).

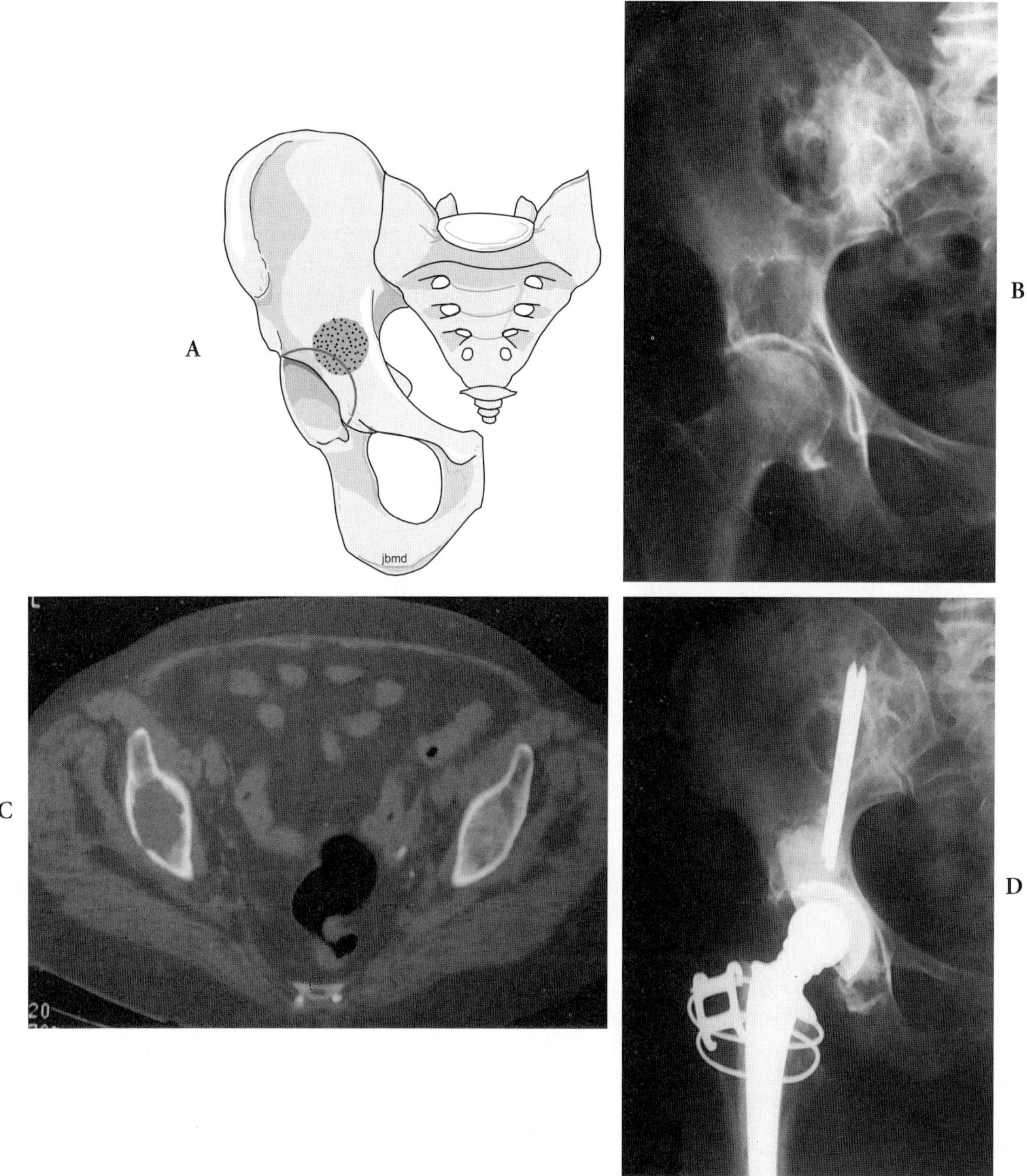

Fig. 31-9 Harrington class I lesion (**A**) with involvement of the supra-acetabular region from metastatic adenocarcinoma of the breast (**B**). CT scan (**C**). Patient had additional lesion in the posterior column and was treated with conventional cemented implants and threaded Steinmann pins (**D**).

neck is osteotomized, and the acetabulum is exposed. Complete exposure is necessary to evaluate the extent of the defect.

The area of the lesion is curetted and burred until structurally healthy bone is reached. The acetabular reamers are then used to enlarge the cup, and appropriate trials are tested. Cemented components are usually used. Metal-backed cups with options for screws and high-profile liners can also be helpful in reconstructing asymmetrical defects (Fig. 31-10). Antibiotics are routinely added to the cement and vacuum-mixed. The acetabular component is inserted first, followed by the femoral component. Immediate weightbearing is encouraged after surgery.

Class II. These defects involve the acetabulum but maintain the integrity of the lateral acetabular rim. Class II defects require reconstruction of the inner acetabulum and medial wall (Fig. 31-11).

A posterior or posterolateral approach is preferred. In addition to the approach for class I defects, the medial wall is reinforced with mesh or bone graft, and the cup is cemented in place.

Trochanteric osteotomy is usually not necessary but can be performed if additional exposure is required. The femoral neck and head is prepared as in class I insufficiency. In patients with longer-standing symptoms the hip capsule and soft tissues may be contracted and must be released before displacement of the femoral head and reduction of the implants. It should be noted that many of these patients have osteopenia or lesions of the femoral shaft; therefore caution should be exercised while the proximal thigh is manipulated to prevent pathologic fracture. When femoral neck osteotomy does not allow exposure or reconstitution of limb length, a four-step process can be performed. This would include (1) release of the *gluteus maximus tendon* insertion on the femur, (2) complete *capsular* release, (3) percutaneous *adductor* release, and (4) *iliopsoas* lengthening. During these soft tissue lengthenings the limb may become more mobile, and lengthening should be limited to 0.5 to 2 cm to avoid traction injury to the sciatic nerve.

Once the acetabulum is exposed, reamers are used to open the acetabulum. The medial wall is deficient, and care should be taken to avoid penetration of the iliacus muscle with the reaming de-

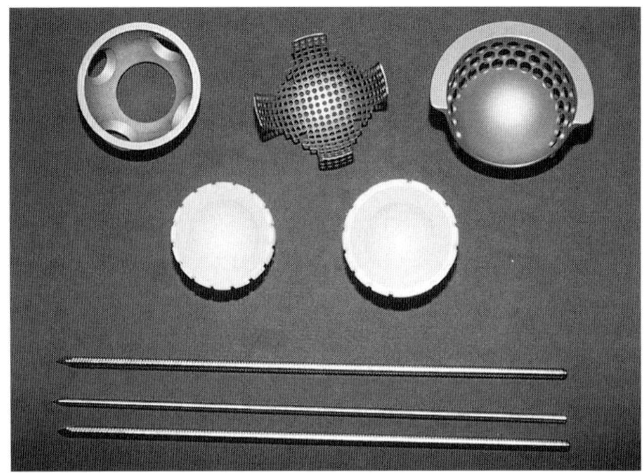

Fig. 31-10   Implants for class I defects are conventional with Steinmann pins, mesh, and cementable acetabular cups.

vice. Small angled curettes and rongeurs can be used to safely resect these areas. The periosteum of the medial acetabulum should be preserved whenever possible to help contain cement and bone graft within the pelvis.

Acetabular cup trials with rim-loading collars should be used. In some instances in which longer-term survival is expected, bone grafting may be considered, but in most instances cement is required to reinforce the medial wall. Metal mesh, either preformed or malleable, should be placed first to help restrict cement. In addition, Steinmann pins can be placed across the ilium into the ischium and pubis to prevent medial displacement of the cup. The Steinmann pins can be inserted via the acetabular exposure or through a separate incision over the iliac crest and angled into the ischium. The pubic pins can be inserted through the anterior wall of the acetabulum. Following this, the cup is again trialed, and the proximal femur is prepared. Trials for the femur and the acetabulum are tested for length and position. When satisfactory trials have been chosen, the acetabulum is cemented first. Cementing techniques are similar to those for the class I lesions, and three packages are usually sufficient.

In instances in which normal acetabular components are insufficient, special cage implants are necessary (Fig. 31-12). These may require additional

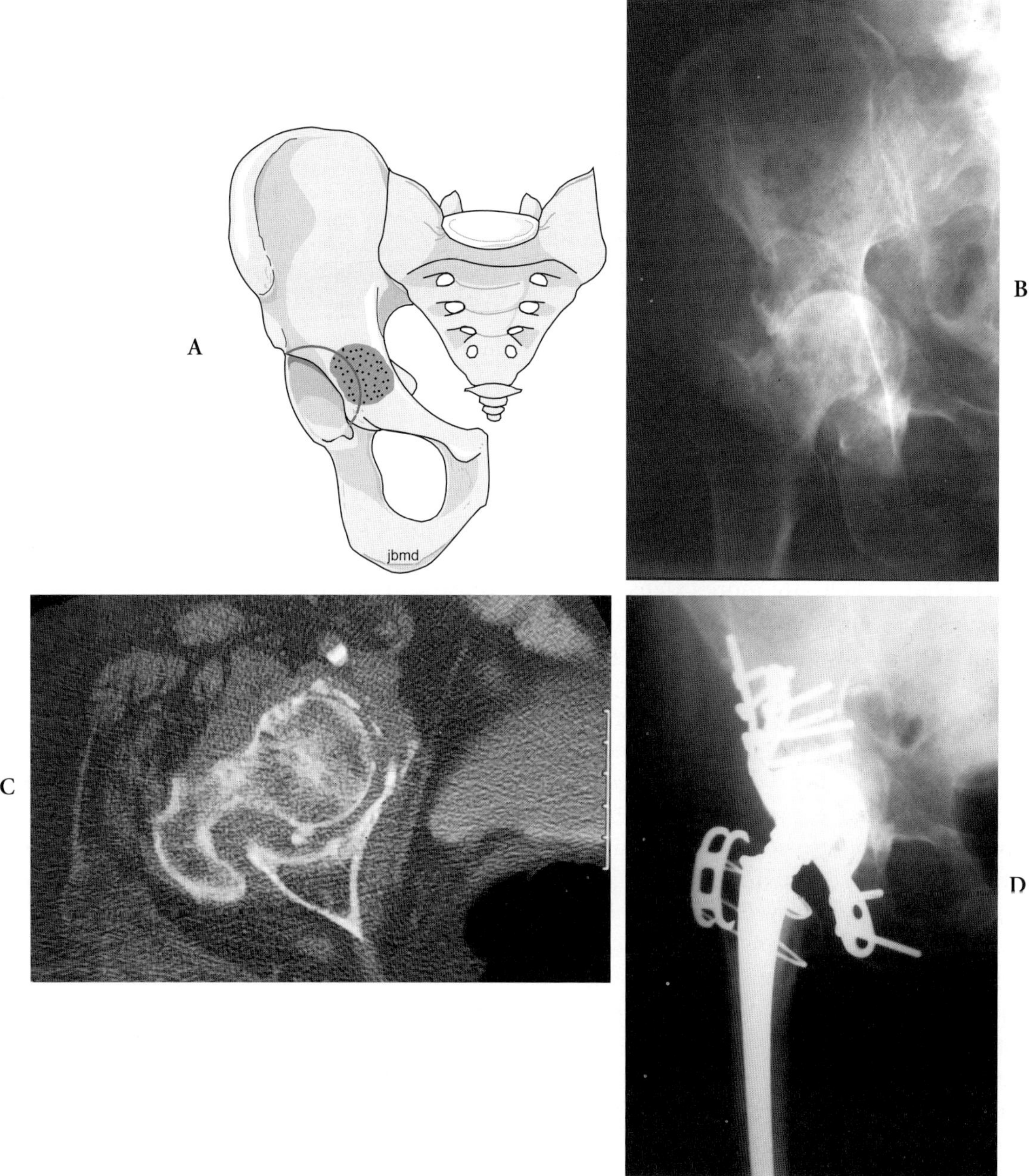

Fig. 31-11 Harrington class II defect with medial wall involvement (**A**), as seen on plain x-ray (**B**), and CT scan (**C**). Reconstruction performed using roof ring (cage) components and poly-methylmethacrylate via posterior approach (**D**).

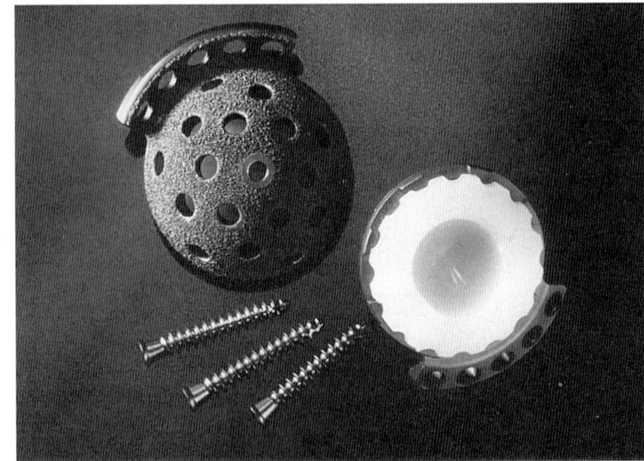
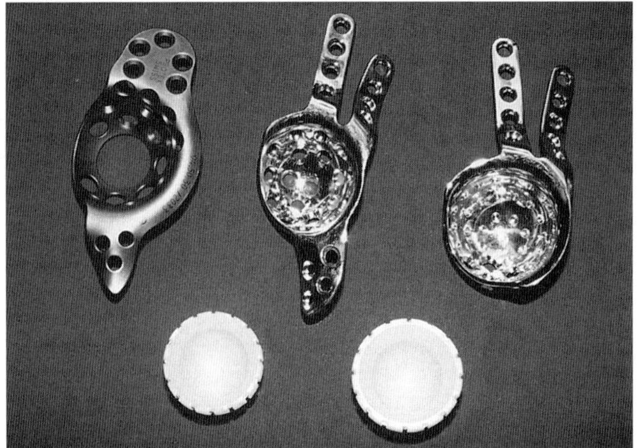

A   B

Fig. 31-12   Implants for class II defects should include rim-loading acetabular prostheses (**A**) and roof ring components (**B**).

exposure of the superior ilium and proximal ischium by trochanteric osteotomy and sciatic nerve mobilization.

Class III. These lesions are more extensive than the class II lesions, with destruction of the lateral cortices, the rim, and the medial wall of the acetabulum. There should be sufficient acetabular rim or wall to support an acetabular protrusio ring or cage-type cup with additional pins and cement. The remaining bone should be reinforced with Steinmann pins and cement in order to transfer the force onto healthier bone, such as the ilium, ischium, pubis, and sacrum. When more than 50% of the acetabular rim is destroyed, this method becomes much more challenging. Anatomic landmarks are lost, and guidelines for accurate cup placement are not available. In these circumstances allografts and roof ring (cage) acetabular components may be used (Fig. 31-13).

The approach to the lesions is similar to that for class II. The lesion is evacuated with curettes and rongeurs. The suction curette used for gynecologic surgeries can be useful. To minimize hemorrhage, the iliacus muscle, always visible with these lesions, should not be violated. Following removal of the gross tumor, the bone edges are assessed. There must be sufficient peripheral bone remaining to allow the roof ring to contact the bone after the central and dome defects are filled with cement. Two or three pins are inserted along the iliac bone of the

sciatic notch into the sacroiliac joint and sacrum. Additional pins are placed superiorly from the iliac crest into the ischium. The ends of the pins are cut off within the acetabular defect deep enough to seat the protrusio ring or cage. The rim flanges should seat against the remaining intact bone of the acetabular rim, and the deep portion should rest along the pins embedded in the bone. The bed is then cleansed with pulse lavage, and acetabular components are trialed. The final position of the construct including the femoral component should be marked on the remaining bone with the cautery or bone cutter to help reproduce the position before cementation. The cement is prepared in the same fashion as for class II defects; three packages are usually required. The femur is then prepared and cemented.

Class IV. According to the Harrington classification system, this type of acetabular insufficiency results when the acetabulum is resected for cure. Treatment of these lesions is similar to more extensive class III defects that result in Enneking-Dunham type II resections. These leave segmental or intercalary defects with resultant pelvic discontinuity. Anatomic landmarks are absent, and preoperative planning is essential if weightbearing is to be restored and postoperative dislocation prevented. Occasionally a portion of the posterior or anterior column is present. Some authors have used the previously described technique for these extensive de-

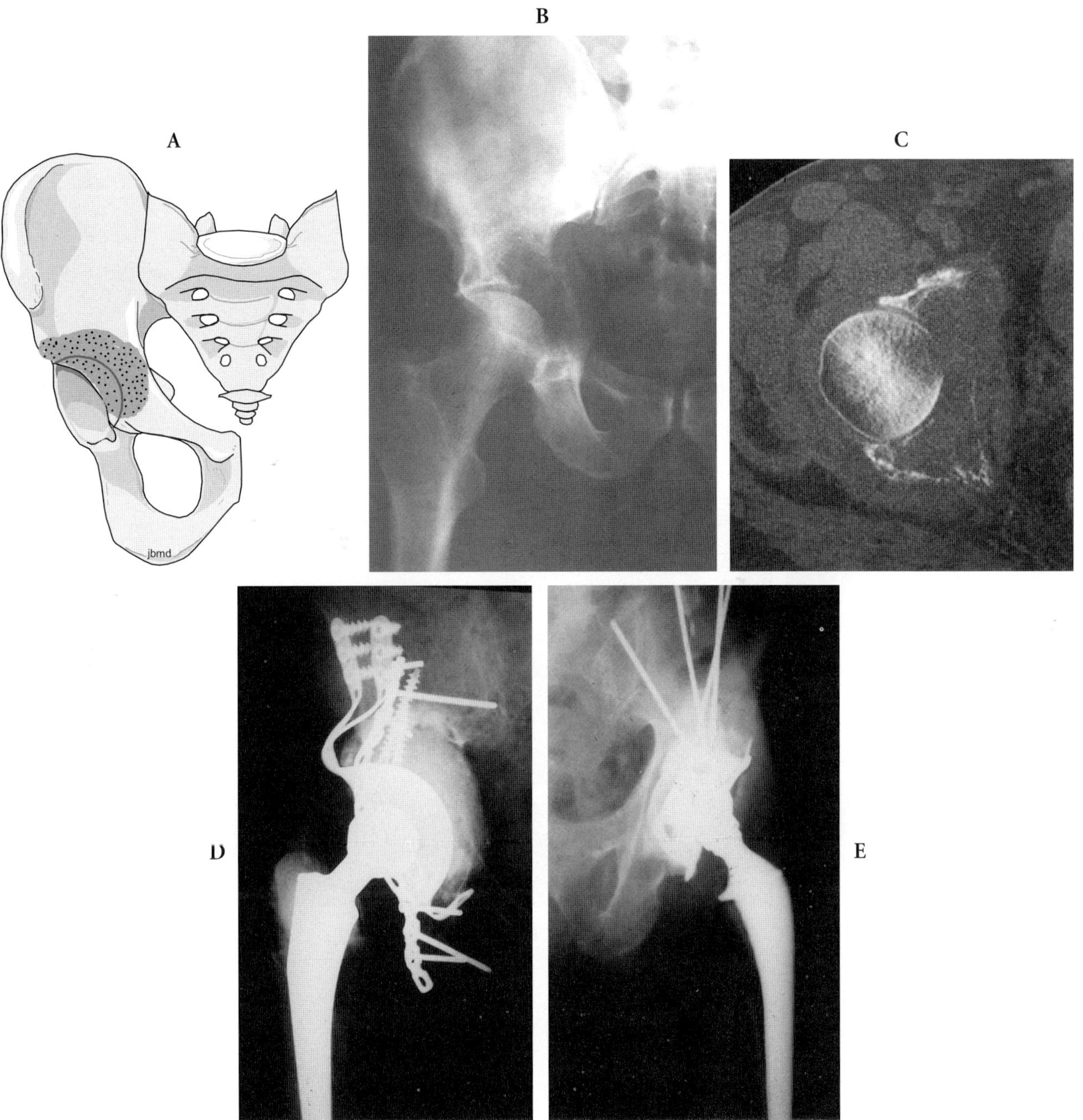

Fig. 31-13   Harrington class III insufficiency with involvement of the medial wall and lateral cortices (**A**), as seen on plain x-ray (**B**), and CT scan (**C**). Reconstruction can be done using polymethylmethacrylate, roof rings, and allograft (**D**), or traditional Steinmann pins (**E**). (**D** courtesy of Dr. David Drucker, Staten Island, N.Y.)

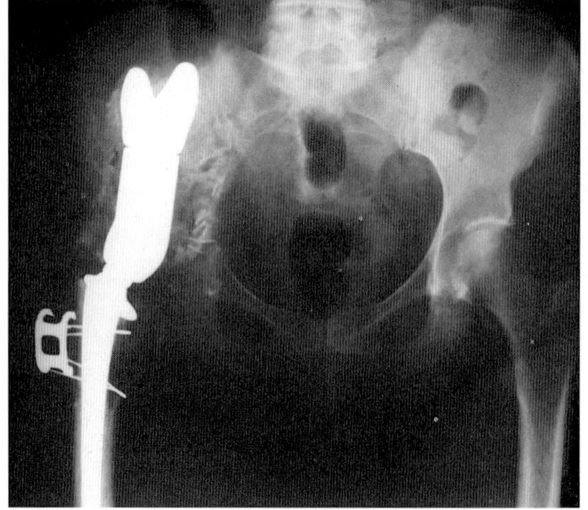

Fig. 31-14 **A,** Harrington class IV insufficiency. **B,** Patient with solitary plasmacytoma. **C,** CT three-dimensional reconstruction showing segmental (intercalary) defect. Reconstruction can be performed using allografts (**D**) and conventional implants (**E**). **F** and **G,** The iliofemoral (saddle) prosthesis can also be used.

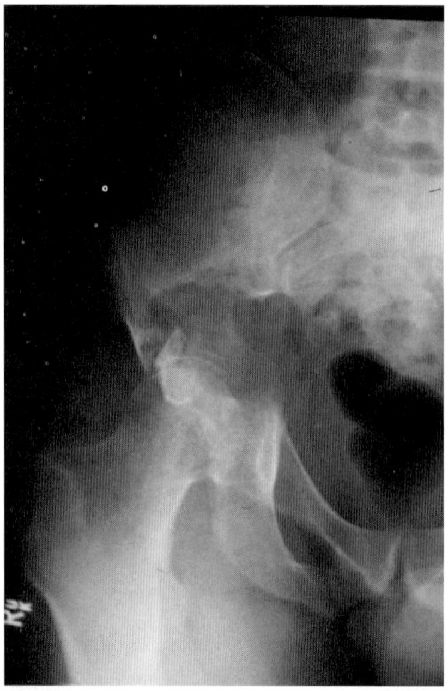

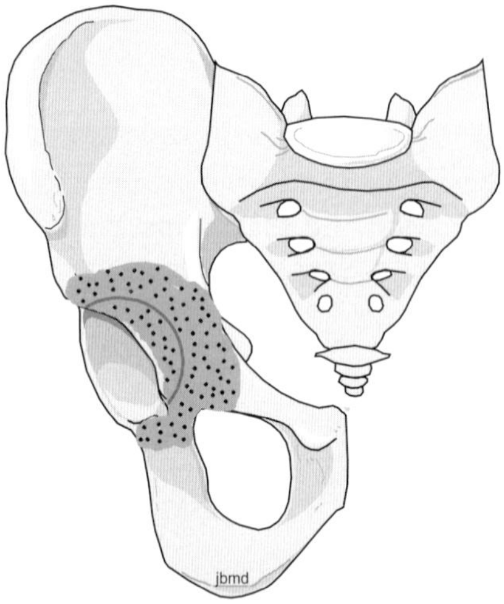

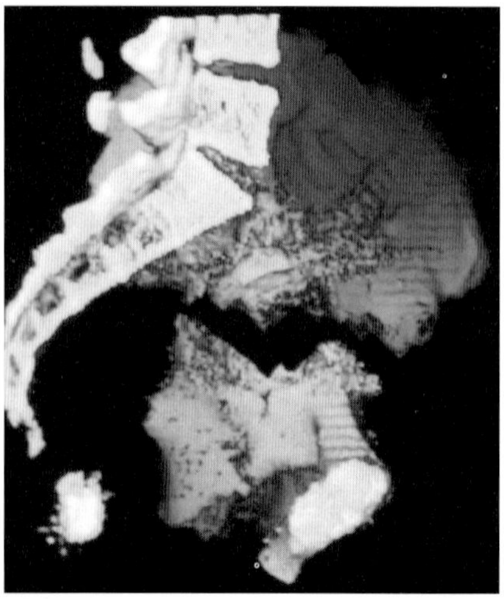

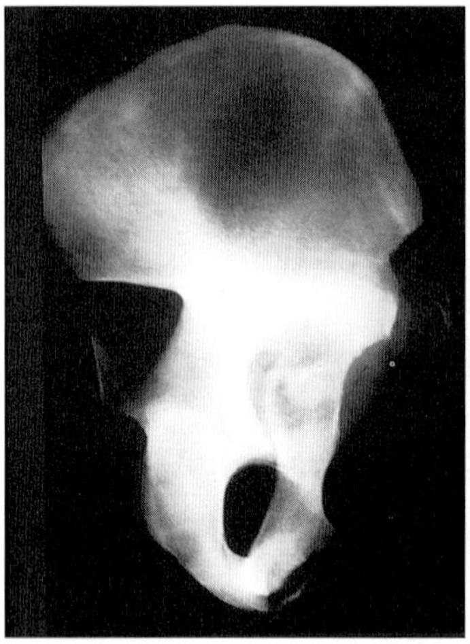

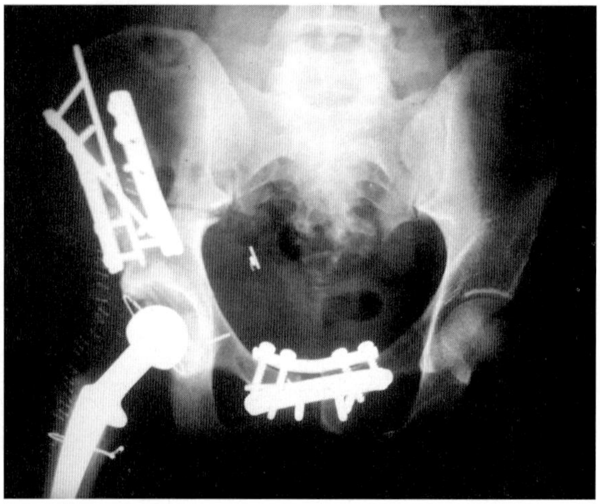

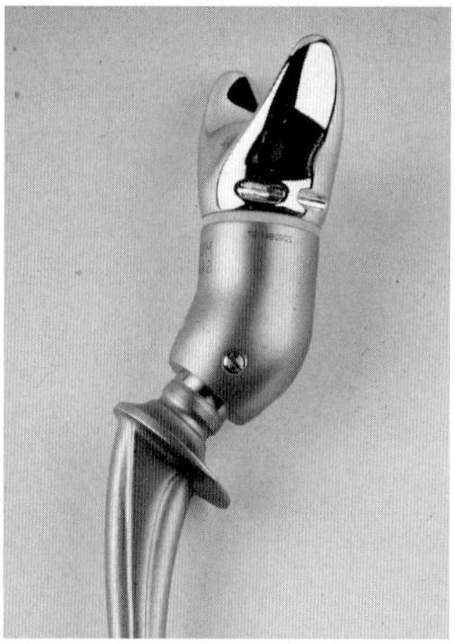

fects, which requires accurate pin and cup placement. In class IV defects, reconstructive methods must address the complex geometry of the acetabulum. The anterior iliofemoral approach may offer extensile exposure of the bone but can be limited for conventional acetabular cup placement. The posterior approach may also be used, but access to the anterior column is limited, and additional trochanteric osteotomy or combined incisions may be required.[24] Once the acetabular region has been resected, reconstruction is accomplished by one of several methods. Custom acetabular components, allografts, and iliofemoral saddle prostheses (Fig. 31-14) can be used. Resection arthroplasty has been described by authors in the past.

Custom acetabular metallic implants can fill defects more accurately and require advanced preoperative planning.[11] Allograft reconstruction of the acetabulum, which is more commonly used for primary tumors, has been used in metastatic disease.[9] The advantage of this material is in its ease of handling, ready availability, and intraoperative flexibility. The disadvantage is in its increased risk of infection and nonunion or fracture. These risks may become significant in the face of limited survival and postoperative radiation treatment.

Iliofemoral saddle reconstruction is also an option for extensive defects.[7] The advantages of this method are the simplicity of the implant design and avoidance of acetabular implant fixation. The disadvantage of this method is the loss of isolated hip flexion and abduction into a single arc of motion and the possibility of postoperative prosthetic dislocation.[7,18]

The anterior approach is the most extensile for pelvic resections. Once the acetabular region is removed, there is complete access to the posterior column. Once the joint is exposed, the lesion is removed as in previously described techniques.

Allograft

The allograft is secured to the host bone by using standard fracture-fixation methods. Whenever possible, a shell of host bone or periosteum should be left to help contain the bone graft. Reconstruction plates can be used to perform the osteosynthesis to the ilium, ischium, and superior pubic ramus. Large cancellous screws are used to secure the grafts to the posterior column and sacroiliac regions. The allograft cup socket can be fashioned

with reamers, and the acetabular components must be cemented to the graft.

Custom Implants (Cage)

Custom hemipelvic implants are secured to the host bone much like allografts are secured, and polyethylene cups must be cemented into the metal shell.

Saddle Prosthesis

The saddle prosthesis can be inserted via the anterior or posterior approach and may be used for Enneking-Dunham type I-II and II-III resections provided there is 6 cm of ilium and 50% sacroiliac joint integrity remaining. The most versatile exposure is the iliofemoral approach to the pelvis. The abductors are released from the outer table of the ilium, and the anterior joint capsule is entered. The posterior extent of the exposure is defined by the sciatic notch, and care must be taken to avoid damage to the superior gluteal vessels. The fascia lata is released transversely at the level of the abductors to allow for posterior visualization. The limb length should be marked on the ilium and femur. The femoral neck is osteotomized, and the posterior aspects of the acetabulum can be accessed. Care is taken not to penetrate the iliacus as the tumor is removed intralesionally. The iliac bone is prepared by fashioning an inverted J-shaped notch with the long end posterior. The anterior portion of the notch should be clear so that the implant will not impinge on the ilium in flexion. As the limb flexes the saddle, it must contact the posterior portion of the bone securely to prevent posterior dislocation. It is helpful to use the saddle trial implant to size the notch. The position of the notch is also important. Care should be taken to place this notch in the thickest bone of the ilium. The ilium should be deepened posteriorly if necessary because the iliac wing becomes thin anteriorly and superiorly. Mersilene tape or Gore-Tex may be used to help secure the saddle around the ilium and prevent dislocation during soft tissue healing. Once this is done, the femur can be prepared and the implant trialed. Soft tissue tensioning is important, and the limb should be assessed for range of motion and stability.

Postoperative Judet views are taken in the operating room to document reduction. The patients who demonstrate instability are kept in balanced suspension for 1 to 2 weeks. Patients with intraoperatively stable implants are allowed to ambulate on the first postoperative day.

FUNCTIONAL OUTCOME OF ACETABULAR RECONSTRUCTIONS

There have been several reports describing the results of surgery for metastatic acetabular lesions (Table 31-1).[7,9-12,25] Harrington's original paper described follow-up functional results in 51 of 58 patients (88%) treated, with an average survival time of 19 months.[16] Thirty patients had class I and II disease, and 28 had class III and IV insufficiency. Patients were treated surgically with conventional implants plus PMMA and Steinmann pins. In addition, patients with class IV insufficiency had bone grafts. Functional results were reported describing pain as minimal, moderate, or severe depending on whether narcotic analgesia was used. Seventy-three percent of patients required no narcotics at 6 months, and 80% had minimal pain at 2 years.[16] Eighty-eight percent of patients were considered ambulatory with or without crutches, cane, or walker at 6 months, and 87% at 2 years.[16] The complication rate was 9% and included one femoral nerve palsy, two superficial infections, one pulmonary embolus, and one lethal hemorrhage.

In another report, Duparc et al.[4] described 42 patients treated and functional with follow-up on 39 (93%). The mean survival was 15 months. Duparc et al. described their own classification system, with 36 of 42 lesions similar to Harrington class I and II. Conventional hip prostheses with PMMA were used in nine cases, and revision implants (Fisher's rings, 13; Miller's ring, 12; and Burch-Schneider, 5) were used in 30, with eight using additional bone graft. Three patients had resection arthroplasty.

Although no specific scoring system was used, functional results were described as relief of pain and ambulation. Thirty-six patients (92%) had satisfactory pain relief, and 36 patients maintained ambulation with or without a cane.

Complications were reported in 10 patients (24%). Three patients died in the perioperative period (0-15 days); three patients had hematomas; one had deep infection with necrosis; one had sciatic nerve palsy; and two had dislocations.

In a report by Allan et al.,[9] 25 patients with Harrington class III insufficiency were studied with a mean follow-up of 14 months. Patients had either roof rings and revision hip components with PMMA (12 patients) or similar components plus bulk allografts (16 patients). Functional scores were available in only nine cases and were rated as one excellent, three good, four fair, and one poor with the MSTS-ISOLS rating system. Scores for relief of pain and ambulation were three excellent, five good, one poor and two excellent, five good, and two fair, respectively. Complications were reported in 10 patients (40%): three had pulmonary emboli (one fatal); three had intraoperative hemorrhages; two had dislocations; one had a re-exploration for postoperative bleeding; and one had wound dehiscence.

In another series of patients by Stark and Bauer,[10] 12 patients with class II and III lesions were treated with protrusio rings, PMMA, and Charnley prostheses. All patients were able to ambulate postoperatively, and the complications included five dislocations and one infection in five patients (42%).

Aboulafia et al.[7] reported on the saddle prosthesis in 17 patients, nine with metastatic malignancies, and a mean follow-up of 15 months. In this group of patients, all had acetabular insufficiencies (class III-IV) requiring minimum Enneking-Dunham type II resections. Functional outcomes were graded according to the MSTS-ISOLS scoring system (30 points) and a modified system.

According to their modified system, six patients had excellent results. These patients maintained community ambulation and did not require narcotic analgesia for pain. Three patients had complications and poor results. These included one patient with a femoral periprosthetic fracture, one with an infection, and one with a wound dehiscence.

In a recent report of saddle prosthesis for class III-IV acetabular insufficiency, 17 patients with metastatic malignancy were followed an average of 22 months.[18] MSTS-ISOLS functional scores for ambulation and pain relief averaged 65% and 82%, respectively, with an overall score of 58% (17 of 30 points).[17] There were four complications in three patients: one had a deep venous thrombosis and hematoma; one had a dislocation of her prosthesis; and one had a fracture-dislocation of the ilium saddle and ilium.

Table 31-1   Literature review

Author	Year	No. patients	No. followed up	I	II	III-IV	Survival (mo)	% Total MSTS	Pain relief	Ambulatory status	% Complications (no. patients)
Harrington[12]	1981	58	51	11	19	25 (3)	19		73% minimal 80% minimal	88% 6 mo 87% 2 yr	9% (5)
Duparc et al.[4]	1989	42	39	20*	16	6 (0)	15		92%	92%	14% (10)
Walker[24]	1993	4	4	0	0	4 (0)	9.3		All	100% walker-cane	25% (1)
Allan et al.[9]	1995	25	9†	0	0	25 (0)	14		89%	78%	40% (10)
Aboulafia et al.[7]	1995	9	9	0	0	9	15	52%	67%	67%	33% (3)
Stark and Bauer[10]	1996	12	12	0	5	7 (0)	9.1		All	Full weight-bearing	42% (65)
Algan and Horowitz[8]	1996	5	5	0	5	0 (0)	12.5		None	100% cane-walker	20% (1)
Uchia et al.[11]	1996	5	5	0	0	0 (5)	17.6		Good	Good	0
Benevenia and Leeson[18]	1997	17	17	0	0	17	22	58%	65%	82%	18% (3)

*Type included 10 superior defects also.
†9 patients with available MSTS F (X) scores.

The evaluation and treatment of patients with metastatic disease involving the hip and femur are an important and common problem for orthopedic surgeons who deal with cancer patients, as well as for medical and radiation oncologists. Although the diagnosis and treatment of metastatic disease in any part of the skeleton is important for the patient, treatment in the area of the hip and femur is especially significant. This is because metastatic disease in this area is relatively common and the morbidity of a fracture in these high-weightbearing areas can be extensive compared with other sites, such as the upper extremities. Decisions made regarding treatment of lesions in the area of the hip and femur tend to have particular significance for the patient's lifestyle. For example, deciding whether a patient should refrain from bearing weight to avoid fracture while undergoing radiation treatment or while prophylactic fixation is being performed has far-reaching implications.

INCIDENCE

In patients who present with skeletal metastases, involvement of the hip and femur with metastatic disease is not uncommon. It has been found that approximately 10% of metastatic lesions are found in the hip.[1] The tumor that metastasizes to the hip and femur with the greatest frequency is carcinoma of the breast.[2-6] Ten percent of patients with disseminated breast cancer and 1% to 2% of all patients with breast cancer will ultimately sustain a pathologic fracture of the hip.[6] In most series, after breast cancer the carcinomas that most frequently metastasize to the hip and proximal femur originate in the lung and then the kidney.[7-9] Because of the relatively long survival of patients with metastatic breast or renal carcinoma, these two tumors are the ones that most frequently require treatment by the radiation oncologist in the area of the hip and femur. They are also the tumors most likely to need operative intervention.

CLINICAL PRESENTATION, PROGNOSIS, AND SURVIVAL

Metastases to the hip and femur may present in several ways. In those patients who have no symptoms, involvement in this area may first be noted on a bone scan, which is used as a screening test to identify sites of metastatic disease in patients with known primary tumors. On occasion, metastatic disease may first be noted when a patient is evaluated for pain from another location, such as the spine, and radiographs that include the hip and pelvis reveal involvement in the hip.

The most common presentation of patients who have metastatic disease of the hip and femur is probably with a symptomatic lesion that has not fractured. Attention is usually drawn to this area by the patient, who will experience pain with weightbearing. Typically, small areas of involvement will be less symptomatic than extensive areas. On some occasions patients may present with a fracture through a metastatic lesion. This is a relatively uncommon presentation because most patients will experience pain before fracture, which draws the attention of a physician. An isolated fracture of the lesser trochanter of the hip may be an indication of more extensive disease involvement in this area.[10]

On occasion a patient may present with an isolated lesion of bone that, upon evaluation, turns out to be a metastasis from an unknown primary tumor. In this case, after biopsy and tissue diagnosis, the patient must be carefully evaluated to determine the origin of the metastatic disease. This evaluation should include a bone scan to look for other sites of skeletal involvement and a computed tomography (CT) scan of the chest and abdomen to look for signs of lung or renal carcinoma. A breast examination in women and a prostate examination and PSA test in men are part of this evaluation.

The survival of patients who present with metastatic disease of the hip and femur varies, depending on the origin of the metastasis and the extent of involvement. In one study by Habermann et al.[2] the overall survival of patients with metastatic disease of the femur was 48% at 12 months. Although there are some differences in the literature as to the overall length of survival, it is generally agreed that of the carcinomas that most frequently metastasize to this area, renal and breast carcinoma are associated with the longest survival and lung cancer with the shortest.

DIAGNOSTIC EVALUATION AND SURGICAL INDICATIONS

When the presence of metastatic disease has been established, the patient should be questioned regarding the severity of pain and the activities that increase the level of discomfort. Lesions that are small and minimally symptomatic can often be treated with radiation therapy, protected weight-bearing, and careful observation. Questions at the time of the initial evaluation should include the need for assistive devices, such as a cane or a walker, and the distance the patient can walk before having to stop to rest.

The radiographic evaluation should include plain radiographs that visualize the hip, pelvis, and femur. A recent bone scan is recommended to assess for other areas in the skeleton that may also be at risk of pathologic fractures. A bone scan that shows multiple lesions is also evidence that the lesion in the hip is metastatic and not a new primary tumor. In certain instances, such as with multiple myeloma, the bone scan may not reveal lesions associated with skeletal destruction. In addition, the patient may be too uncomfortable to tolerate lying supine in the nuclear medicine suite while the bone scan is being performed. In those instances, a skeletal survey may be more useful. Further diagnostic studies in the form of a CT scan or a magnetic resonance imaging (MRI) scan to evaluate the amount of bone destruction may also be helpful.

Guidelines for internal fixation of impending fractures proposed by Harrington et al.[11] in 1976 were based on the evaluation of plain radiographs. It was proposed that lesions at significant risk of causing a pathologic fracture were those that (1) were greater than 2.5 cm in diameter, (2) destroyed 50% of the cortex, or (3) were painful despite treatment with radiation. Added to these guidelines for lesions about the hip are included the presence of an avulsion fracture of the lesser trochanter.[10] These are currently the most commonly used criteria for determining which fractures are in need of internal fixation.

Although all authors agree that larger areas of bone destruction are at higher risk of fracture than smaller areas, defining the amount of risk is difficult. In an article by Menck et al.,[12] it was determined that the ratio of the width of the metastasis to the width of the bone was of particular significance, with 60% being the amount above which internal fixation should be considered. Areas of cortical destruction greater than 13 mm in the femoral neck and 30 mm in the femoral shaft were also considered to be at high risk of fracture.[12] In contrast to the findings of Harrington and Menck, Keene et al.[13] could not find a clear relationship between the

extent of involvement and the risk of fracture in patients who presented with breast carcinoma metastatic to the femur.

Patients who present with lesions that do not meet the criteria for internal fixation should be referred to a radiation oncologist for consideration of radiation therapy. These patients need to be followed by the orthopedic surgeon during and after their radiation treatments. Bone destruction that increases in size or a lesion that remains or becomes symptomatic despite radiation may be an indication for operative intervention. In addition, the weightbearing status of these patients needs to be monitored by the orthopedic surgeon. The majority of these patients need to be restricted to partial weightbearing for at least 6 weeks, and usually until there is evidence that their lesions have healed. If the patient undergoes surgery, the weightbearing status also has to be carefully monitored by the orthopedic surgeon. Most patients are allowed only partial weightbearing for a period of at least 6 weeks after the procedure.

The treatment for a fracture through a lesion is internal fixation or prosthetic replacement similar to that used for impending fractures. If the fracture is through a lesion that has been irradiated and if the patient has a relatively long projected survival, strong consideration should be given to prosthetic replacement. This is because these patients may have fracture nonunion, and if they survive long enough, their internal fixation could fail. It is always preferable to fix impending fractures prophylactically so that the patient can avoid the discomfort and morbidity associated with having a pathologic fracture.

MANAGEMENT, SURGICAL OPTIONS, AND METHODS OF FIXATION
Femoral Head and Neck Fractures

It is recommended that impending and complete fractures of the femoral head and neck be treated by cemented hemiarthroplasty because internal fixation may fail if these lesions progress (Fig. 32-1). A common error in the treatment of pathologic fractures in the femoral head and neck is failure to appreciate distal lesions. This may result in unrecognized perforation during preparation of the femoral canal and placement of the stem of the prosthesis through this perforation. In addition a stem that ends just proximal to a lesion may cause a

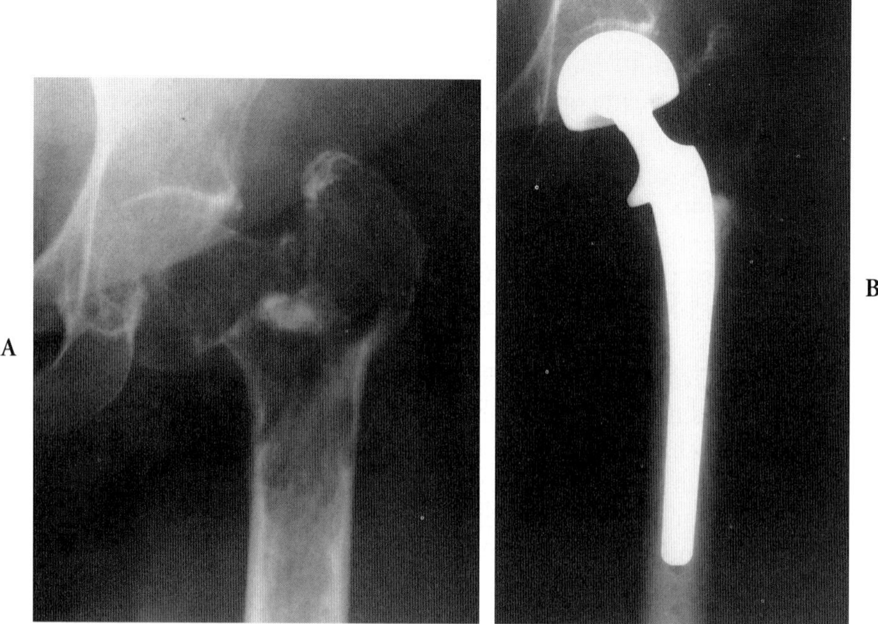

Fig. 32-1 Pathologic fracture in patient with extensive metastatic disease involving the femoral head and subtrochanteric area. Treated with bipolar hip replacement.

stress riser, leading to later fracture. Therefore it is recommended that in all patients radiographs be taken of the entire femur before this procedure is undertaken. In patients who have only proximal disease, a long-stem component can frequently bypass these lesions. If there is a large lesion in the supracondylar area, it may be necessary to place a fixation device, such as a supracondylar screw and side plate, to avoid a stress riser and possible fracture around the tip of the prosthesis.[14]

Postoperatively, patients who undergo bipolar hemiarthroplasty for metastatic disease are treated in much the same way as those patients who undergo this procedure for other conditions. This involves dislocation precautions and partial weight-bearing for 6 weeks after surgery.

Intertrochanteric Fractures

Impending or complete fractures in the intertrochanteric area with a minimal amount of bone destruction can usually be treated with a screw and side plate device (Fig. 32-2). This may be performed with adjunctive bone cement to assist in fixation of the lag screw or proximal screw in the plate. This type of fixation is especially advanta-

geous in patients who present with a solitary lesion in the intertrochanteric area that is suspected of being a metastasis but who have no known primary tumor and no other lesions on bone scan. The lesion can be partially excised and sent to the pathology laboratory for a tissue diagnosis. Because the direct lateral approach is usually used for biopsy of these lesions, if the lesion should turn out to be a primary tumor, an unsalvageable situation has not been created. If a sarcoma is encountered on the frozen section, surgery should stop unless this situation has been considered preoperatively and en bloc resection planned. A biopsy should be performed as a separate procedure on any lesion strongly considered to be a sarcoma.

The disadvantage of using the screw and side plate for these fractures is the significant stress placed on the device during ambulation, which may cause it to eventually fail if the patient becomes a long-term survivor. Progression of the tumor may also interfere with fixation, especially if it is relatively radioresistant. In addition, for patients who have had radiation therapy in this area and who survive for a relatively long period of time, the end of the plate may put stress on the bone weak-

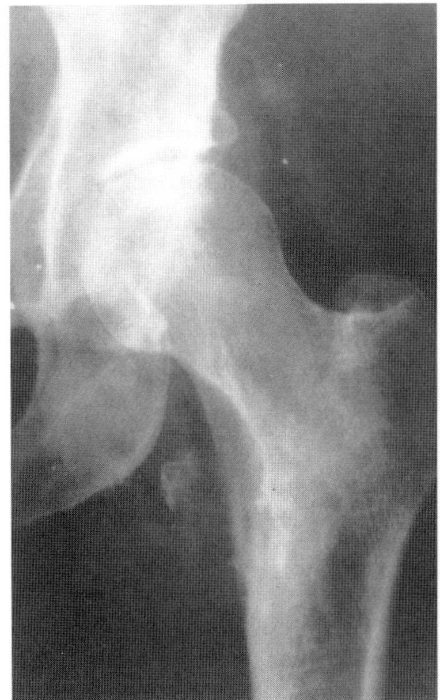
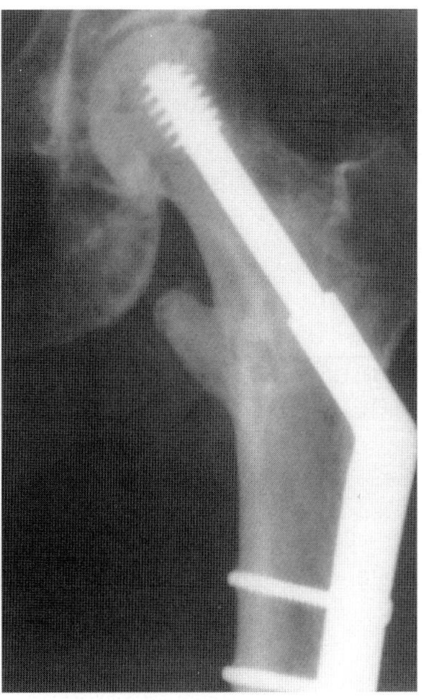

A

B

Fig. 32-2 Patient with metastatic disease involving calcar with avulsion fracture of the lesser trochanter. This fracture healed after treatment with a hip compression screw.

A

B

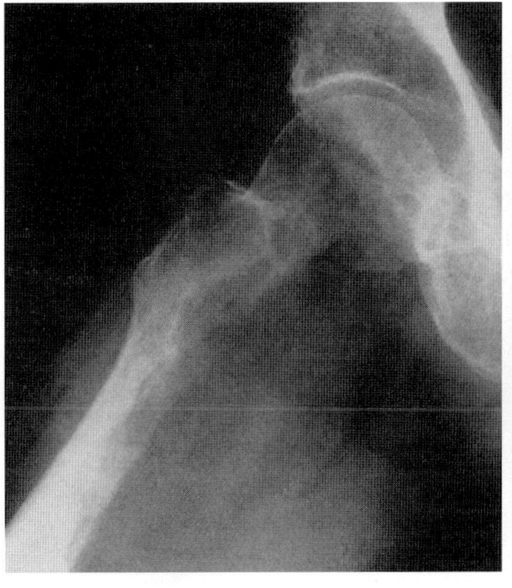
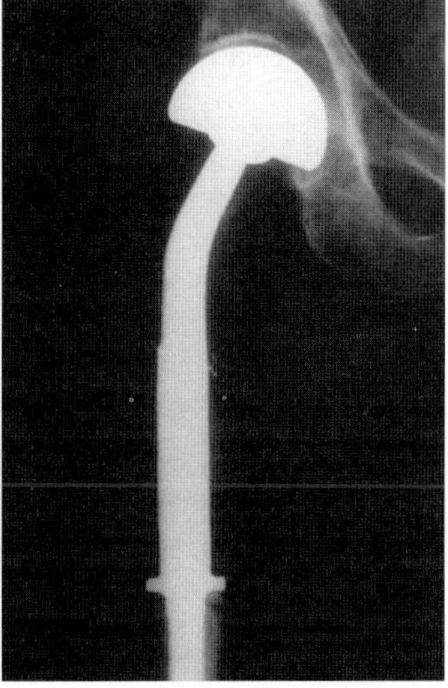

Fig. 32-3 Patient with extensive metastatic disease and bone loss involving the femoral head and neck extending to the subtrochanteric area. Treated with proximal femoral replacement. (From Berman AT, Hermantin FU, Horowitz SM. Metastatic disease of the hip: Evaluation and treatment. J Am Acad Orthop Surg 5[2]:85, 1997. © 1997 American Academy of Orthopaedic Surgeons.)

ened by the radiation and may eventually cause a fracture at the distal aspect of the plate.

If there is extensive destruction in the intertrochanteric area and a complete or impending fracture, a long-stem hip prosthesis or a proximal femoral replacement is recommended (Fig. 32-3). We have had good success with the latter. Proximal femoral replacement prostheses are available in an off-the-shelf format from a variety of manufacturers. The femoral component is usually combined with a bipolar head. The bipolar head reduces the risk of dislocation that would be encountered with a separate acetabular component.[14]

Postoperatively, patients who are treated with a compression screw and side plate do not require dislocation precautions, and their weightbearing status is allowed to progress according to the extent of bone loss and the stability of fixation. Patients who undergo proximal femoral replacement are maintained in a hip-abduction brace with a knee-foot-ankle orthosis extension for 6 to 8 weeks postoperatively to decrease the risk of dislocation.

Subtrochanteric Fractures

For patients with obvious metastatic disease, we recommend intramedullary fixation with screws placed along the femoral neck. This device is biomechanically superior to the screw and side plate and is believed to have a lower probability of mechanical failure. In the past the Zickel nail (Howmedica, Rutherford, N.J.) was the "gold standard" for this type of fixation. At present, most of the manufacturers who produce trauma instrumentation have reconstruction ("recon") nails that can be used. In most of these devices, two screws are directed up the femoral neck, and the nail can be locked distally (Fig. 32-4). Recently Synthes Inc. (Paoli, Pa.) has introduced an unreamed femoral nail that uses a spiral blade rather than screw fixation in the femoral head and neck. The advantage of this device is that it can be inserted without reaming, which makes the surgery faster. In addition, the angle of the blade to the nail can be changed, which gives the surgeon more flexibility.

In the majority of these cases we recommend

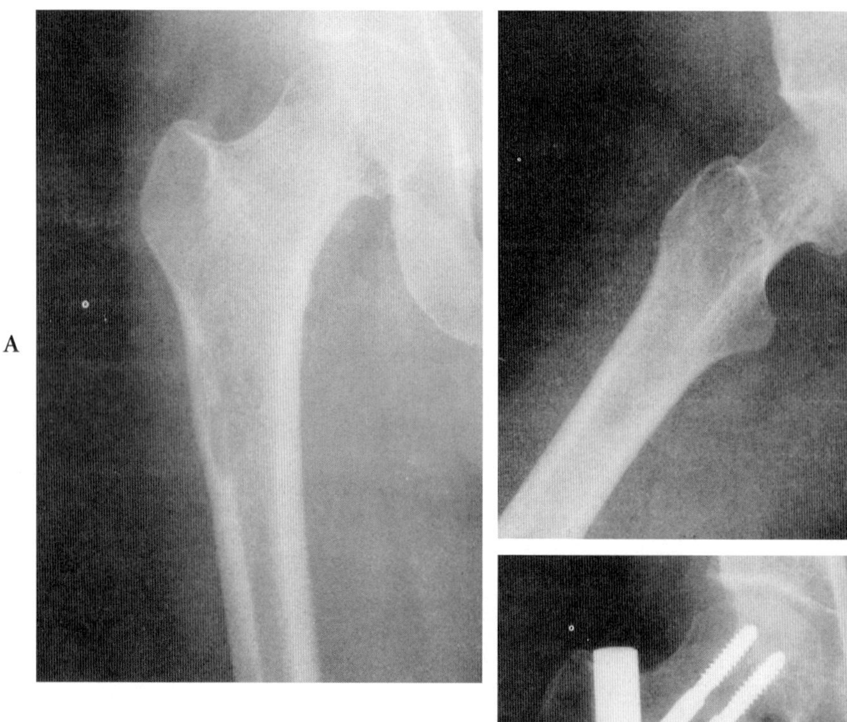

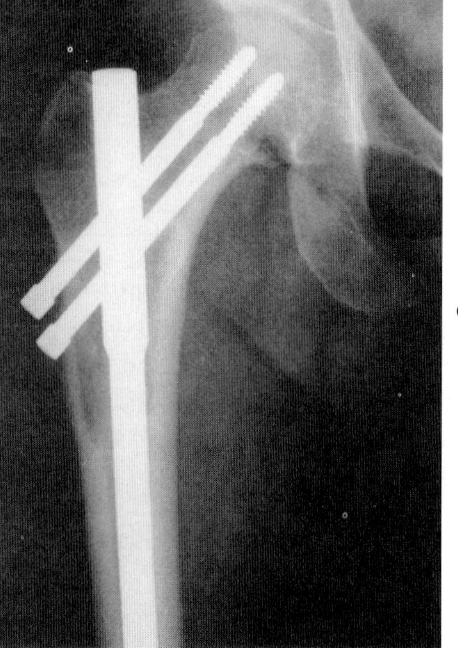

Fig. 32-4 **A** and **B,** Metastatic lesion in the subtrochanteric area. **C,** A reconstruction nail stabilizes this area, the femoral neck, and most of the remaining femur. (From Algan SM, Horowitz SM. Surgical treatment of pathologic hip lesions in patients with metastatic disease. Clin Orthop 332:227, 1996.)

locking the rod both proximally and distally because of the low incidence of complications associated with placement of the distal screws and the potential for loss of stability if they are not used. We use bone cement only in cases in which loss of bone makes the screw fixation tenuous. In those cases, a ¼-inch drill bit is used to make portals in the bone both proximal and distal to the screws. The area is first irrigated with saline solution, and then the polymethylmethacrylate (PMMA) is inserted with a syringe so that it flows around the rod and the screws.

Postoperatively, these patients do not require dislocation precautions. Their weightbearing status is allowed to progress, depending on the extent of bone loss and the stability of fixation. Most patients are bearing full weight or are ambulatory with a cane 6 to 12 weeks postoperatively.

Involvement of Femoral Shaft

If involvement of the femoral shaft is diffuse, extending into the area of the proximal femur and hip, the usual treatment is proximal femoral replacement or hip replacement with a cemented long-stem femoral component. If the hip and subtrochanteric region are not involved and the disease appears confined to the midshaft area, the usual treatment is a femoral rod locked distally and proximally. If the involvement is in the proximal third of the femur or close to the subtrochanteric area, a recon type of nail can be used so that proximal progression of disease after surgery will not affect fixation. In those cases in which disease makes the locking screw fixation poor, we will augment fixation with PMMA.

There are several excellent systems available for intramedullary nails. These include both reamed and unreamed devices. If the canal is large enough for an unreamed nail to be used, operative time may be shortened and blood loss lessened. Postoperatively, most patients will receive radiation therapy. Serial radiographs are obtained to ensure that the disease does not progress to the point where the fixation is compromised.

OUTCOMES

The reported results of internal fixation for impending and pathologic fractures of the hip and femur are good, including an improved ability for the patients to ambulate and relief of pain.[15] These procedures are associated with a low mortality and morbidity and should be performed in patients who would be expected to survive at least a month after surgery. The most commonly reported complication is failure of fixation. This tends to occur more often in patients with longer survival because of the greater stress placed on the reconstruction and the progression of the lesions. Technical recommendations to avoid this problem would be to use a hip replacement rather than a screw and side plate device for impending fractures of the femoral head and neck if the patient is expected to survive more than a few months or if the disease is extensive. Progression of disease in the femoral head or to the end of the plate is a not uncommon cause of loss of fixation in this group. Progression of disease and loss of proximal fixation are also reasons for failures in patients treated for lesions involving the femoral shaft. Another technical recommendation would be to fix the femoral neck internally with a recon type of nail along with fixation of the femoral shaft in patients who have extensive disease of the femur extending into the subtrochanteric region.

REFERENCES

1. Bonarigo BC, Rubin P. Nonunion of pathologic fracture after radiation therapy. Radiology 88:889-898, 1967.
2. Habermann ET, Sachs R, Stern RE, Hirsch DM, Anderson WJ Jr. The pathology and treatment of metastatic disease of the femur. Clin Orthop 169:70-82, 1982.
3. Parrish FF, Murray JA. Surgical treatment for secondary neoplastic fractures. J Bone Joint Surg Am 52:665-686, 1970.
4. Zickel RE, Mouradian WH. Intramedullary fixation of pathological fractures and lesions of the subtrochanteric region of the femur. J Bone Joint Surg Am 58:1061-1066, 1976.
5. Levy RN, Sherry HS, Siffert RS. Surgical management of metastatic disease of bone at the hip. Clin Orthop 169:62-69, 1982.
6. Lane JM, Sculco TP, Zolan S. Treatment of pathological fractures of the hip by endoprosthetic replacement. J Bone Joint Surg Am 62:954-959, 1980.
7. Behr JT, Dobozi WR, Badrinath K. The treatment of pathologic and impending pathologic fractures of the proximal femur in the elderly. Clin Orthop 198:173-178, 1985.
8. Yazawa Y, Frassica FJ, Chao EY, Pritchard DJ, Sim FH, Shives TC. Metastatic bone disease: A study of the surgical treatment of 166 pathologic humeral and femoral fractures. Clin Orthop 251:213-219, 1990.
9. Algan SM, Horowitz SM. Surgical treatment of pathologic hip lesions in patients with metastatic disease. Clin Orthop 332:223-231, 1996.

10. Bertin KC, Horstman J, Coleman SS. Isolated fracture of the lesser trochanter in adults: An initial manifestation of metastatic malignant disease. J Bone Joint Surg Am 66(5):770-773, 1984.

11. Harrington KD, Sim FH, Enis JE, Johnston JO, Dick HM, Gristina AG. The use of methylmethacrylate as an adjunct in internal fixation of pathological fractures. J Bone Joint Surg Am 58:1047-1055, 1976.

12. Menck H, Schulze S, Larsen E. Metastasis size in pathologic femoral fractures. Acta Orthop Scand 59(2):151-154, 1988.

13. Keene JS, Sellinger DS, McBeath AA, Engber WD. Metastatic breast cancer in the femur: A search for the lesion at risk of fracture. Clin Orthop 203:282-288, 1986.

14. Horowitz SM. The management of pathological hip fractures. Operative Techniques in Orthopaedics 4(2):122-129, 1994.

15. van der Hulst RR, van den Wildenberg FA, Vroemen JP, Greve JW. Intramedullary nailing of (impending) pathologic fractures. J Trauma 36(2):211-215, 1994.

Metastatic Disease of the Distal Femur

Patrick J. Getty, M.D., *Azhar M. Awan,* M.D., *and Terrance D. Peabody,* M.D.

INCIDENCE AND PRESENTATION

Bone metastases will develop in approximately one half of the more than 1 million people in the United States in whom carcinoma is diagnosed annually. With effective therapies directed at the primary tumor, these patients have 5-year survival rates that vary between 10% for patients with lung carcinomas and almost 90% for patients with breast or prostate carcinomas.[1] More importantly, in contrast to what may be commonly believed, most patients with metastatic carcinoma who sustain pathologic fractures of the long bones will survive for months, if not years.[2] Obviously, effective treatment of bone metastases and pathologic fractures is important in enhancing the quality and length of these patients' lives.

Metastatic carcinomas are most commonly found in the axial skeleton, that is, in the spine and pelvis, but they also occur frequently in the long bones. The most common among these is the femur.[3] In a study of 399 long-bone fractures secondary to malignant disease, Harrington[2] found that 258, or 65%, of these occurred in the femur. Most metastatic disease and resultant pathologic fractures occur in the proximal femur; however, both Harrington[3] and Habermann et al.,[4] in similar studies, demonstrated that a significant proportion of pathologic femoral fractures occur in the distal femur.

The goals of treatment of metastatic disease of the distal femur are the same as for metastases in other locations in the body. Although cure is often not possible, the physician wishes to provide pain relief, limb stability, and optimal function. In many ways the operative and nonoperative treatments will be the same as those applied to other areas of the body. In some ways, however, the distal femur is unique, and for this reason it is considered separately in this chapter.

ANATOMY AND BIOMECHANICAL CONSIDERATIONS

The diaphysis of the distal femur is a cylindrical bone segment with an anterior bow. The anterior surface is rounded and smooth, but posteriorly the cortex thickens to form a prominent ridge known as the linea aspera. In the supracondylar region the linea aspera divides as the bone expands to three times the diaphyseal diameter, with a corresponding decrease in the ratio of cortical to cancellous bone. Two oblong condyles are separated posteriorly by a deep intercondylar fossa. United anteriorly, these condyles form the trochlear groove.

This anatomy is uniquely adapted for knee function. The distal femur, however, is composed largely of cancellous bone, and the associations of the medial and lateral condyles and the condyles to the femoral diaphysis are tenuous; this leaves that site vulnerable to pathologic fracture in the presence of a metastatic lesion.

The distal femur is subjected to tremendous demands during ambulation. Loads transmitted across the knee can range from 3 to 4 times body weight during heel strike and the preswing phase of gait. The mechanical axis of the limb lies medial to the anatomic axis of the femur. For this reason the distal femur is subjected not only to compression but also to tension and shear loads.

In discussing anatomy, one must also consider the surrounding soft tissues. In contrast to the abundant soft tissue surrounding the proximal femur and pelvis, the distal quadriceps and hamstring muscles do not provide a significant soft tissue envelope, particularly in persons with metastatic carcinoma. Therefore fractures of the distal femur are often associated with instability, frequently threatening the integrity of the skin and subcutaneous tissue. In addition, these fractures may be associated with a higher incidence of neurovascular compromise than are fractures occurring about the hip and pelvis.

PATIENT EVALUATION

The anatomic and biomechanical considerations are important not only in the treatment of patients with pathologic fracture of the distal femur but also in predicting the risk of these fractures and in determining the role of surgery vs. nonoperative means of treatment. Approximately 75% of patients with metastatic disease to bone complain of pain.[5] In other patients the diagnosis may be made on the basis of technetium bone scanning or other imaging modalities. The treatment algorithm will be determined by whether the primary tumor diagnosis is known, by whether single or multiple bone metastases are present, and by the presence or absence of symptoms. The treatment plan will also be determined on the basis of whether bone is the first site of metastasis.

A plain radiograph remains the most valuable

tool in the evaluation of patients with possible metastatic disease. The classic radiographic finding is a permeative radiolucent or mixed radiolucent or radiopaque appearance with associated endosteal scalloping or cortical destruction. When a lesion of the distal femur is noted, it is essential to image the entire femur and proximal tibia so that other areas of involvement are not missed. Because of the lack of a significant amount of cortical bone, because of the overlying patella, and because of at times confusing soft tissue shadows, radiographs of the distal femur may be inadequate for precise evaluation of tumor extent. In these instances, imaging studies such as computed tomography (CT) or magnetic resonance imaging (MRI) may be helpful.

CT is excellent for determining cortical integrity. MRI is capable of showing bone marrow changes and soft tissue extent, which is valuable not only to the surgeon but also to the medical oncologist and the radiation oncologist. Technetium bone scanning is highly sensitive and is useful for demonstrating other lesions in the same or other extremities that should be evaluated; however, its limited resolution makes precise definition of the extent of the tumor impossible.

The next stage in the evaluation is the determination of the need for a diagnostic tissue sample in preparation for treatment. Also, if a fracture has not occurred, the need for prophylactic internal fixation should be assessed.

In patients who have radiographic findings suggestive of a metastatic lesion and no known primary tumor, Rougraff et al.[6] have described a strategy that when used in combination with a bone biopsy identified the primary tumor in 85% of the patients studied. A careful physical examination that includes the breast and prostate, mammography, and serologic tests, such as prostate-specific antigen, serum protein electrophoresis, and urologic protein analysis, are also recommended. If these are nondiagnostic, CT of the chest, abdomen, and pelvis is performed.

Even in patients with a history of carcinoma, biopsy may be important for ruling out a second malignant lesion. This is especially true if the bone lesion is the first site of metastatic disease. It is also advisable to perform a biopsy and a frozen section in cases of pathologic fracture to confirm the diagnosis of metastatic disease before the placement of internal fixation.

After this evaluation the multidisciplinary treatment team can arrive at a rational treatment plan. This will be based on the nature of the primary tumor, the perceived efficacy of nonoperative treatment, an estimate of the proclivity of the bone lesion to fracture, and the operative risks to the patient. Whereas surgery and radiation therapy have traditionally been considered the standard in the treatment of these diseases, newer approaches, including medical therapy directed at the resorptive osteoclasts as well as radiopharmaceuticals and pain therapy, may be beneficial.

MANAGEMENT
Radiation Therapy

The general principles of radiation therapy in the treatment of metastatic disease to the musculoskeletal system have been discussed elsewhere. We will discuss the role of radiotherapy in the palliative management of pain and the prevention and treatment of pathologic fractures, as well as specific principles that apply to radiation therapy for distal femur lesions. There is no body of literature that is specific for the radiation experience in the treatment of lesions in the distal femur. Hence the specific radiation therapy principles for distal femur lesions are derived from the general principles of non-site-specific radiation therapy for metastatic bone disease.

As in other skeletal sites, metastatic lesions in the distal femur often are accompanied by significant bone pain. The efficacy of radiation therapy in providing pain relief has been well documented in several randomized and nonrandomized studies. However, to date there is no standard regimen for treatment of osseous metastases. In fact, a consensus meeting on the topic of treatment of osseous metastases concluded with no significant recommendations and indicated that the relationships between radiotherapy dose and response, duration in terms of pain relief, and bone healing were poorly defined and therefore required further investigation.[7]

In the United States, the Radiation Therapy Oncology Group (RTOG) conducted a large randomized trial testing various dose regimens for solitary and multiple bone metastases. The patients in that study had one or more painful metastases of the femur, humerus, pelvis, or thoracic or lumbar spine. Eligible patients were divided into those with solitary metastases and those who had multiple sites of metastatic disease but only one painful site. The patients with solitary metastases were randomly assigned to receive either 4050 cGy in 3 weeks (270 cGy per fraction $\times$ 15) or 2000 cGy in 1 week (400 cGy per fraction $\times$ 5). Patients with multiple metastatic sites were randomly assigned to four treatment arms. These included 3000 cGy in 2 weeks (300 cGy per fraction $\times$ 10), 1500 cGy in 1 week (300 cGy per fraction $\times$ 5), 2000 cGy in 1 week (400 cGy per fraction $\times$ 5), and 2500 cGy in 1 week (500 cGy per fraction $\times$ 5). All patients were stratified by primary tumor site, site of metastasis, internal fixation, and institution. The patient accrual was completed in February 1980, and the final analysis was presented in 1982.[8] There were 146 evaluable patients in the solitary-metastasis group. In the group with multiple metastases, there were 613 evaluable patients. Of the patients in both groups, close to 90% eventually experienced at least minimal pain relief, whereas 83% achieved partial relief and 54% achieved complete relief. For the solitary-metastasis group, there was no significant difference between the two treatment arms as to frequency of pain relief. Similarly, in the multiple-metastases group, there was no significant difference between the various treatment arms in relation to frequency of pain relief. What was significant in all groups was the fact that patients with primary tumors of the prostate and breast had more frequent complete pain relief than did those with lung or other primary lesions. A total of 62 pathologic fractures occurred at treated sites, comprising 8% of all treated sites. Specifically, in long bones the fracture rate was 13%. For patients with multiple metastatic sites the fracture rate was independent of the radiation dose schedule employed, with an overall fracture rate of 8%. For the group of patients with a solitary metastasis, however, the frequency of fractures was 18% for those treated with 4050 cGy, compared with 4% for those treated with 2000 cGy.

Role of Radiation Therapy in Prevention and Treatment of Pathologic Fractures

There continues to be debate as to the efficacy of radiation therapy in the prevention and treatment of pathologic fractures. Whereas most would favor prophylactic surgical fixation of impending fractures, Cheng et al.[9] reported the outcome of ra-

diation therapy alone in the management of 59 women in whom breast cancer had metastasized to the femur, humerus, and acetabulum. High-risk lesions were not treated with prophylactic internal fixation but, instead, with radiation therapy alone. None of these patients sustained a pathologic fracture. This is in contrast to the RTOG study in which there was a 13% rate of fractures in long bones with radiation therapy alone. With regard to treatment of pathologic fractures, Perez et al.[10] reported on patients with pathologic fractures treated with internal fixation vs. those treated with conservative nonsurgical techniques. Of patients treated with fixation and postoperative radiation therapy, 70% had good to excellent functional outcomes. Of those patients, 80% had good to excellent pain relief. For patients treated nonoperatively, the corresponding rates for functional outcome and pain relief were 30% and 44%, respectively.

Although reports in the orthopedic literature allude to the use of postoperative radiation therapy after internal fixation, details of the radiation therapy and its effect on bone healing are never thoroughly discussed. However, Townsend et al.[11] evaluated postoperative radiation therapy retrospectively in patients who underwent internal fixation for impending pathologic fractures and in those who already had fractures. Of those patients, 91% had femoral lesions. Of the 64 orthopedic stabilization procedures evaluated, 29 patients received no radiation therapy and were treated with surgery alone, whereas the remaining 35 received adjuvant radiation therapy after the surgical procedure. The end points studied were the functional status, subsequent orthopedic procedures to the same site, and survival after surgery. By univariate analysis, surgery plus radiation therapy and prefracture functional status were the only significant predictors of patients achieving normal use of the affected extremity, with or without pain, after treatment. On multivariate analysis, however, only postoperative radiation therapy was significantly associated with obtaining a good functional status. The predicted probability of achieving a good functional status was 52% for the patients undergoing surgery plus radiation therapy vs. 11.5% for the patients who had surgery alone. Similarly, second orthopedic procedures were more common in the surgery-alone patients than in the patients treated with adjuvant radiation therapy despite the fact that the actuarial median survival for the surgery-alone group was 3.3 months, compared with 12.4 months for the combined modality group. However, Townsend et al.[11] comment on the fact that median survival may have been influenced by a possible selection bias in that more favorable patients may have been referred for radiation therapy. For those patients treated with radiation therapy the mean time to the start of radiation therapy after surgery was 2 weeks. Various dose fraction schedules were used, the median dose being 3000 cGy. Of the 25 irradiated sites, 21 included the entire length of the orthopedic device. This study therefore quantitatively supports the benefit of postoperative radiation therapy in patients treated surgically for pathologic fractures or impending pathologic fractures.

Guidelines for Use of Radiation Therapy

At our institution we follow certain general guidelines for patients with distal femoral lesions. Not all patients with metastatic lesions to the distal femur will require radiation therapy. Certainly patients who have generalized metastatic disease from primary tumors generally considered to be chemosensitive and who have no structural concerns may be treated with chemotherapy alone. Patients with metastatic papillary or follicular thyroid carcinomas can be treated successfully with iodine 131 (radioactive iodine). Tumors that are resistant to these treatments, however, may require radiation therapy.

For patients with impending pathologic fracture who undergo prophylactic fixation, postoperative radiation therapy is recommended. The entire surgical bed is treated, including the whole implant and any soft tissue extension that may be present. A dose of 3000 cGy in 10 fractions of 300 cGy each is employed. Symptomatic lesions without impending fractures are treated with radiation therapy alone, with the same dose schedule, and are followed radiographically. Again, care should be employed to include any soft tissue extension that may be present in such lesions. Despite the controversy in the literature regarding dose fractionation schemes, we tend to employ the more protracted course because we believe that this provides a more lasting benefit and because the scheme of 3000 cGy in 10 fractions does not significantly increase the risk of pathologic fracture due to the radiation therapy.

Certain subsets of patients with metastatic disease from favorable primary tumors are being treated with high-dose chemotherapy followed by bone marrow or stem cell rescue. At our institution, if these patients achieve a significant response, most of them then receive radiation therapy to sites of residual gross disease. This consolidative approach to radiation therapy also applies to lesions in the distal femur. If the distal femur lesion is a solitary metastasis or is one of only a few sites of metastatic disease, it may be appropriate to treat these patients with an even more protracted course of radiation therapy that uses a smaller dose per fraction for a higher total dose. This approach is supported by Arcangeli and Micheli,[12] who reported on the responsiveness of bone metastases to doses of radiation therapy beyond 4000 cGy.

The long-term effects of radiation therapy should always be considered in the planning of radiation to the distal femur, especially in patients who have a prolonged expected survival. When radiation therapy alone is employed for nonsurgical patients, it is extremely important to define the extent of the metastatic lesion accurately. Lesions close to the knee joint present a technical challenge. With good MRI a distal femur lesion can be treated with adequate margins without treatment of the knee joint. Avoidance of the knee joint will preserve the synovial structures, and stiff knee and arthritic complications of radiation therapy will be avoided. In lesions that are too distal to allow the knee joint to be avoided, it may be possible to circumvent treatment of the whole knee joint, thereby minimizing the late radiation effects. Finally, care should be taken to avoid treating the entire circumference of the extremity. Sparing a strip of soft tissue, including the cutaneous and subcutaneous tissues, will significantly reduce the likelihood of distal leg edema.

Radiation therapy plays an important role in the treatment of metastatic disease to the distal femur as part of a multidisciplinary approach to the treatment of these patients. The goals of therapy are to provide good palliation of pain, obtain a good functional outcome, and thereby improve the quality of life. In certain patients, it may even lead to prolonged survival and a disease-free interval. Recent and future improvements in the delivery of radiation therapy, such as three-dimensional conformal therapy and intensity-modulation radiation therapy, may soon be used for the treatment of patients with metastatic disease, especially those who have a limited systemic disease burden. It is hoped that these advances will be associated with improved effectiveness of the radiation therapy and improved long-term survival.

Surgical Therapy
Indications for Surgery

The indications for prophylactic fixation of the distal femur remain vague and poorly defined. Hipp et al.[13] demonstrated an inability to reach consensus on this procedure, even among experienced orthopedic oncologists. No prospective studies have been performed in this area. Those studies that have been published have been based on retrospective cohorts and poorly controlled evaluations. In addition, laboratory models of metastatic disease underestimate the permeative nature of these defects and have been of limited usefulness in providing indications for surgery. The indications for prophylactic surgery depend greatly on the surgeon's experience; the patient's functional status, degree of discomfort, and life expectancy; and the size, location, and radiographic appearance (lucent or dense) of the lesion. Mirels[14] described a scoring system for evaluating pathologic lesions that does not specifically address the distal femur (Table 33-1). Other suggested indications, such as a defect of 2.5 cm or larger or 50% cortical involvement, may or may not apply to the distal femur, given the relatively large proportion of cancellous bone. Within the distal femur, location itself may be the single most important variable, because any tumor noted in the intercondylar notch or at the junction of the diaphysis and the condyles is at high risk of fracture. In addition, one must consider that in this location, radiographs frequently underestimate tumor involvement. More extensive involvement is often noted in other imaging studies or intraoperatively. In addition, pain after radiation therapy is an indication for prophylactic fixation.

If a fracture has already occurred, nonoperative treatment should be reserved only for patients who are considered immediately moribund. Ambulation, the ability to transfer, and the ability to perform even the most basic activities of daily living are severely compromised by a supracondylar or intercondylar femur fracture. Fractures of the distal femur are inherently unstable and are unlikely to heal with closed treatment, be it traction, bracing, or casting. Narcotics and immobilization place patients at high risk of hypercalcemia, respiratory depression, and death. For these reasons, open reduction and internal fixation are recommended in almost all cases of pathologic fracture of the distal femur. The precise procedure, however, depends on the tumor location and size, the need for diagnostic tissue, the functional status of the patient, and the surgeon's experience and preference.

Under certain circumstances, en bloc resection of the distal femur with endoprosthetic reconstruction should be considered. For some primary tumors, such as renal cell carcinoma, wide resection of isolated bone metastases has been demonstrated to be associated with prolonged survival.[15] This

---

Table 33-1   Scoring system for radiographs of long bones with pathologic lesions to assess fracture risk

	Score		
Variable	**1**	**2**	**3**
Site	Upper limb	Lower limb	Peritrochanteric
Pain	Mild	Moderate	Functional
Lesion	Blastic	Mixed	Lytic
Size (units)*	$<\frac{1}{3}$	$\frac{1}{3}-\frac{2}{3}$	$>\frac{2}{3}$

Adapted from Mirels H. Metastatic disease in long bones. Clin Orthop 249:256-264, 1989.

*Fraction represents amount of cross-sectional area of bone involved in the lesion. Prophylactic fixation is recommended for scores of 8 or higher.

procedure may also be considered if the primary tumor is thought to be radioresistant, such as adenocarcinoma of the lung and renal cell carcinoma.

Although rarely considered for proximal disease, palliative amputation for distal femoral metastases is indicated in cases of intractable pain in spite of attempts to obtain rigid internal fixation, in cases of local tumor progression threatening surrounding soft tissues, and in cases of sepsis after operative fixation. In addition, transfemoral amputation may be considered as the primary treatment for nonambulatory patients. It is effective in decreasing the metabolic demands placed on the patient and in decreasing the need for narcotic medication. Amputation also improves a patient's mobility and ability to transfer in contrast to the condition with a pathologic fracture.

Surgical Treatment

Open reduction of fractures and internal fixation, most often with the use of plates and screws supplemented by polymethylmethacrylate (PMMA), are recommended for fractures or impending fractures of the distal femur. A lateral approach is preferred; however, in the case of an impending fracture with a medially based lesion, it is better to approach from the medial side, maintaining maximal strength by leaving the lateral cortex intact. The patient is placed in a supine position with a sterile tourniquet applied to the proximal thigh. A laterally based distal thigh skin incision is made, followed by deep dissection that splits the iliotibial band in line with its fibers proximally and curves anterior distally, ending just lateral to the patellar tendon. Exposure of the distal femoral articular surface is gained through a lateral parapatellar arthrotomy. The lesion is identified, subjected to biopsy as required, and curetted, with removal of all visible gross disease. Although debulking may be considered somewhat controversial, it is our belief that curettage minimizes hemorrhage, decreases tumor load, making radiation therapy more effective, and improves the interface between PMMA and bone. Additional mechanical débridement with a pneumatic burr can be performed.

An appropriately sized internal fixation device is

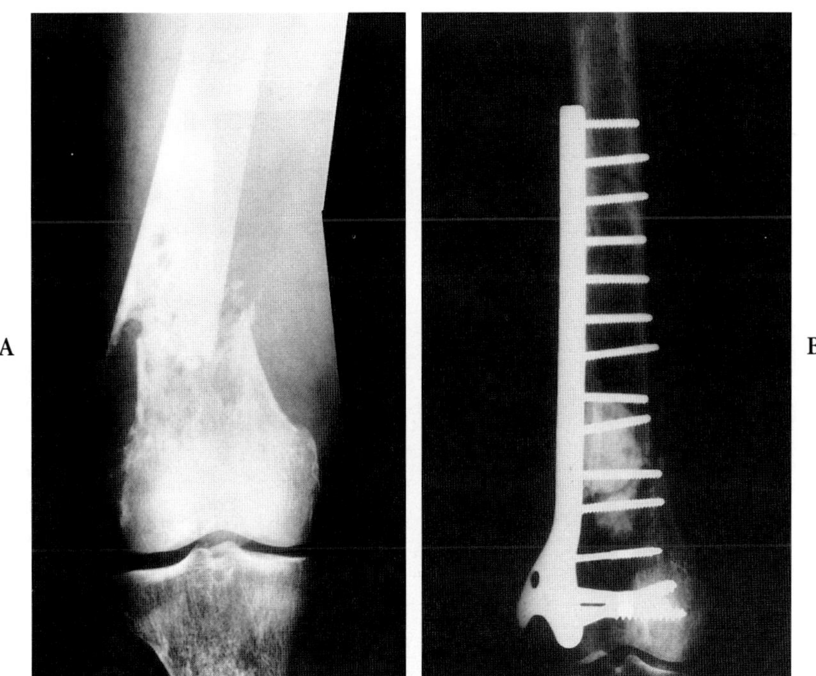

Fig. 33-1   Anteroposterior roentgenogram (**A**) of the right knee of a 66-year-old man with metastatic prostate carcinoma, demonstrating a distal femoral metaphyseal fracture. Note the poor quality of the distal femoral and proximal tibial bone. For that reason, the ankle orthoses supracondylar plate with its multiple distal screw holes was used for internal fixation with polymethacrylate supplementation, as seen on the postoperative anteroposterior roentgenogram (**B**).

CONCLUSION

The proximal femur and femoral shaft are probably the sites of skeletal lesions that most often require surgical intervention. A functional knee joint is crucial to maintenance of the ambulatory status of the patient. Thorough evaluation and intervention before fracture will allow the patient to continue to ambulate and maintain his or her independence.

REFERENCES

1. Landis SH, Murray T, Bolden S, Wingo PA. Cancer statistics. CA Cancer J Clin 48(1):20-23, 1998.
2. Harrington KD. Introduction. In Harrington KD, ed. Orthopaedic Management of Metastatic Bone Disease. St. Louis: CV Mosby, 1988, p 10.
3. Harrington KD. The role of surgery in the management of pathologic fractures. Orthop Clin 8(4):841-858, 1977.
4. Habermann ET, Sachs R, Stern RE, Hirsch DM, Anderson WJ Jr. The pathology and treatment of metastatic disease of the femur. Clin Orthop 169:70-82, 1982.
5. Wagner G. Frequency of pain in patients with cancer. Recent Results Cancer Res 89:64-71, 1984.
6. Rougraff BT, Kneisl JS, Simon MA. Skeletal metastases of unknown origin: A prospective study of a diagnostic strategy. J Bone Joint Surg Am 75:1276-1281, 1993.
7. Bates T, Yarnold JR, Blitzer P, Nelson OS, Rubin P, Maher J. Bone metastasis consensus statement. Int J Radiat Oncol Biol Phys 23:215-216, 1992.
8. Tong D, Gillick L, Hendrickson FR. The palliation of symptomatic osseous metastases: Final results of the study by the Radiation Therapy Oncology Group. Cancer 50:839-899, 1982.
9. Cheng DS, Sietz CB, Eyre HT. Nonoperative management of femoral, humeral, and acetabular metastasis in patients with breast carcinoma. Cancer 45:1533-1537, 1980.
10. Perez CA, Bradfield JS, Morgan HC. Management of pathologic fractures. Cancer 29:684-693, 1972.
11. Townsend PW, Smalley SR, Cozad SC, Rosenthal HG, Hassanein RES. Role of postoperative radiation therapy after stabilization of fractures caused by metastatic disease. Int J Radiat Oncol Biol Phys 31:43-49, 1995.
12. Arcangeli G, Micheli A. The responsiveness of bone metastases to radiotherapy: The effect of site, histology and radiation dose on pain relief. Radiother Oncol 14:95-101, 1989.
13. Hipp JA, Springfield DS, Hayes WC. Predicting pathologic fracture risk in the management of metastatic bone defects. Clin Orthop 312:120-135, 1995.
14. Mirels H. Metastatic disease in long bones. Clin Orthop 249:256-264, 1989.
15. Henriksson C, Haraldsson G, Aldenborg F, Lindberg S, Pettersson S. Skeletal metastases in 102 patients evaluated before surgery for renal cell carcinoma. Scand J Urol Nephrol 26:263-266, 1992.
16. Harrington KD, Johnson JO, Turner RH, Green DL. The use of methylmethacrylate as an adjunct in the internal fixation of malignant neoplastic fractures. J Bone Joint Surg Am 54:1665-1676, 1972.
17. Peabody TD, Finn HA. Femoral diaphysis and distal femur. In Simon MA, Springfield DS, eds. Surgery for Bone and Soft Tissue Tumors. Philadelphia: JB Lippincott, 1998, pp 710-711.
18. Wang HM, Galasko GSB, Crank S, Oliver G, Ward C. Methotrexate loaded acrylic cement in the management of skeletal metastases. Clin Orthop 312:173-186, 1995.

CHAPTER 34

Metastatic Disease of the Tibia, Foot, and Ankle

John P. Heiner, M.D.

The Tibia
Incidence
Management
    Radiation Therapy
    Surgical Therapy

The Foot and Ankle
Incidence
Clinical Presentation
Management
    Radiation Therapy
    Surgical Therapy

Conclusion

Metastatic disease distal to the knee is relatively uncommon. Few series of patients address this area. A wide variety of primary cancers have been described, along with multiple treatment options. Therefore the clinician must use principles learned from other sites to determine the best approach for each patient.

The Tibia

INCIDENCE

Metastatic disease of the tibia is seen more frequently than metastatic disease of the foot. However, the literature is scant regarding the frequency of metastatic lesions in this area. Metastatic lesions involving the knee are covered in the preceding chapter. Leeson et al.[1] reviewed 57 autopsy reports of patients with metastatic disease distal to the elbow and knee. Of 827 autopsies, 33 showed involvement of the tibia, for an incidence of 4%. The fibula was involved in 5 of 827 cases, which makes metastatic lesions there rare (<1% incidence). The article by Leeson et al. may actually underestimate the occurrence of metastasis to the tibia and fibula because many of the patients' records were from the 1970s and earlier, when modern radiographic methods such as magnetic resonance imaging (MRI) were not yet available.

In the 33 cases of tibial involvement, Leeson et al. found five pathologic fractures of the tibia. One of five lesions of the fibula also fractured. Of 233 surgically treated cases of pathologic fractures or impending fractures, Dijkstra et al.[2] operated on only six tibia fractures (5%). In this small series, three of six patients returned to walking at 5 weeks, whereas the others were unable to walk because of the extent of the metastatic disease at other sites. Blood loss for the tibia operations averaged 900 ml, and it was not clear whether a tourniquet was used.

Beauchamp and Sim[3] reported the largest series of tibia metastases: 24 patients treated at the Mayo Clinic from 1970 to 1985. Lung carcinoma was the most common primary cancer. None of the 24 patients presented with a pathologic fracture. Some of the patients had no symptoms, and the disease was found by a screening bone scan. Of the 24 patients, 13 were women. Eight of the 24 patients had lesions involving the patellar tendon's insertion in the proximal tibia.

The presenting symptom in most patients is pain. Asymptomatic lesions seen on bone scan seem to be the second most common diagnostic finding. Pathologic fracture is rare. This may be because patients experience pain in the tibia earlier than in the femur, which is due to the tibia's subcutaneous position.

MANAGEMENT

Metastatic disease may be treated with chemotherapy, hormone therapy, radiation, observation, or bracing. The choice between chemotherapy and hormone therapy depends on the primary tumor. The tibia is much easier to brace than the femur. The proximal tibia may be braced with a long knee brace or a custom hinged knee-ankle-foot orthosis. The distal tibia and ankle may be treated with a removable ankle-foot orthosis or with a removable short-leg walking boot.

Osteoblastic lesions often are due to either breast or prostate carcinoma. These patients often have diffuse bone carcinomatosis, and in these patients surgery is rarely indicated. Chemotherapy or hormone therapy, along with bracing, may relieve symptoms and allow protected weightbearing by the patient (Fig. 34-1).

Radiation Therapy

Most radiation doses to the tibia approach 30 Gy. Some tumors, such as squamous cell carcinoma of the lung and renal cell carcinoma, may require higher doses for local control. The clinician must be careful in radiating the tibia because of its subcutaneous position. Poor soft tissue coverage and marginal blood supply to the tissue put it at much higher risk of soft tissue complications if surgery is required.

Surgical Therapy

Surgical reconstruction of the tibia depends on the exact location of the lesion to be treated. Lesions involving the proximal tibia and knee joint require total joint replacement with resection of the metastatic lesion.[4] In some cases the patella tendon may have to be reconstructed and attached directly to the prosthesis. The construct should be cement-

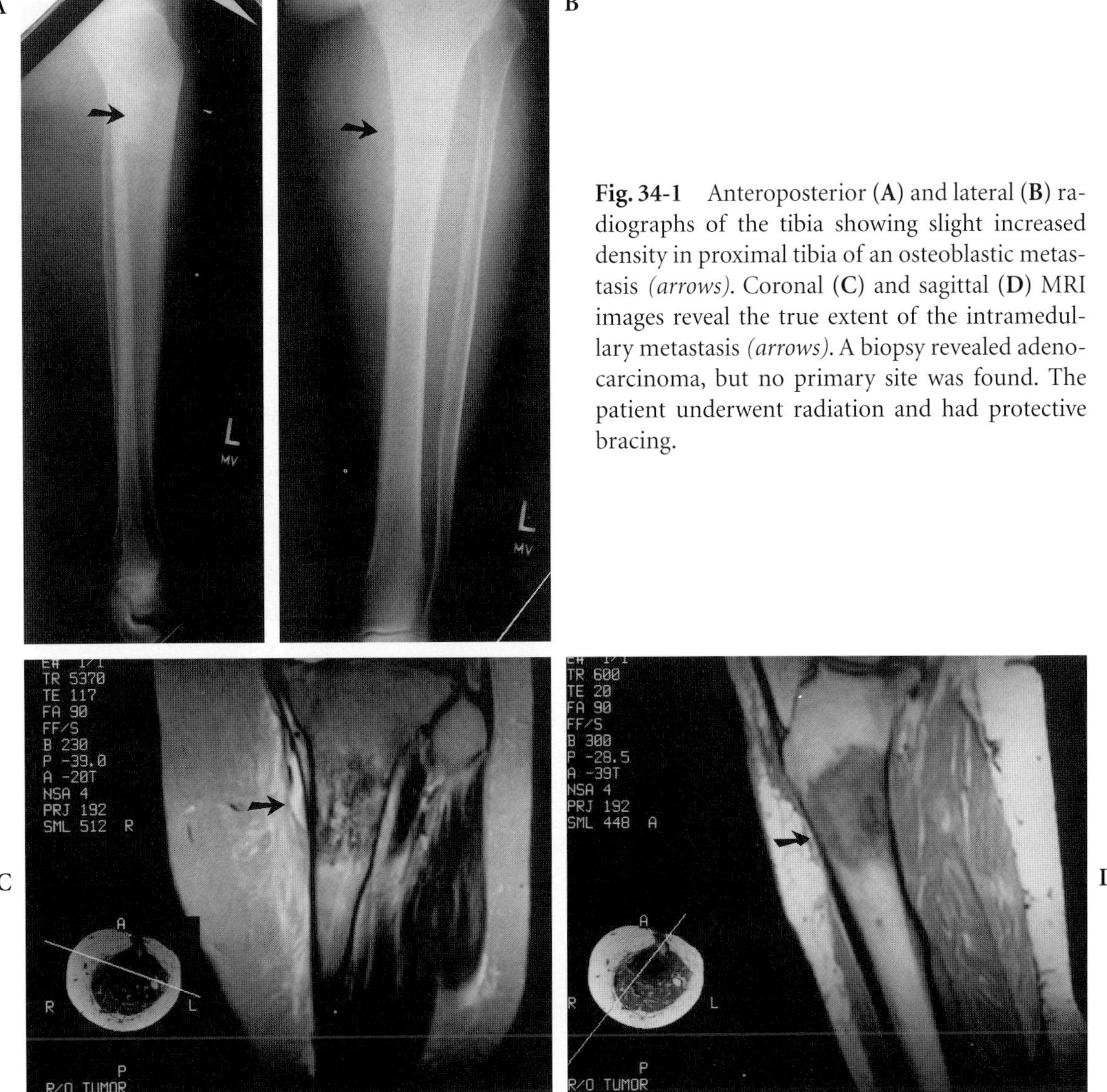

Fig. 34-1 Anteroposterior (**A**) and lateral (**B**) radiographs of the tibia showing slight increased density in proximal tibia of an osteoblastic metastasis *(arrows)*. Coronal (**C**) and sagittal (**D**) MRI images reveal the true extent of the intramedullary metastasis *(arrows)*. A biopsy revealed adenocarcinoma, but no primary site was found. The patient underwent radiation and had protective bracing.

ed to allow immediate motion and progressive weightbearing. Allografts and knee fusions are usually not indicated in metastatic disease.

Metastatic disease of the proximal tibia but distal to the knee joint may be treated with curettage and cementation and supplemented with plate fixation (Fig. 34-2). This allows full weightbearing and rapid rehabilitation. The plate should be inserted on the weakest side of the tibia. Double plating may be necessary. Lesions in the diaphyseal tibia usually do well with an intramedullary nail. The nail should go well past the lesions. Tibial nails should have locking screws to protect the midshaft of the tibia, or methylmethacrylate should be used to augment the stability of the tibia and allow immediate weightbearing (Fig. 34-3).

The distal tibia is treated much the way the proximal tibia is treated. Curettage and cement are used, often in conjunction with a buttress plate. In some cases curettage and cement alone may suffice (Fig. 34-4). Distal tibial lesions that have destroyed the ankle joint may require a below-the-knee amputation. In patients with limited life expectancy, bracing is a better option than amputation.

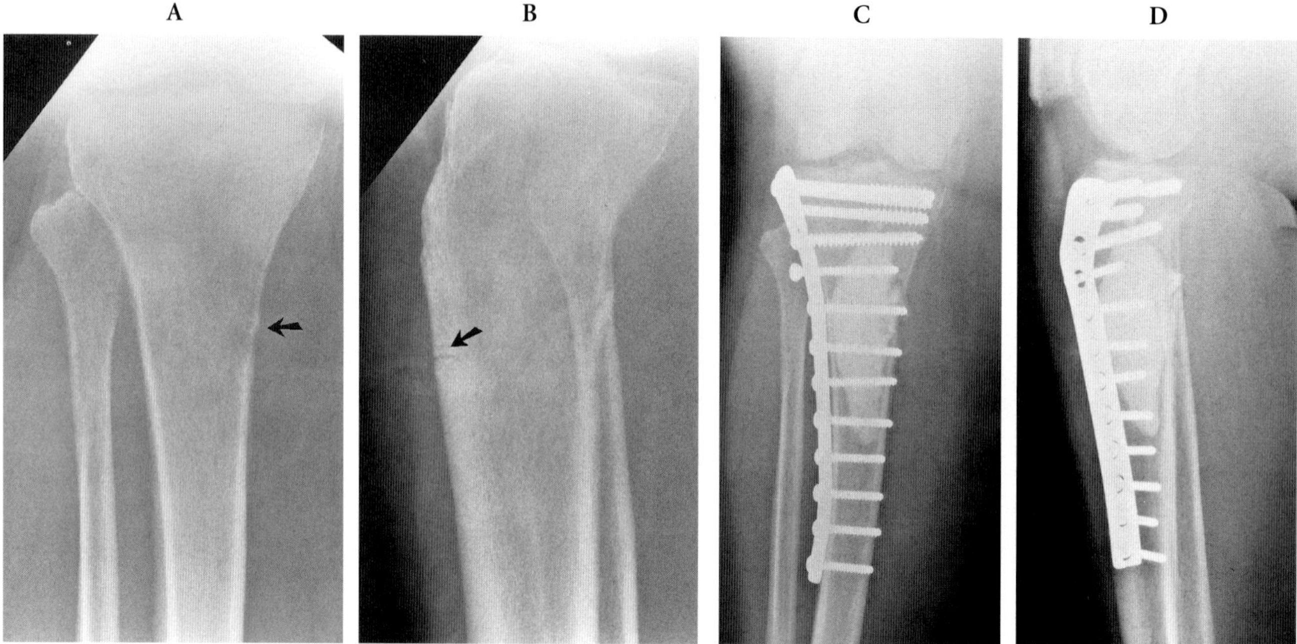

Fig. 34-2 **A,** Anteroposterior proximal tibia radiograph of a 52-year-old white woman with prior history of adenocarcinoma of the uterus who now has progressive, severe pain in the leg with weightbearing. A lytic lesion with cortical destruction is shown *(arrow)*. **B,** Lateral view shows cortical lucency consistent with pathologic fracture *(arrow)*. **C,** Anteroposterior radiograph after surgery shows appearance after open biopsy (which confirmed metastatic adenocarcinoma consistent with original primary lesion), curettage, cementation and stabilization with a buttress plate and screws. **D,** Lateral view after surgical curettage, cementation, and stabilization.

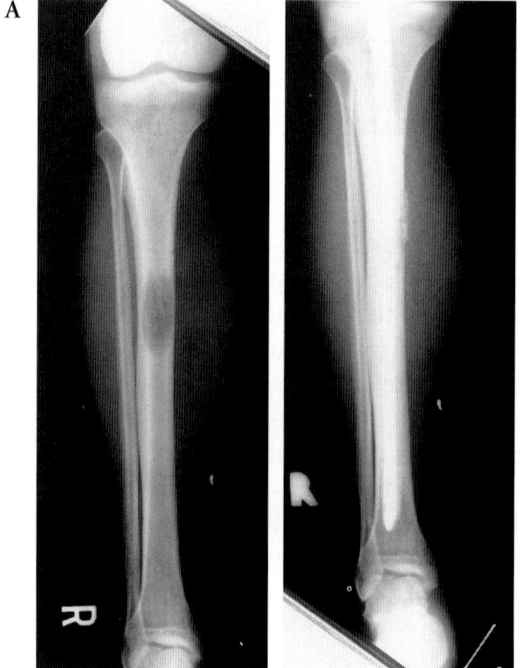

Fig. 34-3 **A,** Anteroposterior radiograph of the tibia demonstrates a large midshaft lytic lesion and a small proximal tibia lesion. The patient had known renal cell carcinoma. **B,** Intramedullary nailing supplemented with methylmethacrylate was performed. Immediate weightbearing was well tolerated. The patient survived 5 more years until death due to widespread metastatic disease to the lungs.

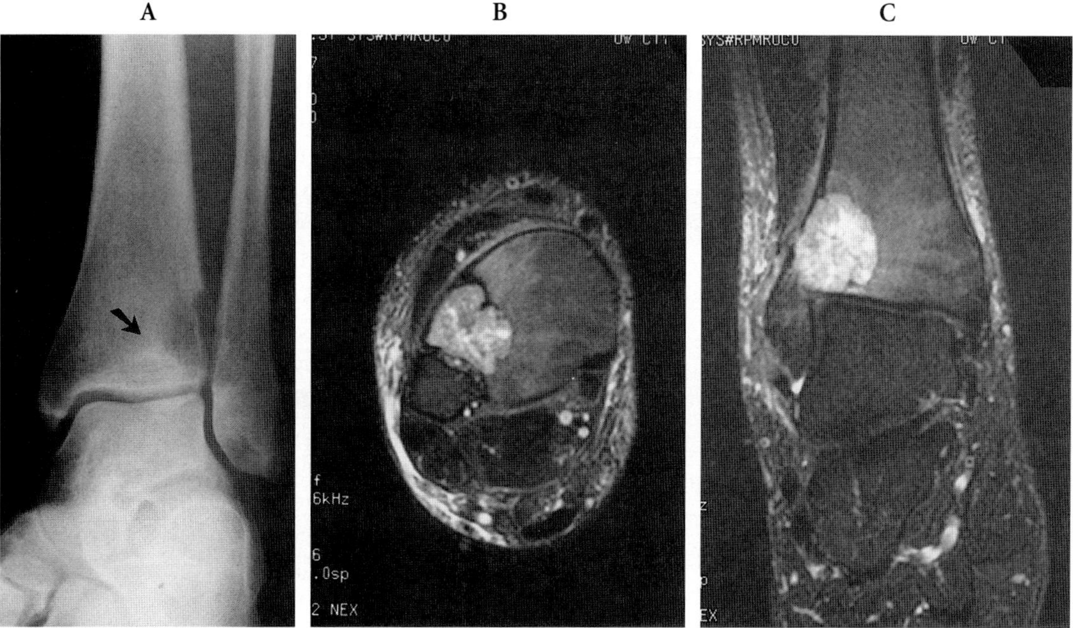

Fig. 34-4   A, Mortise view of the ankle reveals lytic lesion just proximal to the ankle joint *(arrow)*. The patient presented with ankle pain and no known cancer. Coronal **(B)** and transverse **(C)** MRI images reveal preservation of the subchondral bone in the ankle and good containment of the lesion within the distal tibia. A biopsy revealed metastatic renal cell carcinoma. The patient was treated with curettage and methacrylate insertion. The ankle continues to perform well 4 years after surgery.

The Foot and Ankle

INCIDENCE

The ankle joint and foot are uncommon sites of metastatic disease. Wu and Guise[5] found only four cases among 41,833 patients with cancer. As with the tibia, little is written about metastases in these sites, with several small series and a variety of case reports making up most of the literature.[6-9]

A number of case reports of metastases to the synovium of joints have appeared over the years.[10-12] Munn et al.[13] reviewed 27 cases of metastatic disease of the synovium, and four patients presented with ankle synovitis. Each patient had a different type of primary tumor. In the entire group of 27 patients, 14 had lung carcinoma as the primary tumor. The effusions could be due to either periarticular lesions or synovial metastases without adjacent bone involvement. Hypertrophic osteoarthropathy may also present with effusions, which is most commonly seen in patients with lung carcinoma. Nine of fourteen patients in the series respond-

ed to radiation, but specific data for the patients with ankle effusions were not available. Koss and Johnson[11] reported a patient with lung carcinoma metastatic to the ankle synovium who had intractable pain. A below-the-knee amputation was performed, but the patient survived only several months.

Metastatic disease of the foot can be extremely disabling, and treatment should be directed at maintaining the patient's ability to ambulate. The lesions can occur anywhere in the foot, and some patients, especially those with long-standing disease, can have diffuse involvement of multiple bones in the foot. Hattrup et al.[14] reported 21 cases of metastases to the foot and ankle. In nine patients this was the first evidence of metastatic disease. The calcaneus was involved in 8 of 21 cases, and six metastases were in the phalanges. Two patients had only soft tissue involvement. Lung carcinoma was responsible for six of the patients; renal carcinoma was found in four patients; and colon carcinoma was found in an additional four patients.

Table 34-1   Incidence of specific bones of the foot involved with metastatic disease as described in the literature

Bones involved	Percent of cases
Tarsals	50
Calcaneus	23
Talus	8
Cuneiform	7
Cuboid	5
Navicular	4
Tarsals unspecified	3
Metatarsals	23
Phalanges	17
Foot unspecified	10
TOTAL	100

From Zindrick MR, Young MP, Daley RJ, Light TR. Metastatic tumors of the foot: Case report and literature review. Clin Orthop 170:219-225, 1982.

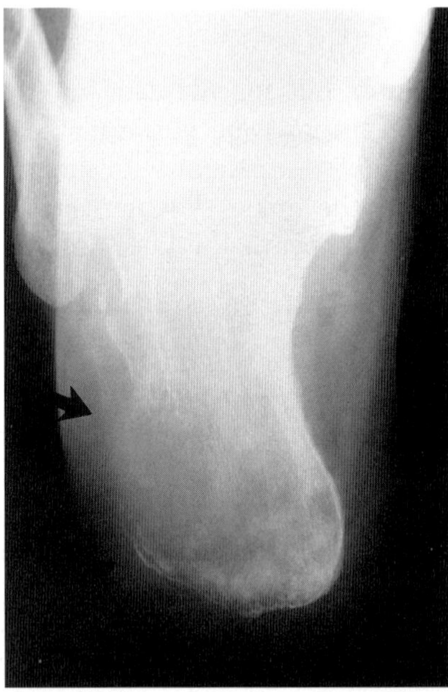

Fig. 34-5   An elderly woman presented with severe heel pain. Axial view of the calcaneus revealed destruction of the lateral body *(arrow)*. Open biopsy and curettage were performed. Biopsy revealed transitional cell carcinoma of the bladder. The patient died of widespread metastatic disease.

Zindrick et al.[15] reviewed reports of metastatic tumors of the foot in 1981. Seventy-two cases were located, with 38 having histologic confirmation. Colon, kidney, and lung carcinomas were found to be the most common primary tumors. The tarsal bones were involved most often, with the calcaneus being involved 23% of the time (Table 34-1). The hindfoot is also mentioned most frequently in case reports. Healey et al.[16] reported 20 lesions involving the foot, with five calcaneal lesions and no talar lesions. Petru et al.,[17] Groves and Stiles,[18] Clarke and Smith,[9] and Litton et al.[19] all recently reported calcaneal metastatic disease from widely varying primary sites (Fig. 34-5). Lombardi and Amadio[20] reviewed the Mayo Clinic experience with metastases to the foot. Mean survival was 11 months after diagnosis of the lesion. However, several patients did survive more than 2 years.

CLINICAL PRESENTATION

In the hindfoot as well as in the forefoot the presenting complaint is usually pain. Many of the patients present with foot pain as the primary complaint or as the first evidence of metastasis. Diffuse swelling of the foot seems to accompany both hindfoot and forefoot lesions. In many cases the pain and swelling are disproportionate to the findings on standard radiography. The swelling can be mistaken for infection. Multiple bones may be involved, and a biopsy may be required.[21] In the absence of x-ray abnormalities, a technetium bone scan, computed tomography (CT), or MRI can give much additional information[9,17,18] (Fig. 34-6).

MANAGEMENT

As in most cases of metastatic skeletal disease, the treatment depends on the specific needs of the patient. Nonoperative treatment may consist of chemotherapy, hormone therapy, radiation, or bracing. Chemotherapy and hormone therapy are most effective for relief of pain in responsive tumors, such as breast cancer. Bracing and protection of the involved foot may be done with several off-the-shelf devices. Protective shoes and boots are available in different designs (Fig. 34-7). Many of these were developed to protect the diabetic foot. The boots are well padded and have insoles that can be customized for individual patients. Pressure relief shoes have cutouts in the sole to relieve any pres-

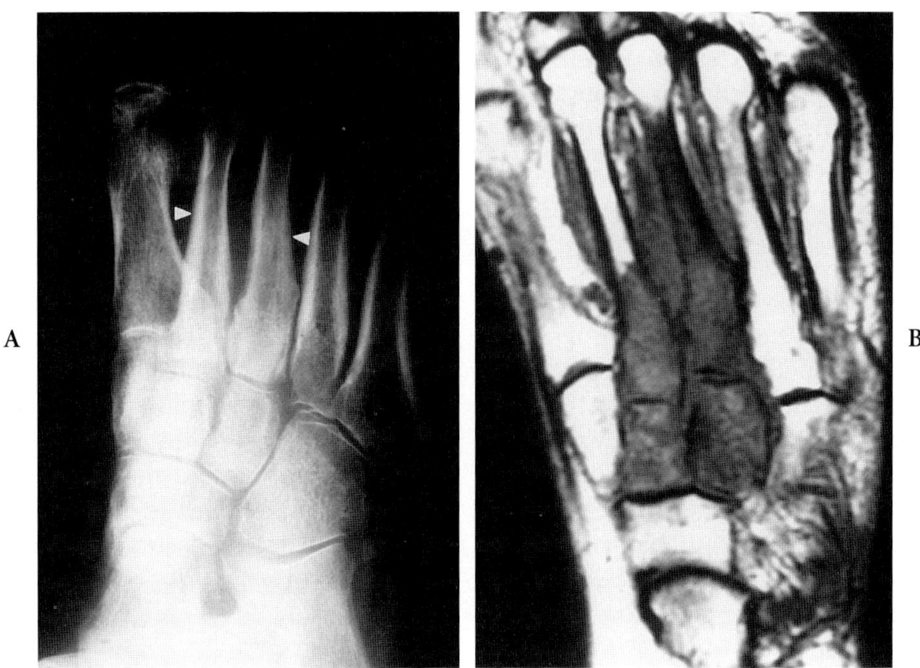

Fig. 34-6 **A,** An elderly woman with known breast cancer presents with severe foot pain. Oblique radiograph reveals mild intramedullary osteoblastic disease in the second and third metatarsals *(arrowheads)*. **B,** T1-weighted MRI reveals extensive disease in the second and third cuneiforms and second and third metatarsals. An open biopsy revealed metastatic breast cancer. Radiation therapy gave symptomatic relief.

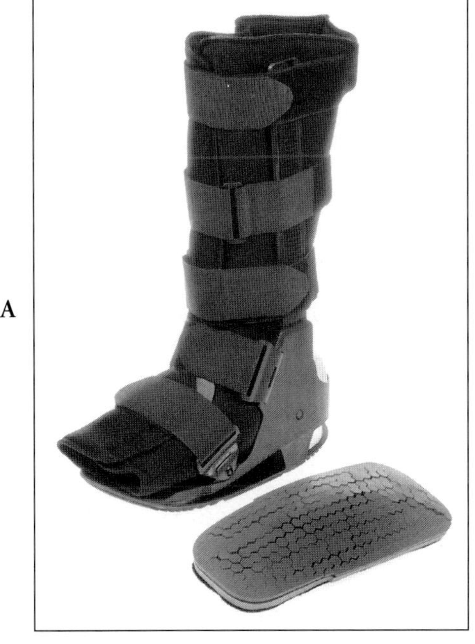

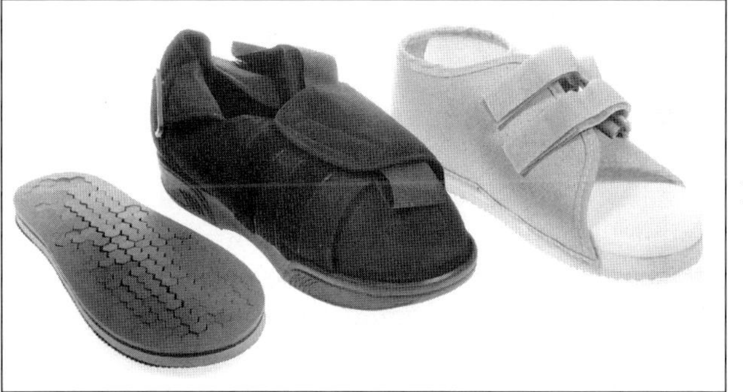

Fig. 34-7 **A,** Short leg boot (Centec Pressure Relief Boot, Centec, Camirillo, Calif.) with removable insole that is used for metastatic disease as well as the neuropathic foot. The insole has removable cutouts for pressure relief to the sole of the foot. **B,** Two removable pressure relief shoes are illustrated. On the left is the Centic pressure relief shoe (Centec, Camirillo, Calif.). This is used for metastatic disease of the foot when immobilization of the ankle is not required. This shoe features the removable pressure relief insole. Another option is the E24 wrap diabetic shoe (Professional Products, Inc., Defuniak Springs, Fla.) with a foam insole. In this shoe, the sole will mold to the foot, but it does not have the removable cutouts to the sole.

sure points in the foot. Custom molded shoes can also be used but they are much more expensive to make and often do not fit well after a short while because of the changing nature of the neoplasm in the foot.

Radiation Therapy

Radiation to the foot is usually reasonably well tolerated. Approximately 50% of the patients reported in all studies seem to have achieved relief of symptoms with radiation to the foot. Menon et al.[12] treated breast cancer that metastasized to the talus with 20 Gy of radiation and tamoxifen, with good local control. Healey et al.[16] reported a good clinical response with radiation in multifocal disease of the foot, but no dose was specified in their article. Hattrup et al.[14] reported that 12 of 21 cases of foot metastases were treated with radiation. Four of the twelve patients had good functional relief, but five had a poor response to radiation. Almost all of these patients had adenocarcinoma of the lung or colon or had a primary kidney carcinoma, all of which tend to respond poorly to radiation. The doses of radiation mentioned were 27 to 30 Gy, but not all of the radiated cases were discussed. Schwartz et al.[8] gave 40 Gy for multifocal disease of the foot, with a good clinical result.

Surgical Therapy

Surgical treatment of metastatic disease of the foot is used for pain relief or when other treatment modalities have failed. Often a biopsy is required to rule out other diagnoses, such as infection.[22] Debulking of large multifocal tumors has been reported, but it is not clear whether debulking a large area improves function or survival. Curettage can be done with insertion of methylmethacrylate in isolated lytic lesions of the hindfoot. Most reported cases of surgical treatment of foot metastases involve some type of amputation. Baran and Tosti[23] reported an amputation for a phalangeal lesion that achieved good relief. Hattrup et al.[14] reported three digital amputations out of 21 cases. For multifocal and hindfoot lesions, larger amputations are frequently reported. Dripchack and Roberson[24] reported a below-the-knee amputation for a metastasis from an extremely aggressive multifocal breast carcinoma. The patient survived more than 6 months. Hattrup's group reported four limb amputations for local disease control. One amputation

followed an unsuccessful curettage and radiation. These patients survived for an average of 24 months; three had adenocarcinoma, and one had renal cell carcinoma.

Conclusion

Metastatic disease distal to the knee is relatively unusual when compared with the number of lesions seen in the axial skeleton. Many patients present with distal lesions later in the course of their disease. Treatment should allow patients to maintain their ambulatory status and allow weightbearing if possible. Bracing and radiation can be used with success in many cases. In advanced cases, or if radiation is unsuccessful, surgery may be necessary for local control.

REFERENCES

1. Leeson MC, Makley JT, Carter JR. Metastatic skeletal disease distal to the elbow and knee. Clin Orthop 206:94-99, 1986.
2. Dijkstra S, Wiggers T, Van Geel BN, Boxma H. Impending and actual pathological fractures in patients with bone metastases of the long bones: A retrospective study of 233 surgically treated fractures. Eur J Surg 160:535-542, 1994.
3. Beauchamp CP, Sim FH. Lesions of the tibia. In Sim FH, ed. Diagnosis and Management of Metastatic Bone Disease: A Multidisciplinary Approach. New York: Raven Press, 1988, pp 207-212.
4. Tillman RM, Smith RB. Total knee replacement for metastatic destruction of the proximal tibia. J Bone Joint Surg Br 73:516-617, 1991.
5. Wu KK, Guise ER. Metastatic tumors of the foot. South Med J 71:807-808, 1978.
6. Tuteja A, Owings M, Pulliam J, Elzinga L. Adenocarcinoma of the colon metastasizing to the foot masquerading as osteomyelitis. J Am Podiatr Med Assoc 88(2):84-86, 1998.
7. Gauntt K, Boykoff TJ, Danna AT. Adenocarcinoma: A case of metastasis to the foot. J Am Podiatr Med Assoc 80(12):657-659, 1990.
8. Schwartz ED, Donahue FI, Bromson MS, Blaise JF. Metastatic prostate carcinoma to the foot with magnetic resonance imaging and pathologic correlation. Foot Ankle Int 19(9):594-597, 1998.
9. Clarke SJ, Smith TP. Metastatic endometrial carcinoma of the foot: A case report. J Am Podiatr Med Assoc 86(7):331-333, 1997.
10. Thompson KS, Reyes CV, Jensen J, Gattuso P, Sacks R. Synovial metastasis: Diagnosis by fine-needle aspiration cytologic investigation. Diagn Cytopathol 15(4):334-337, 1996.
11. Koss SD, Johnson KH. Metastatic lung cancer to ankle synovium: A case report. Foot Ankle Int 17(1):51-53, 1996.
12. Menon S, Smith CR, Baum M. Monoarthritis of the ankle: An unusual presentation of metastatic breast carcinoma. Eur J Cancer 30A(4):563-564, 1994.

13. Munn RK, Pierce ST, Sloan D, Weeks JA. Case report: Malignant joint effusions secondary to solid tumor metastasis. J Rheumatol 22(5):973-975, 1995.

14. Hattrup SJ, Amadio PC, Sim FH, Lombardi RM. Metastatic tumors of the foot and ankle. Foot Ankle 8(5):243-247, 1988.

15. Zindrick MR, Young MP, Daley RJ, Light TR. Metastatic tumors of the foot: Case report and literature review. Clin Orthop 170:219-225, 1982.

16. Healey JH, Turnbull AD, Miedema B, Lane JM. Acrometastases: A study of twenty-nine patients with osseous involvement of the hands and feet. J Bone Joint Surg Am 68(5):743-746, 1986.

17. Petru E, Malleier M, Lax S, Lahousen M, Ehall R, Pickel H, Winter R. Solitary metastasis in the tarsus preceding the diagnosis of primary endometrial cancer: A case report. Eur J Gynaecol Oncol 16(5):387-391,1995.

18. Groves MJ, Stiles RG. Metastatic breast cancer presenting as heel pain. J Am Podiatr Med Assoc 88(8):400-405, 1998.

19. Litton GJ, Ward JH, Abbott TM, Williams HJ Jr. Isolated calcaneal metastasis in a patient with endometrial adenocarcinoma. Cancer 67:1979-1983, 1991.

20. Lombardi RM, Amadio PC. Acrometastases. In Sim FH, ed. Diagnosis and Management of Metastatic Bone Disease: A Multidisciplinary Approach. New York: Raven Press, 1988, pp 237-243.

21. Sebag-Montefiore DJ, Lam KS, Arnott SJ. Case report: Tarsal metastases in a patient with rectal cancer. Br J Radiol 70:862-864, 1997.

22. Delgadillo LA, Nichols DE. Oat cell carcinoma metastasis to the foot. J Foot Ankle Surg 37(1):55-62, 1998.

23. Baran R, Tosti A. Metastatic carcinoma to the terminal phalanx of the big toe: Report of two cases and review of the literature. J Am Acad Dermatol 31(2-1):259-263, 1994.

24. Dripchack PO, Roberson JR. Breast cancer metastatic to the foot with massive bone loss. Orthop Rev 19(10):877-879, 1990.

CHAPTER

35

Metastatic Disease of the Humerus and Shoulder Girdle

Alan W. Yasko, M.D.

Bone destruction secondary to metastatic disease, with or without an associated fracture, can result in significant limitation of upper extremity function. Although considered by many to be less problematic than disease involving the lower extremities, the consequences of tumor-induced bone destruction, mechanical insufficiency, and pain can be quite debilitating. Simple activities of daily living, self-care tasks, bed-to-chair transfers, and ambulation with an assistive device are easily compromised, which adversely affects a patient's quality of life. Contemporary management of shoulder girdle lesions has focused on an aggressive approach to upper extremity metastases to provide expeditious and durable pain relief and restoration of function in the context of increasing patient longevity.

EVALUATION

The bones of the shoulder girdle are particularly vulnerable to metastatic disease. Approximately 20% of metastases to bone arise in the upper extremity.[1] The primary tumors most frequently responsible for bone metastases of the upper extremity are the same as for other sites (e.g., breast, prostate, kidney, and lung carcinomas). Approximately one half of metastatic lesions in the upper extremity are in the humerus. Most of the remaining metastases involving the upper extremity are to the scapula and the clavicle.

The evaluation and treatment of metastatic disease arising in the shoulder girdle depend on the setting in which the lesion is brought to the attention of the clinician. For a patient with a newly diagnosed primary carcinoma, skeletal screening by a technetium 99m bone scan or a skeletal survey provides an effective way to identify asymptomatic foci of disease in the bones of the shoulder girdle. Plain radiography is the single most valuable imaging modality for delineation of the characteristics of any abnormality detected on a bone scan that is a suspected site of metastases (Fig. 35-1). For patients with established cancer the subsequent emergence of localized shoulder girdle pain or functional limitation should prompt radiographic evaluation of the affected region for the presence of a metastatic lesion. If symptoms are temporally associated with a known primary disease and charac-

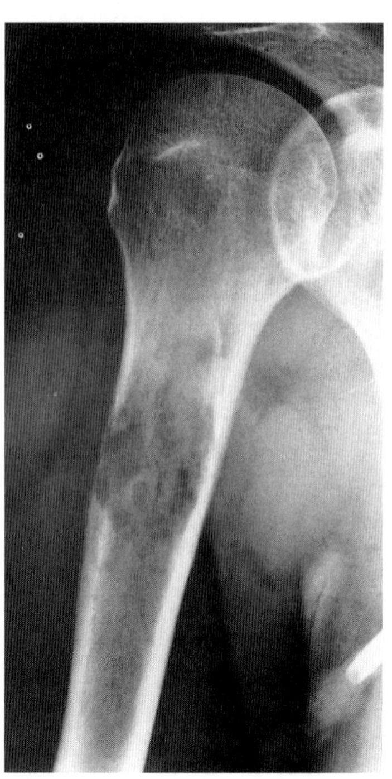

Fig. 35-1 Plain radiograph demonstrates the focal, lytic destructive lesion in the proximal diaphysis of the humerus secondary to metastatic renal cell carcinoma.

teristic of a metastatic focus radiographically, no additional testing is needed to establish the diagnosis prior to treatment.

In far fewer patients, a painful bone lesion may be the initial manifestation of an occult malignancy, a primary sarcoma of bone, a secondary sarcoma associated with prior irradiation, or a marrow cell tumor. In patients with a prolonged disease-free interval after radiation treatment for a remote cancer, secondary radiation-induced sarcomas may arise and may be overlooked as a diagnosis, leading to inappropriate treatment. This is a particularly important consideration for the upper extremity bone lesions that involve the clavicle and scapula in patients for whom breast, lung, and head and neck cancers have been treated with irradiation after initial tumor resection.

If the relationship of a bone lesion to a known primary carcinoma is not obvious, a careful workup, including staging studies and an expedient biopsy for histopathologic diagnosis, is warranted before treatment is undertaken.[2] A solitary focus of metastatic disease in the absence of a known primary carcinoma must be distinguished from a pri-

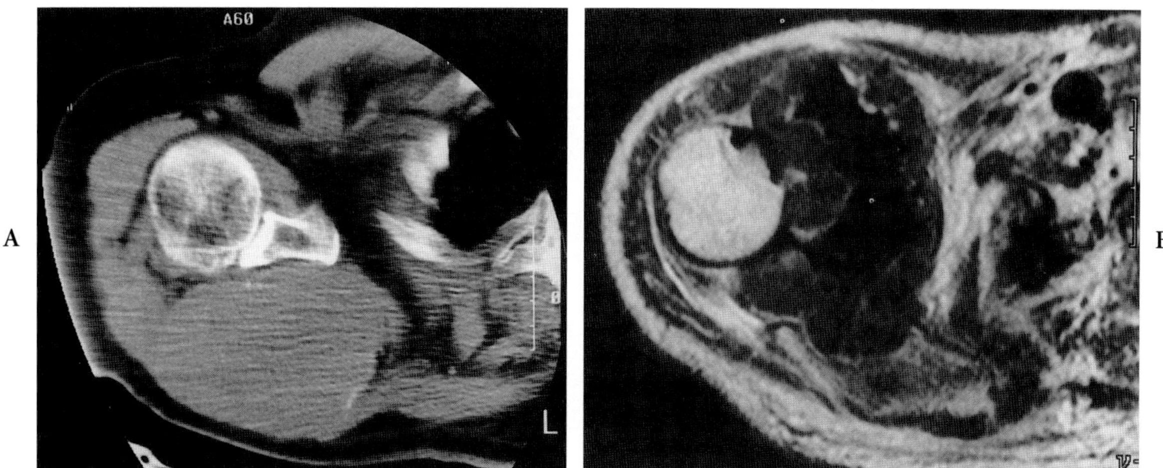

Fig. 35-2   A, CT scan of the scapula in a patient with an established diagnosis of renal cell carcinoma and new onset of shoulder pain. The extent of osseous destruction of the scapula and the associated soft tissue mass are demonstrated. **B,** MRI of the shoulder delineates the extent of involvement of the periscapular tissues from a locally advanced metastatic lesion of the scapula secondary to a rectal carcinoma. The acromion, coracoid, glenoid, and scapular neck were destroyed by tumor that also involved the axillary nerve and abutted the musculocutaneous nerve.

mary or secondary bone sarcoma, marrow cell tumor, or a nonneoplastic process (e.g., Paget's disease, osteitis). Plain radiographs of the entire affected bone should be made to determine the site of disease, the pattern and extent of bone destruction, the presence of pathologic fracture, and the presence of synchronous lesions. Any biopsy method that provides adequate tissue sampling and minimizes sampling error is acceptable; however, percutaneous biopsy is preferred if confirmation of a suspected metastatic lesion is required. Fine-needle aspiration with or without core-needle biopsy under fluoroscopic or computed tomography (CT) guidance with local anesthesia should provide sufficient tissue in the overwhelming majority of patients to establish the diagnosis of metastatic carcinoma.

CT and magnetic resonance imaging (MRI) have specific roles in the diagnostic evaluation of metastatic disease of the shoulder girdle. Although rarely indicated for the overwhelming majority of patients with bone metastases, the limitations of conventional radiographs to image the scapula and clavicle, together with the complex relationship of the adjacent brachial plexus and proximal extremity vasculature to these bones, makes these imaging modalities particularly useful when one is planning surgery (Fig. 35-2). Arteriography has a limited role in the diagnosis of metastatic lesions, but it has a significant role in the management of selected tumors.

MANAGEMENT
General Considerations

The primary treatment of any patient with skeletal metastases is disease-specific systemic chemotherapy, hormonal therapy, or immunotherapy. Systemic pharmacologics and radiotherapeutics, such as bisphosphonates and strontium, recently have emerged as effective adjuncts to standard antineoplastic therapies for the treatment of patients with advanced disease involving bone.[3-5]

Local treatment may not be necessary for small asymptomatic lesions. Painful lesions that do not put a bone at risk of fracture, that are in non-load-bearing sites (i.e., the scapular body), or that represent tumors known to be responsive to contemporary systemic therapies may not require local treatment. Failure to respond to systemic therapies, lesions that are large at presentation, and tumors arising in sites at risk of fracture usually are addressed with local treatment involving radiation, surgery, or both.

Management of symptomatic upper extremity

lesions includes both nonsurgical and surgical strategies and must be individualized. For the overwhelming majority of patients, treatment is palliative. The goals of treatment include relief of pain, prevention of fractures, stabilization of established fractures, and restoration of function. Rarely is local treatment initiated with curative intent. Patients with a solitary metastasis, usually secondary to a renal cell or thyroid primary carcinoma, should be considered candidates for a curative resection. Although there are no conclusive data to support such a procedure, definitive resection may be the most appropriate treatment for this subset of patients to extend overall disease-free survival.[6] Resection may also be considered for patients who present with (1) massive local bone destruction that precludes stabilization with internal fixation or conventional joint arthroplasty, (2) failure of fixation associated with persistent or recurrent tumor, (3) unremitting pain despite stabilization, (4) active neuroendocrine tumors, (5) tumor involving an expendable bone, and (6) an atypical, protracted clinical course (Yasko, unpublished data).

The management approach to metastatic lesions in the upper extremity is influenced by a number of tumor- and site-specific factors. These include tumor histology, extent of osseous and nonosseous disease, prior therapies, effectiveness of systemic and local adjuvant therapies, the site of disease, degree of local bone destruction, extent of disease within the affected bone, quality of uninvolved bone, and impending or established fracture. These factors play a major role in the determination of the nature and scope of the approach taken to achieve the treatment objectives.

Patient-related factors also influence the management approach to these tumors. These include the general health status of the patient, comorbid medical conditions, level of functional debilitation, functional demands of the patient, hand dominance, and life expectancy. These latter factors determine the appropriateness of any treatment strategy within the clinical context at presentation. In general, for patients who have an expected survival of less than 1 month, for whom the risks of surgical treatment outweigh the potential benefit, or for whom the state of health and level of disability preclude operative intervention, conservative therapy is recommended.

Nonsurgical Therapy

Shoulder girdle metastases are treated nonsurgically more commonly than are metastases involving the lower extremities. Nonsurgical management involves local radiation therapy, orthotics, and analgesics. For symptomatic lesions, radiation therapy is the treatment of choice. Most patients tolerate radiation therapy well and experience some degree of, if not complete, pain relief.[7,8] For large, symptomatic lesions that place a bone at risk of fracture or that have resulted in fracture, radiotherapy can have a primary or adjuvant role in local management. The radiosensitivity of the lesion is the major determinant of the success of this treatment modality.

Appropriate splinting or immobilization of the upper extremity may be necessary to protect the bone at risk of fracture during radiotherapy if a nonsurgical approach is recommended or if surgery is planned after radiation therapy. The scapula and clavicle may be immobilized with a shoulder immobilizer or figure-of-eight splint, respectively. Diaphyseal humeral lesions can be supported with a functional humeral brace. A deltoid extension can be used if the lesion is in the proximal metaphyseal region.

Bones identified at risk of fracture usually prompt orthopedic evaluation. As with lower extremity lesions, the criteria for upper extremity bones at risk of fracture are imprecise.[9,10] This is particularly true of lesions in the upper extremity that have been evaluated less rigorously than lesions involving the long bones of the lower extremity. Although nonsurgical treatment of an impending fracture may be effective in selected cases, contemporary treatment of impending or established fractures generally reflects a more aggressive approach.

Pathologic fractures of the humerus, scapula, and clavicle have the potential to heal if responsive to systemic and local radiotherapy if the patient's lifespan is sufficiently long. Union of a pathologic fracture is affected to a large extent by the histologic character of the tumor, with the best results observed in metastases from prostate, breast, and myeloma, which usually heal with conservative therapy.[11] Despite this observation, closed treatment of pathologic fractures of the upper extremity is associated with a period of immobilization and often results in incomplete pain relief, subopti-

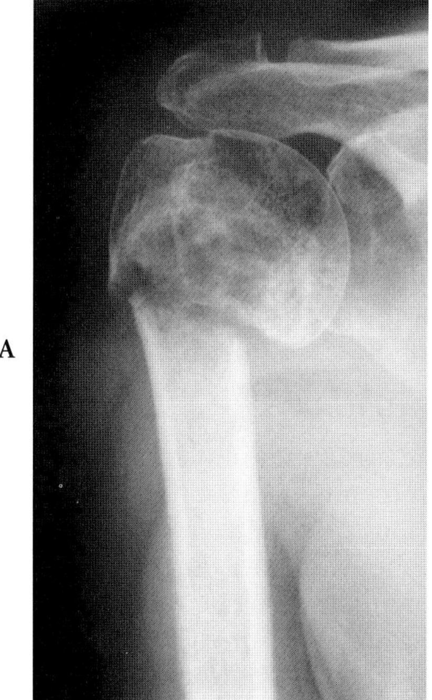

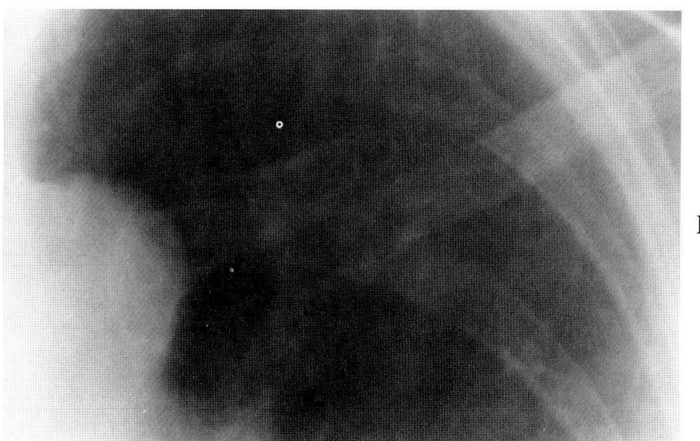

Fig. 35-3   **A,** A pathologic fracture nonunion is demonstrated in a patient with metastatic lung carcinoma treated with radiation to the humerus. Pain and limited range of motion of the shoulder compromised upper extremity function. **B,** Breast carcinoma in a 59-year-old woman treated with surgery and local irradiation. Plain radiograph demonstrates a midclavicle fracture. The affected extremity was immobilized in a sling. Pain was minimal with moderate doses of analgesics.

mal function, protracted physical therapy, unpredictable healing, and refracture. In cases of established fracture involving the upper extremity, bracing techniques as noted previously may be used when a decision is made to treat a patient nonoperatively. Serial radiographs are important to document healing of the metastatic lesion and to rule out local tumor progression.

No randomized studies have established the superiority of surgical treatment over nonsurgical management of metastatic fractures of the upper extremity; however, it is generally maintained that durable pain control and function of the arm are optimized by surgery, irrespective of the site of involvement, in several reported series of patients with impending or established fractures.[12,13] Fracture, refracture after healing, or nonunion can be a consequence of failure of nonsurgical treatment to control the local tumor. Sufficient stability must be achieved to allow healing to occur and to reconstitute sufficient bone to support unrestricted use of the arm after nonsurgical therapy (Fig. 35-3, *A*). Surgery may be indicated to salvage failed nonsurgical therapy for the humerus; however, for most treated lesions of the clavicle and scapular body, functional compromise may be limited and a toler-

able level of resultant pain responsive to oral analgesics may be an acceptable result for certain patients, particularly when the nondominant arm is involved (Fig. 35-3, *B*).

Surgical Therapy

Currently, surgical intervention is recommended for impending fractures, established fractures, and symptomatic lesions that have failed to respond to nonsurgical therapy. The principal goal of surgery is to achieve stability of the affected bone in order to relieve mechanical pain and restore function. A secondary objective is to control local tumor to reduce tumor-associated pain, slow local progression of disease, and preserve fixation.

Operative intervention addresses the pain associated with both local tumor advancement and mechanical insufficiency of the affected bone. The surgical approach depends on the location and the nature of the lesion, the extent of local bone destruction, the presence of a fracture, the presence of multifocal involvement within a given bone, the quality of the uninvolved bone, the risks and potential complications attendant with a given surgical procedure, and the general condition of the patient. The goals of surgery for humeral metastases are achieved most consistently by curettage and internal stabilization or replacement of the affected region of bone. Although, in general, few patients with metastatic lesions of the humerus should be considered for true resection, this is not so with metastases arising in the scapula and clavicle, where resection of the tumor-bearing portion of the bone or the entire bone is more routinely performed.

Indications for prophylactic fixation have to be extrapolated from nonvalidated, observational criteria and include the location, size, and nature of the lesion as well as the presence of pain.[12] Although the bones of the upper extremity are considered nonloaded, nonweightbearing bones, a substantial number of patients with advanced disease need full, unrestricted use of the upper extremity for successful transfers and ambulation. For these patients, a nonsurgical approach can delay resumption of normal function and compromise their quality of life.

For patients with an established fracture of the humerus, stable fixation is essential to optimize function and minimize pain.[13] Adequate bone stock is a requisite for successful long bone fixation. Given current advances in the treatment of patients with metastatic disease, patient longevity has increased substantially; therefore the orthopedic procedure and the method of fixation should provide a rigid construct that should exceed the life expectancy of the patient. Maximum-length stabilization of the humerus augmented with polymethylmethacrylate (PMMA) cement reduces the risk of fixation failure and provides stabilization of synchronous lesions.[13,14] Newer devices that permit interlocked fixation proximal and distal to the lesion provide additional flexibility to the surgical management of humerus metastases.

Local tumor control is a secondary but extremely important objective of surgical intervention for metastatic disease to the upper extremity. The single most frequent cause of treatment failure is local progression of disease.[15] Thorough curettage of focal disease, intramedullary reaming, administration of local surgical adjuvants,[16] long bone stabilization augmented with PMMA, and adjuvant radiotherapy help to reduce tumor progression and minimize pain and risk of fixation failure. Occasionally, controlling local disease by resection with immediate skeletal reconstruction can be the best option to preserve function and relieve pain, particularly when the patient has a significant chance of a prolonged survival or presents with a radioresistant tumor. Expendable bones or bones not easily amenable to internal fixation (e.g., the clavicle and the scapula) are suitable for resection.

Rarely is amputation indicated for metastatic disease. However, in patients with massive extent of disease, fungating tumor, or intractable pain due to brachial plexus infiltration, palliative amputation may be indicated.

CLAVICULAR LESIONS

Clavicular lesions are less common than those involving the scapula, accounting for only 4% of osseous metastatic lesions. A painful lesion arising from the clavicle in the setting of a known radiosensitive primary cancer may be treated with radiation therapy. A sling or figure-of-eight shoulder immobilizer can provide substantial symptomatic relief for most patients, even if a pathologic fracture develops. Nonunion may be tolerated if pain is minimal. For patients with tumors that are associated with uncontrollable pain (with or without fracture), proximal vasculature compromise from local tumor progression, or plexopathy from extrinsic compression on the brachial plexus, surgical treatment is recommended. Surgical stabilization after intralesional excision of the tumor by curettage is often difficult and fraught with potential complications. Any construct for stabilization of the clavicle is at risk of infection because of the subcutaneous location of the bone. Moreover, frequently the lesions are irradiated before fracture, thus compromising wound healing and placing the construct at an even greater risk of infection. Resection of the clavicle is recommended if surgery is indicated for pain palliation or local tumor control (Fig. 35-4). A transverse approach along the long axis of the clavicle provides excellent exposure for partial or total claviclectomy. Reapproximation of the pectoral and anterior deltoid muscles to the trapezius and sternocleidomastoid muscles assists in reducing dead space and promoting wound healing. Functional compromise is minimal with partial or total claviclectomy.

SCAPULAR LESIONS

The scapula accounts for approximately 6% of observed osseous metastases. Renal cell carcinoma has a demonstrated predilection for this bone, of-

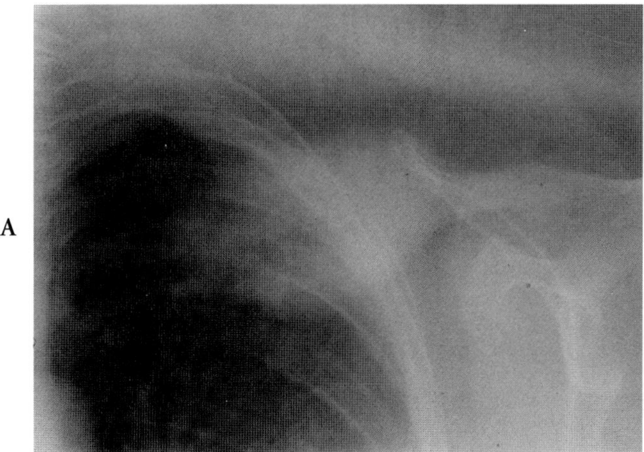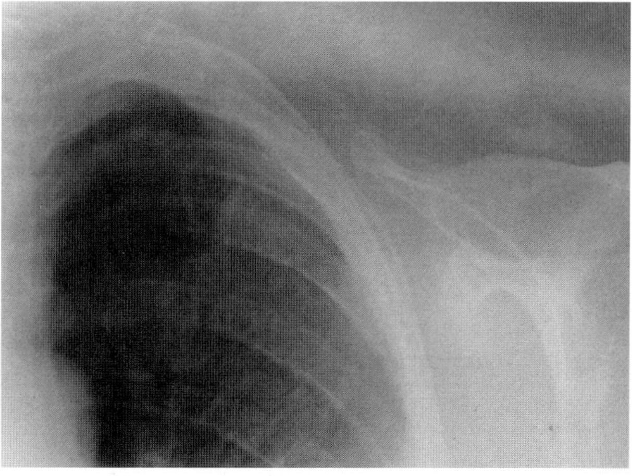

Fig. 35-4 Metastatic osteosarcoma involving the clavicle 7 years after treatment of the pelvic primary tumor. The painful mass was associated with swelling of the affected arm secondary to compression of the subclavian vein. **A,** Preoperative radiograph demonstrates the osteoblastic lesion in the midsubstance of the clavicle. **B,** Radiographic appearance after total claviclectomy. After healing, the patient resumed full, unrestricted use of the affected upper extremity.

ten as a solitary metastasis.[17] Pain is the most common complaint associated with lesions at this site. Pathologic fracture is rare, except when the glenoid and the scapular neck are involved. Most of the lesions of the body of the scapula can be managed adequately with nonsurgical treatment. Surgical resection of the tumor-bearing portion of the scapula body can be performed if pain persists with little or no functional deficit (Fig. 35-5). Myodesis of the adjacent periscapular muscles is important to optimize function and reduce dead space that results after scapular resection.

Scapular neck and glenoid fractures are problematic. Internal fixation can be accomplished, but with difficulty. More often they are treated nonoperatively with radiation. Acromial lesions are treated aggressively because of their subcutaneous location and their potential for fungation. Coracoid lesions can place the brachial plexus and axillary vessels at risk of compromise if the tumor is left uncontrolled.

Total or subtotal scapulectomy is indicated for large symptomatic lesions. The approach to the scapula can vary, but scapulectomy commonly is performed through a posterior longitudinal midscapular incision, which can be extended anteriorly over the shoulder to gain access to the acromion and coracoid regions as necessary. Postoperative function is compromised when the glenoid region

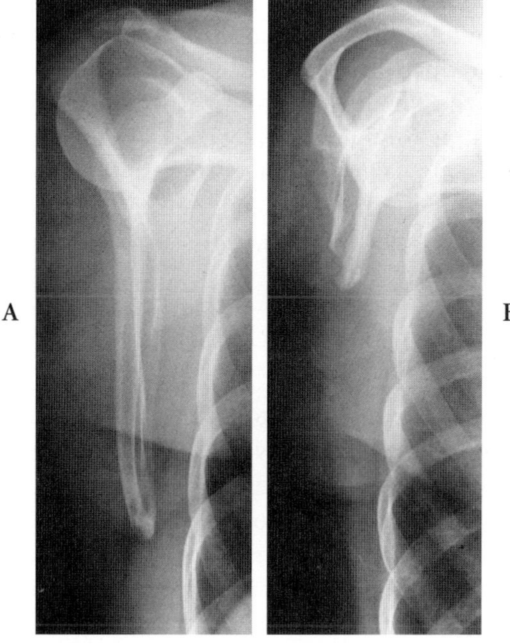

Fig. 35-5 Radiograph of a 47-year-old woman with a history of breast carcinoma, who had been free of disease for 3 years, with new-onset upper back pain about the scapula. **A,** Plain radiographs demonstrate localized destruction of the infraspinatus fossa of the scapula. **B,** Postoperative radiograph after partial scapulectomy. Upper extremity function was not compromised.

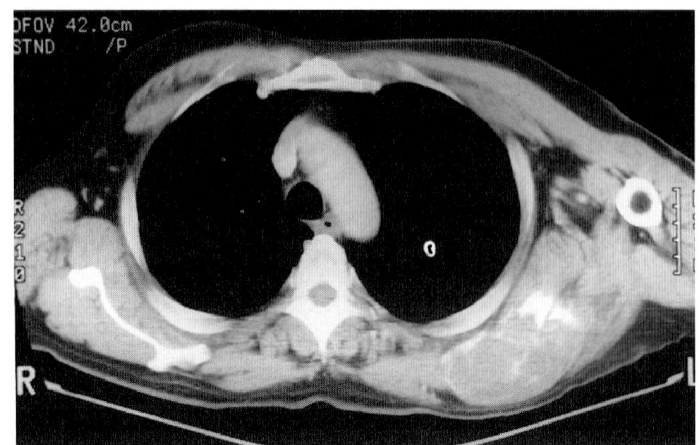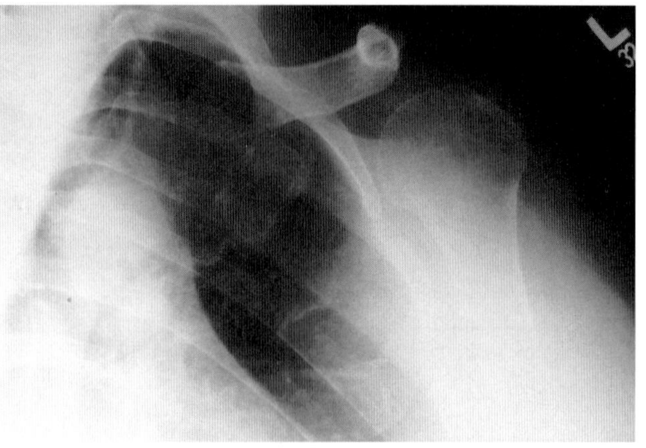

Fig. 35-6   CT of the scapula demonstrating a large metastatic lesion of the scapula secondary to Hürthle cell carcinoma of the thyroid. **A,** Bone destruction involves the body and neck of the scapula. **B,** Postoperative radiograph of the shoulder after total scapulectomy.

is resected. When a total scapulectomy is performed, the humerus is suspended from the clavicle or ribs by means of nonabsorbable sutures or 5 mm Mersilene or Dacron tape (Fig. 35-6). Soft tissue reconstruction is important to provide maximal stability of the motor-compromised shoulder and to reduce dead space after resection. Postoperatively the shoulder is immobilized for comfort with a sling for approximately 6 weeks to allow soft tissue healing. Gentle, limited motion at the shoulder is permitted for hygiene. Active range-of-motion exercises for the elbow, wrist, and hand are encouraged.

PROXIMAL HUMERUS LESIONS

The proximal humerus is a common site for metastatic lesions. Symptomatic metastases of the proximal humerus usually are associated with a significant loss of cancellous bone in the head and surgical neck. Bone support of the insertion of the rotator cuff is compromised frequently, limiting meaningful active range of motion without pain.

The primary objective of surgery in this region of the humerus is pain palliation. Restoration of shoulder stability will facilitate elbow and hand function, but loss of full range of motion of the shoulder is anticipated after surgery. Rarely is there sufficient bone stock to permit stabilization of pathologic fractures with plate fixation for lesions arising in this area. Poor proximal bone purchase of unicortical screws, coupled with the stresses experienced across the shoulder through a full range of

activities of daily living, places this type of construct at high risk of failure. If internal fixation is considered feasible, an intramedullary device with the capability of multidirectional proximal locking screw fixation may be more appropriate as a stabilization device. In the absence of fracture healing in this region of the humerus, any fixation device inserted, with or without PMMA augmentation, is at risk of failure. Moreover, local tumor progression in the humeral head and surgical neck regions can readily compromise any construct.

Hemiarthroplasty reconstruction of the proximal humerus is the recommended treatment for metastatic disease involving the proximal humerus because it provides pain relief and shoulder stability while being a more predictable and durable construct. Mobilization can commence early, and radiation therapy can be administered upon wound healing. For pathologic fractures, it obviates the concerns regarding fracture healing because the segment proximal to the fracture usually is excised. Construct durability is excellent. A long-stem hemiarthroplasty should be used in the majority of cases to support as much of the humeral diaphysis as technically can be achieved (Fig. 35-7).

A deltopectoral approach is appropriate to expose the proximal humerus and provide an extensile approach if more distal regions of the diaphysis are to be addressed. When the tumor involvement is isolated to the metaphyseal region of the proximal humerus, the tuberosities and rotator cuff attachments may be retained with a collar of bone af-

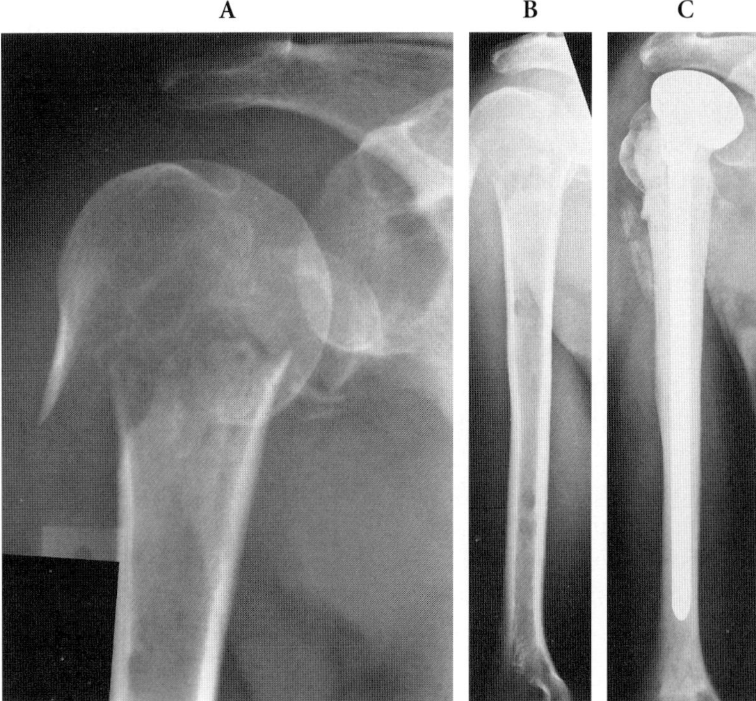

Fig. 35-7 Plain radiograph demonstrated a comminuted pathologic fracture of the proximal humerus in a 48-year-old man without a known cancer. **A,** Lytic destruction within the head and tuberosities was associated with synchronous rounded lesions in the proximal diaphysis, suggesting the diagnosis of multiple myeloma. **B,** Whole-bone radiograph established the presence of diffuse involvement of the humerus. **C,** Long-stem hemiarthroplasty stabilization of the humerus was performed after the diagnosis of multiple myeloma was established by bone biopsy.

ter curettage while the humerus distal to the fracture is skewered with the prosthesis. If a fracture of the head or tuberosities occurs, the humeral head is excised and the rotator cuff is reattached directly to the prosthesis.

A custom or modular proximal humeral replacement may be appropriate for those patients in whom extensive tumor involvement has destroyed the substance of the head and proximal metaphysis of the humerus. In cases of shoulder arthroplasty where the rotator cuff has been released and reattached, function is compromised, although pain palliation usually is achieved and stability of the shoulder is adequate to optimize elbow and hand function.

Not infrequently, a lesion of the proximal humerus represents a solitary deposit of disease and may be the only manifestation of advanced cancer (Fig. 35-8). These solitary lesions commonly are hypervascular tumors secondary to metastatic renal cell or thyroid carcinoma. It is recommended that one consider wide resection of the proximal humerus in an attempt at a cure for these patients. Selective transcatheter arterial embolization should be performed preoperatively to interrupt the blood flow to the tumor so as to reduce intraoperative blood loss.

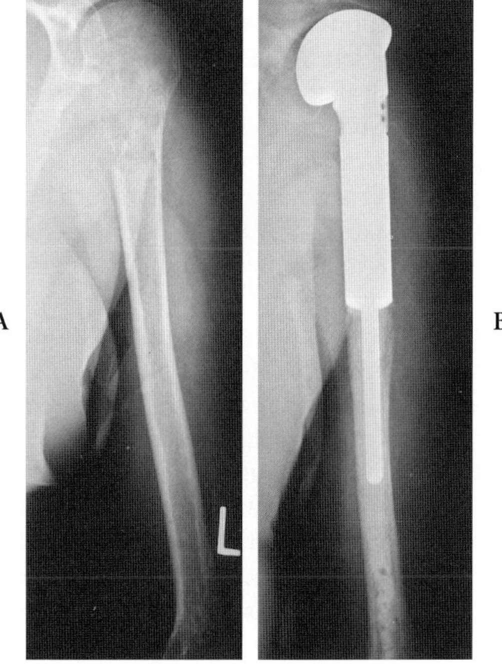

Fig. 35-8 Radiograph of a 58-year-old woman with shoulder pain 5 years after nephrectomy for renal cell carcinoma. **A,** Radiographs demonstrated a solitary metastasis in the proximal humerus with an impending fracture. **B,** Custom shoulder endoprosthesis was inserted after wide excision of the metastatic deposit was performed.

Postoperative management includes sling immobilization as needed for comfort and support. Pendulum exercises and passive range of motion of the shoulder, avoiding forced abduction and external rotation, can commence immediately postoperatively. Active elbow flexion and extension strengthening exercises are encouraged and can be performed as tolerated. Hospitalization is usually 2 to 3 days in duration. Wound drains are discontinued on discharge.

HUMERAL SHAFT LESIONS

The majority of symptomatic metastases of the humeral shaft compromise the mechanical integrity of the bone and place it at risk of fracture.[9] Most of these lesions and those resulting in pathologic fracture are best managed by internal stabilization augmented with PMMA.[18] Lesions distal to the surgical neck and proximal to the olecranon fossa are amenable to this treatment approach. Standard nonlocking rigid or flexible nails can be inserted in an antegrade or retrograde fashion. Interlocking nails provide enhanced fixation capability to provide additional stability to the construct.[19] Relief of pain and functional restoration commonly result from appropriately applied techniques using any commercially available nail for stabilization.

There are two general approaches to diaphyseal lesions. One involves an open technique that exposes the tumor site, and one allows for closed reduction and stabilization of the humerus without direct visualization of the tumor. The open procedure is recommended for patients with segmental bone loss. This technique is routinely used when plate fixation is applied for stabilization. It allows direct excision of the tumor, thereby reducing local tumor burden, and establishes a more favorable interface for the bone cement augmentation, resulting in improved rigidity of fixation constructs. The open technique can be applied for pathologic fractures to facilitate reduction and direct inspection of local bone quality. Physical adjuvants to control local tumor, such as liquid nitrogen, can be applied directly to the bone. PMMA can be inserted proximal and distal to the lesion under controlled conditions to minimize extrusion of cement into the soft tissues.

The standard surgical technique appropriate for insertion of any one of a variety of currently available intramedullary nails is used. The open technique may be performed through one or two incisions, depending on the site of the tumor. To minimize blood loss, the starting point for insertion of the nail is established under fluoroscopic guidance before exposure of the tumor site. The tumor is then excised by thorough curettage. The guide wire is passed across the compromised or fractured region into the distal region of the humerus. An anterolateral approach to the humerus is recommended to provide exposure of the tumor site. Through a separate incision, the proximal humerus is approached in the standard fashion to develop the entry site for the intramedullary device at or just distal to the rotator cuff insertion on the greater tuberosity. The canal is reamed to the appropriate diameter. A nail that fills the canal should be advanced across the tumor site or at the fracture site under fluoroscopic guidance while reduction is

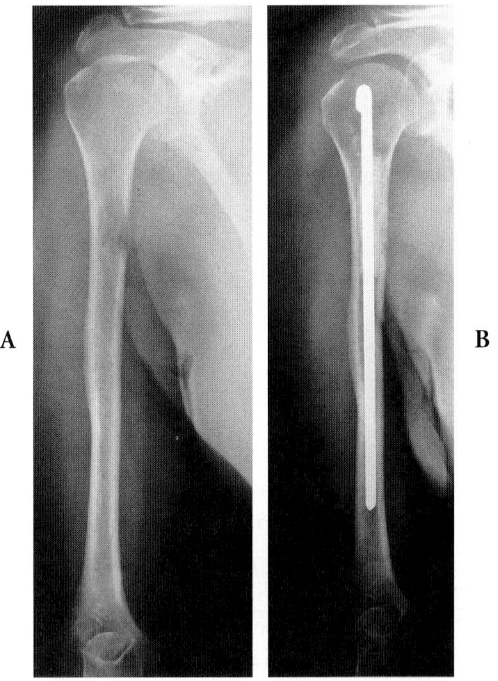

Fig. 35-9   Plain radiographs of a 52-year-old woman with metastatic squamous cell carcinoma of the cervix presenting with onset of progressive pain and restricted use of the dominant upper extremity. **A,** Lytic lesion destroying the medial cortex of the proximal diaphysis of the humerus. **B,** Prophylactic fixation was performed by an open technique to facilitate excision of the tumor by curettage and fixation of the humerus with a single Rush rod (because of the small diameter of the medullary canal) augmented with polymethylmethacrylate cement.

maintained (Fig. 35-9). The nail can be backed out to facilitate adequate cement placement into the canal distally and proximally and then reinserted. The nail should be buried deep to the rotator cuff to avoid postoperative acromial impingement. Cement should be inserted as far proximal and distal to the fracture as possible to assure firm fixation (Fig. 35-10). All extruded cement should be removed, with special attention paid to the region of the radial nerve as it passes intimately along the posterior aspect of the mid humerus so as to avoid injury. For more distal diaphyseal lesions, the nail may be inserted retrograde to gain better fixation and avoid disrupting the rotator cuff. Additional stability may be achieved by inserting interlocking screws proximally or distally if deemed necessary.[19,20] The tumor site is closed over a drain. Exploration of the subacromial space may prove beneficial to disrupt adhesions that may have formed secondary to painful restricted range of motion if the surgical exposure of more proximal diaphyseal lesions permits. Overnight hospitalization is usually required for intravenous analgesic administration. A sling is used for comfort and support. Patients are encouraged to perform pendulum and passive range-of-motion exercises of the shoulder for 6 weeks to allow the rotator cuff to heal. Thereafter progressive active range of motion is encouraged. Resistive exercises involving the shoulder are discouraged. Passive and active range of motion of the elbow, wrist, and hand as tolerated is encouraged.

Closed techniques for intramedullary nail stabilization may be useful in selected patients in whom there is no segmental loss of bone, with or without fracture (Fig. 35-11).[21] The availability of intramedullary nails capable of being locked proximally

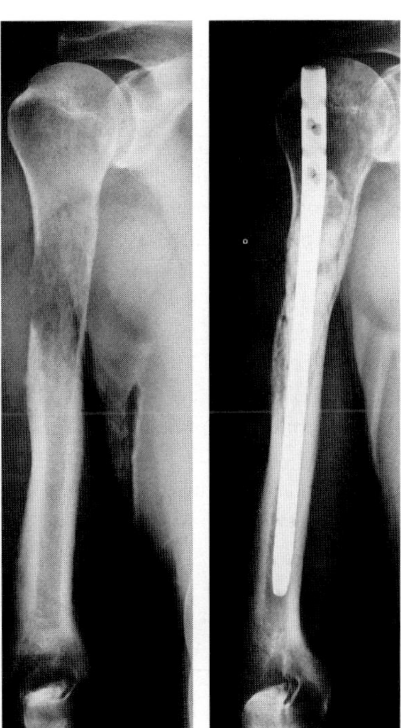

Fig. 35-10   Renal cell carcinoma metastasis involving the humerus. **A,** Large permeative destruction with cortical thinning and focal disruption in the proximal diaphysis of the humerus places the bone at risk of fracture. **B,** Local tumor control and rigid stabilization were achieved with curettage of the tumor followed by intramedullary nail insertion augmented with polymethylmethacrylate cement. Transcatheter arterial embolization of the tumor was performed preoperatively to reduce intraoperative bleeding.

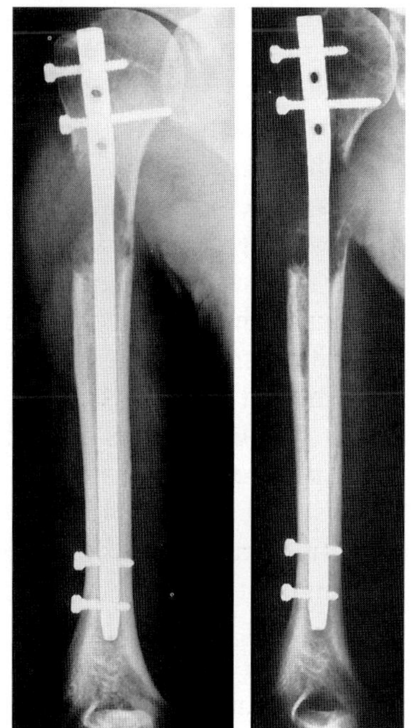

Fig. 35-11   Impending fracture of the proximal humerus through a metastatic lesion secondary to renal cell carcinoma. **A,** Closed intramedullary nail with proximal and distal interlocking screws inserted to provide stability across the large hypervascular tumor in a patient with extensive visceral disease. **B,** Interval progression of tumor locally before the patient's death did not compromise fixation.

and distally has made this approach more appealing. Statically locked nails may be used with or without cement augmentation to achieve improved rotational and axial stability.[22,23] These nails are most applicable for patients with radiosensitive tumors. The limited incisions are ideal for patients who have undergone radiation to minimize soft tissue dissection through compromised tissues. Although blood loss can be minimized and operating time reduced, a thorough excision of tumor is compromised by this technique, and only indirect reduction of fractures is achievable.

Plate fixation may also be used for stabilization of a humeral diaphyseal lesion or fracture. Since bone quality adjacent to the tumor is poor, plate fixation must also be augmented by cement to gain adequate screw purchase both proximal and distal to the poor-quality bone stock. The humerus may be shortened to facilitate stability without adverse functional consequences. An anterolateral approach is used commonly to expose the humeral diaphysis. This technique involves a larger exposure and stripping of soft tissues from the humerus. It requires good bone stock both proximal and distal to the lesion. The plate does not support the humerus when synchronous lesions are present, and it is more likely to fail if conditions are not optimal and the patient's survival is prolonged. Plate fixation has been associated with less total energy absorbed to failure and stiffness than intramedullary nailing in bone defects simulating metastatic lesions in the humerus.[19] With the more widespread availability of a variety of intramedullary devices, there is no particular advantage to this technique.

Both intramedullary nail and plate or screw constructs confer immediate stability to the extremity, thereby allowing early motion of the shoulder and elbow while facilitating use of the extremity to assist in weightbearing.[24] Intramedullary nails have a significant advantage over plates in that they are load-sharing devices that can support a maximal length of the humerus beyond the level of the tumor site and appear to be superior to plates at maintaining bone stability more consistently. Postoperative irradiation should be directed at the entire length of the humerus because tumor cells contaminate the entire bone after nailing.[25]

Prosthetic devices also are available to reconstruct the humeral diaphysis compromised by met-

astatic disease. The principal indication for their use is large diaphyseal segmental bone loss with preservation of adequate bone stock at the proximal and distal ends to allow cement fixation.[26] Postoperative management includes a sling for support and early passive and active range of motion exercises for the elbow and shoulder.

CONCLUSION

Metastatic disease in the shoulder girdle and proximal humerus can be extremely painful, especially if there is involvement of the brachial plexus. In extreme cases, amputation may be necessary. In disease of the humeral shaft, early intervention with radiation therapy, bracing, or surgery will often give a stable, pain-free arm so that the patient can resume independent activities.

REFERENCES

1. Clain A. Secondary malignant disease of bone. Br J Cancer 19:15, 1965.
2. Rougraff BT, Kneisl JS, Simon MA. Skeletal metastases of unknown origin: A prospective study of a diagnostic strategy. J Bone Joint Surg Am 75:1276-1281, 1993.
3. Hortabagyi GN, Theriault RL, Porter L, et al. Efficacy of pamidronate in reducing skeletal complications in patients with breast cancer and lytic bone metastases: Protocol 19 Aredia Breast Cancer Study Group. N Engl J Med 335:1785-1791, 1996.
4. Berenson JR, Lichtenstein A, Porter L, et al. Efficacy of pamidronate in reducing skeletal events in patients with advanced multiple myeloma. N Engl J Med 334:488-493, 1996.
5. Robinson RG, Preston DF, Shiefelbein M, et al. Strontium 89 therapy for the palliation of pain due to osseous metastases. JAMA 274:420-424, 1995.
6. Takashi M, Takagi Y, Sakata T, et al. Surgical treatment of renal cell carcinoma metastases: Prognostic significance. Int Urol Nephrol 27:1-8, 1995.
7. Tong D, Gillick L, Hendrickson FR. The palliation of symptomatic osseous metastases: Final results of the study by the Radiation Therapy Oncology Group. Cancer 50:893-899, 1982.
8. Price P, Hoskin PJ, Easton D, Austin D, Palmer SG, Yarnold JR. Prospective randomized trial of single and multifraction radiotherapy schedules in the treatment of painful bony metastases. Radiother Oncol 6:247-255, 1986.
9. Hipp JA, McBroom RJ, Cheal EJ, at al. Structural consequences of endosteal metastatic lesions in long bones. J Orthop Res 7:828-837, 1989.
10. Hipp JA, Springfield DS, Hayes WC. Predicting pathologic fracture risk in the management of metastatic bone defects. Clin Orthop Rel Res 312:120-135, 1995.
11. Gainor BJ, Buchert P. Fracture healing in metastatic bone disease. Clin Orthop Rel Res 178:297-302, 1983.

12. Mirels H. Metastatic disease in long bones: A proposed scoring system for diagnosing impending pathologic fractures. Clin Orthop Rel Res 249:256-264, 1989.

13. Sim FH, Daugherty TW, Ivins JC. The adjunctive use of methylmethacrylate in fixation of pathological fractures. J Bone Joint Surg Am 56:40-48, 1974.

14. Harrington KD, Sim FH, Enis J, Johnston JO, Dick HM, Gristina AG. Methylmethacrylate as an adjunct in internal fixation of pathologic fractures. J Bone Joint Surg Am 58: 1047-1055, 1976.

15. Vail TP, Harrelson JM. Treatment of pathologic fracture of the humerus. Clin Orthop Rel Res 268:197-201, 1991.

16. Marcove RC, Miller TR. Treatment of primary and metastatic bone tumors by cryosurgery. JAMA 207:1890-1894, 1969.

17. Gurney H, Larcos G, McKay M, et al. Bone metastases in hypernephroma: Frequency of scapular involvement. Cancer 64:1429-1431, 1989.

18. Lewallen RP, Pritchard DJ, Sim FH. Treatment of pathologic fractures or impending fractures of the humerus with rush rods and methylmethacrylate: Experience with 55 cases in 54 patients. Clin Orthop Rel Res 166:193-198, 1982.

19. Damron TA, Rock MG, Choudhury SN, et al. Biomechanical analysis of prophylactic fixation for middle third humeral impending pathologic fractures. Clin Orthop Rel Res 363: 240-248, 1999.

20. Tome JL, Carsi B, Garcia-Fernandez C, et al. Treatment of pathologic fractures of the humerus with Seidel nailing. Clin Orthop Rel Res 350:51-55, 1998.

21. Kunec JR, Lewis RJ. Closed intramedullary rodding of pathologic fractures with supplemental cement. Clin Orthop Rel Res 188:183-186, 1984.

22. Redmond BJ, Biermann JS, Blasier RB. Interlocking intramedullary nailing of pathologic fractures of the shaft of the humerus. J Bone Joint Surg Am 78:891-896, 1996.

23. Thomsen NOB, Mikkelsen JB, Svendsen RN, et al. Interlocking nailing of humeral shaft fractures. J Orthop Sci 3:199-203, 1998.

24. Dijkstra S, Stapert J, Boxma H, Wiggers T. Treatment of pathological fractures of the humeral shaft due to bone metastases: A comparison of intramedullary locking nail and plate osteosynthesis with adjunctive bone cement. Eur J Surg Oncol 22:621-626, 1996.

25. Townsend P, Smalley S, Cozad S, et al. Role of postoperative radiation therapy after stabilization of fractures caused by metastatic disease. Int J Radiat Oncol Biol Phys 31:43-49, 1995.

26. Damron TA, Sim FH, Shives TC, et al. Intercalary spacers in the treatment of segmentally destructive diaphyseal humeral lesions in disseminated malignancies. Clin Orthop Rel Res 324:233-243, 1996.

Metastatic Disease of the Distal Humerus, Forearm, and Hand

Timothy A. Damron, M.D., and Jesse Aronowitz, M.D.

The distal upper extremity is an unusual but interesting region of metastatic disease involvement. The infrequency with which metastasis to this region is encountered has been noted in numerous reviews on the subject and underscored by the many case reports but relatively few series of patients with such sites of metastasis.

However, each site covered in this chapter—distal humerus, forearm, and hand—presents a unique challenge to the clinician and surgeon. Metastatic disease to the *distal humerus* presents a technical challenge to the surgeon confronted with a pathologic fracture of the distal humerus because of the unique anatomy that limits fixation options. Involvement of the *forearm* challenges clinical decision making in determining whether patients with fractures here are best treated operatively or nonoperatively. Metastatic carcinoma to the *hand* presents a diagnostic challenge because metastatic disease in this site frequently mimics such infectious conditions as paronychia, felon, and osteomyelitis, which are much more common.

DISTAL HUMERUS METASTASES
Epidemiology

The distal third is the humeral segment least commonly affected by metastatic disease.[1,2] Despite the frequency with which humeral metastatic disease in general is encountered, there are no reported series of patients specifically with distal third involvement. Most of these patients have been included in larger series of patients with all sites of humeral metastatic disease.[1,3-6]

Pathophysiology

The infrequency of distal humeral involvement by metastatic carcinoma, relative to that of the proximal humerus, may be attributed to various factors. Because the distal humerus is less likely than the proximal humerus to have persistent red marrow, it is perhaps less favorable "soil"[7] for growth of transplanted tumor cells. The unique anatomy of the humerus, with a diminishing medullary canal distally, also diminishes the potential marrow space and small vascular channels available as soil for metastases.

In addition, only the head of the humerus was demonstrated by Batson[8] to be involved in the ver-

tebral venous plexus after injection of the small mammary veins in cadavers. More distal humeral venous communication may occur by retrograde venous embolism in the major venae vasorum of the extremity vessels, also claimed as a part of Batson's plexus, by entry into the arterial circulation via invasion of the pulmonary venous system, by paradoxical embolism through a patent foramen ovale, or by transpulmonary passage via systemic visceral disease.[9]

Unique Anatomy of the Distal Humerus

The distal humerus is unusual for a long bone in that the central intramedullary canal ends 3 to 4 cm proximal to the distal articular surface, well proximal to the olecranon fossa. In addition, the diameter of the distal canal typically tapers over the final centimeters. This anatomy precludes standard locked intramedullary nail fixation of impending or actual distal third humeral pathologic fractures because of lack of distal canal access in all but the most unusual circumstances.

The best surfaces for application of plates in fixation of distal humerus fractures are the posterior (either medial or lateral columns) and lateral surfaces. Plates in these positions allow the most distal placement possible without interfering with elbow flexion. Longer plates extending more proximally on the humeral shaft, as may be considered when more extensive areas of bone are involved, are difficult to apply on either the posterior or lateral surfaces because of the limitations of normal anatomy here. Application of a long plate posteriorly requires mobilization of the radial nerve from the spiral groove with the inherently higher risk of radial neuropraxia. Application of a long plate laterally is limited by the deltoid insertion over the large portion of the middle third of the humerus which embodies the deltoid tuberosity.

Evaluation

Patients with metastatic deposits in the distal humerus may present with arm, elbow, or more distal referred pain, swelling, or pathologic fracture, or they may be without symptoms but with abnormal findings on bone scans or skeletal surveys. Plain radiographs of the entire humerus, shoulder, and elbow in two planes are usually sufficient to confirm clinical suspicion, assess risk of fracture, and allow for adequate preoperative planning when necessary. As for other sites of bone metastatic disease, a bone scan or a skeletal survey is important to assess the extent of bone involvement. For the occasional solitary lesion of the humerus without a known primary tumor, the differential diagnosis of a sarcoma should be considered. In the latter instance, magnetic resonance imaging (MRI) to assess soft tissue and intramedullary extent may be advisable before biopsy.

Nonoperative Treatment

The usefulness of radiotherapy for palliation of skeletal metastases has long been recognized[10,11] and has been demonstrated by prospective trials[12-14] and departmental reviews.[15] These studies do not evaluate effectiveness by site, but the available evidence does not suggest that upper extremity lesions respond less well than metastases elsewhere. Because there are no viscera in the treated volume, the toxicity of judicious use in the distal upper extremity should be negligible.

Nonoperative radiotherapy for metastatic disease in the distal humerus is usually advisable for small but symptomatic lesions, particularly when the primary tumor is known to be radiosensitive. Each lesion, however, should be considered from the standpoint of its potential to lead to a pathologic fracture. In a biomechanical study of defects in the distal third of the humerus, a laterally based model defect involving 50% of the cortex resulted in statistically significant reductions in torsional rigidity, peak torque, and total energy absorbed to failure when compared with the intact paired con-

tralateral humerus[16] (Table 36-1). According to Mirels' clinicoradiographic scale for assessing impending pathologic fracture risk, however, a lytic lesion that occupies more than one half the canal diameter in the upper extremity must be accompanied by at least moderate pain to qualify as an impending fracture.[17] Painful, purely lytic lesions of at least 50% of the canal diameter should be given consideration for prophylactic stabilization, particularly if pain persists after radiotherapeutic management.

Pathologic fractures of the distal humerus are usually best dealt with operatively. Exceptions include those in the patient who has less than 4 to 6 weeks of anticipated survival, has a medical contraindication to operative intervention, or is unwilling to undergo surgery. In these unfortunate circumstances, distal humeral fracture stability and symptoms may be improved with the use of a posterior splint or custom-hinged elbow orthosis while the patient undergoes palliative radiation.

Radiotherapy is generally recommended as an adjunct to surgical fixation for pathologic fracture or impending pathologic fracture, although documentation of benefit is limited.[6,12,18-20] Theoretically, ionizing radiation has the potential to inhibit bone repair by inhibiting osteogenesis and chondrogenesis. In practice, bone union of properly stabilized fractures is usual after moderate doses of x-irradiation.[21] The optimal dose, timing, and even sequence of modalities is unknown. Doses of between 2000 and 4000 cGy have been recommended, with radiotherapy commencing between 1 and 2 weeks after surgery.[12,21,22]

Table 36-1   Biomechanical properties for intact humerii compared to those with distal third 50% cortical defect

Biomechanical properties	Intact specimens*	Defect specimens*	P value
Peak torque (nm)	81.5 ± 22.8	20.6 ± 8.2	0.001
Torsional stiffness (nm per degree)	2.67 ± 0.37	2.07 ± 0.39	0.004
Total energy absorbed (J)	1608 ± 780	104 ± 68	0.001

Excerpted with permission from Damron TA, Heiner JP, Freund EMN, Damron LA, McCabe R, Vanderby R. A biomechanical analysis of prophylactic fixation for pathological fractures of the distal third of the humerus. J Bone Joint Surg Am 76:839-847, 1994.
*Values are given as mean and standard deviation.

A few caveats regarding upper extremity irradiation are in order. Patients with arm pain who have radiologic documentation of humeral metastasis are often referred to radiation oncologists. The presence of a lesion in a painful extremity should not be accepted as prima facie evidence that the imaged lesion is the source of pain. It must be appreciated that the pain of nerve root or brachial plexus infiltration or compression by tumor may be referred into the arm. Examination should be performed to consider this latter possibility, particularly when the site of patient's pain is nontender or when there is evidence of an upper extremity neurologic deficit. Conversely, after supraclavicular irradiation (as in patients with breast cancer), upper extremity pain is often inappropriately attributed to radiation-induced brachial plexopathy. This diagnosis should be viewed with skepticism because this entity is extremely rare and generally follows doses much higher than are commonly employed in prophylactic supraclavicular irradiation.[23] A far more likely explanation of such pain is an occult tumor deposit, which should be sought aggressively and treated appropriately.

Operative Treatment

Operative treatment of impending and pathologic fractures of the distal third of the humerus poses the greatest challenge in the treatment of metastatic disease at this site. When the disease is truly within the distal third of the humerus, standard locked intramedullary nail fixation is inadequate, as it will not provide adequate fixation distally within the insufficient to nonexistent intramedullary canal. In these instances the two best options to consider are rigid plate fixation, either dual 90:90 (Fig. 36-1) or

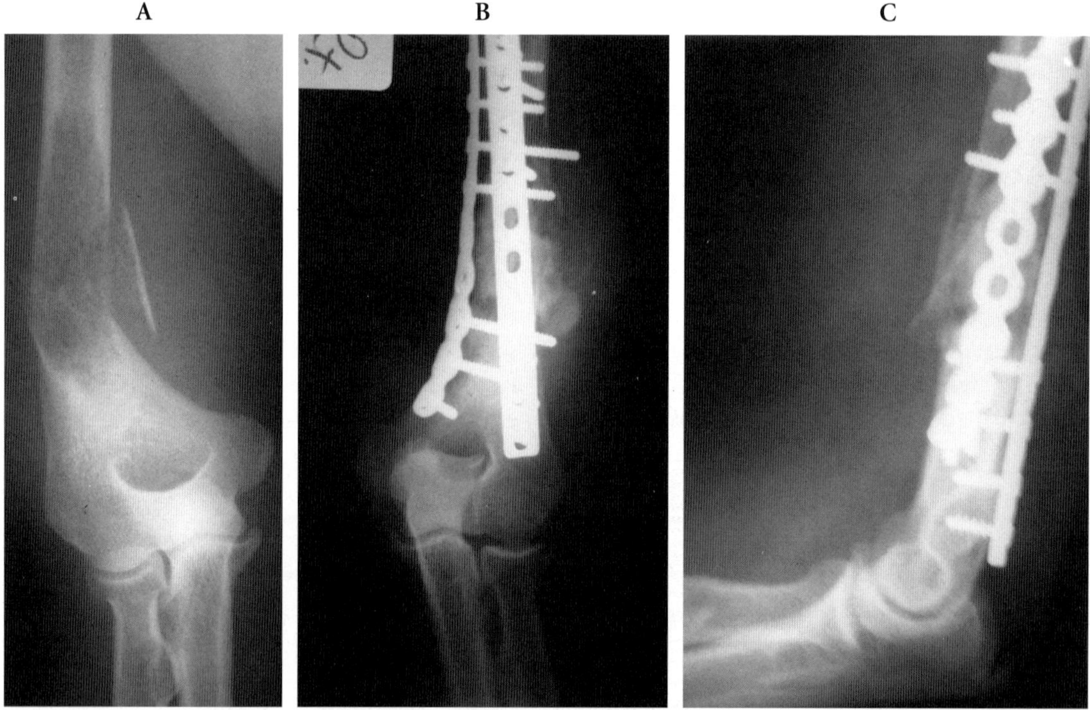

Fig. 36-1　Dual plating of distal humerus pathologic fracture. **A,** Anteroposterior radiograph of elbow shows displaced pathologic distal third humeral fracture through a myeloma deposit. Postoperative anteroposterior (**B**) and lateral (**C**) radiographs of elbow and distal humerus after open reduction internal fixation with dual 90:90 plating using a posterior narrow dynamic compression plate and a medial pelvic reconstruction plate. At 3 months' follow-up the anteroposterior radiograph demonstrates significant callus formation. The patient was free of symptoms, with elbow range of motion from 5 to 135 degrees. (Case presented courtesy of Brian Davison, M.D., Columbus, Ohio.)

single, or dual retrograde Rush rods (Fig. 36-2) introduced through the epicondyles.[1,2,16,24,25] In rare situations in which these options are not feasible because of inadequate distal bone, a custom distal humeral replacement total elbow arthroplasty has been used as a salvage procedure.[2,25,25a] Finally, when distal humeral involvement is combined with more substantial proximal shaft lesions, intramedullary rod fixation may be combined with distal plate fixation (Fig. 36-3).

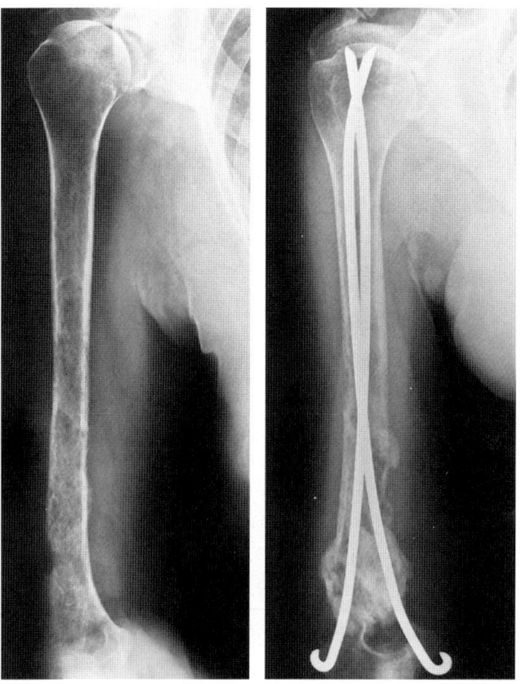

Fig. 36-2 Retrograde Rush rod fixation of distal humerus fracture. **A,** Anteroposterior radiograph of the humerus of a woman who presented with arm pain and a previously unrecognized breast carcinoma. Extensive involvement of the distal three fifths of the humerus by metastatic breast disease is evident, with particularly lytic areas within the distal third of the humerus extending to the olecranon fossa. **B,** Postoperative anteroposterior humerus radiograph after retrograde stabilization with dual Rush rods introduced through the epicondyles and supplemented with cementation and postoperative radiotherapy.

Fig. 36-3 Combined plate and locked intramedullary rod fixation of distal humeral disease. **A,** Anteroposterior humerus radiograph of a woman with extensive skeletal-extraskeletal lymphangiomatosis in whom functionally limiting pain had developed in the arm. Note the diffuse humeral involvement with lesions extending beyond the end of the intramedullary canal of the distal humerus. Postoperative anteroposterior (**B**) and lateral (**C**) radiographs after antegrade locked humeral intramedullary nail fixation supplemented distally with dynamic compression plating, including screws through both the plate and distal interlocking nail holes. This should not be considered standard fixation for potentially progressive metastatic disease.

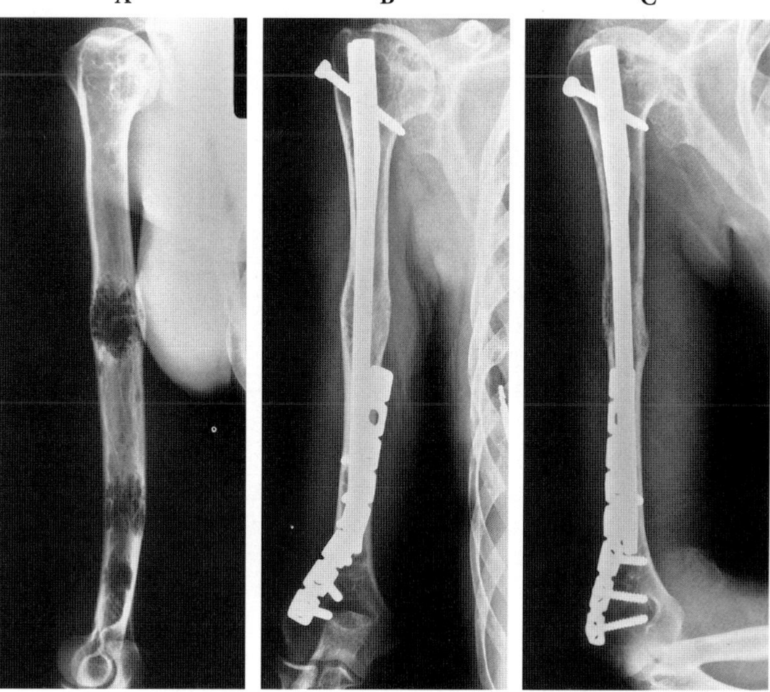

Each patient's case must be evaluated individually with respect to biomechanics, size of the region involved by the pathologic process, fracture configuration, quality of the proximal and distal bone stock, vascularity of the tumor, condition of the soft tissues from any prior radiation, overall patient condition, and cost of the implants.

From a purely biomechanical point of view, for disease isolated to the distal third of the humerus,

dual 90:90 plating with bone cement is the preferred construct, followed by dual retrograde Rush rods with cement, and finally by single plate fixation with cement.[16] Dual 90:90 plate with cement fixation yields statistically significantly greater peak torque and total energy absorbed than either of the other two constructs (Fig. 36-4). The biomechanical testing on which this was based employed fresh frozen cadaveric distal humeral bone without

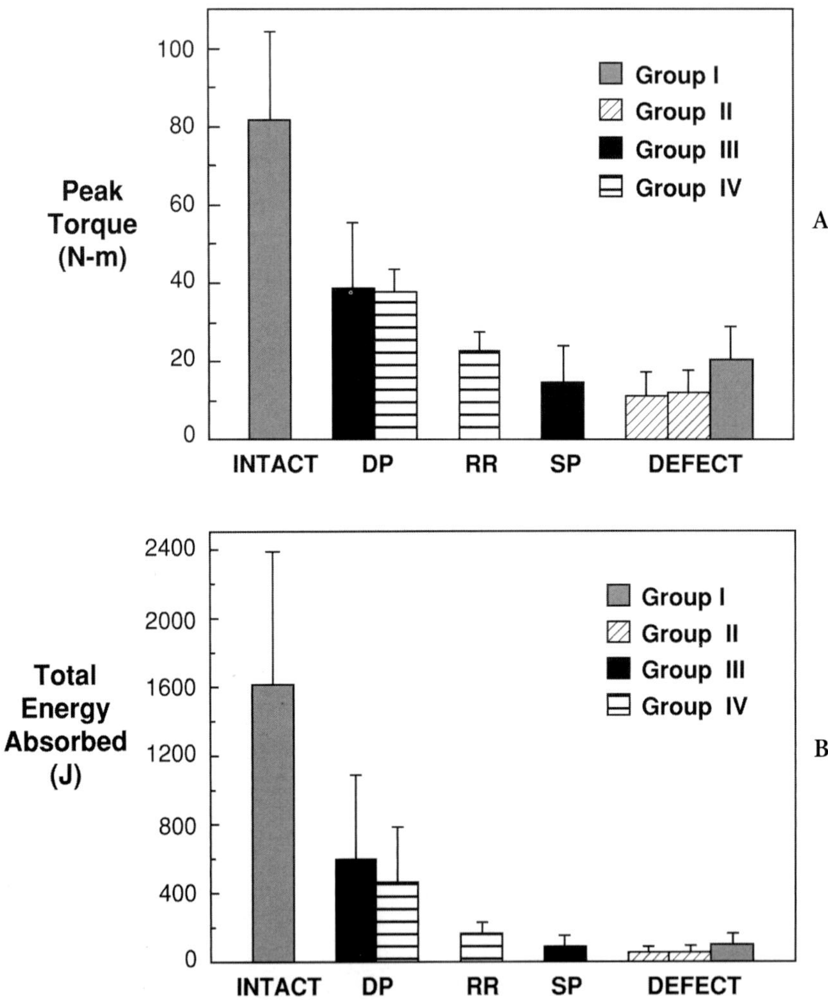

Fig. 36-4   Results of biomechanical analysis of prophylactic fixation for distal third humeral impending pathologic fracture model. **A,** Graph showing the peak torque for intact humerus, dual 90:90 plating *(DP)* of 50% lateral distal third cortical defect, Rush rod *(RR)* fixation of defect, single plate *(SP)* fixation of defect, and defect alone. **B,** Graph showing the total energy absorbed for the same sets of humeral specimens. Error bars represent standard deviations. (Printed with permission from Damron TA, Heiner JP, Freund EMN, Damron LA, McCabe R, Vanderby R. A biomechanical analysis of prophylactic fixation for pathologic fractures of the distal third of the humerus. J Bone Joint Surg Am 76:839-847, 1994.)

structural compromise above or below the model defect, allowing secure screw or Rush rod fixation proximally and distally.[16]

In situations in which a more extensive area of the mid and distal humerus is involved by metastatic disease, plating becomes less feasible because achievement of adequate fixation proximally would require continuation of at least one plate beyond the middle third of the humerus. Proximal extension of a plate to this level is limited posteriorly by the radial nerve in the spiral groove and laterally by the deltoid insertion at the tuberosity. In these situations of extensive distal humeral·involvement including the distal third, dual retrograde Rush rod fixation with cement may be the better, although more technically challenging, alternative (see Fig. 36-2). A second alternative here is the combination of an intramedullary rod and a distal plate, with

use of the distal interlocking screw holes for screws that pass through both the plate and the rod and extension of the plate fixation more distally (see Fig. 36-3). For each of these alternatives, adequate distal bone stock must be present. Polymethylmethacrylate (PMMA) should generally be employed in this difficult location of metastatic bone disease.

When hypernephroma is known or suspected to be the primary tumor, consideration should be given to preoperative embolization to minimize intraoperative blood loss. The extensive exposure required for dual plating may be difficult when the area has been previously radiated, increasing the risk of neuropraxia (Fig. 36-5). Cost should not be a major factor in choosing between standard means of fixation for this site. However, the cost of custom distal humeral replacement total elbow arthroplas-

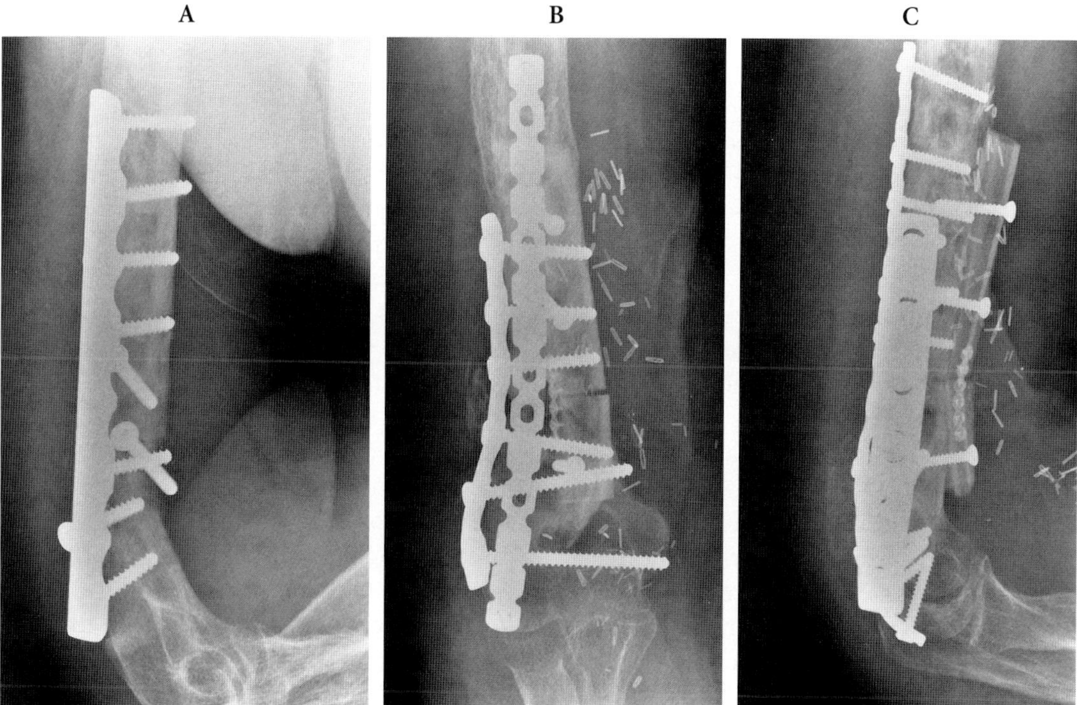

Fig. 36-5   Failure of single-plate fixation salvaged with dual plating. **A,** Lateral radiograph of the elbow and distal humerus shows loss of fixation 6 months after open reduction for internal fixation of a distal humeral pathologic fracture through weakened, radiated bone years after surgical and radiotherapy treatment of a soft tissue sarcoma. Postoperative anteroposterior (**B**) and lateral (**C**) radiographs show 90:90 plate fixation of the lateral column with a posterior pelvic reconstruction plate and a lateral dynamic compression plate. A vascularized fibular onlay graft has been added medially. Mobilization of the radial nerve in the previously radiated, multiply operated field was difficult.

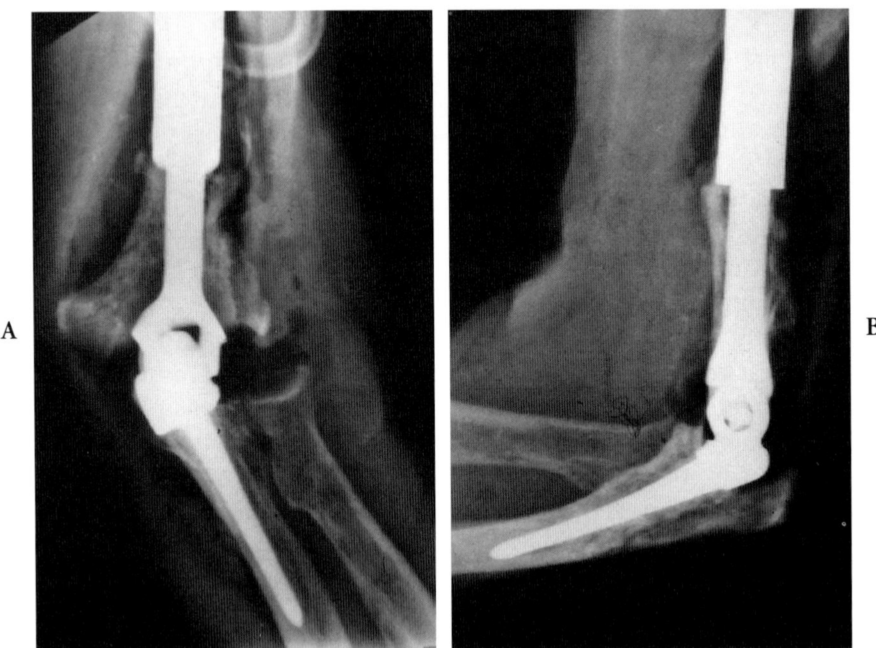

Fig. 36-6   Distal humeral replacement, total elbow arthroplasty. Anteroposterior (**A**) and lateral (**B**) elbow radiographs after placement of a custom-hinged elbow arthroplasty because of failure of prior reconstruction of a distal metastatic deposit with an intercalary spacer device.

ty should be weighed carefully when one is considering that option (Fig. 36-6).

FOREARM METASTASES
Epidemiology

The radius and the ulna are often neglected sites of metastatic disease. In fact, metastases to the forearm are more common than the more frequently reported hand metastases. In a series of 827 autopsies on patients with proven metastatic carcinoma to the skeleton, 11 patients (1.3%) had forearm involvement (7 radius, 4 ulna) compared with only 5 (0.6%) with hand metastases.[26] Only seven cases of radial metastatic lesions and four cases of ulnar metastatic lesions were identified among 2001 patients with bone metastases in another review.[27] Those 11 lesions accounted for 0.3% of all bone metastases and occurred in a total of 0.6% of the 2001 patients.[27] In another series of 334 patients with osseous metastases, forearm metastases were similarly rare but still more frequent than the metastasis to a hand bone found in a single patient.[28] One metastasis to the radius was identified among 100 patients with metastatic breast carcinoma in yet another series.[29]

Despite their apparently greater prevalence, metastases to the forearm have not generated the interest that hand metastases have. There are no published series devoted exclusively to metastatic disease of the forearm. Hence little is known regarding the patterns of primary carcinomas that involve the forearm. In Copeland's series of 334 patients with osseous metastases from more than 20 known primary malignant tumors, the only forearm metastases observed were in patients with breast carcinoma.[28] The most common primary tumors metastasizing to bones distal to the knee and elbow, 11 forearm bones inclusive, were reported to be carcinomas of the lung, breast, and kidney.[26] Unfortunately the origins of metastases to the forearm bones themselves were not specifically described. Primary tumors reported in case reports to have metastasized to the forearm include those of the prostate, breast, lung, kidney, thyroid, larynx, pancreas, and retinoblastoma and malignant mixed tumor of the parotid gland.[30-42] Forearm involvement by myeloma has been well documented (Fig. 36-7). Meyerding[43] identified radius and ulnar involvement in 2 of 13 cases of multiple myeloma.

The risk of pathologic forearm fracture is also

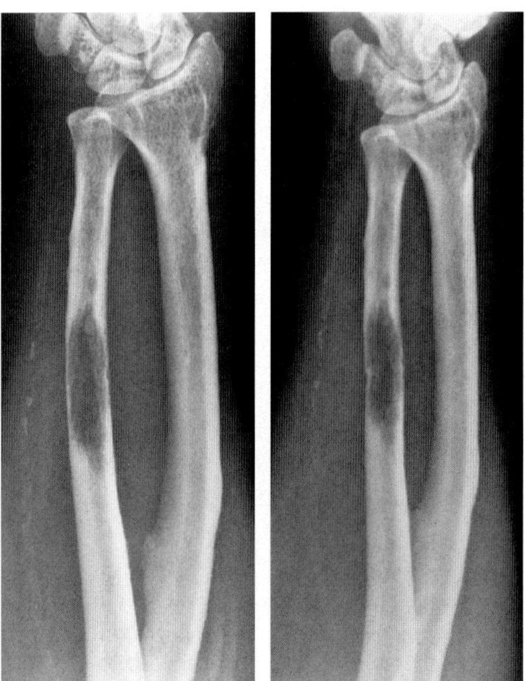

Fig. 36-7   Myeloma involvement of forearm. **A,** Initial posteroanterior forearm radiograph shows a large lytic myelomatous area involving the ulnar shaft picked up on skeletal survey. **B,** Later posteroanterior forearm radiograph after acute increase in ulnar forearm pain shows a minimally displaced pathologic fracture. The patient was treated with an ulnar gutter brace.

difficult to assess but would appear to be low, according to most of the available literature. In Copeland's series, no forearm fractures were observed.[28] In the series reported by Leeson et al.[26] none of the seven radial lesions resulted in fracture whereas one of the four ulnar lesions did. The highest reported rate of pathologic forearm fracture is 43% (three of seven) for radial metastatic deposits.[27] The risk of ulnar fracture from the same series was 25% (one of four).[27] Other ulnar pathologic fractures have also been reported.[25,34]

Pathophysiology

The rarity of forearm metastases, the lack of active red marrow in the forearm bones of the elderly population (which has a higher prevalence of metastatic disease), and the distal position of the radius and ulna in the upper extremity all suggest that, similar to the distal humerus, the forearm is relatively poor "soil" for growth of metastatic disease.

Nonoperative Treatment

Metastatic disease to the radius and ulna traditionally has been treated with palliative radiotherapy and bracing. Most forearms are very amenable to application of a custom-molded ulnar-gutter orthosis, which may be extended proximally with hinges at the elbow or distally across the wrist for more proximal or distal forearm lesions, respectively. Such treatment is no doubt best for the smaller forearm lesions without significant risk of fracture and for those with minimal symptoms. The efficacy of such treatment, however, has not been evaluated well, particularly for those patients with fractures. Some authors have indicated limited use of the arm and a generally poor result with nonoperative treatment of pathologic forearm fracture.[26]

Operative Treatment

The rarity of reported cases of operatively treated pathologic forearm fractures is illustrated by a report that included 70 operatively treated upper extremity pathologic fractures, 68 of which were located in the humerus.[3] Only two proximal ulnar fractures had been treated operatively in that series. Pathologic fractures of the radius or ulna may be fixed with plate and screws, intramedullary devices, or a combination (Fig. 36-8). The addition of PMMA is advisable.[3] Unfortunately, there are no biomechanical or clinical series to guide the choice of fixation in this site. Successful intramedullary rod and plate fixations, each accompanied by bone cement, have been reported for proximal ulnar

9. Marten ME, Meyer LM. Carcinoma of the pancreas with cardiac and cutaneous metastases. Am J Cancer 27:106-110, 1936.

10. Ritchie G. Metastatic tumors of the myocardium: A review of sixteen cases. Am J Pathol 17:483, 1941.

11. Mignani G, McDonald D, Boriani S, Avella M, Gaiani L, Campanacci M. Soft tissue metastasis from carcinoma: A case report. Tumori 75:630-633, 1989.

12. Munk PL, Gock S, Gee R, Connell DG, Quenville NF. Case report 708: Metastasis of renal cell carcinoma to skeletal muscle (right trapezius). Skel Radiol 21:56-59, 1992.

13. Buerger LG, Monteleone PN. Leukemic-lymphomatous infiltration of skeletal muscle. Cancer 19:1416-1421, 1966.

14. Chandler RW, Shulman I, Moore TM. Renal cell carcinoma presenting as a skeletal muscle mass: A case report. Clin Orthop Rel Res 145:227-229, 1979.

15. Laurence AE, Murray AJ. Metastasis in skeletal muscle secondary to carcinoma of the colon: Presentation of two cases. Br J Surg 57:529-530, 1970.

16. McKeown PP, Conant P, Auerbach LE. Squamous cell carcinoma of the lung: An unusual metastasis to pectoralis muscle. Ann Thorac Surg 61:1525-1526, 1996.

17. Mulsow FW. Metastatic carcinoma of skeletal muscles. Arch Pathol 35:112, 1943.

18. Porile JL, Olopade OI, Hoffman PC. Gastric adenocarcinoma presenting with soft tissue masses. Am J Gastroenterol 85:76-77, 1990.

19. Rosenbaum LH, Nicholas JJ, Slasky BS, Obley DL, Ellis LD. Malignant myositis ossificans: Occult gastric carcinoma presenting as an acute rheumatic disorder. Ann Rheum Dis 43:95-97, 1984.

20. Schultz SR, Bree RL, Schwab RE, Raiss G. CT detection of skeletal muscle metastases. J Comput Assist Tomogr 10:81-83, 1986.

21. Steinbaum S, Liss A, Tafreshi M, Alexander LL. CT findings in metastatic adenocarcinoma of the skeletal muscles. J Comput Assist Tomogr 7:545-546, 1983.

22. Hattrup SJ, Amadio PC, Sim FH, Lombardi RM. Metastatic tumors of the foot and ankle. Foot Ankle 8:243-247, 1988.

23. Stener B, Henriksson C, Johansson S, Gunterberg B, Pettersson S. Surgical removal of bone and muscle metastases of renal cancer. Acta Orthop Scand 55:491-500, 1984.

24. Weigensberg IJ. The many faces of metastatic renal carcinoma. Radiology 98:353-358, 1971.

25. Bennington JL, Kradjian RM. Distribution of metastases from renal carcinoma. In Renal Carcinoma. Philadelphia: WB Saunders, 1967, pp 156-169.

26. Hedju SI, Antoinette GT. Renal cell carcinoma at autopsy. J Urol 97:978, 1967.

27. Ochsner MB, Brannan W, Pond HS III, Goodier EH. Renal cell carcinoma: Review of 26 years experience at the Ochsner Clinic. J Urol 110:643-646, 1973.

28. Alburquerque TL, Ortin A, Cacho J. Metastasis in deep calf muscles as first manifestation of bronchus adenocarcinoma. [Letter.] Am J Med 83:606-607, 1987.

29. Araki K, Kobayashi M, Ogata T, Takuma K. Colorectal carcinoma metastatic to skeletal muscle. Hepatogastroenterology 41:405-408, 1994.

30. Avery GR. Metastatic adenocarcinoma masquerading as a psoas abscess. Clin Radiol 39:319-320, 1988.

31. Bibi C, Benmeir P, Maor E, Sagi A. Hand metastasis from renal cell carcinoma with no bone involvement. Ann Plast Surg 31:377-378, 1993.

32. Bordy Z, Pasztarak E, Bansagi G, Sik E. Soft-tissue involvement by adenocarcinoma imaged during bone scintigraphy. Clin Nucl Med 22:508, 1997.

33. Chang PC, Low HC, Mitra AK. Colonic carcinoma with metastases to the tibialis anterior muscle—A case report. Ann Acad Med Singapore 23:115-116, 1994.

34. Di TF, Rigon R, Capizzi G, Bucca D, Di PR, Zennari R. Solitary metastasis in the gluteus maximus from renal cell carcinoma 12 years after nephrectomy: Case report. Scand J Urol Nephrol 27:143-144, 1993.

35. Fusco MA, Paluzzi MW. Abdominal wall recurrence after laparoscopic-assisted colectomy for adenocarcinoma of the colon: Report of a case. Dis Colon Rectum 36:858-861, 1993.

36. Nash S, Rubenstein J, Chaiton A, Morava-Protzner I. Adenocarcinoma of the lung metastatic to the psoas muscle. Skel Radiol 25:585-587, 1996.

37. O'Keefe D, Gholkar A. Metastatic adenocarcinoma of the paraspinal muscles. Br J Radiol 61:849-851, 1988.

38. Pellegrini AE. Carcinoma of the lung occurring as a skeletal muscle mass. Arch Surg 114:550, 1979.

39. Potter GK, Strauss H, Potter RC. Delayed appearance of metastatic renal cell carcinoma subcutaneously in the left fifth toe after ipsilateral nephrectomy. J Foot Surg 30:147-150, 1991.

40. Ruiz JL, Vera C, Server G, Osca JM, Boronat F, Jimenez CJF. Renal cell carcinoma: Late recurrence in 2 cases. Eur Urol 20:167-169, 1991.

41. Sarma DP, Kovac A, Socorro N. Metastatic carcinoma of the skeletal muscle. South Med J 74:484-485, 1981.

42. Sidhu PS, Lewis M, Nicholson DA. Soft tissue metastasis from a renal cell carcinoma. Br J Urol 74:799-801, 1994.

43. Sridhar KS, Rao RK, Kunhardt B. Skeletal muscle metastases from lung cancer. Cancer 59:1530-1534, 1987.

44. Stabler J. Case report: Ossifying metastases from carcinoma of the large bowel demonstrated by bone scintigraphy. Clin Radiol 50:730-731, 1995.

45. Suto Y, Yamaguchi Y, Sugihara S. Skeletal muscle metastasis from lung carcinoma: MR findings. J Comput Assist Tomogr 21:304-305, 1997.

46. Torosian MH, Botet JF, Paglia M. Colon carcinoma metastatic to the thigh: An unusual site of metastasis. Report of a case. Dis Colon Rectum 30:805-808, 1987.

47. Amano Y, Kumazaki T. Gastric carcinoma metastasis to calf muscles: MR findings. Radiat Med 14:35-36, 1996.

48. Gleeson NC, Nicosia SV, Mark JE, Hoffman MS, Cavanaugh D. Abdominal wall metastases from ovarian cancer after laparoscopy. Amer J Obstet Gynecol 169:522-523, 1993.

49. Hoshi S, Orikasa S, Suzuki K, Saitoh T, Takahashi T, Yoshikawa K, Kuwahara M, Nose M. High-energy underwater shock wave treatment for internal iliac muscle metastasis of prostatic cancer: A first clinical trial. Jpn J Cancer Res 86:424-428, 1995.

50. Kambouris A. Full thickness abdominal wall resection for recurrent and metastatic neoplasms: A report of three cases. Am Surg 54:356-360, 1988.

51. Kanematsu M, Hoshi H, Takao H, Sugiyama Y. Abdominal wall tumor seeding at sonographically guided needle-core aspiration biopsy of hepatocellular carcinoma. [Letter.] AJR Am J Roentgenol 169:1198-1199, 1997.

52. Khajuria A, Karmakar T, Srinivasan R. Fine needle aspiration cytology of a subcutaneous metastasis of a malignant Brenner tumor of the ovary: A case report. Acta Cytologica 39: 246-248, 1995.

53. La FA, Di MEM, Preda L, Schifino MR, Campani R. Infiltrative subcutaneous metastases from ovarian carcinoma after paracentesis: CT findings. Abdom Imaging 22:522-523, 1997.

54. Masters JG, Cumming JA, Jennings P. Psoas abscess secondary to metastases from transitional cell carcinoma of the bladder. Br J Urol 77:155-156, 1996.

55. Rodgers WB, Mankin HJ. Metastatic malignant chondroblastoma. Am J Orthop 25:846-849, 1996.

56. Sahai S, Leigh D. Metastasis of adenocarcinoma of breast to gluteus medius. Iowa Med 85:369-370, 1995.

57. Swartjes JM, de BS, Blaauwgeers JL. Abdominal wall metastases after surgical resection of an immature teratoma of the ovary. Eur J Obstet Gynecol Reprod Biol 74:41-43, 1997.

58. Varma DG, Godiwala T. Unusual metastases from esophageal carcinoma: Computed tomography demonstration. J Comput Tomogr 11:205-207, 1987.

59. Warde P, Gospodarowicz M. Carcinoma of the prostate: Case report. Can J Surg 36:89-90, 1993.

60. Williams JB, Youngberg RA, Bui-Mansfield LT, Pitcher JD. MR imaging of skeletal muscle metastases. AJR Am J Roentgenol 168:555-557, 1997.

61. Oates KM, Malicki D, Shabaik A, Vaughan LM, Botte MJ. Right thigh mass in a 59-year-old man. [Clinical conference.] Clin Orthop 342:248-253, 1997.

62. Bansal R, Pai RR, Nayak R, Raghuveer CV. Metastatic chondrosarcoma in soft tissue diagnosed by fine needle aspiration (FNA) cytology. Cytopathology 7:70-72, 1996.

63. Khalili K, White LM, Kandel RA, Wunder JS. Chondroblastoma with multiple distant soft tissue metastases. Skel Radiol 26:493-496, 1997.

64. Meyer CA, Kransdorf MJ, Moser RPJ, Jelinek JS. Case report 716: Soft-tissue metastasis in synovial sarcoma. Skel Radiol 21:128-131, 1992.

65. Silvestri E, Bertolotto M, Perrone R, Neumaier CE, Derchi LE. Case report: US detection of tendinous metastasis from malignant melanoma. Clin Radiol 49:288-289, 1994.

66. Kohr RM. Primary cardiac angiosarcoma with disseminated bone and soft tissue metastases: A reassessment of diagnostic criteria based upon a review of the literature. Indiana Med 80:20-23, 1987.

67. Sunita, Kapila K, Singhal RM, Verma K. Extracranial metastasis of an astrocytoma detected by fine-needle aspiration: A case report. Diagn Cytopathol 7:290-292, 1991.

68. Kondo H, Kainuma O, Itami J, Minoyama A, Nakada H. Extramedullary plasmacytoma of maxillary sinus with later involvement of the gall bladder and subcutaneous tissues. Clin Oncol (R Coll Radiol) 7:330-331, 1995.

69. Stevens MJ, Gonet YM. Malignant psoas syndrome: Recognition of an oncologic entity. Australas Radiol 34:150-154, 1990.

70. Slatkin DN, Pearson J. Intramyofiber metastases in skeletal muscle. Hum Pathol 7:347-349, 1976.

71. Falkinburg LW, Fagan JH. Malignant mixed tumor of the parotid gland with a rare metastasis. Am J Surg 91:279-282, 1956.

72. Kerin R. Metastatic tumors of the hand. J Bone Joint Surg Am 40:263-278, 1958.

73. Bell JL, Mason ML. Metastatic tumors of hand: A report of two cases. Quart Bull Northwestern University Med School 27:114-116, 1953.

74. Mohanty S, Federowicz TE, Uehara H. Metastatic lesions of the fingers. Surgery 64:411-415, 1968.

75. Rose BA, Wood FM. Metastatic bronchogenic carcinoma masquerading as a felon. J Hand Surg Am 8:325-328, 1983.

76. Vinod SU, Gay RM. Adenoid cystic carcinoma of the minor salivary glands metastatic to the hand. Southern Med J 72:1483-1485, 1979.

77. Wheelock MC, Frable WJ, Urnes PD. Bizarre metastases from malignant neoplasms. Am J Clin Pathol 37:475-490, 1962.

78. Pedersen L, Balslev I, Guldhammer B, Rose C. Repeated fine needle aspirations in the diagnosis of soft tissue metastases in breast cancer. Eur J Cancer Clin Oncol 24:1039-1040, 1988.

79. Weiss L. Biochemical destruction of cancer cells in skeletal muscle: A rate regulator for hematogenous metastasis. Clin Exp Metastasis 7:483-491, 1989.

80. Seely S. Possible reasons for the high resistance of muscle to cancer. Med Hypoth 6:133-137, 1980.

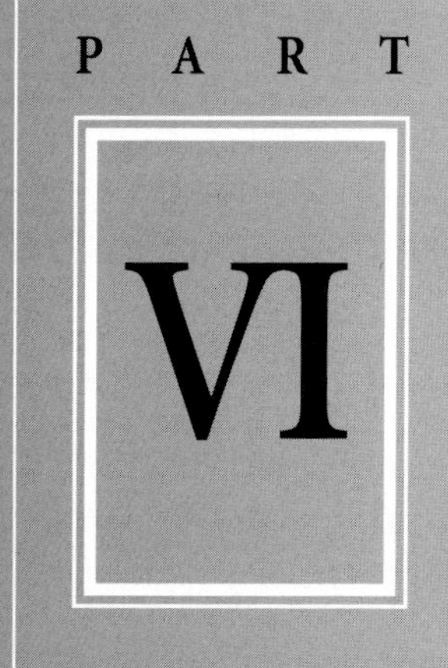

Special Problems

Effect of Radiation Therapy on Tissue and Wound Healing

David L. Larson, M.D.

There is little question that Roentgen's discovery of the x ray in 1895 was a seminal event in the history of medicine. It not only provided a way to document normal structures but also gave invaluable diagnostic information about pathologic conditions of the body not visible to the human eye. Following closely on Roentgen's achievement, however, was the Curies' discovery in 1898 that these same "x rays" could somehow have a surprisingly destructive effect on both normal and abnormal tissue. In fact, in these early days it was this reaction of the skin to radiation that offered the only guide to a patient's ability to tolerate this new treatment.

In this chapter we review the basic biology of radiation therapy, the rationale of the clinical application of the modality as both a primary and an adjunctive treatment, the expected positive results with proper use, and the untoward responses to radiation therapy when given in the treatment of metastatic disease to the musculoskeletal system.

BIOLOGY OF RADIATION PHYSICS[1,2]

When radiation comes in contact with tissue, it causes the release of an orbiting electron from an atom, thereby causing ionization. The energy thus released is sufficient to break strong chemical bonds. This has a biologic effect on the DNA bond in both normal and abnormal tissue. The amount of energy absorbed per unit mass is measured in joules per kilogram. One joule per kilogram is 1 Gy, and one hundredth of a gray is called a centigray, formerly known as a rad. The gray and the centigray are the major units used in describing the amount of radiation that a patient receives.

Electromagnetic energies of more than 1 MeV are used to penetrate skin and have an effect on the deeper tissues. With an increase in the dosage the skin is spared, and the full effect of the radiation dose is received at varying depths below the skin. The absorption in bone of high-energy photons, which are discrete quanta of electromagnetic radiation energy, differs from that in soft tissue. Although radiation at low energies (125 to 250 KeV) dissipates mostly at the level of the skin and is therefore used to treat skin cancers, radiation at higher energies (million electron volts) is used to treat deeper tissue tumors. Very low energies are best absorbed by bone, a quality that makes low-energy radiation best suited for diagnostic purposes.

Radiation Delivery

Radiation may be administered clinically in a number of different ways. A sealed radioactive source may be placed directly into a tumor or into tissue potentially containing a tumor. This technique, called brachytherapy, delivers a high dose of radiation to the tumor locally with a relatively rapid falloff of energy into the surrounding tissues. This minimizes destruction of normal tissues. The other and most common method of administering radiation is teletherapy, which makes use of an external beam, with either radioactive sources placed remotely from the patient or machines that generate x rays aimed at the patient's tumor. Obviously there are specific clinical settings in which each technique may be used most effectively. Brachytherapy can deliver high doses of radiation to a tumor but is of little use in treating the nodal echelons of metastatic disease from the primary tumor, whereas teletherapy can be used both locally and regionally. The two techniques can be used in the same patient to complement each other. Administering appropriate doses of radiation is a highly sophisticated aspect of radiation therapy, requiring direct measurements made in tissue equivalents and employing a computerized treatment plan. Details of dosage determination are beyond the scope of this chapter.

Radiation and the Cell

The most important target of the radiation beam is the DNA molecule, which is altered in a way that compromises its ability to reproduce. Although a tumor or normal cell may continue to reproduce once its DNA has been altered, the products of that activity are not the same. Tumor cells affected by radiation are eventually destroyed and phagocytosed by macrophages. One can appreciate how the effect of radiation is directly dependent on the reproductive cycle of cells and the number of cells in cycle at the time of a given radiation treatment. Because all the cells of the body are in different reproductive cycles at any one time and treatments are given for a number of weeks, the effects of the radiation are cumulative rather than immediate. Although the effects are the same on both normal and

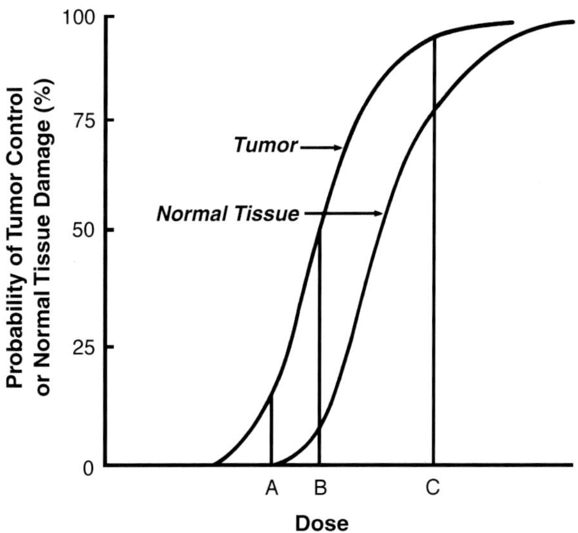

Fig. 38-1   Probability of tumor control or damage to normal tissue vs. dose of radiation therapy. At the low radiation dose, *A*, there is little to no effect on normal tissue and minimal effect on the tumor. At dose *B*, there is a nominal effect on normal tissue but a substantial impact on tumor tissue. As dose *C* is approached, normal tissue may have complications, but there is near eradication of the tumor. The radiation therapist must administer the dose of radiation that maximally affects the tumor without irreversibly damaging the normal tissue.

tumor cells, the normal cells have the ability to "rebound" more effectively than tumor cells; thus the desired effect of tumor cell ablation is obtained.

Balance must be achieved in determining the proper dose of radiation to control the tumor and yet not damage normal tissue beyond its ability to repair itself (Fig. 38-1). The dose-response ratio can be plotted as a sigmoid curve. A minimal dose of radiation is required to obtain any response; once that level is reached, additional radiation produces a positive exponential effect, but only up to a point. By an increase in the dose, tumor control can be achieved; in fact, all tumor eventually can be ablated with enough radiation. The problem arises when that dose exceeds a certain level. Radiation then has an increasingly negative effect on normal tissue surrounding the tumor, producing the complications of therapy. It is therefore the technique and skill of the radiotherapist in judging when to administer the radiation, how much radiation to administer, for what period, and in what fractions, that produce a favorable balance between cure and complications.

Obviously, tissues that have a greater cell turnover (e.g., skin, hair follicles, mucosa) will sustain a greater acute effect and, to an extent, limit the dose and fractionation of radiation. Most acute effects are self-limiting once the radiation is reduced or stopped. It is the long-term, late effects of treatment that are significant clinical problems and produce morbidity. These effects, which include soft tissue necrosis, fibrosis, fistula formation, ulceration, and bone viability compromise, will be discussed later in this chapter.

Radiation Fractionation

Total doses are given in fractions administered on a regular basis (usually daily for 5 days with a 2-day rest) in increments of 1.8 to 2 cGy/d for a 5- to 7-week period. Depending on the tumor type and location, there may be more or less total radiation given in more than one fraction per day (hyperfractionation) or only two or three times per week (hypofractionation). Cells irradiated in the presence of oxygen are two to three times more sensitive to a given dose of radiation than those with little or no oxygen. Fractionated doses allow the tissue to repair sublethal damage between doses because hypoxic cells are less sensitive to ionizing radiation therapy.

In summary, four factors must be considered when one is attempting to identify the results of a given radiation treatment in a patient: the total dose, the fractionation of that dose, the total volume of tissue treated, and the time elapsed during treatment. All these factors must be considered in a given clinical application.

A well-known adage related to radiation therapy demonstrates the interrelationship of these factors: "The effects of surgery are immediately visible, but those of radiation therapy are continuous and progressive during the patient's entire life." Changes in

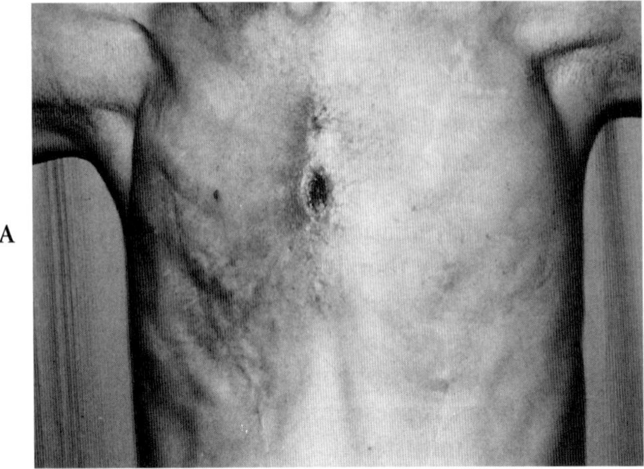

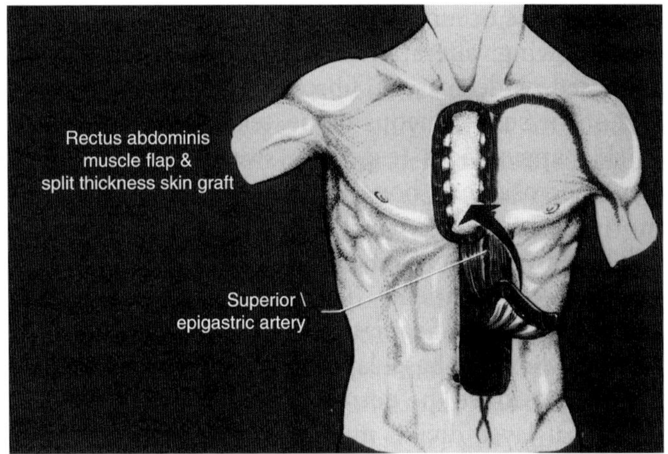

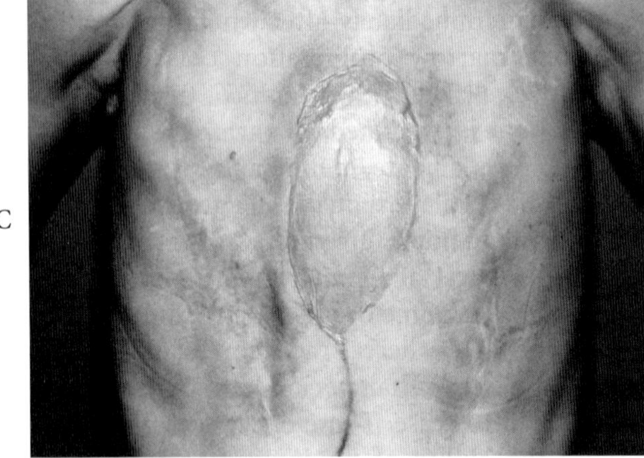

Fig. 38-2 **A,** Patient was given two postoperative radiation doses—one to each chest wall after mastectomy—at two different times. This wound will never heal because of the radiation necrosis incurred where the two doses of radiation overlapped each other. **B,** Method used to reconstruct radiation defect. New, nonirradiated tissue must be transposed into the debrided wound. The rectus muscle covered by a skin graft is used in this instance. **C,** Result is a healed wound and freedom from the pain of the open wound.

which occurs locally. Even though there is no good animal model for the late effects of radiation therapy, some assumptions can be made in the acute phase based on our knowledge of collagen remodeling in the wounded patient. We know that radiation will have a toxic effect on the fibroblast, the cell that produces collagen and thereby provides strength to any healing wound. The integrity of a given wound can be determined by measurement of its wound-burst strength. By radiating the skin of animals and subjecting it to these model systems, one can study the effects of alterations of dose, fractionation, and other parameters of radiation therapy. Wound healing in mouse skin was evaluated by wound-burst strength, and it was found that the threshold dose for a decrease in wound healing was 8 Gy administered in a single dose, but strength increased significantly with small daily doses.[7] This finding documents the potential effect in the human being and justifies the rationale for giving daily fractions of 1.8 to 2 Gy.

We also know that irradiation of skin produces changes in tissue that will persist long after the dose is given. A large dose (e.g., 18 Gy) given to a mouse up to 95 days before wounding will significantly alter wound healing.[8] If a wound is allowed to heal for at least 7 days[9] before radiation is administered, however, the normal wound-healing process is not altered.

To study chronic radiation effects, researchers harvested fibroblasts from human irradiated wounds previously treated with radiation at 2, 13, 15, and 18 years. These fibroblasts were cultured, and normal fibroblasts from another site on the same patient were used as controls. In all cases the fibroblasts from the irradiated skin grew more slowly than controls.[10] It thus appears that there is a definite alteration at the cellular level that in some way links wound-healing impairment to changes in the fibroblast.

When radiation has been administered before surgery, it is best to wait 3 to 6 weeks before proceeding with a surgical procedure. Of course, fewer problems will arise when radiation is given in a postoperative setting, and larger doses can also be given. Often, when one is forced to operate in a clinical setting where a large dose of radiation was received years earlier, it is best to plan on replacing irradiated skin with new, healthy tissue by using a local or distant flap of tissue. This approach eliminates the morbidity associated with poor healing in an irradiated wound (Fig. 38-2).

The deleterious effects of radiation are nowhere more clearly evident than in children who have received radiation therapy as a necessary treatment of tumor. The severity of the physical changes are directly related to the age at administration and the dose of therapy. The earlier in life and the greater the dose, the more telling the long-term effects. Because more than two thirds of children now treated for cancer will be cured and will survive into adulthood, the challenge for treating physicians today is to learn how to keep these effects to a minimum and yet maintain the high cure rate.[5,11]

SPECIAL PROBLEMS
Radiation-Induced Neoplasia

Since the early 1900s, occupational hazards involving tissue exposed to radiation have been observed. Osteosarcomas were noted in the bones of radium-dial painters, who ingested between 15 and 125 µg of radioactive material weekly.[12] Once such hazards were recognized, appropriate measures were taken to minimize exposure. Ironically, large therapeutic doses of radiation have been implicated in many reports, most of which are anecdotal and poorly documented. Strict criteria should be used to suggest a causal relationship between a course of radiation and subsequent tumor development. These criteria include (1) documented proof of radiation dose and fields, (2) an adequate latent period of at least 3 years and preferably 5 years from the time of irradiation to onset of tumor, (3) occurrence of the tumor within the irradiated field, and (4) unequivocal evidence that the tumor is different from that originally treated.[4]

The most frequent cancers arising within an irradiated field are skin tumors associated with an area of radiodermatitis. These tumors may be basal or squamous cell cancers. The latter can be highly malignant, with a tendency to metastasize.[13]

The incidence of high-dose radiation-induced tumor is unknown, but it is certainly low and varies with the tissue irradiated, the patient's age at the time of radiation therapy, and the type of radiation used. The resulting neoplasms are not necessarily different from those that might occur spontaneously within the tissue, but when sarcomas arise, they can be bizarre and aggressive,[14,15] which suggests that they are from previously altered tissue. It is this potential to develop life-threatening tumors in the latency period after radiation therapy that mandates follow-up of the patient long after the threat of recurrent tumor is past.

Management of Radiation Complications

The most effective management of negative sequelae of radiation therapy is to make certain that the therapy is not used capriciously, that excellent technique is applied, and that the patient is not only followed up rigorously by his or her physicians but also is made aware of the potential problems that may occur if protection from the elements and from trauma is not maintained.

When there is a nonhealing wound within an irradiated area, it may be only a nuisance, requiring a dressing change. However, it could be life-threatening if it overlies a major vessel, such as the carotid or femoral artery, or an organ, such as the brain, lung, or abdominal viscera. Because these wounds rarely heal spontaneously, the usual therapy is surgical resection not only of the wound but also of all the irradiated tissue surrounding the area. Once resection is accomplished, new, healthy, nonirradiated tissue must be introduced to cover the wound. Until the late 1970s, dependable, reproducible reconstructive tools for this therapy were not available. With the advent of musculocutaneous flaps and free tissue transfer, the management of the soft tissue defect resulting from radiation necrosis has become routine. Details of these methods of tissue transfer will be presented in the next chapter.

When radionecrosis involves bone, the use of hyperbaric oxygen has been advocated, particularly when the mandible is affected. The rationale has been that the periodic elevation of the oxygen tension (2.4 atm for 90 minutes once a day for 5 or 6 weeks) will support capillary angiogenesis[16] and collagen synthesis[17] and will enhance leukocyte bacterial killing.[18] Some randomized, prospective studies have reported the use of hyperbaric oxygen in soft-tissue flap survival[19] and in the prevention of infection of the mandible after tooth extraction from irradiated bone.[20] The reader is referred to a definitive review of the use of hyperbaric oxygen in radiation necrosis by Kindwall.[21]

ACKNOWLEDGMENT

The author wishes to acknowledge the assistance of Beth Kaczmarek in the preparation of this manuscript.

REFERENCES

1. Bernstein EF, Sullivan FJ, Mitchell JB, Salomon GD, Glatstein E. Biology of chronic radiation effect on tissues and wound healing. Clin Plast Surg 20:435-453, 1993.
2. Eisbruch A, Lichter AS. What a surgeon needs to know about radiation. Ann Surg Oncol 4:516-522, 1997.
3. Sanders CL, Katthren RL. Bone marrow. In Sanders CL, Katthren RL, eds. Ionizing Radiation: Tumorigenic and Tumoricidal Effects. Columbus, Ohio: Battekke Press, 1983, p 125.
4. Berthrong M. Pathologic changes secondary to radiation. World J Surg 10:155-170, 1986.
5. Goldwein JW, Meadows AT. Influence of radiation on growth in pediatric patients. Clin Plast Surg 20:455-464, 1993.
6. Mustoe TA, Prudy J, Gramates P. Reversal of impaired wound healing in irradiated rats by platelet-derived growth factor-BB. Am J Surg 158:345-350, 1989.
7. Gorodetsky R, Mou X, Fisher DR. Radiation effect in mouse skin: Dose fractionation and wound healing. Int J Radiat Oncol Biol Phys 18:1077-1081, 1990.
8. Gorodetsky R, McBride WH, Withers HR. Assay of radiation effects on mouse skin as expressed in wound healing. Radiat Res 116:135-144, 1988.
9. Devereux DF, Kent H, Brennan MF. Time dependent effects of adriamycin and x-ray therapy on wound healing in the rat. Cancer 45:2805-2810, 1980.
10. Rudolph R, Vande Berg J, Schneider JA. Slowed growth of cultured fibroblasts from human radiation wounds. Plast Reconstr Surg 82:669-677, 1988.
11. Kroll SS, Woo S, Santin A, Zietz H, Reid HS, Jaffee N, Larson DL. Long-term effects of radiotherapy administered in childhood for the treatment of malignant disease. Ann Surg Oncol 1:473-479, 1994.
12. Martland HS. Occupational poisoning in manufacture of luminous watch dials. JAMA 92:452-466, 1929.
13. Lever WF, Schambaugh-Lever G. Inflammatory diseases due to physical agents and foreign substances. In Lever WF, ed. Histopathology of the Skin, 3rd ed. Philadelphia: JB Lippincott, 1990, pp 9-44.
14. Seo IS, Warner TF, Warren JS, Bennett JE. Cutaneous postirradiation sarcoma: Ultrastructure evidence of pluripotential mesenchymal cell derivation. Cancer 56:761-767, 1985.
15. Souba WM, McKenna RJ Jr, Meis J. Radiation-induced sarcomas of the chest wall. Cancer 57:610-615, 1986.
16. Knighton DR, Silver IA, Hunt TK. Regulation of wound healing, angiogenesis: Effect of oxygen gradient and inspired oxygen concentrations. Surgery 90:262-270, 1981.
17. Touhey JE, Davis JC, Workman WT. Hyperbaric oxygen. Orthop Rev 16:41-46, 1987.
18. Hunt TK, Pai MP. Effect of varying ambient oxygen tensions on wound metabolism and collagen synthesis. Surg Gynecol Obstet 13:561-564, 1872.
19. Marx RE. Radiation injury to tissue. In Kindwall EP, ed. Hyperbaric Medicine Practice. Flagstaff, Ariz.: Best Publishing, 1994, p 500.
20. Marx RE, Johnson RP, Kline SN. Prevention of osteoradionecrosis: A randomized prospective clinical trial of hyperbaric oxygen versus penicillin. J Am Dent Assoc 111:49-54, 1985.
21. Kindwall EP. Hyperbaric oxygen's effect on radiation necrosis. Clin Plast Surg 20:473-483, 1993.

Reconstructions in Delayed Wound Healing

Stephen P. Hardy, M.D.

curred in the dissection, rather than to the intrinsic radiation changes in the vein.[14] A study using a rabbit free-flap model demonstrated a higher flap failure rate when irradiated recipient vessels were used.[8]

Despite the conflicting results in animal models, clinical evaluation has shown that with careful handling of the recipient vessels, the flap failure rate is not significantly increased. In a large prospective multicenter study of free-flap surgery and its outcome, it was determined that reconstruction in an irradiated recipient bed was a statistically significant risk factor for flap failure.[15-18] As with any clinical situation, each case must be evaluated on its own merits, and, if possible, nonirradiated recipient vessels should be used. Clearly these reconstructions should be handled by surgeons well experienced with microsurgical techniques.

The lack of readily accessible large-caliber recipient vessels for microvascular anastomosis in the back, upper abdomen, and epigastrium make the need for vein grafting likely to obtain additional pedicle length. Rather than struggling with a difficult dissection with small, potentially damaged recipient vessels, judicious planning and preparation for vein grafting will improve the likelihood of success.

Free Flap Choices

The rectus abdominis and latissimus dorsi muscles are the workhorses of microvascular free tissue transfer. These two muscles both have very reliable anatomy, with large-caliber arteriovenous pedicles. Neither leaves a major functional deficit after harvest.

The rectus abdominis muscle has the advantage of ease of harvest with the patient in the supine position. The straplike nature of the muscle makes it well suited for reconstruction in the extremities. One can take advantage of the length of the muscle to effectively add length to the vascular pedicle. The latissimus dorsi muscle's broad, flat architecture makes it ideally suited for scalp reconstruction and wounds with a large surface area. The gracilis muscle is also a reliable unit for microvascular free tissue transfer. Advantages include reliable anatomy and vascular pedicle and the minimal morbidity of harvest in terms of postoperative pain, scar, and functional deficit.

Regarding fasciocutaneous units, the scapular-parascapular flap is often used. The disadvantages of a short vascular pedicle and relatively more technically challenging dissection, in comparison with the rectus abdominis or latissimus dorsi muscles (with or without an overlying cutaneous unit or skin graft), make the scapular-parascapular flap less popular. It is probably much simpler to use a large, highly reliable muscle flap and a skin graft than a more challenging fasciocutaneous flap. Simplicity and the maximal likelihood of success are always preferred over style and aesthetics of reconstruction when one is dealing with an irradiated wound.

Ideally a single flap should be used for a reconstruction. On some occasions, this is not possible because of the requirements of the reconstruction. Composite flaps consisting of two or more tissue units have been especially helpful in head and neck reconstruction.[19] With extensive forethought, the intricacies of the reconstructive requirements can be predicted and built into the flap. Nowhere is this principle better illustrated than with the subscapular arterial system flaps used for reconstruction of complex craniofacial defects.[20,21] The branching of the subscapular artery into the thoracodorsal and circumflex scapular arteries permits two large blocks of tissue—latissimus dorsi muscle with or without bone from the scapula via the angular branch from the thoracodorsal artery plus a scapular-parascapular fasciocutaneous unit—to be transferred on a singular large-caliber vascular pedicle for microanastomosis. The three-dimensional freedom of movement of the subunits enables the surgeon to meet several requirements with a single flap. For example, skin and mucosal defects, bone structural needs, and vascularized coverage of the skull base to separate the intracranial contents from the paranasal sinuses or external environment can all be components of extirpative craniofacial wounds. This type of reconstruction can be exceedingly complex, time-consuming, and technically demanding, requiring an experienced team of surgeons.

One's comfort level with the complexity of the surgical situation may limit the "elegance" of a reconstruction, and there is nothing wrong with this limitation. As is often stated, "perfect is the enemy of good." The important concept is to prioritize the needs of a given wound. Coverage of the dura or major vascular structure obviously takes precedence over facial contour or skin match. Secondary procedures to address perhaps the less important functional elements or cosmetic aspects of a reconstruction may be necessary. The goal is to return the patient to as comfortable and functional an existence as possible given the overall prognosis and his or her general state of health.

Bone Reconstruction

Osteonecrosis of the mandible is a relatively uncommon and difficult problem. Bone reconstruction is not essential after adequate débridement, and at times either a titanium reconstruction plate or no bone reconstruction at all is the only reasonable option. When bone is used for mandible reconstruction, however, the fibula free flap is generally the first choice.[22-25] Its vascular anatomy provides a relatively long pedicle and allows multiple segmental osteotomies to aid in precision of the bone reconstruction.[23] On rare occasions a second flap is necessary to provide adequate soft tissue for the reconstruction.

The iliac crest free flap, because of difficulty in dissection and morbidity of the donor defect, has fallen to a distant second choice for microvascular transfer when bone is required. Other possibilities include the lateral portion of the scapula, depending on the circumflex scapular artery, or the thoracodorsal angular branch, which has the advantage of potentially including a large cutaneous element in the scapular or parascapular fasciocutaneous unit. The need to reposition the patient and a tedious pedicle dissection are disadvantages. The radial forearm free flap, with a segment of radius included, carries a potentially significant donor-site morbidity and may not be able to provide adequate bone in the setting of osteonecrosis. A segment of rib, vascularized via the pectoralis major flap, can have problems reaching the reconstruction site and is less reliable than other osseous free flaps. Non-vascularized bone grafts run an extremely high likelihood of failure in a radiation-damaged wound bed and in general should not be used in this setting.

The high incidence of breast cancer and lung cancer and the use of radiation therapy in their treatment results in a relatively high occurrence of osteonecrosis of rib bone or cartilage. Although there may be concern for the potential paradoxical chest wall motion and its effect on respiratory effort, alloplastic or bone reinforcement of the thorax has been shown to be unnecessary in most cases.[10,26] If necessary, reinforcement of the thorax with Prolene mesh under tension and a well-vascularized flap cover is simple and efficacious.

ADJUVANT THERAPIES
Hyperbaric Oxygen

The use of hyperbaric oxygen (HBO) treatment to augment healing in the irradiated wound has been well documented.[27-30] The process involves placing the patient in an isolated pressurized environment, or "chamber," at 2.4 atm, so that he or she breathes pure oxygen for 20 to 40 treatment sessions, each lasting up to 90 minutes. The high-pressure O_2 environment increases blood O_2 tension. It is suggested that the mechanism of benefit of HBO is the creation of a steep O_2 gradient between the irradiated tissue and the surrounding normal tissue; this gradient is otherwise gradual and is thought to be inadequate for the stimulation of angiogenesis.[31,32] HBO therapy, despite its ability to improve the overall healing environment, is probably, by itself, inadequate for the complete treatment of osteonecrosis. It is best used as an adjunct to aggressive surgical treatment.[33] The major drawbacks of HBO therapy are the unavailability of treatment facilities at most hospitals and the labor-intensive nature of the therapy. It seems that the skepticism (or enthusiasm) regarding HBO treatment is best correlated with the availability of hyperbaric facilities at one's institution.

Tissue Expansion

The use of tissue expanders for local reconstruction in radiation-damaged areas is mentioned only to be condemned. An attempt to dissect an expander pocket in the fibrotic ischemic bed will further damage tissue, eventually leading to expander exposure, infection, and overlying skin necrosis. Even if the irradiated region seems relatively normal in terms of appearance and tissue consistency, tissue expansion is not looked on favorably.[34,35]

One potential use of expanders, however, would be in the preexpansion of a flap, such as the parascapular fasciocutaneous unit, before transfer. Ex-

40. Thaller SR, Lee TJ, Armstrong M, Tesluk H, Stern JS. Effect of insulin-like growth factor type I on critical-size defects in diabetic rats. J Craniofac Surg 6:218-223, 1995.

41. Pierce GF, Mustoe TA, Lingelbach J, Masakowski VR, Gramates P, Deuel TF. Transforming growth factor β reverses the glucocorticoid-induced wound healing deficit in rats: Possible regulation in macrophages by platelet-derived growth factor. Proc Natl Acad Sci USA 86:2229-2233, 1989.

42. Mustoe TA, Pierce GF, Thomason A, Gramates P, Sporn MB, Deuel TF. Accelerated healing of incisional wounds in rats induced by transforming growth factor β. Science 237:1333-1335, 1987.

43. Bishop JB, Phillips LG, Mustoe TA, VanderZee AJ, Wiersema L, Roach DE, Heggers JP, Hill DP, Taylor EL, Robson MC. A prospective randomized evaluator-blinded trial of two potential wound healing agents for the treatment of venous stasis ulcers. J Vasc Surg 16:251-257, 1992.

44. Knighton DR, Ciresi K, Fiegel VD, Schumerth S, Butler E, Cerra F. Stimulation of repair in chronic, nonhealing, cutaneous ulcers using platelet-derived wound healing formula. Surg Gynecol Obstet 170:56-60, 1990.

45. Bernstein EF, Harisiadis L, Salomon G, Norton J, Sollberg S, Uitto J, Glatstein E, Glass J, Talbot T, Russo A. Transforming growth factor-beta improves healing of radiation-impaired wounds. J Invest Derm 97:4430-4434, 1991.

46. Cromock DT, Purdy JA, Porras-Reyes B, Mustoe TA. Acceleration of tissue repair by transforming growth factor β: In vivo mechanism of action by selective radiotherapy impaired healing. Surg Forum 4:630-632, 1990.

47. Cromack DT, Porras-Reyes B, Purdy JA, Pierce GF, Mustoe TA. Acceleration of tissue repair by transforming growth factor β: Identification of in vivo mechanism of action with radiotherapy-induced specific healing deficits. Surgery 113:36-42, 1993.

48. Mustoe TA, Purdy J, Gramates P. Reversal of impaired wound healing in irradiated rats by platelet-derived growth factor β. Am J Surg 158:345-350, 1989.

49. Mustoe TA, Porras-Reyes BH. Modulation of wound healing response in chronic irradiated tissues. Clin Plast Surg 20:465-472, 1993.

50. Thaller SR, Salzhauer MA, Rubinstein AJ, Thion A, Tesluk H. Effect of insulin-like growth factor type I on critical size calvarial bone defects in irradiated rats. J Craniofac Surg 9:138-141, 1998.

51. Würzler KK, DeWeese TL, Sebald W, Reddi AH. Radiation-induced impairment of bone healing can be overcome by recombinant human bone morphogenetic protein-2. J Craniofac Surg 9:131-137, 1998.

52. Eppley BL, Connolly DT, Winkelmann T, Sadove AM, Heuvelman D, Feder J. Free bone graft reconstruction of irradiated facial tissue: Experimental effects of basic fibroblast growth factor stimulation. Plast Reconstr Surg 88:1-11, 1991.

53. Khouri RK, Brown DM, Koudsi B, Deune EG, Gilula LA, Cooley BC, Reddi AH. Repair of calvarial defects with flap tissue: Role of bone morphogenetic proteins and competent responding tissues. Plast Reconstr Surg 98:103-109, 1996.

54. Zhao LL, Davidson JD, Wu L, Mustoe TA. Total reversal of hypoxic wound healing deficit by hyperbaric oxygen plus growth factors. Surg Forum 43:711-714, 1992.

55. Hohn DC. Oxygen and leukocyte microbial killing. In Dani JC, Hunt TK, eds. Hyperbaric oxygen therapy. Bethesda, Md.: Undersen Medical Society, 1977, pp 101-110.

56. Girod DA, McCulloch TM, Tsue TT, Weymuller EAJ. Risk factors for complications in clean-contaminated head and neck surgical procedures. Head Neck 17:7-13, 1995.

57. Kurul S, Dincer M, Kizir A, Uzunismail A, Darendeliler E. Plastic surgery in irradiated areas: Analysis of 200 consecutive cases. Eur J Surg Oncol 23:48-53, 1997.

Extremity Fixation in Metastatic Disease

Gerald J. Lang, M.D., and Ray Vanderby, Jr., Ph.D.

Metastatic cancers are the most common osteolytic lesions in the adult population.[1] As survival times for patients with primary organ tumors increase, management of skeletal metastases and their potential complications becomes even more important. Patients with the most common cancers (breast carcinoma, prostate carcinoma, lymphomas, and myelomas) survive three times longer after their first pathologic long bone fracture than they did 25 years ago.[2] Five-year survival rates are 20% for breast cancer and 25% for prostate cancer.[2] Survival times, however, can vary widely depending on the type of primary tumor, the stage of disease, and the location of the lesion. For example, patients with breast cancer survive for an average of 21.4 months after identification of the first skeletal metastasis, vs. only 3.5 months for patients with primary lung tumors.[3] The extended time frames are critical issues when one is treating metastatic lesions in the extremities.

The biomechanical consequence of an osteolytic metastatic lesion is a weakened bone, which can become at risk of fracture or can fracture under normal physiologic loading. The goal of the surgeon is to stabilize or reconstruct the pathologic fracture or to prophylactically stabilize the bone at risk of fracture, ultimately relieving pain and maintaining or restoring function.

Several biomechanical challenges become apparent when pathologic fractures are treated. First, the appropriate use of prophylactic stabilization requires an accurate assessment of fracture risk. This relatively simple objective has been difficult to realize in clinical practice.[4] Second, the fixation construct (i.e., the bone and orthopedic implant together) must provide immediate stability and last the lifetime of the patient. Because of the limited healing potential of many pathologic fractures, the fixation techniques used may differ from those of nonpathologic fracture fixation. The surgical techniques discussed here have provided good or excellent pain relief and restored function to the majority of patients.[2,5] This chapter reviews important biomechanical considerations associated with surgical reconstruction of patients with metastatic disease.

BIOMECHANICAL CONSIDERATIONS FOR PATHOLOGIC FRACTURE RISK

When metastatic lesions create osseous defects in long bones, the objective of surgery is to maintain a patient's ability to walk. Operative treatment is clearly indicated when a patient has a pathologic fracture and is otherwise medically stable. Predicting which lesions will cause a fracture without prophylactic operative treatment, however, is extremely difficult.

Factors for Fracture Prediction

A host of confounding biomechanical and biologic factors diminish the veracity of any specific prediction for pathologic fracture. For a single, high-level loading the risk of fracture depends on the structural strength of the bone, which in turn depends on the bone's geometry and material properties. This includes information about the normal portions of the bone and about the size, geometry, material properties, and location of the lesion. For repetitive, lower-level loadings (a more likely scenario), subfailure damage accumulates until the weakened bone fractures. The risk of fracture then depends on the fatigue strength of the residual normal bone, its ability to repair damage, and the fatigue-related characteristics of the osseous defect. In all cases the risk of fracture depends on loading. Even a substantially compromised bone will not fracture if it is sufficiently guarded from loading. The loads applied to a bone depend on its location in the body, the activity level of the patient, and the pain or other complications tending to reduce the level and frequency of physiologic loadings. Loadings are often complex combinations of loading modes, such as bending, torsion, or compression. With loadings difficult to predict and with structural and biologic compromise hard to estimate, predicting the risk of fracture is particularly problematic.

The effects of lesions on bones have been simulated in a laboratory setting by creating endosteal deficiencies in the diaphysis or metaphysis of long bones.[6-10] These studies have given us some insight into the biomechanical effects of metastatic lesions. The shape and size of a defect and its anatomic location affect the ability of a bone to carry load. A cylindric long bone, for example, is efficient at bearing torsional loads. A structure that is not circular in cross section is less efficient and will warp. If a defect is sufficiently long in the axial direction (an "open section"), the bone begins to warp and becomes more susceptible to torsional failure. If a long bone is being loaded in bending, a defect at or near the neutral axis will be of less consequence than one at the extremes of tension or compression. A periosteal defect will therefore be of greater structural concern than an endosteal defect because stress levels increase linearly in a radial direction for bending or torsion. In addition, a defect creates a stress concentration, or "stress riser," the intensity of which is dependent on its shape. A small circular hole in a hollow cylinder increases local stresses three to four times.[7] A biopsy hole with sharp corners reduces a bone's torsional strength more than a hole with rounded ends.[11] The sharper the corners on the defect, the higher the stress riser. It is clear, then, that a single parameter, such as the diameter of a defect, cannot predict the likelihood of fracture with confidence.

Two cortical defects are commonly discussed in the biomechanical literature: "stress risers" and "open section" defects.[12] Stresses are concentrated near any sudden geometric or material change in the bone cortex that increases the nominal stress. Stress risers are often used to describe the effect of perforations in the cortex that are much smaller than the cross-sectional diameter of the bone, typically less than 20%. Open section defects are either larger (approaching the diameter of the bone) or, if the defect runs in an axial direction, long enough to create an open section. A single longitudinal saw cut, for example, reduced the torsional load capacity of human tibias by 58% and their energy storage capacity by 80%.[13] In reality, these two defects, stress risers and open sections, are more of a continuum than a binary set of behaviors. In vitro mechanical testing has shown that increases in defect size decrease the torsional strength in a continuous and almost linear manner (Fig. 40-1).[7] This study tested sheep femora in pure torsion with circular holes and found a 62% reduction in strength and an 88% reduction in energy storage capacity for a 50% circular defect. A companion study showed that these results could be reasonably well predicted with an inelastic computer model.[14]

Many other biomechanical studies echo the profound consequence of osteolytic metastases. Brooks et al.[15] reported a 55% decrease in energy storage capacity for canine femora in torsion with 2.8 or 3.6 mm drill holes. McBroom et al.[16] reported a 62% reduction in bending strength for canine femora with drill holes 20% of their diameter. They also showed that a nonlinear finite element model could simulate this behavior. Hipp et al.,[17] using both in vitro experimental data and computer modeling, reported a reduction of the bending strength of canine femora that was linearly related to the remaining wall thickness. When a symmetrical endosteal defect removed 50% of the intact bone, bending strength decreased by 55%.

Changes in material properties within and adjacent to a metastatic defect affect the ability of a bone to carry load. Data are limited, however, that describe these changes biomechanically. For trabecular bone, Hipp et al.[18] suggested that osteolytic defects reduce both strength and stiffness in uniaxial compression but that osteoblastic metastases reduce only stiffness. Behavior for other modes of loading, for combined loadings, and for bone within or surrounding cortical defects remains largely undefined.

The healing or repair ability of bone surrounding a metastatic defect is another factor that affects the risk of pathologic fracture. The cycle of subfailure damage and biologic repair that comes from repeated mechanical loadings is normally homeostatic. A defect of any type will concentrate stresses and cause physiologic loadings to produce local damage bone at a higher rate. This is particularly a problem for patients with osteolytic lesions, who are often older and have osteomalacia or osteoporosis. In addition, adjuvant therapy for cancer, such as local radiation or systemic chemotherapy, may also attenuate the repair processes, allowing microdamage to grow, coalesce, and eventually catastrophically weaken the bone. Tong et al.[19] found that patients receiving higher levels of radiation in their therapy (40 Gy vs. 20 Gy) had a higher rate of fracture (18% vs. 4%).

The size of a defect is certainly an important factor for predicting the risk of fracture. Unfortunately, radiographic estimates of defect size can be highly inaccurate. Galasko[20] estimated that bone

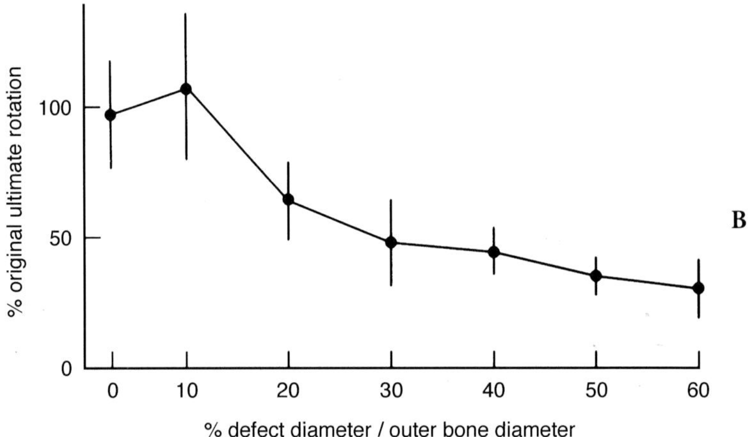

Fig. 40-1   Changes in ultimate torque (**A**) and ultimate deformation (**B**) of sheep femora with holes of different diameters, as measured in percentage of intact values. (From Edgerton BC, An KN, Morrey BF. Torsion strength reduction due to cortical defects in bone. J Orthop Res 8:851-855, 1990.)

destruction approaching 50% must occur before a lesion can be identified. In a more recent study using 10 pairs of human cadaveric femora with simulated intertrochanteric metastatic defects, three orthopedic oncology surgeons evaluated defect size on plain radiographs and computed tomography scans. There was only modest agreement among the surgeons with regard to the size of the lesions.[21] In a study with simulated defects in the mid-diaphyseal cortex of canine femora, measurement errors as large as 100% were reported when the size was taken from radiographs that were not optimally aligned with respect to the defect.[22]

Theoretic estimates of structural compromise are, at best, only qualitatively accurate. The biomechanical experiments noted here and the corresponding computer models use normal cortical bone with idealized defects produced by sharp instruments. The structural consequence of a single overload is estimated from a single mode of loading, and the models are optimized to fit the data set. Even when these well-constructed computer models are used with well-designed and controlled in vitro experiments, it is difficult to determine the risk of fracture precisely.[23] Additional uncertainties, such as complex, variable, and repeated loadings, three-dimensional biomechanical properties for strength and fatigue, osteogenic potential for repair and healing of subfailure damage, and an imprecise knowledge of the defect geometry diminish the value of any specific prediction, even if it is produced with great technical rigor. Hipp et al.[21] suggested that if our knowledge of load-bearing capacity were to be combined with estimated loads for activities of daily living, it would be possible to calculate a factor for the risk of pathologic fractures. Although biomechanically sound, this approach is currently lacking the detailed data required for implementation. The prognostic accuracy and validity of this approach remain to be demonstrated in either a prospective or a retrospective study.

Guidelines

Because of the current limitations and qualitative nature of biomechanical predictions for risk of fracture, surgeons usually use simpler, clinical guidelines for prophylactic fixation. These guidelines, discussed in greater detail below, recommend stabilization of metastatic defects in long bones of functional significance if the defects are painful, greater than 2.5 cm in diameter, or greater than 50% of the bone diameter.

Pain from bone damage often precedes a pathologic fracture; hence it is sometimes used as an indication for prophylactic fixation. This is not, however, a selective criterion. Pain is the most frequent clinical symptom of metastatic bone disease. Winchester et al.[24] reported that pain was symptomatic in 32 of 33 patients with breast cancer and osseous metastases. There is no conclusive evidence that pain is a reliable predictor of risk for pathologic fracture.[21] Pain, regardless of its efficacy as a predictor, is typically attenuated or relieved with fracture fixation in patients thought to have impending fractures from metastatic defects.[25,26]

Two radiographic measurements have been commonly suggested to predict impending fractures; hence they are guidelines for operative treatment. First, a defect greater than 2.5 cm should be considered at risk of fracture, and second, a defect greater than 50% of the cortical cross-sectional area should also be considered at risk.[27,28] These guidelines arose from retrospective clinical studies, and neither has been tested by in vitro experimentation. In a study by Fidler[29] the radiographic parameter of 50% cortical destruction predicted that 33 lesions should have fractured. Fracture occurred in 20. Thus this criterion was correct for 61% of the fractures, but the other 39% were falsely positive. The alternative hypothesis, that bone lesions larger than 2.5 cm are predictive of pathologic fractures, was used to study 19 femoral pathologic fractures.[27] Of these, 8 fractures occurred in patients who did not meet this criterion. This study therefore had a false-negative rate of 42%.

A retrospective study of 203 patients with 516

metastatic defects in the proximal portion of the femur was unable to determine any radiographic measurement that clearly discriminated those defects that resulted in fracture from those that did not.[30] Several problems were discussed. First, lesions were permeative. They did not have clear boundaries and therefore were difficult to measure. The measured size of a lesion could vary on two radiographs of the same patient. Second, 54% of the fractures occurred through lesions that were not measurable. Third, measurable lesions that fractured had defect sizes that overlapped those that did not fracture.

In an attempt to overcome these problems with radiographically based measurements, Mirels[31] proposed a more complex system to predict the risk of fracture with metastatic defects. With this system a composite score, which included the size of the defect, the location of the defect, the lesion type, and pain, would be used to predict impending fracture. When this system was used to evaluate 38 patients with 78 metastases, there were still 22% false-positive findings and 4% false-negative findings.

Summary of Fracture Risk Prediction

The inconsistencies discussed here clearly show that predicting fracture on the basis of radiographic criteria (even if augmented with other information) is problematic. Application of the guidelines discussed in the preceding section requires measurements that have inherent inaccuracies (up to 100% according to Hipp et al.[22]). False-negative and false-positive results are common with every current radiographic guideline. This unfortunately is to be expected because the size of a defect, even if it could be accurately measured, is only one of the biomechanical parameters essential for predicting fracture. The other parameters have the same level or even greater levels of uncertainty. There is a confounding level of variability among patients with regard to osseous quality in a specific region, local stress concentrations, and the ability of bone to repair microdamage and arrest crack propagation. The diminution of a bone's osteogenic potential because of age, disease, and treatments is typically unknown for a given patient. Another essential biomechanical parameter not considered at all by radiographic criteria is loading.

It is conceptually appealing and logical that biomechanical information about lesions in bone could be applied in a clinical setting for correct diagnosis and recommendation of surgical treatment for an impending pathologic fracture. In a practical sense and at the present time, this information cannot be so applied with a high degree of confidence.

CONCEPTS OF FIXATION IN PATHOLOGIC FRACTURES

Many of the implants and surgical techniques used to treat acute pathologic fractures due to metastatic disease[32] have been adapted from the treatment of nonpathologic fractures. Pathologic fractures, however, have many variables that may make techniques used in routine fracture care inadequate. For example, a bone lesion, if extensive, may require reconstruction of the bone rather than fracture fixation for subsequent healing. The patient's overall prognosis, degree of metastatic disease, and anticipated survival time must be considered, in addition to the ability of the pathologic fracture to heal. Adaptations in the treatment of pathologic fractures must be made on an individual basis.

Patient Survival

Many patients have short life expectancies after pathologic fracture. Survival time is difficult to predict; therefore short-term function and pain management should be emphasized. It is unreasonable to undertake procedures that require significant recovery times or lengthy weightbearing restrictions in patients with advanced disease. However, if a patient has limited disease with a more favorable prognosis, efforts at healing, reconstruction, or both are warranted.

Location of Pathologic Fracture

The location of a pathologic fracture is also important when one is deciding on a treatment strategy. In general, most epiphyseal and many metaphyseal lesions are treated with excision and prosthetic replacement. Pathologic femoral neck fractures almost never heal[2] and are therefore excellent candidates for prosthetic replacement. Humeral diaphyseal fractures have shown good healing rates[33] and generally undergo fixation.

Pathologic fractures of the upper extremities are more amenable to nonoperative treatment with external immobilization than are fractures of the lower extremities. Upper extremities can be shielded from normal physiologic loadings with less functional debilitation than the lower extremities. Because the upper extremities are not needed for weightbearing, forces generated in their long bones are less than in those of the lower extremities. The risk of fracture failure in the upper extremities also is less than in the lower extremities.[34]

Lesion Size

Treatment options for pathologic fractures are affected by the size of the surrounding metastatic lesion. Fixating a pathologic fracture that has occurred in an area of extensive bone destruction would cause the fixation device to take on much of the limb load, resulting in a greater likelihood of fixation failure. Rather, large osteolytic defects need to be excised and replaced with allograft or polymethylmethacrylate (PMMA). These large lesions are unlikely to heal, so rigid fixation that is able to withstand high limb loads is often selected. Alternatively, prosthetic replacement can be considered.

Fracture Healing

The healing ability of fractures caused by metastatic disease varies and must therefore be considered when choosing a method of treatment. The bone in the area of the fracture is already undergoing a primary pathologic process, which alters its healing potential. Often radiation or systemic chemotherapy, which is further detrimental to fracture healing, is added to the treatment plan. Several authors have recommended that radiation doses of less than 30 Gy will minimize the impairment of fracture healing but will still have an impact on most tumors.[35,36] Gainor and Burnhert[37] found that pathologic fractures due to multiple myeloma had a 6-month healing rate of 67%, compared with a 0% healing rate in fractures due to lung cancer. They also noted that internal fixation and a life expectancy of >6 months were associated with an increased healing rate.

With expectations for fracture healing downgraded, implants that stabilize pathologic fractures may be required to bear physiologic loads for a prolonged period. The strength and fatigue properties of the bone-implant construct are then important. A common treatment complication of a pathologic fracture is a fixation failure of the implant hardware and of its connection to the bone. This is more common in the lower extremities because of increased loads on the implants. Fixation failures in the lower extremities also can increase with increased survival time.[34] Treatment decisions can limit the failures to some degree. With this discussion as a backdrop, a review follows on the pertinent biomechanical information on fracture fixation and its adaptation to fractures caused by skeletal metastases.

BIOMATERIALS OF PATHOLOGIC FRACTURE FIXATION

Stainless steel and titanium alloys are the biomaterials used for the majority of fixation implants. Stainless steel, cobalt-chrome-molybdenum alloys, and titanium alloy are used for prosthetic devices. PMMA is often used in pathologic fractures to secure prosthetic devices, enhance the bone-implant interface, or fill a void caused by a pathologic lesion. The most common stainless steel alloy used for fixation devices is 316L, which consists primarily of iron (58%), chromium (17% to 20%), and nickel (13% to 16%). Small amounts of carbon (which can increase strength), molybdenum (which decreases corrosion and hardens the alloy), and other elements are also present. The strength of stainless steel can be greatly altered by the method of manufacturing. It is a popular material because the base materials are relatively inexpensive and can be manufactured in a way to achieve optimal mechanical qualities.[38-40]

Titanium used in the manufacturing of fixation devices either is pure (>99%) or is part of an alloy with 6% aluminum, 4% vanadium, and traces of other elements. Titanium is relatively resistant to corrosion and biologically inert in comparison with most other metals. In general the modulus (or material stiffness) of titanium and its alloys is half that of stainless steel, but the failure stress and fatigue stress compare favorably (Table 40-1).[38-40] Because the implants are less stiff, they have a theoretical advantage in sharing loads with the bone and may thereby improve the biomechanical environment for healing.

Patients with impending or pathologic fractures in weightbearing long bones who are expected to survive at least 3 months are candidates for surgical

Table 40-1   Typical properties of materials associated with metastatic fracture (or impending fracture) fixation*

Material	Modulus (GPa)	Poisson's ratio	Failure stress (MPa)	Fatigue stress (MPa at 10^6)
Stainless steel (316L)	193	0.30	480-1,300	240-700
Titanium alloy (Ti-6A1-4V)	110	0.32	800-1,500	350-600
Cobalt-chrome-molybdenum alloy (Co-Cr-Mo)	220	0.30	800-1,000	310-950
PMMA	2-3	0.35	25-40 (tension) 90-100 (compression)	14
Cortical bone	10-20	0.39	51-133 (tension) 33-195 (compression)	60-100
Cancellous bone (porous structure)	0.5-1.5	0.32	3-10 (compression)	
PMMA-bone interface			7-10 (tension) 2-4 (shear)	0.06
PMMA-metal interface			5-10 (tension) 5-8 (shear)	2
UHMWPE	1			
Fiberous tissue	0.001			

PMMA, polymethylmethacrylate; UHMWPE, ultrahigh molecular weight polyethylene.
*Variations in failure stress and fatigue stress for metals arise from how the material was formed (e.g., cast, cold worked, hot forged), the surface condition, surface treatment, and other factors.

stabilization. Such stabilization can relieve pain, reduce nursing care, restore reasonable mobility, and minimize hospitalization costs. In some cases, however, there is so much bone destruction that secure internal fixation is not possible by conventional methods. In such cases, diseased bone is resected. Bone cement (PMMA) is then used with fixation devices or prostheses to fill in areas of resected bone. The stiffness and strength of PMMA are similar to those of cortical bone, and, like cortical bone, PMMA is particularly well suited to bearing compressive loads. The weakest link in the PMMA-augmented construct, however, is its adhesion to bone and metal. If patients are likely to survive a longer time after fixation, the fatigue strength of PMMA can be a concern (see Table 40-1). In a biomechanical study simulating metastatic fracture fixation in the femoral diaphysis, PMMA-augmented nails consistently failed during torsional loading at the bone-PMMA interface and therefore were much weaker than double-plated fixation systems.[41] The degree to which the PMMA interfaces must bear tension or shearing loads in fracture fixation is a limiting factor in the structural integrity of PMMA constructs. Pugh et al.[42] recommend choosing devices that maximize the PMMA-metal interface. These concerns are mild, however, because the adjunctive use of PMMA has been successful in the management of metastatic fractures. Harrington et al.[26] reported on a large series of patients who required PMMA to supplement the internal fixation of their fractures. The ability to walk was regained by 94% of 323 patients who were ambulatory before fracture. In addition, 84% reported excellent or good pain relief. Sim et al.[25] also reported success with the adjunctive use of PMMA. Their series included 35 metastatic fractures and 16 imminent fractures. They reported good pain relief and good functional improvement in 75%.

PROSTHETIC REPLACEMENT

In the geriatric population, prosthetic replacement is commonly used for treatment of nonpathologic displaced fractures of the femoral neck and is occasionally used for comminuted nonpathologic fractures of the proximal humerus or the humeral head and neck. Prosthetic replacement has gained favor over open reduction and internal fixation (ORIF) because the results are more predictable.

The nonunion, avascular necrosis, and fixation failures sometimes associated with ORIF are generally avoided by using prosthetic replacement.

These general principles of prosthetic replacement have been expanded and applied to patients with pathologic fractures in periarticular locations. As in geriatric nonpathologic fractures, prosthetic replacement is a common form of treatment for pathologic fractures in the proximal portions of the femur and humerus.[34] Because of the significant bone loss and poor surrounding bone quality associated with pathologic fractures, ORIF is a less attractive treatment option. Prosthetic replacement eliminates the need to achieve fracture healing and often allows early, unrestricted use of the limb as well as a decrease in pain.

Once the lesion and pathologic fracture are excised, the prosthesis must be coupled to the remaining bone. This can be accomplished with an interference fit, a bioingrowth implant, or the use of bone cement. Coupling the implant to bone with cement is most common in the treatment of pathologic fractures. The bone cement provides excellent stability and allows immediate weightbearing.

All pathologic femoral head and neck fractures can be treated with standard cemented hemiarthroplasties. If other foci of metastatic disease in the femoral diaphysis are a concern, a long-stemmed component should be considered (Fig. 40-2). The tip of the prosthetic stem should bypass any distal metastatic foci. Prosthetic replacement for intertrochanteric and selected subtrochanteric pathologic fractures may require a calcar-replacing prosthesis with large cement mantles to fill bone defects.

When loss or involvement of the proximal portion of the femur is extensive, a replacement can be considered (Fig. 40-3). A large area of the proximal portion of the femur must be excised and the prosthesis fixed into the remaining femur with cement. Custom implants can be used in a similar manner to replace the distal portion of the femur (Fig. 40-4).

Prosthetic replacements are also indicated in the treatment of pathologic fractures of the proximal portion of the humerus. Again, the diseased bone must be completely removed and the proximal portion of the humerus replaced with a prosthetic device.

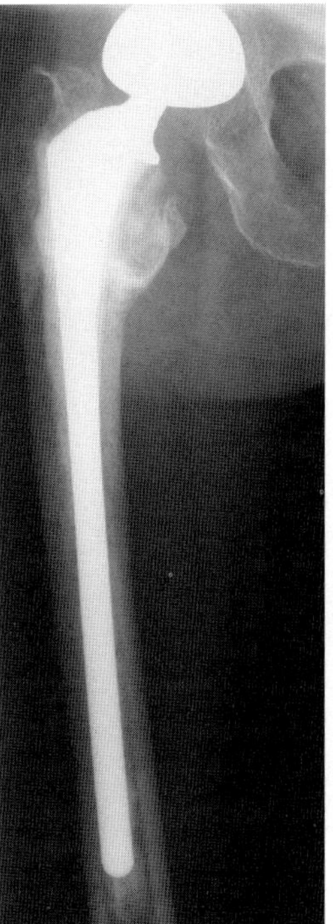

Fig. 40-2   Anteroposterior radiograph of a long-stemmed bipolar hemiarthroplasty for a pathologic fracture of the proximal portion of the femur. The patient had carcinoma of the prostate. Extension of the stem well into the femur will protect other areas of metastatic involvement.

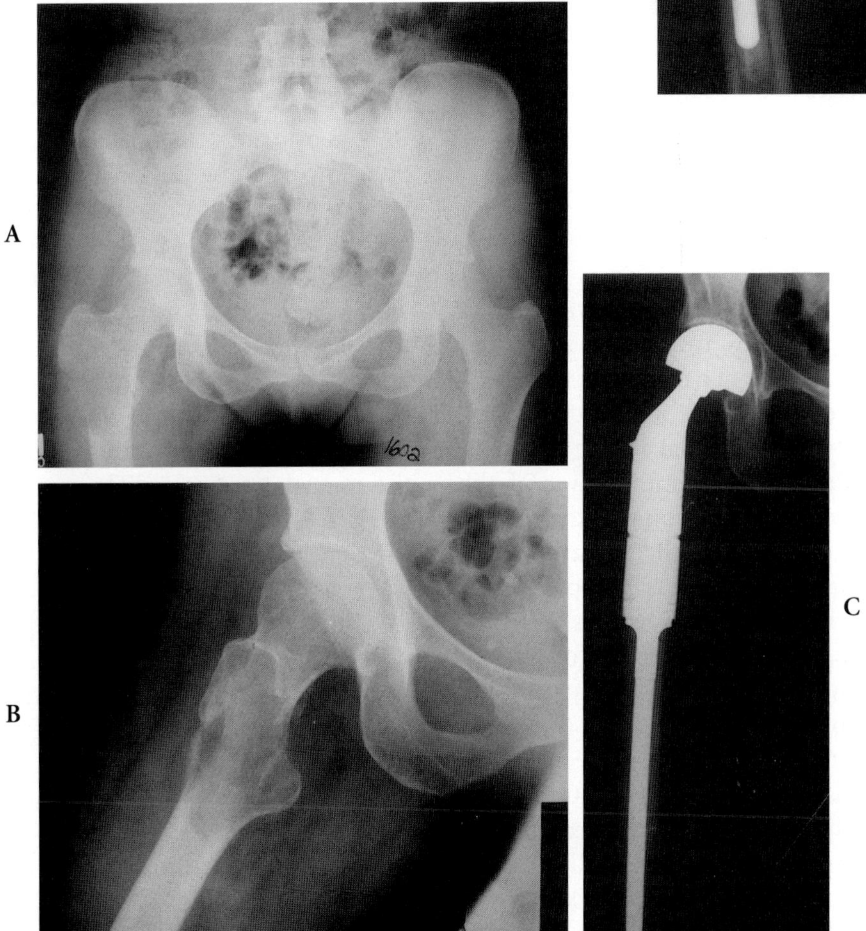

Fig. 40-3   **A** and **B,** Anteroposterior and lateral x-ray films, revealing extensive bony destruction of the proximal portion of the femur. **C,** Patient was treated surgically with excision and prosthetic replacement of the entire proximal third of the femur. (From Edgerton BC, An KN, Morrey BF. Torsion strength reduction due to cortical defects in bone. J Orthop Res 8:851-855, 1990.)

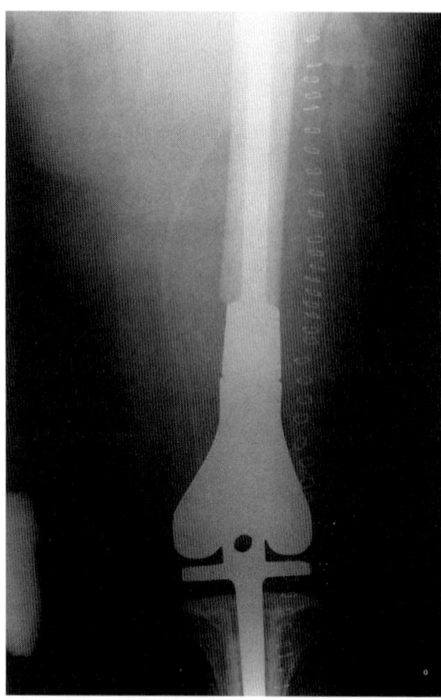

Fig. 40-4 Extensive involvement of the distal portion of the femur was managed with excision and a custom replacement.

FRACTURE FIXATION
Plate Fixation

Plates are attached to the bone surface with screws or, occasionally, with cables around the bone and plate. The bending stiffness of a plate (i.e., the transverse force required to produce a unit of angular bending) is linearly proportional to the width of the plate, proportional to the third power of the thickness, and inversely proportional to the second power of the unsupported length.[41] Fixation with plates generally produces more rigid constructs than fixation with intramedullary splints and thus promotes healing by primary bone formation. When bone-to-bone contact exists at a fracture site, the plate is able to share the load with the bone. When no bone contact exists, the plate bears the entire load, which is an undesirable situation.[43]

Plates commonly used for fracture fixation are available in stainless steel and titanium alloy. Stainless steel has a long track record and has many compatible implants, including cables and screws. Titanium alloy has the potential advantage of increased biocompatibility, favorable fatigue properties, and a stiffness that is closer to that of bone. When the two materials are compared, stainless steel plates are similar in strength and fatigue

strength but are noticeably stiffer[44] (see Table 40-1). Design features have been added to decrease the amount of cortical contact with the plate and more uniformly distribute the amount of material along the entire length of the plate. Thus the plate is easier to contour but does not have added strength or improved rigidity. A so-called low-contact plate, which decreases necrosis beneath the bone and the plate, may further the long-term function of the bone. The low-contact feature is less important in this patient population, in whom fixation is of primary importance and healing is problematic.

Dynamic compression plates come in a variety of sizes—large, small, and mini—and are coupled with 6.5/4.5 mm, 4.0/3.5 mm, and 2.7 mm screws. Tubular plates, which are much thinner and weaker, are also available in three sizes. Specialty plates are available for metaphyseal fixation and are generally coupled with the 4.5 mm screws (Fig. 40-5).

Plates can function to compress, neutralize, buttress, or bridge. They have relatively good resistance to torsion and tension but are relatively poor at handling compression. Plates are designed to compress the fracture surfaces together to enhance stability, although this goal is often not possible with metastatic lesions. Many fixation failures that occur with screw-plate constructs are at the screw-bone interface and not in the plate itself.[43] This type of failure is of considerable concern in pathologic fractures because of the underlying incidence of senile osteoporosis and alteration of the bone due to the metastatic disease. The use of PMMA to augment a fracture site and to stabilize the screws in the bone has been shown to be beneficial[26] (Fig. 40-6). A potential limitation of a plate, however, is that in a long bone the pathologic process can extend beyond the plate's boundaries, causing a second fracture distal from or proximal to the plate. A stress riser effect at the end of the plate can also contribute to a second fracture.

Intramedullary Nails

Intramedullary nailing devices have been used extensively for acute femoral, tibial, and, increasingly, in humeral fracture fixation. They are generally considered internal splints that provide relative stability. All modern femoral and tibial, and most humeral, nailing systems have interlocking capabilities with proximal and distal locking nails. The locking nails couple the implant to the bone, main-

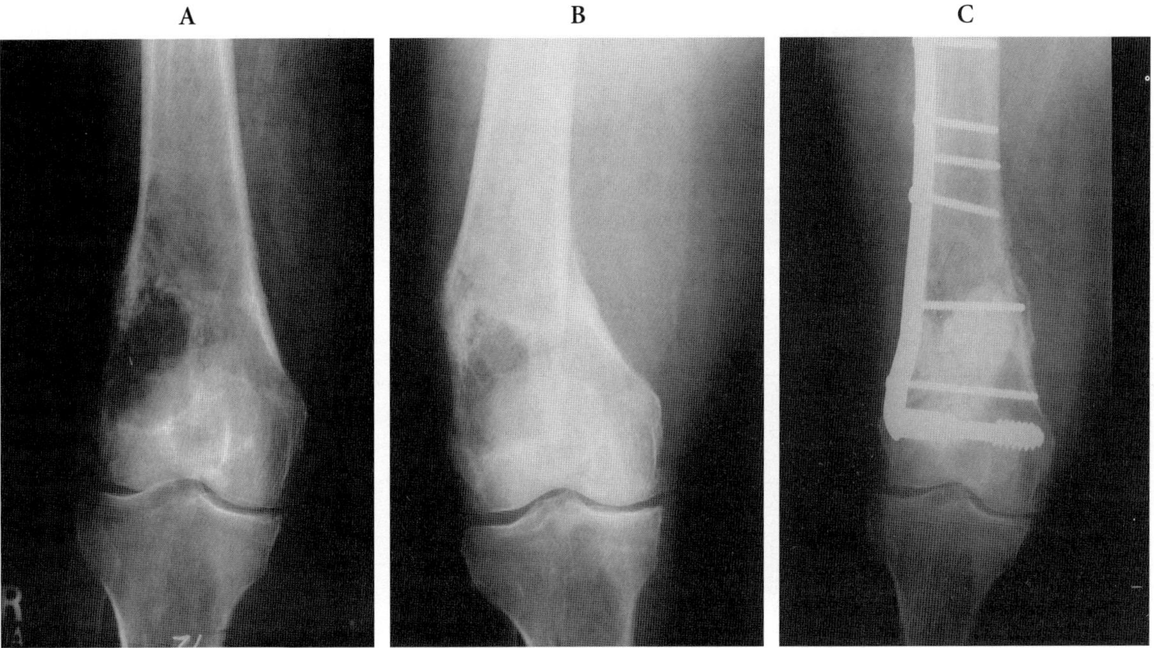

Fig. 40-5   Distal femoral metaphyseal lesion caused by multiple myeloma, **A,** that went on to fracture, **B.** The fracture was stabilized with a fixed-angle device (95-degree dynamic condylar screw) and PMMA augmentation, **C.**

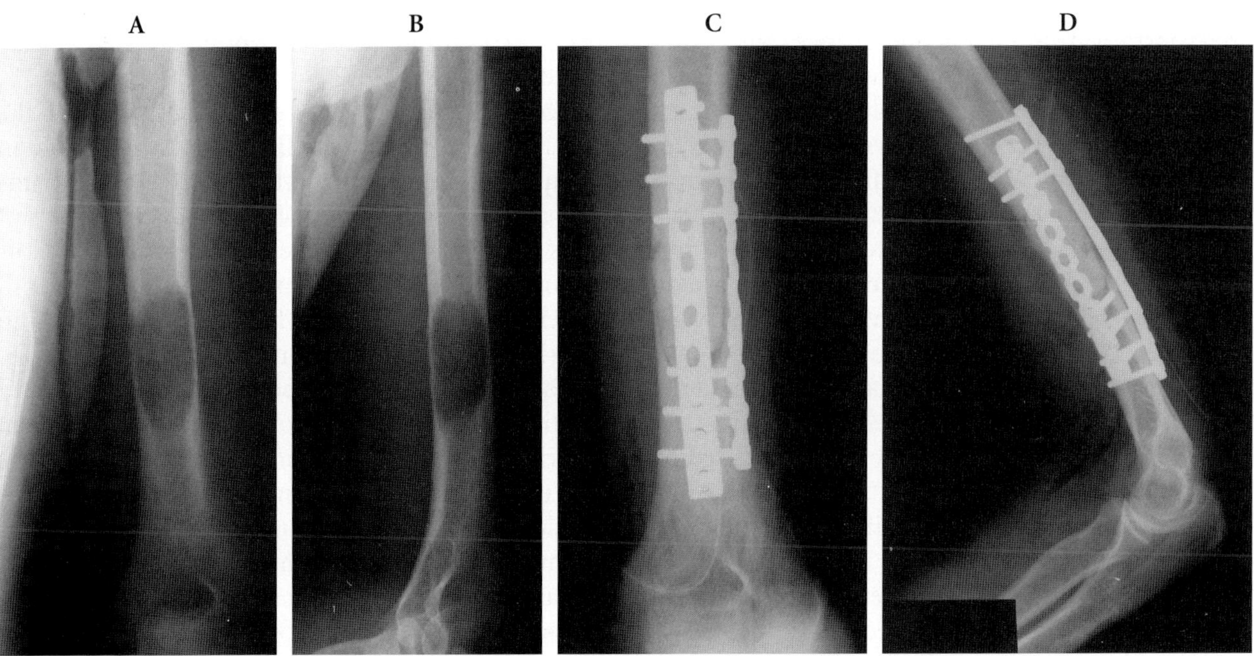

Fig. 40-6   Anteroposterior (**A**) and lateral (**B**) x-ray films showing a lytic lesion of the distal third of the humerus. Anteroposterior (**C**) and lateral (**D**) x-ray films showing fixation achieved with methylmethacrylate and two plates at 90-degree angles to one another. One plate was a 3.5 mm reconstruction plate, and the other was a 3.5 mm dynamic compression plate.

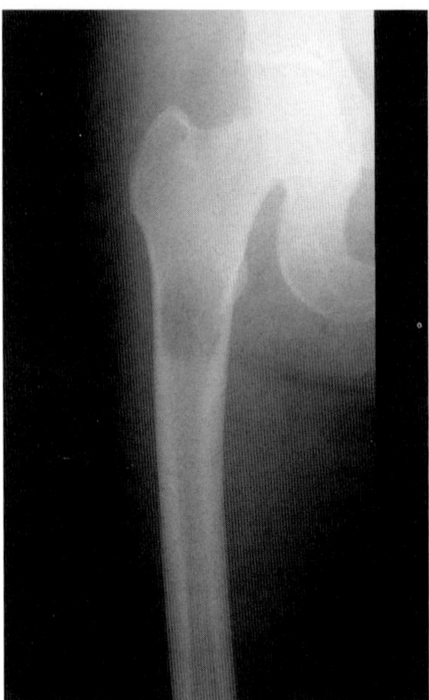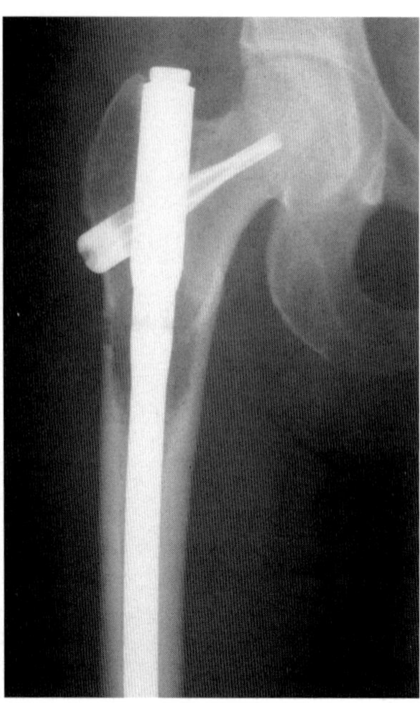

A

B

Fig. 40-7   A, Lytic subtrochanteric lesion. Prophylactic fixation was performed with an intramedullary nail with a proximal spiral blade. **B,** Distal interlocking screws were also used.

taining length in axially unstable fractures and contributing to the torsional stiffness of the bone-implant construct (Fig. 40-7).

Nail Properties

The mechanical properties of intramedullary nails are determined by their material, size, and cross-sectional design. Intramedullary nails are made of stainless steel or a titanium alloy, both of which appear to have acceptable physical properties to meet their structural demands. Intramedullary nail length varies, but generally nails run the entire length of the diaphysis of the femur, tibia, or humerus. Nail diameter has a significant influence on the strength and rigidity of an implant. Bending and torsional stiffness increase by the fourth power of the intramedullary device's radius, provided the wall thickness remains the same.[45] Larger-diameter nails therefore have significantly increased bending stiffness and lower stresses and hence better resistance to fatigue failure. As with plates, bending stiffness as previously defined diminishes by the second power of the unsupported length. Torsional stiffness (i.e., the torque required to produce a unit rotation) is inversely proportional to the unsupported length.

Cross-sectional designs are variable. Most devices are hollow and have variable wall thickness. Smaller-diameter nails tend to have an increased wall thickness for maintenance of minimal requirements of strength and resistance to mechanical failure. Some nails are solid and can be thought of as having a wall thickness equivalent to the radius of the nail. Cross-sectional geometries range from cylindric to triangular to I-beam configurations; in addition, Küntscher popularized a cloverleaf design (Table 40-2).

The presence of a slot down the length of the nail reduces torsional rigidity as much as 40-fold in comparison with a nonslotted nail of similar diameter and wall thickness.[45] The presence of the slot does not significantly affect bending rigidity. Slotted nails, however, are often designed to be less stiff, which may be of benefit when they are placed into long intact segments of bone.

Together, a nail and bone can be thought of as a fixation construct. The "working length" of the nail is defined as the unsupported length between the two contact points of the implant bone construct.[46] A relatively long working length will be more flexible and will also result in more bending stress over the unsupported segment of the nail. In a short transverse fracture with good bone apposition between the rod and the bone, the working length will be short and the construct more rigid. Working length is less critical in torsion, where compliance increases only linearly with increasing working length.

Table 40-2   Description of femoral nails

Femoral nail	Material	Radius of curvature (m)	Cross-sectional design	Second generation (reconstruction nails)
Synthes Universal	Stainless steel	1.5	◗	No
Grosse Kempf	Stainless steel	3	◖	No
Russell Taylor	Stainless steel	2	◯	Yes
ZMS	Stainless steel	2.74	⬒	Yes
Alta	Titanium alloy	1.8	⬡	Yes
UniFlex	Titanium alloy	2.3	◯	Yes
Synthes titanium	Titanium alloy	1.5	●	Yes

Femoral Nails

Femoral interlocking nails range from the slotted, more flexible older designs made of stainless steel (Grosse Kempf and Synthes Universal) to the unslotted, stiffer modern designs made of either stainless steel (Russell Taylor) or titanium (Alta, Synthes). The radius of curvature of a nail also varies, from relatively straight (Grosse Kempf, 3 m radius of curvature) to relatively curved (Synthes, 1.5 m radius of curvature). The relative shape and flexibility of the nail have implications when nails are used in long segments of intact bone. For example, when a subtrochanteric lesion is stabilized or a nail is used prophylactically for an impending fracture in the femoral diaphysis, a relative mismatch between the radius of curvature of the human femur (1.1 m)[47] and that of the nail could cause severe difficulties with insertion and potential iatrogenic complications. These difficulties are more likely when stiff, relatively straight nails are used. To lessen this risk, most manufacturers recommend overreaming the canal by 1.5 to 2 mm before inserting the nail into a long segment of intact bone.[48,49]

All available femoral nailing systems interlock the bone to the proximal and distal ends of the nail. Standard proximal interlocking systems have screws placed in the subtrochanteric area either obliquely (proximal to distal) or transversely. "Second generation" interlocking nails (also termed reconstruction nails) have proximal interlocking devices that go into the head and neck of the proximal portion of the femur. These nails tend to have more fatigue resistance and more strength built into their proximal section than their more distal sections.[50] Again, the choice of nails has implications when lesions or fractures are stabilized in the subtrochanteric area, which is subject to high bending loads.

Femoral nails are generally inserted in an antegrade fashion through the piriformis fossa, although retrograde insertion through the knee joint is gaining some interest.[51] Coupling the implant to the bone is generally done with locking screws, both proximally and distally, and at times can be augmented with PMMA. Bone cement enhances stability by improving the coupling of the nail to the bone; it is also used to fill osteolytic bone defects. However, despite an ability to enhance fixation, PMMA may have some deleterious effects on the healing of a pathologic fracture.

Comparison of Plates and Nails

Intramedullary devices provide relative stability, whereas compression plates provide absolute stability. Intramedullary devices help maintain length and alignment and can be inserted without exposing the fracture. They allow moderate interfragmentary motion, which promotes fracture healing by secondary bone formation. Use of compression plates, on the other hand, often requires direct exposure of the fracture site, which can have a negative effect on healing. Compression plates provide more rigid stability at the fracture site, which promotes healing by primary bone formation.

Plates are fastened to the exterior of a bone, and nails are inserted into the central portion of the bone. With nails, the entire length of the bone is supported, whereas with a plate a limited portion of the bone is supported. Central placement of the nail allows it to resist bending forces in all directions. In some diaphyseal osteotomy models, intramedullary nails resist bending better than plates, but torsion rigidity is greater with a plate.[52] Stiffness, however, is not as great a concern as failure strength and fatigue strength of the construct.

CONCLUSION

Managing pathologic fractures from metastatic disease and predicting fracture risk from bone metastases are challenging. A firm understanding of the pertinent biomechanical considerations for treatment will aid the physician in decision making. Many factors, such as the type of primary malignancy, the degree of metastatic disease, the patient's expected survival time, and the fracture's ability to heal, must be considered before deciding on a treatment plan. Treatment is intended to provide immediate stability and to last the lifetime of the patient.

Many of the concepts, implants, and techniques commonly used to treat nonpathologic fractures are adapted to treat pathologic fractures; however, there are unique technical problems associated with pathologic fractures. PMMA, for example, is frequently used to augment hardware fixation and to fill osteolytic defects. Pain relief and preservation of function remain the primary goals of treatment and ones that are usually achieved. Careful selection of treatment can limit, but not eliminate, complications such as fixation failure, progression of disease, and loss of limb.

REFERENCES

1. Aaron AD. Treatment of metastatic adenocarcinoma of the pelvis and the extremities. J Bone Joint Surg Am 79:917-932, 1997.
2. Harrington KD. Orthopedic surgical management of skeletal complications of malignancy. Cancer 80(Suppl 8):1614-1627, 1997.
3. Coleman RE. Skeletal complications of malignancy. Cancer 80(Suppl 8):1588-1594, 1997.
4. Hipp JA, Springfield DS, Hayes WC. Predicting pathologic fracture risk in the management of metastatic bone defects. Clin Orthop 312:120-135, 1995.
5. Perez CA, Bradfield JS, Morgan HC. Management of pathological fractures. Cancer 29:684-693, 1972.
6. Clark CR, Morgan C, Sonstegard DA, Mathews LS. The effects of biopsy-hole shape and size on bone strength. J Bone Joint Surg Am 59:213-217, 1997.
7. Edgerton BC, Ank N, Morrey BF. Torsion strength reduction due to cortical defects in bone. J Orthop Res 8:851-855, 1990.
8. Hipp JA, McBroom RJ, Cheal EJ, Hayes WC. Structural consequences of endosteal metastatic lesions in long bones. J Orthop Res 7:828-837, 1989.
9. Hipp JA, Edgerton BC, An KN, Hayes WC. Structural consequences of transcortical holes in long bones loaded in torsion. J Biomech 23:1261-1268, 1990.
10. McBroom RJ, Cheal EJ, Hayes WC. Strength reduction from metastatic cortical defects in long bones. J Orthop Res 6:369-378, 1988.
11. Clark CR, Morgan C, Sonstegard DA, Matthews LS. The effect of biopsy-hole shape and size on bone strength. J Bone Joint Surg Am 59:213-217, 1977.
12. Chao EYS, Sim FH, Shives TC, Pritchard DJ. Management of pathologic fracture: Biomechanical considerations. In Sim FH, ed. Diagnosis and Management of Metastatic Bone Disease. New York: Raven Press, 1988, pp 171-181.
13. Frankel VH, Burstein AH. Load capacity of tubular bone. In Kenedi RM, ed. Biomechanics and Related Bio-Engineering Topics. Oxford: Pergamon Press, 1965, pp 381-396.
14. Hipp JA, Edgerton BC, An KN, Hayes WC. Structural consequences of transcortical holes in long bones loaded in torsion. J Biomech 23:1261-1268, 1990.
15. Brooks DB, Burstein AH, Frankel VH. The biomechanics of torsional fractures. J Bone Joint Surg Am 52:507-514, 1970.
16. McBroom RJ, Cheal EJ, Hayes WC. Strength reductions from metastatic cortical defects in long bones. J Orthop Res 6:369-378, 1988.
17. Hipp JA, McBroom RJ, Cheal EJ, Hayes WC. Structural consequences of endosteal metastatic lesions in long bones. J Orthop Res 7:828-837, 1989.
18. Hipp JA, Rosenberg AE, Hayes WC. Mechanical properties of trabecular bone within and adjacent to osseous metastases. J Bone Miner Res 7:1165-1171, 1992.

19. Tong D, Gillick L, Hendrickson FR. The palliation of symptomatic osseous metastases: Final results of the study by the Radiation Therapy Oncology Group. Cancer 50:893-899, 1982.

20. Galasko CS. The detection of skeletal metastases from mammary cancer by gamma camera scintigraphy. Br J Surg 56:757-764, 1969.

21. Hipp JA, Springfield DS, Hayes WC. Predicting pathologic fracture risk in the management of metastatic bone defects. Clin Orthop 312:120-135, 1995.

22. Hipp JA, Katz G, Hayes WC. Local demineralization as a model for bone strength reductions in lytic transcortical metastatic lesions. Invest Radiol 26:934-938, 1991.

23. Cheal EJ, Hipp JA, Hayes WA. Evaluation of finite element analysis for prediction of the strength reduction due to metastatic lesion in the femoral neck. J Biomech 26:251-264, 1993.

24. Winchester DP, Sener SF, Khandekar JD, Oviedo MA, Cunningham MP, Caprini JA, Burkett FE, Scanlon EF. Symptomatology as an indicator of recurrent or metastatic breast cancer. Cancer 43:956-960, 1979.

25. Sim FH, Daugherty TW, Ivins JC. The adjunctive use of methylmethacrylate in fixation of pathological fractures. J Bone Joint Surg Am 56:40-48, 1974.

26. Harrington KD, Sim FH, Enis JE, Johnston JO, Dick HM, Gristina AG. Methylmethacrylate as an adjunct in internal fixation of pathological fractures: Experience with three hundred seventy-five cases. J Bone Joint Surg Am 58:1047-1055, 1976.

27. Beals RK, Lawton GD, Snell E. Prophylactic internal fixation of the femur in metastatic breast cancer. Cancer 28:1350-1354, 1971.

28. Parrish FF, Murray JA. Surgical treatment for secondary neoplastic fractures: A retrospective study of ninety-six patients. J Bone Joint Surg Am 52:665-686, 1970.

29. Fidler M. Incidence of fracture of metastases in long bones. Acta Orthop Scand 52:623-627, 1981.

30. Keene JS, Sellinger DS, McBeath AA, Engber WD. Metastatic breast cancer in the femur: A search for the lesion at risk of fracture. Clin Orthop 203:282-288, 1986.

31. Mirels H. Metastatic disease in long bones. Clin Orthop 249:256-264, 1989.

32. Springfield D, Jennings C. Pathological fracture. In Rockwood CA, Green DP, Bucholz RW, Heckman JD, eds. Fractures in Adults, 42nd ed. Philadelphia: Lippincott-Raven, 1996, pp 513-537.

33. Redmond BJ, Biermann JS, Blasier RB. Interlocking intramedullary nailing of pathologic fractures of the shaft of the humerus. J Bone Joint Surg Am 78:891-896, 1996.

34. Yazawa Y, Franssica FJ, Chao EYS, et al. Metastatic bone disease: A study of the surgical treatment of 166 pathologic humeral and femoral fractures. Clin Orthop Rel Res 251:213-219, 1990.

35. Bonarigo BC, Rubin P. Nonunion of pathologic fractures after radiation therapy. Radiology 88:889-898, 1967.

36. Douglas HO Jr, Shukla SK, Mindell E. Treatment of pathological fractures of long bones excluding those due to breast cancer. J Bone Joint Surg Am 58:1055-1061, 1976.

37. Gainor BJ, Burnhert P. Fracture healing in metastatic bone disease. Clin Orthop 178:297-302, 1983.

38. Tencer AF, Johnson KD. Basic concepts in biomechanics of fractures and fixation. In Biomechanics in Orthopedic Trauma. Philadelphia: JB Lippincott, 1994, pp 1-17.

39. Tencer AF, Johnson KD. Factors affecting the strength of bone. In Biomechanics in Orthopedic Trauma. Philadelphia: JB Lippincott, 1994, pp 18-32.

40. Tencer AF, Johnson KD. Biomaterials used in fracture fixation. In Biomechanics in Orthopedic Trauma. Philadelphia: JB Lippincott, 1994, pp 84-115.

41. Anderson JT, Erickson JM, Thompson RC, Chao EY. Pathologic femoral shaft fractures comparing fixation techniques using cement. Clin Orthop 131:273-278, 1978.

42. Pugh J, Sherry HS, Futterman B, Frankel VH. Biomechanics of pathologic fractures. Clin Orthop 169:109-114, 1982.

43. Tencer AF, Johnson KD. General biomechanical principles of some common fracture fixation devices. In Biomechanics in Orthopedic Trauma. Philadelphia: JB Lippincott, 1994, pp 118-157.

44. Disegi JA, Cesarone DM. Metallurgical properties of limited contact dynamic compression plates. In Harvey G Jr, Gaines RF, eds. Clinical and Laboratory Performance of Bone Plates. Philadelphia: American Society for Testing and Materials, 1994, pp 34-41.

45. Russell TA, Taylor JC, LaVelle DG, Beals ND, Brumfield DL, Durham AG. Mechanical characteristics of femoral interlocking intramedullary nailing systems. J Orthop Trauma 5:332-340, 1991.

46. Tencer AF, Johnson KD. Lower extremity fixation. In Biomechanics in Orthopedic Trauma. Philadelphia: JB Lippincott, 1994, pp 269-270.

47. Harper MC, Carson WL. Curvature of the femur and the proximal entry point for an IM nail. Clin Orthop 220:155-161, 1987.

48. Uniflex Femoral Nail Surgical Technique. Warsaw, Ind.: Biomet, 1992, p 8.

49. Russell TA, Taylor JC, LaVelle DG. Surgical technique. In The Smith & Nephew Richards Family of Reconstruction Interlocking Nails. Memphis: Smith & Nephew Richards, 1992, p 10.

50. Wilkey KD, Mehserle W. Mechanical characteristics of eight femoral intramedullary nailing systems. J Orthop Trauma 12:177-185, 1998.

51. Miller GJ, Vander Griend RA, Blake WP, Springfield DS. Performance evaluation of a cement-augmented intramedullary fixation system for pathologic lesions of the femoral shaft. Clin Orthop 221:246-254, 1987.

52. Henley MB, Monroe M, Tencer AF. Biomechanical comparison of method of fixation of a midshaft osteotomy of the humerus. J Orthop Trauma 5:14-20, 1991.

Failure of Fixation to the Pelvis and Extremities

Richard D. Lackman, M.D.

The treatment of pathologic fractures is one of the most challenging aspects of modern orthopedic surgery. These lesions involve many variables that are not encountered in the treatment of nonpathologic injuries. As such, many of these considerations can be easily overlooked by physicians who treat these problems infrequently. For a discussion of the issues associated with loss of fixation in pathologic fractures, some of the basic concepts of pathologic fracture treatment should be reviewed.

The treatment of pathologic fractures bears little resemblance to the treatment of ordinary posttraumatic injuries. Ordinary fractures are often amenable to closed treatment. Internal fixation, when used, is best when it results in a solid construct, but frequently, even less rigid fixation is adequate because fracture healing will augment the mechanical fixation of the device in time. Pathologic fractures, on the other hand, are much less forgiving. Closed treatment is rarely sufficient if the patient is to return to a high level of function. Internal fixation, when used, must provide rigid fixation so that the patient can use the part immediately. In the treatment of ordinary fractures it is frequently not essential that the patient use the extremity immediately because healing eventually will allow subsequent rehabilitation and return to function. Patients with pathologic fractures frequently have little time because of the prognosis associated with their malignant disease. As such, the only rationale for performing internal fixation in these patients is to plan for a construct that will allow immediate mobilization and use of the limb.

Healing is frequently irrelevant to the treatment of a pathologic fracture because many such fractures will never actually heal, and many patients will die before healing is completed. One must also consider, however, that many patients undergoing internal fixation for metastatic bone disease will live long and active lives. This is especially true for patients with metastatic tumors such as breast or renal cell carcinoma, who commonly survive 5 to 10 years or even longer after the diagnosis of bone metastasis. In these patients the rigidity and quality of internal fixation are especially important if later complications are to be avoided.

CLINICAL ANALYSIS

When asked to evaluate any patient with an actual or impending pathologic fracture, the orthopedic surgeon's first consideration should be to deal with the state of disease of the patient in question. The best source for this information is usually the oncologic "captain of the ship," typically the treating medical oncologist or radiation oncologist. The clinical information to be obtained from these sources includes the rapidity of progression of the patient's underlying malignancy, especially as it relates to major organ system involvement. Brain, lung, kidney, and liver metastases have the most bearing both on the patient's ability to undergo surgery and on the immediate prognosis. Further data regarding the patient's level of activity, nutritional status, other bone involvement or pain, and history of prior chemotherapy or radiation therapy are also essential elements in the decision-making process for the orthopedist considering surgical intervention.

The nutritional status of patients with pathologic fractures is probably one of the most overlooked elements in modern medicine. Orthopedic surgeons are frequently faced with patients who were minimal ambulators before a major fracture and who expect to return to their former level of function after internal fixation. A 2-week period of poor nutrition during preoperative and postoperative treatment can be enough to diminish muscle mass to such a critical level that the patient's return to previous functional status is not possible. Consultation with a nutrition support team is essential in these situations and will greatly facilitate the patient's welfare and return to preoperative function. The history of recent adjuvant treatments is also paramount in terms of considering the timing and appropriateness of surgical intervention. Patients with a pathologic fracture in close proximity to an expected white blood cell count or platelet count nadir cannot safely undergo surgery until after the period of greatest risk has passed. In terms of impending fractures, immobilization until marrow suppression diminishes may be necessary, whereas bed rest, traction, or both are occasionally still necessary for the patient with a major pathologic fracture of a lower extremity during this period of greatest marrow suppression. Radiation doses given to areas of metastatic bone involvement rarely exceed 45 cGy and typically are more likely to be in the range of 30 cGy. These radiation doses usually have no significant effect on wound healing and can be ignored in terms of surgical planning. Not infrequently, patients undergoing radiation for bone lesions will experience fracture either during or immediately after the course of radiation. Again, these treatments can be ignored in terms of surgical planning, and typically radiation therapy can be restarted within a few days of surgical treatment.

CLASSIFICATION OF PATHOLOGIC FRACTURES AND TYPES OF FIXATION

To understand the revision of failed internal fixation, the surgeon must have a clear concept of the types of mechanical constructs available and must understand their application to the various clinical situations that may be encountered.

Long Bone Diaphyseal Lesions With Good Bone Continuity

As typified in Fig. 41-1, *A*, long bone diaphyseal lesions are areas of tumor involvement that are large enough to create a mechanical problem in the cor-

tical bone of the diaphysis but not large enough to preclude bone continuity. With these lesions, as well as with all pathologic lesions, the surgeon must ask not whether to use cement but, rather, where to put the cement. In these cases there typically is no room for cement application, and either a simple intramedullary rod or an intramedullary rod with proximal and distal locking usually will suffice and provide enough support for immediate function (Fig. 41-1, *B*). Rarely will failure occur in these situations, and healing is typically the norm after appropriate tumoricidal treatment.

Patients who are predisposed to nonunion will have received high-dose radiation to an area that subsequently fractured. In such cases, little reparative potential remains in the bone, and so failure of stable fixation is not uncommon. Figure 41-2, *A*, shows a pathologic fracture of the femur that occurred 7 years after high-dose radiation therapy for a large soft tissue sarcoma of the thigh. Initial treatment with an intramedullary rod gave a satisfactory reduction (Fig. 41-2, *B*). With time, however, the fracture collapsed on itself (Fig. 41-2, *C*), requiring repeat fixation with a locked rod and bone graft substitute because there was no place to add bone cement (Fig. 41-2, *D* and *E*).

A 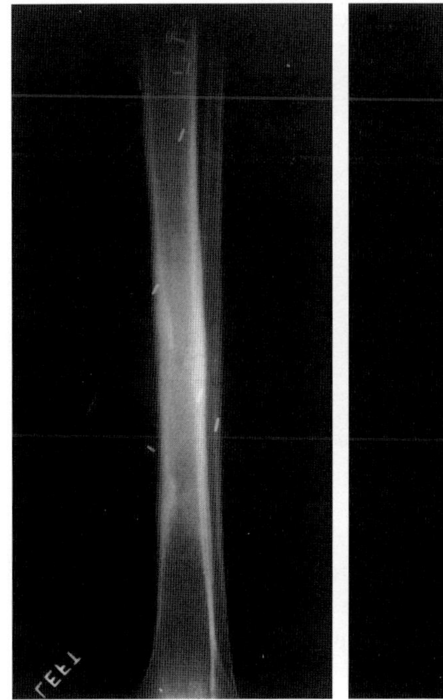 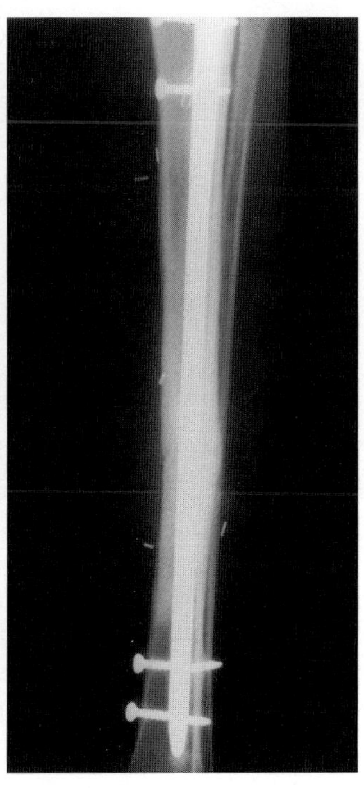 B

Fig. 41-1   A, Femoral shaft osteolytic lesion due to metastatic breast carcinoma; the patient had mechanical pain. **B,** Locked intramedullary rod is sufficient fixation if there is no loss of bone continuity.

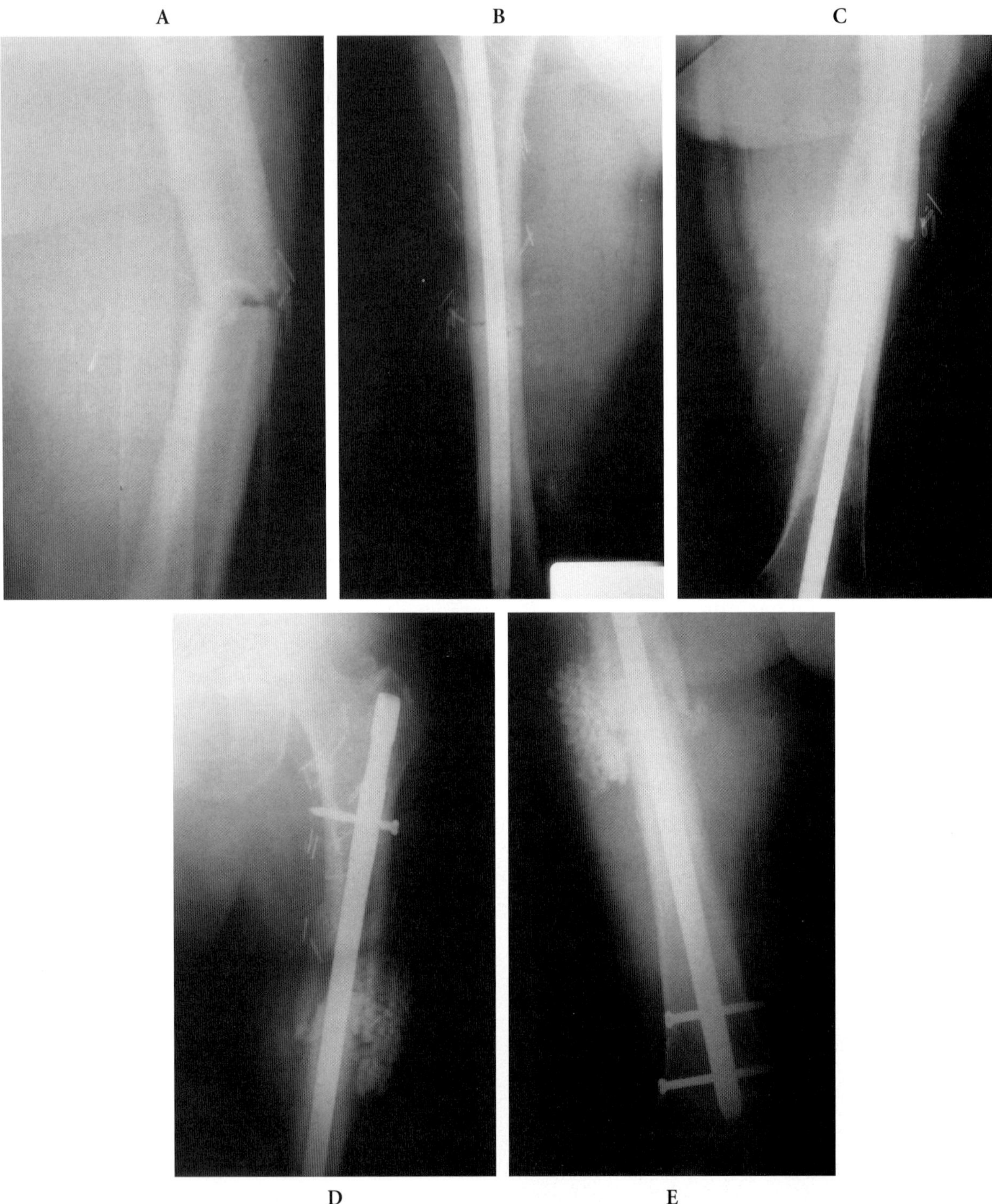

Fig. 41-2 **A,** Transverse femoral shaft fracture, which occurred several years after high-dose radiation therapy for a soft tissue sarcoma. **B,** Intramedullary nail yielded an anatomic reduction so that the fracture could impact on itself. **C,** Loss of reduction resulted as the fracture collapsed on itself. **D** and **E,** Repeat fixation was performed with a larger-diameter locked intramedullary nail and bone graft substitute.

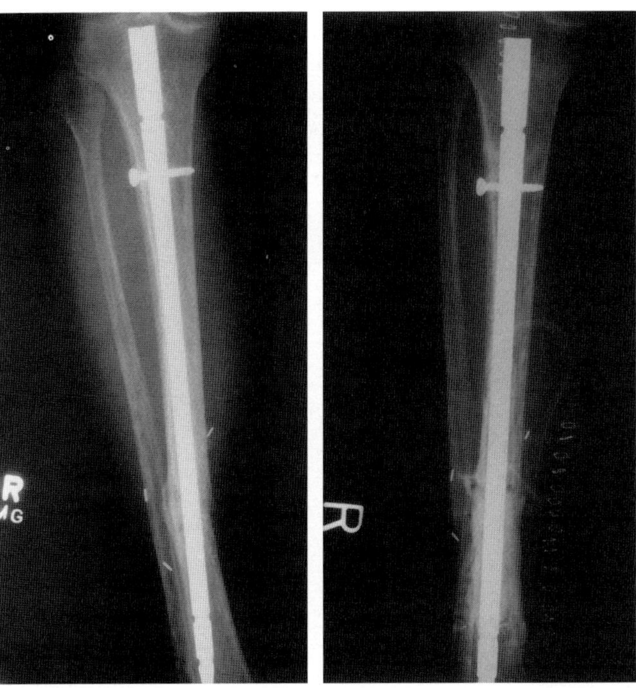

Fig. 41-3   **A,** Pathologic fracture of previously irradiated tibia. **B,** After failure of initial fixation, a stable reconstruction was accomplished by filling the distal fragment with bone cement.

Figure 41-3, *A,* shows a pathologic tibia fracture in previously irradiated bone. Despite adequate fixation the intramedullary rod eventually fractured because of prolonged but asymptomatic nonunion. The broken rod was removed, and a new rod was placed by means of cement augmentation in the distal fragment (Fig. 41-3, *B*).

Long Bone Diaphyseal Lesions With Poor Bone Continuity

Lesions such as those seen in Fig. 41-4, *A,* frequently are encountered with the more aggressive bone metastatic tumors such as those seen with metastasis from the lung or kidney. In these cases, application of an intramedullary rod, with or without locking, is not sufficient because the fixation will not allow weightbearing or return to function without pain. If the locking screws do provide enough immediate support to allow painless use of the limb, the screws will soon fail because they are not designed to bear the stresses of weightbearing for long periods. The essential aspect of fixation in these injuries is the application of bone cement to bridge the gap and restore weightbearing continuity along the length of the bone. This unweights the fixation device and provides solid mechanical stability so that weightbearing is comfortable. Because

bone cement is strong in compression, it can provide support for long periods, regardless of whether the fracture actually heals, if fixation is solid (Fig. 41-4, *B*). Figure 41-5, *A,* shows a pathologic fracture of the tibial shaft with some loss of cortical continuity. Seemingly adequate fixation failed (Fig. 41-5, *B*) because of chronic nonunion. This was then treated with repeat fixation and the application of bone cement to the nonunion site (Fig. 41-5, *C*).

Metaphyseal Fractures

For a metaphyseal lesion to be seen as an impending or actual fracture, it must usually be relatively large and involve osteolysis of the majority of the metaphyseal cancellous bone in the area in question. One must remember that the normal anatomy of long bones is such that in the metaphyseal region the cortex thins and weightbearing is transferred from the thick diaphyseal cortex to the abundant cancellous bone of the metaphysis. Internal fixation that augments the cortex of the metaphysis but ignores the medullary canal therefore is doomed to fail. Specifically, plate and screw constructs or intramedullary rods by themselves are typically poor options for the fixation of metastatic metaphyseal fractures. Again, the surgeon must ask

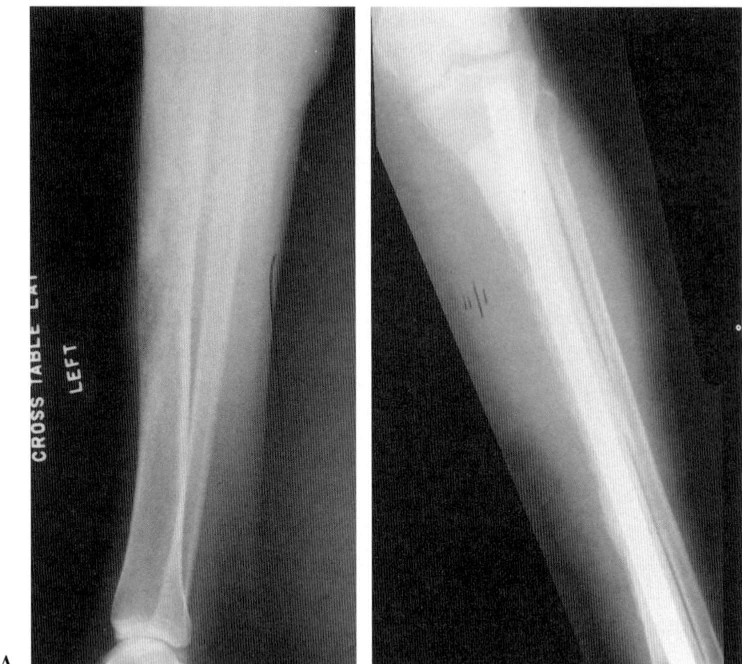

Fig. 41-4 **A,** Diaphyseal osteolytic lesion with loss of bone continuity. **B,** Solid fixation was achieved by augmenting the metallic device with bone cement to reestablish bone continuity.

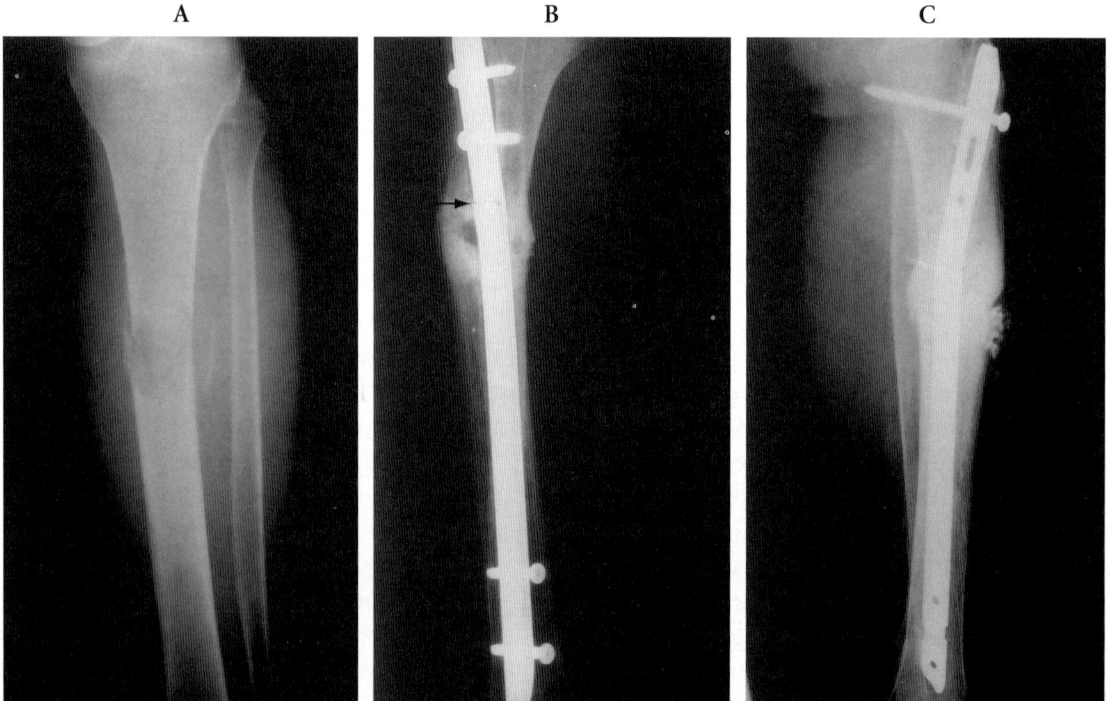

Fig. 41-5 **A,** Pathologic fracture of the tibia, with loss of cortical continuity through the fracture site. **B,** Internal fixation failed because it did not reestablish weightbearing continuity throughout the fracture site. **C,** Repeat fixation augmented with bone cement achieved a stable reconstruction.

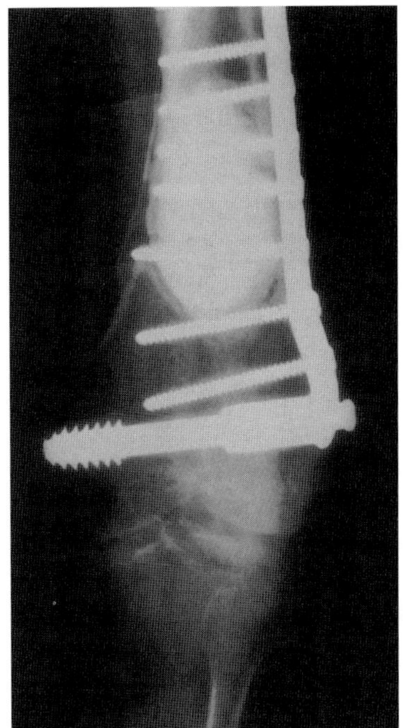

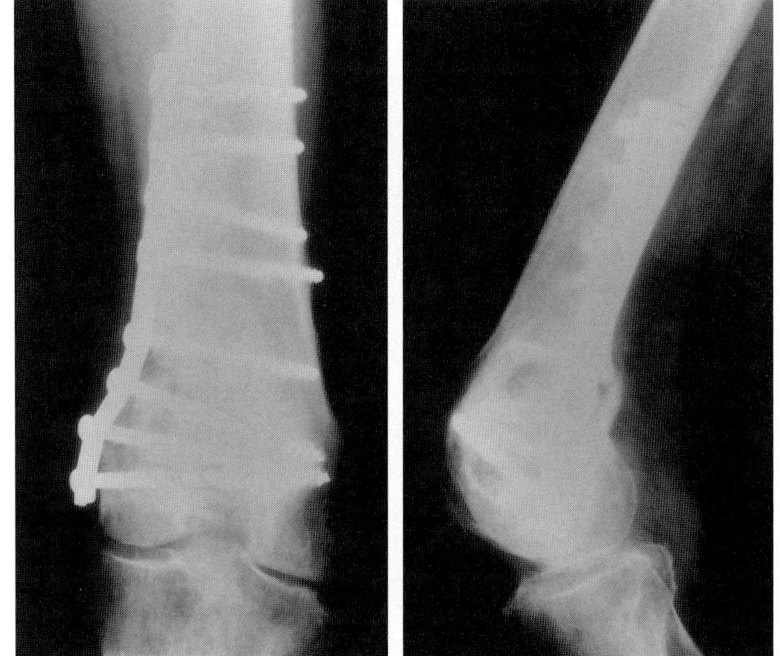

Fig. 41-6 Reconstruction of metaphyseal defects requires complete filling of the bone defect with bone cement before placement of the fixation device.

Fig. 41-7 Distal femoral intra-articular pathologic fracture treated with a side plate (**A**), which went on to nonunion and loss of fixation (**B**).

the critical question of where to put the cement. In cases such as that shown in Fig. 41-6, metallic fixation devices alone would be entirely inadequate, but when they are combined with bone cement to replace the weightbearing function of the destroyed metaphyseal medullary bone, a composite construct is formed that allows for effective weightbearing transfer along the length of the bone. Patients can easily detect when fixation is rigid and also when it is not. A lack of rigidity of internal fixation will cause mechanical pain, and the patient will be unable to return to acceptable levels of function.

Epiphyseal (Intra-articular) Fractures

Pathologic fractures that extend into the major joint surfaces are occasionally amenable to internal fixation but frequently require resection and segmental replacement prostheses. For example, it is difficult to restore the continuity and integrity of the distal portion of the femur or the proximal portion of the tibia when pathologic fractures have disrupted the articulating surfaces. Again, healing that would assist in convalescence from nonpathologic injuries may never occur in the context of pathologic fractures. In the absence of fracture healing, even fairly rigid initial fixation in the metaphyseal and epiphyseal bone typically will fail under the stresses of continued weightbearing.

Figure 41-7 shows a distal femoral intra-articular fracture treated with a side plate and screws in a patient given two courses of radiation and chemotherapy for a recurrent lymphoma. Nonunion of the intra-articular fragments led to the gradual onset of a valgus deformity and pain. Severe postradiation fibrosis precluded reoperation.

Occasionally these fractures can be treated with internal fixation and cement augmentation, such as one would do for metaphyseal fractures. This possibility assumes that there is still adequate bone to hold the fracture fragments together. Frequently, however, these attempts will fail and will require segmental resection and prosthetic replacement. In the treatment of pathologic fractures, it should always be the surgeon's desire to perform the last operation first. This is especially true in consideration of the limited survival time many of these patients have. It is less than desirable to have a patient with progressive metastatic cancer spend a significant portion of his or her remaining lifespan recovering from numerous surgical interventions, especially when a more effective early surgical procedure could have precluded the need for further surgeries and their associated periods of recuperation.

REASONS FOR FAILURE OF FIXATION
Inadequate Bone

In approaching internal fixation for pathologic fractures, a surgeon must ask first whether the bone is adequate to accept internal fixation. Some situations will not allow the return of weightbearing function after internal fixation, and some lesions may require a more aggressive initial surgical approach, such as resection and segmental prosthetic replacement or even amputation. Unfortunately these issues are often difficult to assess preoperatively. Even after careful preoperative planning, surprises can certainly occur when bone stock that appeared adequate on preoperative imaging is found to be of poor quality in the course of the operation. The most effective imaging studies for the purposes of preoperative assessment are x-ray films and computed tomography (CT). Although x-ray films do show bone detail, large areas of bone loss may be easily overlooked. CT scanning, on the other hand, clearly shows loss of both cortical and cancellous bone. Even the CT scan, however, cannot confirm the quality of bone in metaphyseal areas where the cortex is already typically thin. As an example, in the acetabulum the bone content may look dense and the integrity of the anterior, posterior, superior, and medial aspects may seem to be intact on CT scanning, but in reality the bone may be soft and of poor mechanical quality. Magnetic

resonance imaging (MRI) gives little information as to bone quality because bone is typically dark on all MRI scans, and assessment of the quantity and quality of bone is therefore difficult.

Figure 41-8, *A*, shows a radiograph of a patient with breast carcinoma metastatic to the acetabulum. At the time of presentation the acetabular bone stock was thought to be inadequate for reconstruction. As is frequently the case with breast cancer, the bone stock reappeared after radiation (Fig. 41-8, *B*). The patient was then able to undergo uneventful cemented total hip replacement.

In all cases of disease metastatic to bone that appears equivocal from the start in terms of the ability of the remaining bone to accept internal fixation, it is critical to have a plan to deal with the possible need for resection. The planning needed for such a contingency is complicated even in the relative calm of the physician's office. It is much more difficult in the context of an open wound and ongoing anesthesia. However, planning for contingencies on the basis of possible intraoperative findings will prevent the consternation associated with the surgeon's inability to handle unforeseen surgical problems.

Adequate Bone but Inadequate Fixation

Adequate bone but inadequate fixation is the most common scenario encountered in patients with failed fixation. The most common error in the original procedure usually relates to a lack of understanding of the differences between pathologic and nonpathologic fractures. Typically, again, this translates to a lack of cement application in situations in which bone cement would have elevated the quality of fixation from inadequate to adequate. Figure 41-9, *A*, shows a proximal humeral pathologic fracture fixed with a locked rod. The lack of bone continuity caused a failure of fixation (Fig. 41-9, *B*). This was treated with repeated intramedullary rodding, humeral shortening, and the application of bone cement in the gap to reestablish cortical continuity (Fig. 41-9, *C*).

Regarding the use of intramedullary rods, even in cases where the fixation would be adequate by nonpathologic standards, the lack of healing in pathologic situations frequently produces stresses on hardware and fracture fragments that would

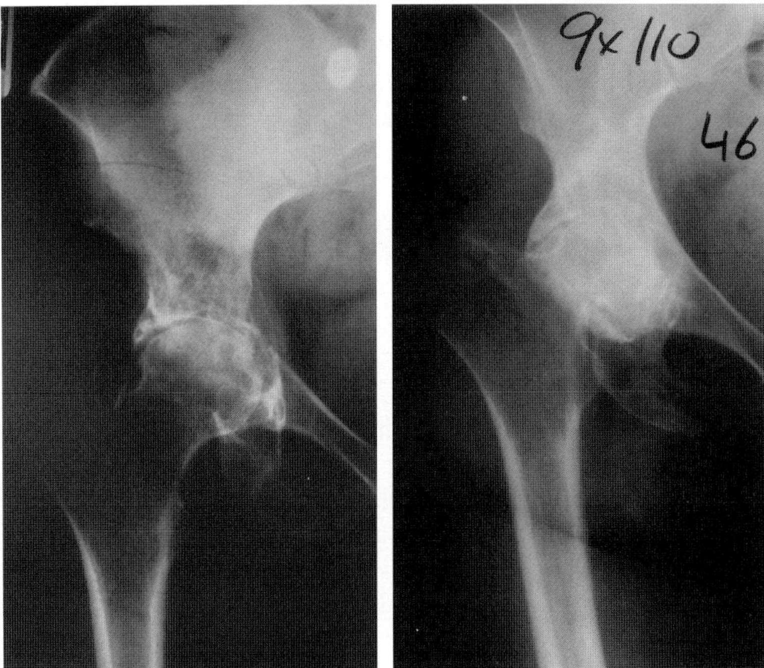

Fig. 41-8 **A,** Diffuse loss of acetabular bone due to metastatic breast carcinoma. **B,** After external beam radiation the acetabular bone stock reappeared.

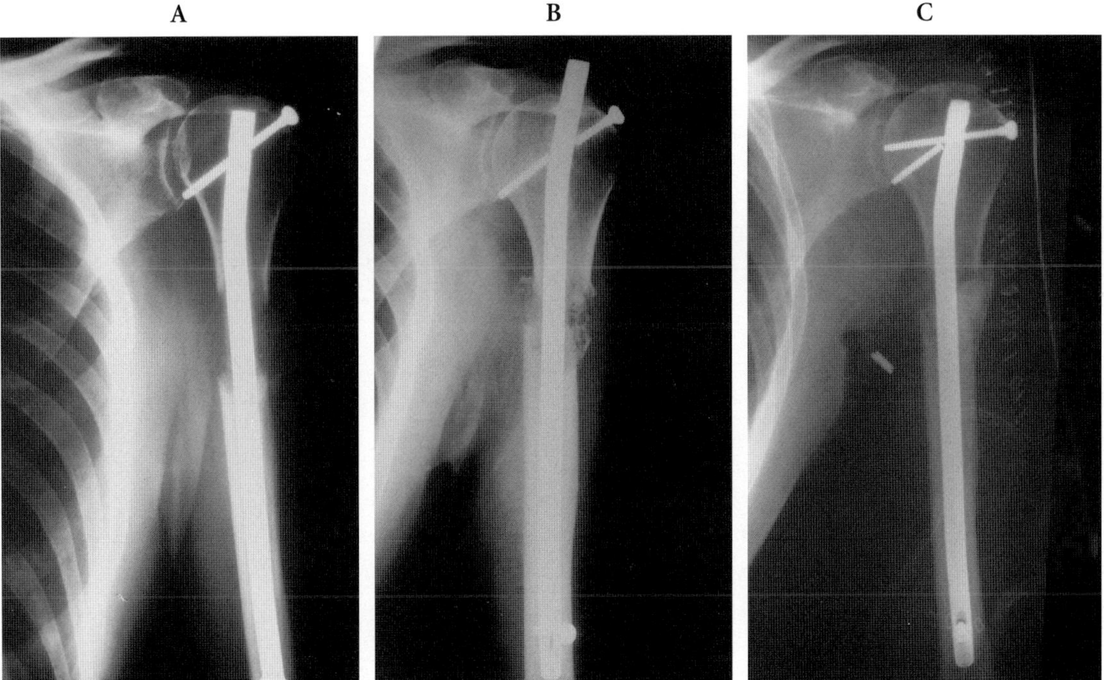

Fig. 41-9 **A,** Proximal humeral pathologic fracture fixed with a locked intramedullary nail. **B,** Internal fixation failed because the initial operation did not address the loss of bone continuity. **C,** Fixation device was revised, and bone defect was packed with bone cement, resulting in a stable reconstruction.

have been precluded by the healing process in normal fractures. Oblique femoral shaft fractures, for example, may be treated with delayed weightbearing until healing occurs in nonpathologic states. In the presence of a pathologic fracture, however, these injuries will frequently never compress to a stable configuration. The result may be eventual failure of fixation.

Another point to be made is that bulk allograft cortical struts, although commonly used in nonpathologic conditions, have no real application in the context of metastatic lesions. Figure 41-10, *A*, shows a metastatic lesion of the distal portion of the femur fixed with an intramedullary rod and allograft cortical struts. The allograft does not rectify the loss of bone continuity as well as would bone cement. Fixation of the fractured bone failed (Fig. 41-10, *B* and *C*). Failure necessitated resection and reconstruction with a distal femoral segmental replacement hinged total knee prosthesis (Fig. 41-10, *D*).

Adequate Bone and Adequate Fixation but Failure Due to Nonunion

Nonunion typically is a late-onset complication often occurring 1 year or longer after appropriate fixation that establishes a stable configuration. Again, a lack of healing will continue to place significant stresses on the fracture site and will lead to eventual failure of fixation. The two major options in these cases are the use of repeated fixation with cement augmentation and the use of segmental replacement prostheses.

Figure 41-11, *A*, shows intramedullary rod fixation for a low, pathologic subtrochanteric fracture. Painful nonunion ensued, and in reoperation a locked intramedullary nail was used (Fig. 41-11, *B*). Nevertheless the patient had continued pain at the nonunion site. This fixation was then converted to a proximal femoral replacement bipolar prosthesis, which achieved good relief of pain and a return to a high level of function (Fig. 41-11, *C*). Figure 41-

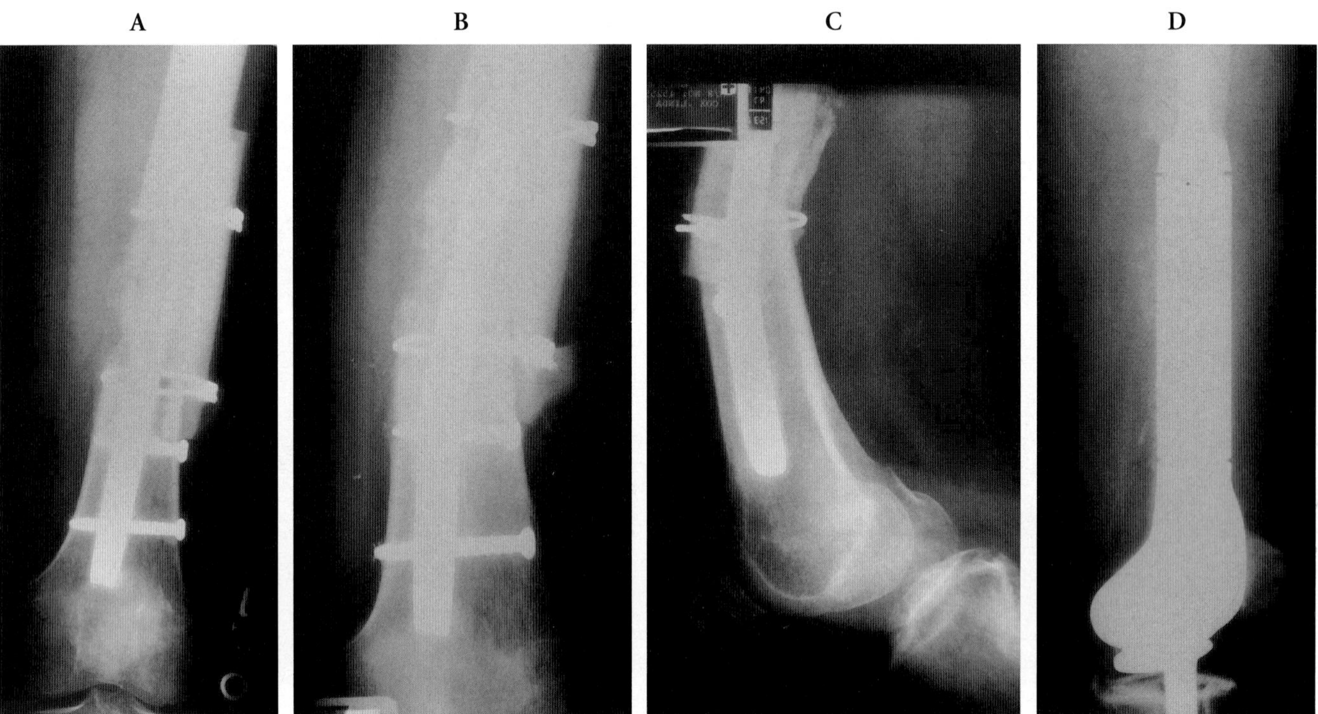

A   B   C   D

Fig. 41-10 **A,** Distal femoral osteolytic lesion due to metastatic carcinoma was fixed with an intramedullary nail and allograft cortical struts. **B** and **C,** Fixation failed, and collapse ensued. **D,** Distal femur was then salvaged by using a segmental replacement hinged total knee prosthesis.

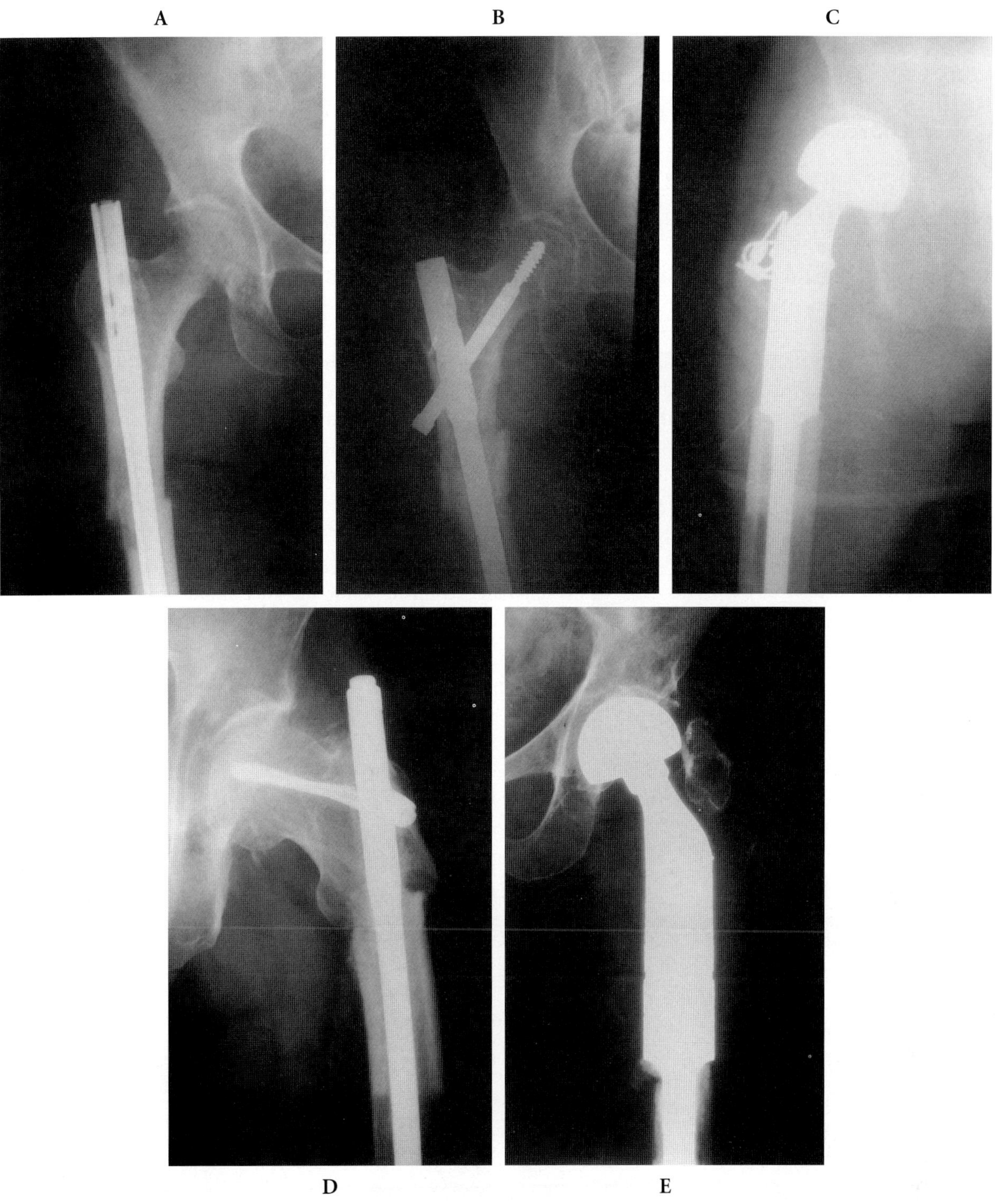

Fig. 41-11 **A,** Intramedullary nail fixation of low subtrochanteric pathologic femur fracture, with subsequent painful nonunion. **B,** Problem was corrected by using locked reconstruction nail, but the patient remained unable to bear weight because of mechanical pain. **C,** Persistent symptoms resulted in removal of hardware and conversion to a proximal femoral segmental replacement prosthesis. **D,** Subtrochanteric pathologic fracture of the femur, with development of fatigue fracture of the spiral nail. **E,** Conversion to a proximal femoral segmental replacement prosthesis was therefore required.

11, *D,* shows a subtrochanteric pathologic femoral fracture with nonunion and fracture of the spiral nail. This patient was also treated with resection and prosthetic replacement (Fig. 41-11, *E*).

CONDITIONS REQUIRING RESECTION OR AMPUTATION

Conditions do arise, although infrequently, in patients with metastatic disease in which amputation or resection, rather than internal fixation, is the appropriate treatment option. Figure 41-12 shows an x-ray film of a patient with diffuse renal cell metastases to the distal portions of the tibia and fibula and to the talus. For several months, this patient had been treated with a short leg cast, which did little to alleviate the severe pain associated with this lesion. A below-the-knee amputation dramatically relieved the patient's symptoms.

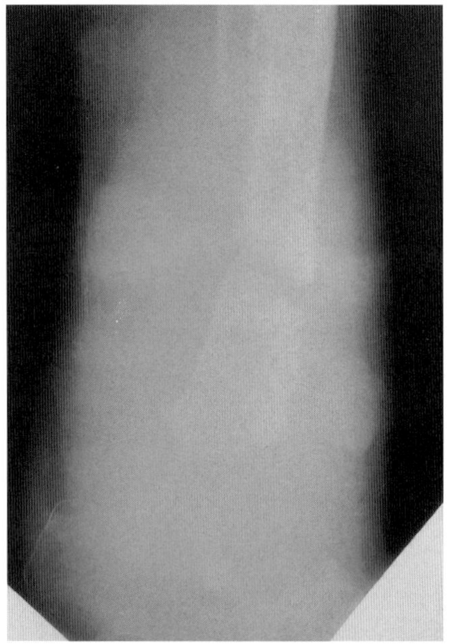

Fig. 41-12   Diffuse renal cell metastasis to the tibia, fibula, and talus, requiring below-the-knee amputation.

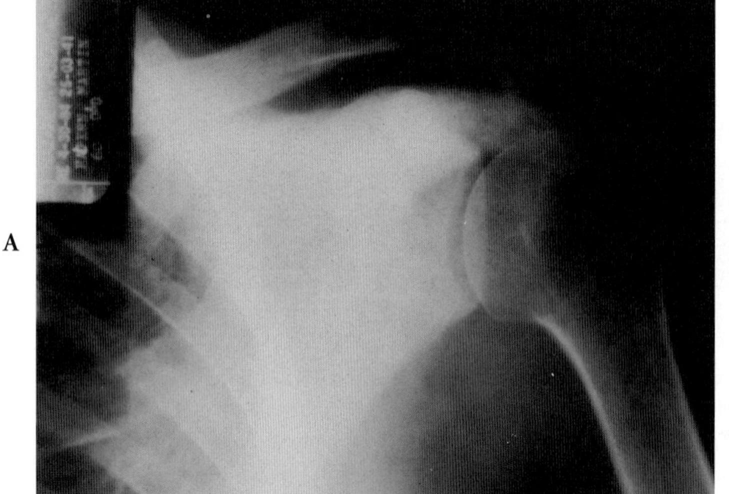
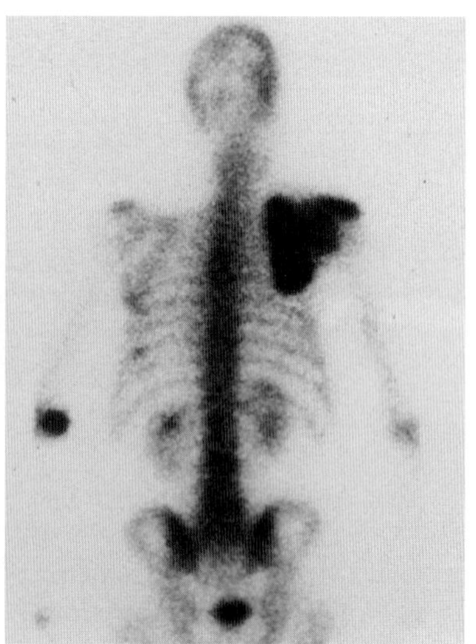

Fig. 41-13   **A,** Roentgenogram of patient with metastatic prostate carcinoma and severe recalcitrant pain despite chemotherapy and two courses of radiation. **B,** Bone scan showing scapulectomy, which was needed for pain control.

Figure 41-13 shows an x-ray film and a bone scan of a patient with metastatic prostate carcinoma confined to the scapula. The patient had severe pain in the scapula despite chemotherapy and two courses of radiation. He was treated with scapulectomy, which gave him dramatic relief of pain.

CONCLUSION

In patients with metastatic disease to bone, surgical intervention is often required. Patients should have the optimal procedure to restore their functional status. Fixation failures are often due to stabilization inadequate to allow immediate weightbearing. Bone quality and the amount of bone loss are key variables in deciding which type of fixation is necessary.

Paraneoplastic Syndromes

James A. Stewart, M.D.

Skeletal Syndromes
    Hypercalcemia
    Hypertrophic Osteoarthropathy
    Polymyositis-Dermatomyositis
    Pemphigus
Neurologic Syndromes
Hematologic Complications
Fat Embolism
Additional Syndromes
Conclusion

Clinical cancer care and the understanding of cancer biology have progressed rapidly in recent years. We are better at tumor imaging and symptom control. A well-developed system of clinical trials has enhanced steady progress in the evaluation of new treatments. Knowledge of the genetic changes that result in the diseases we call cancer has been dramatically expanded in just the past decade. Although invasion and metastasis remain the hallmark processes of the cancer phenotype, many of the effects of cancer are not related to simple organ replacement or blockage and destruction of critical anatomy by tumor mass. Rather, the production of systemically released molecules, including cytokines, hormonal peptides, or antibodies, often results in effects anatomically remote from tumor masses. These mechanisms produce a number of so-called paraneoplastic syndromes.

Paraneoplastic syndrome is defined by Tannock and Hill[1] as "signs or symptoms occurring in a patient with cancer that are not due directly to the local effects of the tumor cells." *Para* refers to the Greek preposition meaning "along the side of" or "during."[2] *Paraneoplastic* is the term commonly used for a wide range of findings and symptoms that may predate the diagnosis of cancer or may occur after an established diagnosis of malignancy. Some paraneoplastic syndromes can be treated by treating the cancer, some need syndrome-specific noncancer treatment approaches, and some have no effective treatment. All, however, provide interesting diagnostic and management challenges for clinicians.

Increasingly, patients are studying their diagnoses in consumer-oriented books and in information sites and discussion groups on the Internet. More than ever, they are asking questions about how the cancer causes changes in their bodies. It is important for us to understand the common paraneoplastic syndromes and be able to explain them to our patients.

Various classification approaches have been developed for paraneoplastic syndromes, including molecular mechanism (e.g., cytokine, antibody, hormonal), target organ (e.g., skin, nervous system, bone), or clinical outcome (e.g., fever, cachexia, dementia). With a more detailed understanding of the molecular products of cancer cells and the resulting host response, all the syndromes will in time be classified according to biologic chemistry.

SKELETAL SYNDROMES

Much cancer-related morbidity involves the skeleton. Pain and fracture are frequent outcomes of breast, lung, and prostate cancers as a direct consequence of tumor metastasis to the bone. These complications are particularly distressing in their reduction of quality of life in patients with limited survival time.

Hypercalcemia

Hypercalcemia is a common problem in patients with bone metastases, as well as in some patients whose cancers have no direct bone involvement. Some refer to the former type of hypercalcemia as local osteolytic hypercalcemia and to the latter as humoral hypercalcemia of malignancy.[3] It is important to identify hypercalcemia for the treatment of symptoms and for prognosis. In many medical settings, routine chemical studies are not done as they were in the past; therefore the symptoms of weakness, frequent urination, thirst, nausea, and constipation, which are common in a cancer population may not trigger the measurement of serum calcium. In addition, the clinician must be aware that many patients have a low albumin level; because calcium is often reported as an "uncorrected" value, a total serum calcium value in the normal range may actually represent an elevated ionized calcium value.

The pathophysiology of cancer-related hypercalcemia in many patients with carcinoma is mediated by parathyroid hormone–related protein (PTHrP). Despite the historical use of the term *ectopic PTH,* actual PTH production by tumors is rare.[4] The *PTHrP* gene, on chromosome 12, is expressed at low levels in many normal tissues, with overexpression occurring with malignant transformation.[5,6] Most neoplastic hypercalcemia involves increased bone resorption and decreased renal clearance of calcium from the blood. Most patients with carcinoma and hypercalcemia have detectable peripheral levels of PTHrP.[7] Both PTHrP and PTH bind to the same receptor, so biochemical effects such as hypophosphatemia and hypercalciuria are similar.

Most patients with cancer and hypercalcemia

will have demonstrable bone involvement by tumor. Occasional patients with squamous cell cancer of the lung or the head and neck, with kidney cancer, or with ovarian cancer will have PTHrP-mediated hypercalcemia without significant or any bone metastasis. In lung cancer, hypercalcemia is a poor prognostic finding, even though the calcium value may return to normal after tumor resection.[8] Recent studies suggest that even in patients with extensive bone metastases an important mediator of osteoclast stimulation and bone resorption is PTHrP, which is perhaps produced by tumor cells as a product of other growth factor stimulators, such as transforming growth factor beta.[9]

Multiple myeloma deserves special mention because it is generally an osteolytic process without the "blastic" reaction of bone formation seen so often in breast and prostate cancer metastases. Multiple mediators of osteolysis, such as interleukin 6 and tumor necrosis factor beta, are produced by myeloma cells and may be involved in both bone destruction and hypercalcemia.[10] In hypercalcemia associated with T-cell lymphomas and with some cases of Hodgkin's disease and other non-Hodgkin's lymphomas, vitamin D may play a role. Only modest elevations of 1,25-hydroxyvitamin D are seen, however, and the importance of this mechanism is unclear.[11]

Treatment of cancer-related hypercalcemia first requires a diagnosis. As mentioned earlier, clinicians caring for patients with cancer need to be wary of the subtle symptom complex that suggests an elevated calcium level and to have a low threshold for ordering calcium and albumin serum levels or an ionized calcium determination. Significant hypercalcemia can go undiagnosed in the face of sedation from analgesia for bone metastases, from nausea associated with bowel or liver disease or chemotherapy, or from fatigue caused by disease or cancer treatment. Symptoms vary with the calcium level and the rate of serum calcium elevation. Volume depletion can increase calcium resorption and rapidly worsen symptoms. Because most patients are dehydrated at presentation, simple volume repletion with sodium chloride solution will alleviate symptoms in the short term. Previously used agents such as corticosteroids, plicamycin, and phosphate are usually not needed. The most useful treatment after rehydration is with a bisphospho-

nate such as the second-generation agent pamidronate, which is effective in the majority of patients with hypercalcemia and has few toxic effects.[12] It can be used even in patients with underlying renal failure.[13] Prolonged hypocalcemia is possible with pamidronate use, particularly if parathyroid function is abnormal.[14] Pamidronate is now routinely used in patients with myeloma and osteolytic breast cancer for preservation of bone structure and prevention of pain.[15] Bisphosphonates are being evaluated not only for their bone preservation properties in malignancy but also for possible anticancer effects. Given their effect on a variety of growth factors, there is optimism that bisphosphonates may play a role in true prevention of metastasis.

Hypertrophic Osteoarthropathy

The major manifestations of hypertrophic osteoarthropathy (HOA) are clubbing of the digits and periostosis of the tubular bones.[16,17] The syndrome is no longer prefaced by the term *pulmonary*, because it is now recognized that a variety of conditions, such as cirrhosis, inflammatory bowel disease, chronic infections, and cardiac disease with cyanosis, are associated with HOA. Nevertheless, lung cancer is among the most common causes of HOA (Fig. 42-1).

Clubbing is an outcome of a proliferative reaction with edema in the tissues of the distal portions of the digits. The hallmark finding is loss of the acute angle between the base of the nail and the nail fold, often giving the distal segment of the finger a bulbous appearance.[18] The cause is unclear but likely relates to changes in tissue oxygenation and humoral substances.[19] Lung cancer and mesothelioma are the most common neoplasms associated with clubbing. A recent prospective assessment detected clubbing in 32 (29%) of 111 patients with lung cancer, with non-small-cell cancer being the dominant cancer type.[20]

The other components of HOA include arthralgia, often with synovitis and periosteal change, with tenderness near the large joints and radiologic findings of periosteal elevation with underlying new bone formation.[21] Treatment of the syndrome involves therapy for the underlying cancer, which for pulmonary neoplasms can often be difficult. Analgesic and anti-inflammatory agents can be

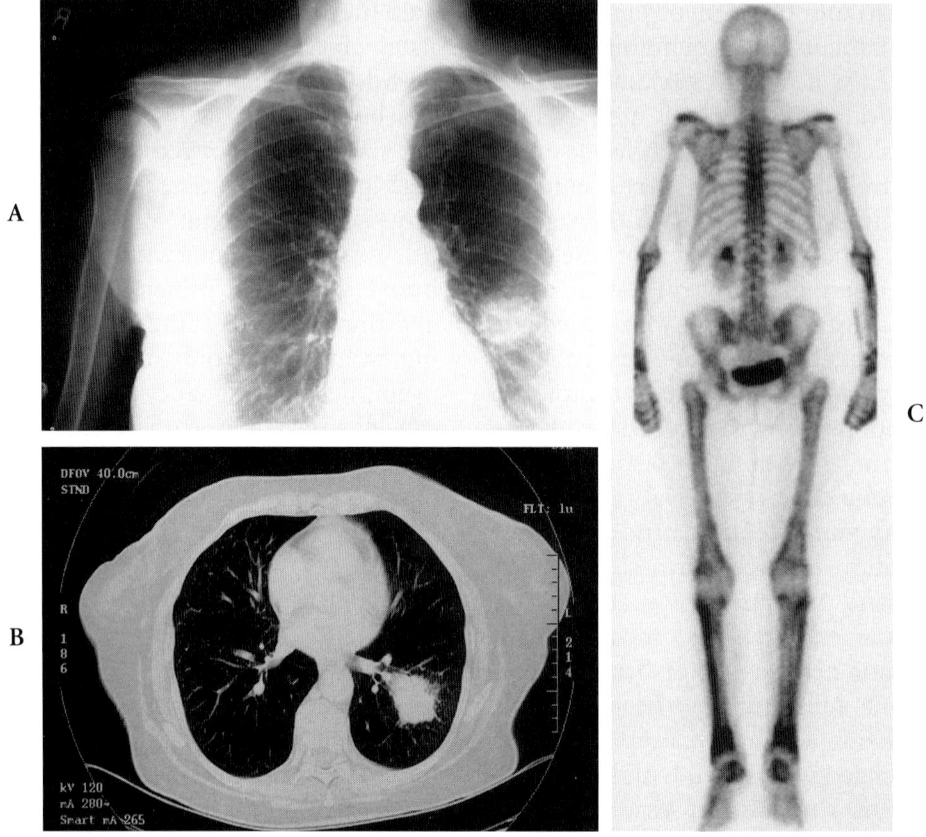

Fig. 42-1 **A,** Adult man with widespread bone pain. Initial diagnostic study revealed a large mass in the left lobe, consistent with lung carcinoma. **B,** Computed tomography scan confirmed large primary lung carcinoma. **C,** Bone scan revealed diffuse periostitis, consistent with hypertrophic osteoarthropathy. The changes are best seen in both tibiae and radii. (Figures courtesy of Jannette Collins, M.D.)

useful. Some reports have suggested that pamidronate or irradiation of the painful areas can be useful.[22,23]

Polymyositis-Dermatomyositis

Inflammatory myopathies are another category of syndromes occasionally associated with neoplasms but most commonly seen without a diagnosis of cancer. Because they may occur before the diagnosis of cancer, there has been a long-standing controversy about the importance of doing a thorough cancer evaluation for anyone with polymyositis-dermatomyositis (PD). A retrospective, matched-control Mayo Clinic study did not find a clinically significant relationship between cancer and PD.[24] A much larger study in Sweden concluded that the risk of cancer is increased in patients with PD compared with the general population; the investiga-

tors suggested that a search for cancer in patients with PD would be reasonable.[25] Other reports suggest that generalization to all cancers may be misleading because strong correlations may hold for specific cancers or certain populations. In Singapore, for example, investigators reported nasopharyngeal carcinoma in 38% of a group of patients with dermatomyositis.[26]

Polymyositis is a syndrome of proximal muscle weakness often associated with muscle pain. PD is clinically characterized by symmetric proximal muscle weakness and elevated serum muscle enzyme values, with inflammatory and myopathic changes seen on muscle biopsy.[27] In dermatomyositis there is also a characteristic skin rash with erythema over the knuckles and possible purplish rash on the eyelids, hands, or knees.

The cause of PD is not known. A wide variety of

diseases other than cancer are associated with PD, including connective tissue disorders, endocrinopathies, and infections. It is likely that immunologic factors such as interleukin 1, perhaps with some genetic predisposition, are involved in the pathogenesis.[28,29] Immunosuppressive treatments are commonly used.

Pemphigus

Numerous skin disorders have been associated with cancer not involving the skin. An excellent review of the many syndromes, including informative photographs, is provided by Cohen and Kurzrock.[30] A recently described syndrome with a poor prognosis is paraneoplastic pemphigus.[31] Criteria include mucosal ulcerations, with polymorphous skin eruptions that can resemble erythema multiforme or toxic epidermal necrolysis. Deposition of IgG in the epidermal intercellular spaces is associated with loss of cell-to-cell adhesion and cell necrosis.[32] Related neoplasms include non-Hodgkin's lymphoma, chronic lymphocytic leukemia, and thymoma.

Patients with paraneoplastic pemphigus have a poor prognosis. One mechanism of death is progressive respiratory failure with antibody-mediated disruption of the bronchial epithelium.[33]

NEUROLOGIC SYNDROMES

Current immunologic techniques provide the opportunity for pathophysiologic characterization of many paraneoplastic syndromes. Neurologic disorders related to cancer are well studied; some are examples of antibody-mediated syndromes, with tumor-stimulated antibodies cross-reacting with antigens on normal tissue. When neurologic syndromes occur, it is common for them to antedate the diagnosis of the associated cancer. Lung cancer, particularly small-cell cancer, is the most common type of malignancy to be associated with syndromes affecting the nervous system. In a series of 162 patients seropositive for type I antineuronal nuclear antibody (ANNA-1, or anti-Hu), 128 patients had a small-cell lung cancer diagnosed after the appearance of a variety of the neurologic syndromes.[34] These disorders are important in terms not only of the diagnostic sequence but also of the morbidity inflicted. Significant reduction in quality of life, including dementia and loss of motor function, can occur. Several excellent reviews have described in more detail the immunologic and clinical features of the large category of paraneoplastic syndromes involving the central and peripheral nervous systems.[35-39]

These syndromes can be grouped by the associated cancer (with lung, ovarian, and lymphoproliferative cancer being the most common), the proven or purported pathogenetic mechanism (type of antibody involved), or the anatomic part of the nervous system affected (peripheral or central). The syndromes are relatively uncommon but nevertheless are often overlooked by clinicians because of the frequency of neuromuscular symptoms and findings related to direct invasion by tumor or to toxic effects of radiation or chemotherapy. Three specific syndromes are mentioned here.

Lambert-Eaton myasthenic syndrome is often associated with small-cell cancer of the lung and is characterized by progressive weakness of the trunk, proximal portion of the limb, and ocular muscles, as well as by autonomic dysfunction, including dry mouth and orthostatic hypotension.[40] The syndrome can have a rapid course and be associated with other neurologic syndromes such as polyneuropathy or cerebellar degeneration. A characteristic feature is that weakness is greatest in rested muscles, with strength improved after repeated contraction. It is likely that the pathophysiology involves production of antibodies to calcium channels on the cancer that cross-react with channels at the neuromuscular junction.[41] Treatment results are poor, although cases in which weakness has improved with successful treatment of the cancer have been reported.

Central nervous system dysfunction is common in a population with cancer. Clinically evident brain metastases have become increasingly common as treatment of systemic cancer has improved. Spinal cord or nerve plexus compression occurs in breast, prostate, and lung cancer, with frequent metastases to nodal areas and bone. A less common but significantly disabling problem is immunologically mediated inflammation, often linked with the ANNA-1 or anti-Yo antibody. Henson et al.[42] used the term *encephalomyelitis* with carcinoma more than 30 years ago, and they and other investigators have characterized the clinical and pathologic changes describing what is now known as paraneoplastic encephalomyelitis–paraneoplastic sensory neuronopathy.[39]

The clinical picture varies with the part of the

central nervous system most affected. Mental status changes with dementia, ataxia, hyporeflexia, and sensory changes can all be seen. Again, small-cell lung cancer is commonly associated with these syndromes. Prognosis is poor, but occasionally therapy for the underlying cancer results in significant neurologic improvement.[43]

Paraneoplastic cerebellar degeneration is associated with small-cell cancer of the lung, with breast and ovarian cancer, and with lymphoma. As with other syndromes discussed earlier, the cancer is usually diagnosed after manifestation of diffuse cerebellar dysfunction, which can be of sudden onset. Vertigo, nausea, and gait ataxia and dysarthria are common.[44] Women with breast and ovarian cancers dominated a series from the Mayo Clinic; half of these women were seropositive for Purkinje cell cytoplasmic antibody.[45] This antibody, now called anti-Yo, is found in both the serum and the cerebrospinal fluid and is associated with breast and gynecologic cancers.[46]

HEMATOLOGIC COMPLICATIONS

Hematologic complications in patients with cancer are common. Reduction or elevation of multiple hematopoietic cell lines are seen in a variety of cancers. Marrow damage from radiation and chemotherapy is the most likely cause, but paraneoplastic erythrocytosis and thrombocytosis can occur as a result of tumor production of erythropoietin, thrombopoietin, or similar substances. Renal cancer and primary liver cancer have long been known to cause erythrocytosis. Bone marrow changes are seen in patients with cancer without demonstrated marrow metastases. Castello et al.[47] noted changes in bone remodeling and stromal modifications in 40 patients with cancer not involving the marrow.

Venous thrombosis causes considerable morbidity in patients with cancer. In the general population it is estimated that venous thrombosis occurs in about 1 in 1,000 people per year in developed countries.[48] In patients with cancer, venous access devices are common, and clots related to central lines are now a fairly common cause of superior vena cava syndrome. The hypercoagulable state associated with many cancers, most notably adenocarcinomas, presents a difficult management problem. Patients with cancer of the pancreas, stomach, and lung have a high incidence of thrombosis, which is a common cause of death.[49] The pathophysiology is complex and involves release of procoagulant activators of thrombosis.[50] Simple screening tests for cancer patients likely to have deep venous thrombosis (DVT) are not available. Coagulation profiles and screening for DVT were done in a series of 98 patients with advanced malignancy.[51] Although patients with DVT had a lower level of fibrinogen, the wide variation in the measurement of coagulation factors offered little predictive value.

The considerable controversy regarding the need to search for cancer in anyone with DVT but without obvious risk factors has continued. Investigators in Padua evaluated the incidence of subsequent cancer in such patients and found a significant correlation between thrombosis without well-recognized risk factors and an eventual diagnosis of cancer, in comparison with a population with risk factor–associated thrombosis.[52] Most of the cancers were detected after a second episode of thrombosis. Screening for cancers in such a population may be appropriate.

Emboli to the lungs and brain are underappreciated causes of morbidity and death in a population with cancer. Pulmonary emboli can be a lethal result of DVT. Most clinicians are sensitive to the association between DVT and the risk of emboli; nevertheless, autopsy evaluation commonly finds unsuspected pulmonary emboli. A less common cause of systemic embolization often associated with major brain morbidity is nonbacterial thrombotic endocarditis, previously known as marantic (from marasmus, or wasting) endocarditis.[53] In this condition, left-sided cardiac valvular vegetations may embolize, with resulting hemorrhagic or thrombotic complications. The spleen, kidney, and brain are the most common sites of emboli. Echocardiography is the most useful diagnostic tool, and a high index of suspicion is needed to make the diagnosis before death.[54]

FAT EMBOLISM

Another cause of systemic emboli resulting in significant morbidity is fat embolism, which is associated with both traumatic and nontraumatic disorders.[55] Patients with cancer often undergo the trauma of long-bone fracture or the placement of pins and rods to stabilize or repair a femur with metastatic cancer (Fig. 42-2). Fat embolism syndrome is manifested by the classic triad of pulmonary distress, cerebral dysfunction, and petechial rash.

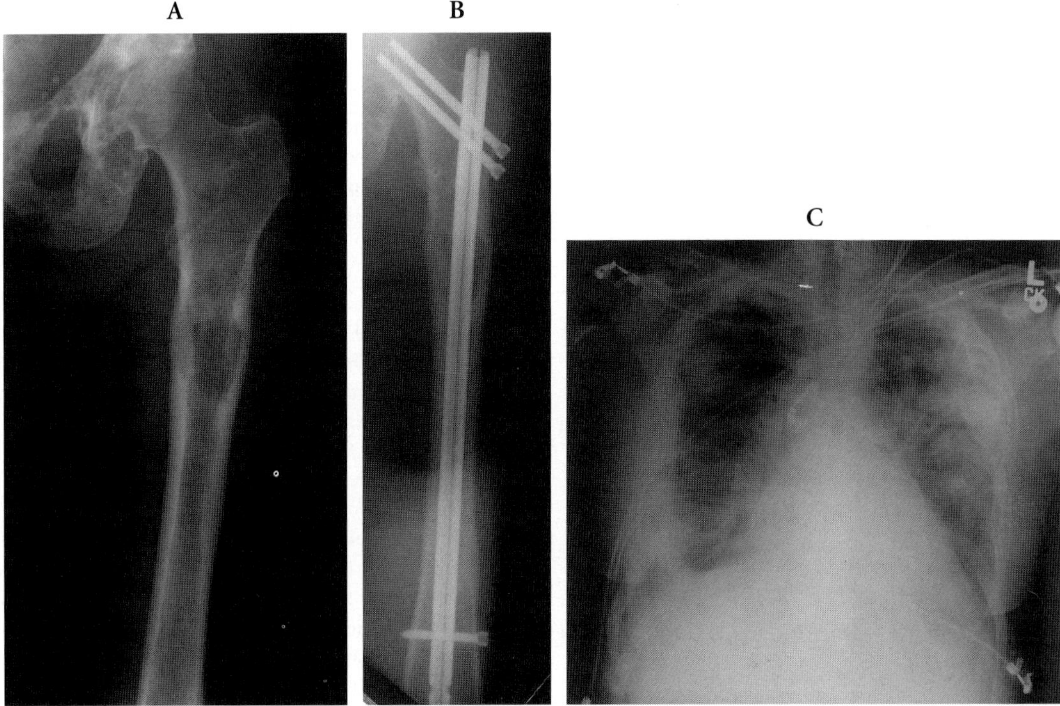

Fig. 42-2   A, Painful osteolytic lesion in proximal third of femur, in a patient with widespread breast carcinoma. **B,** Locked intramedullary nail. During preparation of the medullary canal the patient's oxygen saturation acutely dropped and increased resistance to ventilation developed. **C,** Upright chest x-ray film taken after surgery, showing increased interstitial markings with peripheral changes consistent with an intraoperative embolization from the marrow of the femoral canal. Several peripheral pulmonary metastatic lesions can be seen.

Nontraumatic causes of fat emboli include intravenous administration of lipid emulsion for nutritional support; reports of bone marrow necrosis in lymphoma with resulting fat embolus have also been made.[56] No specific treatment has been found for fat embolus, but most patients do well with vigorous supportive care. Although fat embolism is not traditionally thought of as a paraneoplastic syndrome, the frequency of skeletal involvement in cancer should keep the clinician aware that it can result from bone fracture or repair.

ADDITIONAL SYNDROMES

Numerous other syndromes can be considered paraneoplastic. The language of classification is complex, and many syndromes are considered truly paraneoplastic only if the pathophysiology has a humoral component. Tumor fever, for example, has long been a diagnosis of exclusion, competing with infection (which is usually the cause of fever) for therapeutic attention. Cytokines produced by the tumor or host in response to the tumor are the cause, and nonsteroidal anti-inflammatory agents are often useful in treatment.[57] Endocrinologic syndromes include tumor production of adrenocorticotropic hormone or antidiuretic hormone, each with the resulting metabolic outcomes that one would expect with excessive hormone production.[58,59] Successful treatment of these syndromes is related to therapy for the cancer. Proinflammatory cytokines such as tumor necrosis factor and interleukin 1 are likely related to the anorexia-cachexia syndrome seen in patients with advanced cancer.[60] Tissue wasting, weight loss, and decrease in muscle mass and performance status are common in patients with advanced cancer despite an intact gastrointestinal tract. Some gain in appetite and weight is achieved with the use of the progestational agent megestrol acetate, although support for improvement in performance status or survival is lacking.[61]

The study of clinical cancer and the care of patients with these diseases are challenging in part because of the numerous biologic effects of the neoplastic process. Humoral effects of tumor-related hormones, cytokines, and antibodies generated by the host or the cancer itself can create striking changes in all organs of the body. There continues to be considerable discussion about the definition of the term *paraneoplastic* because it is unclear whether, in some neurologic syndromes, the production of the identified antibodies is causative or epiphenomenal.[62] Definitions, language, and treatment options will continue to evolve as each syndrome is better characterized on a molecular and cause-and-effect basis.

CONCLUSION

1. Paraneoplastic syndromes are common and often undiagnosed.
2. Small-cell cancer of the lung is one of the most common cancers associated with paraneoplastic syndromes.
3. Bone is a common target organ associated with cancer-related syndromes (osteoarthropathy, hypercalcemia).
4. Effective treatment of cancer is the ultimate best therapy for these syndromes.

Cancer-associated syndromes make the field of oncology not only interesting but also challenging. Greater understanding of the molecular nature of these problems will diminish some of their mystery but will enhance our ability to effectively treat them. Clinicians must be thoughtful regarding a differential diagnosis in patients with cancer and symptoms remote from the obvious sites of tumor.

REFERENCES

1. Tannock IF, Hill RP. The Basic Science of Oncology, 3rd ed. New York: McGraw-Hill, 1998, p 504.
2. Haubrich WS. Medical Meanings: A Glossary of Word Origins. Philadelphia: American College of Physicians, 1997, p 160.
3. Wysolmerski JJ, Broadus AE. Hypercalcemia of malignancy: The central role of parathyroid-related protein. Ann Rev Med 45:189-200, 1994.
4. Mundy GR, Guise TA. Hypercalcemia of malignancy. Am J Med 103(2):134-145, 1997.
5. Odell W. Endocrine/metabolic syndromes of cancer. Semin Oncol 24:299-317, 1977.
6. Thiede MA, Rodan GA. Expression of a calcium-mobilizing parathyroid hormone–like peptide in lactating mammary tissue. Science 242:278-280, 1988.
7. Burtis WJ, Brady TF, Orloff JJ, Ersbak JB, Warrell RP Jr, Olson BR, Wu TL, Mitnick ME, Broadus AE, Stewart AF. Immunochemical characterization of circulating parathyroid hormone–related protein in patients with humoral hypercalcemia of cancer. N Engl J Med 322:1106-1112, 1990.
8. Hiraki A, Ueoka H, Segawa Y, et al. Hypercalcemia-leukocytosis syndrome in lung cancer. Proc Am Soc Clin Oncol 18:508, 1999.
9. Pfeilschifter J, Mundy GR. Modulation of transforming growth factor beta in bone cultures by osteotropic hormones. Proc Natl Acad Sci USA 84:2024-2028, 1987.
10. Garrett IR, Durie BG, Nedwin GE, Gillespie A, Bringman T, Sabatini M, Bertolini DR, Mundy GR. Production of lymphotoxin, a bone-resorbing cytokine, by cultured human myeloma cells. N Engl J Med 317:526-532, 1987.
11. Schweitzer DH, Hamdy NA, Frolich M, Zwinderman AH, Papapoulos SE. Malignancy-associated hypercalcemia: Resolution of controversies over vitamin D metabolism by a pathophysiological approach to the syndrome. Clin Endocrinol 41:251-256, 1994.
12. Nussbaum SR, Younger J, Vandepol CJ, Gagel RF, Zubler MA, Chapman R, Henderson IC, Mallette LE. Single-dose intravenous therapy with pamidronate for the treatment of hypercalcemia of malignancy: Comparison of 30-, 60-, and 90-mg dosages. Am J Med 95:297-304, 1993.
13. Machado CE, Flombaum CD. Safety of pamidronate in patients with renal failure and hypercalcemia. Clin Nephrol 45:175-179, 1996.
14. Sims EC, Rogers PB, Besser GM, Plowman PM. Severe prolonged hypocalcaemia following pamidronate for malignant hypercalcemia. Clin Oncol (R Coll Radiol) 10:407-409, 1998.
15. Hortobagyi GN, Theriault RL, Lipton A, Porter L, Blayney D, Sinoff C, Wheeler H, Simeone JF, Seaman JJ, Knight RD, Heffernan M, Mellars K, Reitsma DJ. Long-term prevention of skeletal complications of metastatic breast cancer with pamidronate. J Clin Oncol 16:2038-2044, 1998.
16. John WJ, Patchell RA, Foon KA. Paraneoplastic syndromes. In DeVita VT Jr, Hellman S, Rosenberg SA: Cancer: Principles and Practice of Oncology, 5th ed. Philadelphia: JB Lippincott, p 2417.
17. Martinez-Lavin M, Matucci-Cerinic M, Jajic I, Pineda C. Hypertrophic osteoarthropathy: Consensus on its definition, classification, assessment and diagnostic criteria. J Rheumatol 20:1386-1387, 1993.
18. Cohen PR. Cutaneous paraneoplastic syndromes. Am Fam Physician 50:1273-1282, 1994.
19. Dickinson CJ. The aetiology of clubbing and hypertrophic osteoarthropathy. Eur J Clin Invest 23:330-338, 1993.
20. Sridhar KS, Lobo CF, Altman RD. Digital clubbing and lung cancer. Chest 114:1535-1537, 1998.
21. Burstein HJ, Janicek MJ, Skarin T. Hypertrophic osteoarthropathy. J Clin Oncol 15:2759-2760, 1997.
22. Speden D, Nicklason F, Francis H, Ward J. The use of pamidronate in hypertrophic pulmonary osteoarthropathy. Aust NZ J Med 27:307-310, 1997.
23. Roos DE. Hypertrophic pulmonary osteoarthropathy: Is there a role for radiotherapy to symptomatic sites? Case report and literature review. Acta Oncol 35(1):101-103, 1996.

24. Lakhanpal S, Bunch TW, Ilstrup DM, Melton LJ. Polymyositis-dermatomyositis and malignant lesions: Does an association exist? Mayo Clinic Proc 61:645-653, 1986.

25. Sigurgeirsson B, Lindelöf B, Edhag O, Allander E. Risk of cancer in patients with dermatomyositis or polymyositis: A population-based study. N Engl J Med 326:363-367, 1992.

26. Leow YH, Goh CL. Malignancy in adult dermatomyositis. Int J Dermatol 36:904-907, 1997.

27. Bunch TW. Polymyositis: A case history approach to the differential diagnosis and treatment. Mayo Clinic Proc 65:1480-1497, 1990.

28. Kovacs SO, Kovacs SC. Dermatomyositis. J Am Acad Dermatol 39:899-920, 1998.

29. Lundberg IE, Nyberg P. New developments in the role of cytokines and chemokines in inflammatory myopathy. Curr Opin Rheumatol 10:521-529, 1998.

30. Cohen PR, Kurzrock R. Mucocutaneous paraneoplastic syndromes. Semin Oncol 24:334-359, 1997.

31. Anhalt GJ, Kim SC, Stanley JR, Korman NJ, Jabs DA, Kory M, Izumi H, Ratrie H III, Mutasim D, Ariss-Abdo L, et al. Paraneoplastic pemphigus: An autoimmune mucocutaneous disease associated with neoplasia. N Engl J Med 323:1729-1735, 1990.

32. Anhalt GJ. Paraneoplastic pemphigus. Adv Dermatol 12:77-96, 1997.

33. Nousari HC, Deterding R, Wojtczack H, Aho S, Uitto J, Hashimoto T, Anhalt GJ. The mechanism of respiratory failure in paraneoplastic pemphigus. N Engl J Med 340:1406-1410, 1999.

34. Lucchinetti CF, Kimmel DW, Lennon VA. Paraneoplastic and oncologic profiles of patients seropositive for type I antineuronal nuclear antibodies. Neurology 50:652-657, 1998.

35. Dalmau JO, Posner JB. Paraneoplastic syndromes affecting the nervous system. Semin Oncol 24:318-328, 1997.

36. Nath U, Grant R. Neurologic paraneoplastic syndromes. J Clin Pathol 50:975-980, 1997.

37. Dropcho EJ. Principles of paraneoplastic syndromes. Ann NY Acad Sci 841:246-261, 1998.

38. Amato AA, Collins MP. Neuropathies associated with malignancy. Semin Neurol 18(1):125-144, 1998.

39. Hinton RC. Paraneoplastic neurologic syndromes. Hematol Oncol Clin North Am 10:909-925, 1996.

40. Smith RG, Appel SH. The Lambert-Eaton syndrome. Hospital Pract 27:101-106, 111-113, 116, 1992.

41. Boonyapisit K, Kaminski HJ, Ruff RL. Disorders of neuromuscular junction ion channels. Am J Med 106:97-113, 1999.

42. Henson RA, Hoffman HL, Urich H. Encephalomyelitis with carcinoma. Brain 88:449-464, 1965.

43. Batson OA, Fantle DM, Stewart JA. Paraneoplastic encephalomyelitis: Dramatic response to chemotherapy alone. Cancer 69:1291-1293, 1992.

44. Andersen NE, Rosenblum MK, Posner JB. Paraneoplastic cerebellar degeneration: Clinical immunological correlations. Ann Neurol 24:559-567, 1988.

45. Hammack JE, Kimmel DW, O'Neill BP, Lennon VA. Paraneoplastic cerebellar degeneration: A clinical comparison of patients with and without Purkinje cell cytoplasmic antibodies. Mayo Clinic Proc 65:1423-1431, 1990.

46. Furneaux HM, Rosenblum MK, Dalmau J, Wong E, Woodruff P, Graus F, Posner JB. Selective expression of Purkinje-cell antigens in tumor tissue from patients with paraneoplastic cerebellar degeneration. N Engl J Med 322:1844-1851, 1990.

47. Castello A, Coci A, Magrini U. Paraneoplastic marrow alterations in patients with cancer. Haematologica 77:392-397, 1992.

48. Rosendaal FR. Venous thrombosis: A multicausal disease. Lancet 353:1167-1173, 1999.

49. Schafer AI. The hypercoagulable states. Ann Intern Med 102:814-828, 1985.

50. Green KB, Silverstein RL. Hypercoagulability in cancer. Hematol Oncol Clin North Am 10:499-530, 1996.

51. Johnson MJ, Walker ID, Sproule MW, Conkie J. Abnormal coagulation and deep venous thrombosis in patients with cancer. Clin Lab Haematol 21(1):51-54, 1999.

52. Prandoni P, Lensing AW, Büller HR, Cogo A, Prins MH, Cattelan AM, Cuppini S, Noventa F, ten Cate JW. Deep-vein thrombosis and the incidence of subsequent symptomatic cancer. N Engl J Med 327:1128-1133, 1992.

53. Rosen P, Armstrong D. Nonbacterial thrombotic endocarditis in patients with malignant neoplastic diseases. Am J Med 54:23-29, 1973.

54. Joffe II, Jacobs LE, Owen AN, Ioli A, Kotler MN. Noninfective valvular masses: Review of the literature with emphasis on imaging techniques and management. Am Heart J 131:1175-1183, 1996.

55. Richards RR. Fat embolism syndrome. Can J Surg 40:334-339, 1997.

56. Case records of the Massachusetts General Hospital, Weekly clinicopathological exercises. Case 23-1998: Tachypnea, changed mental status, and pancytopenia in an elderly man with treated lymphoma. N Engl J Med 339:254-261, 1998.

57. Johnson M. Neoplastic fever. Palliat Med 10:217-224, 1996.

58. Wajchenberg BL, Mendonca BB, Liberman B, Adelaide M, Pereira A, Kirschner MA. Ectopic ACTH syndrome. [Review.] J Steroid Biochem Mol Biol 53:139-151, 1995.

59. Schwartz WB, Bennet W, Curelop S, et al. A syndrome of renal sodium loss and hyponatremia probably resulting from inappropriate secretion of antidiuretic hormone. Am J Med 23:529, 1957.

60. Tisdale MJ. Cancer cachexia: Metabolic alterations and clinical manifestations. Nutrition 13(1):1-7, 1997.

61. Vadell C, Segui MA, Gimenez-Arnau JM, Morales S, Cirera L, Bestit I, Batiste E, Blanco R, Jolis L, Boleda M, Anton I. Anticachectic efficacy of megestrol acetate at different doses and versus placebo in patients with neoplastic cachexia. Am J Clin Oncol 21:347-351, 1998.

62. Fathallah-Shaykh HM. Paraneoplastic neurological syndromes: Paraneoplastic or neurological? Arch Neurol 56:151-152, 1999.

Index